Intelligent Systems Reference Library

Volume 211

Series Editors

Janusz Kacprzyk, Polish Academy of Sciences, Warsaw, Poland

Lakhmi C. Jain, KES International, Shoreham-by-Sea, UK

The aim of this series is to publish a Reference Library, including novel advances and developments in all aspects of Intelligent Systems in an easily accessible and well structured form. The series includes reference works, handbooks, compendia, textbooks, well-structured monographs, dictionaries, and encyclopedias. It contains well integrated knowledge and current information in the field of Intelligent Systems. The series covers the theory, applications, and design methods of Intelligent Systems. Virtually all disciplines such as engineering, computer science, avionics, business, e-commerce, environment, healthcare, physics and life science are included. The list of topics spans all the areas of modern intelligent systems such as: Ambient intelligence, Computational intelligence, Social intelligence, Computational neuroscience, Artificial life, Virtual society, Cognitive systems, DNA and immunity-based systems, e-Learning and teaching, Human-centred computing and Machine ethics, Intelligent control, Intelligent data analysis, Knowledge-based paradigms, Knowledge management, Intelligent agents, Intelligent decision making, Intelligent network security, Interactive entertainment, Learning paradigms, Recommender systems, Robotics and Mechatronics including human-machine teaming, Self-organizing and adaptive systems, Soft computing including Neural systems, Fuzzy systems, Evolutionary computing and the Fusion of these paradigms, Perception and Vision, Web intelligence and Multimedia.

Indexed by SCOPUS, DBLP, zbMATH, SCImago.

All books published in the series are submitted for consideration in Web of Science.

More information about this series at http://www.springer.com/series/8578

Chee-Peng Lim · Ashlesha Vaidya · Kiran Jain ·
Virag U. Mahorkar · Lakhmi C. Jain
Editors

Handbook of Artificial Intelligence in Healthcare

Vol. 1—Advances and Applications

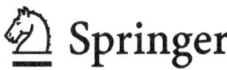

Springer

Editors
Chee-Peng Lim
Institute for Intelligent Systems Research
and Innovation
Deakin University
Waurn Ponds, VIC, Australia

Kiran Jain
St. Joseph's Hospital and Medical Center
Stockton, CA, USA

Lakhmi C. Jain
KES International
Shoreham-by-Sea, UK

Ashlesha Vaidya
Royal Adelaide Hospital
Adelaide, SA, Australia

Virag U. Mahorkar
Avanti Institute of Cardiology
Nagpur, Maharashtra, India

ISSN 1868-4394   ISSN 1868-4408 (electronic)
Intelligent Systems Reference Library
ISBN 978-3-030-79160-5   ISBN 978-3-030-79161-2 (eBook)
https://doi.org/10.1007/978-3-030-79161-2

© The Editor(s) (if applicable) and The Author(s), under exclusive license to Springer Nature Switzerland AG 2022

This work is subject to copyright. All rights are solely and exclusively licensed by the Publisher, whether the whole or part of the material is concerned, specifically the rights of translation, reprinting, reuse of illustrations, recitation, broadcasting, reproduction on microfilms or in any other physical way, and transmission or information storage and retrieval, electronic adaptation, computer software, or by similar or dissimilar methodology now known or hereafter developed.

The use of general descriptive names, registered names, trademarks, service marks, etc. in this publication does not imply, even in the absence of a specific statement, that such names are exempt from the relevant protective laws and regulations and therefore free for general use.

The publisher, the authors and the editors are safe to assume that the advice and information in this book are believed to be true and accurate at the date of publication. Neither the publisher nor the authors or the editors give a warranty, expressed or implied, with respect to the material contained herein or for any errors or omissions that may have been made. The publisher remains neutral with regard to jurisdictional claims in published maps and institutional affiliations.

This Springer imprint is published by the registered company Springer Nature Switzerland AG
The registered company address is: Gewerbestrasse 11, 6330 Cham, Switzerland

Preface

Artificial intelligence (AI) has undergone a rapid growth in recent years, covering advances in both theoretical and practical aspects. In the healthcare sector, AI-based methods and tools have played a critical role in solving a variety of medical and healthcare-related issues, saving time, costs, and lives as well as fostering economic resilience particularly under the COVID-19 pandemic environments. Research and development (R&D) initiatives to enhance AI capabilities covering a variety of areas, from big data analytics, text mining, natural language processing, to signal, image, video processing continue unabated.

This edition on *Handbook of Artificial Intelligence in Healthcare* has two volumes. The first volume is dedicated to advances and applications of AI methodologies in specific healthcare problems, while the second volumes are concerned with general practicality issues and challenges and future prospects in the healthcare context. In this first volume, a total of 17 chapters are presented in two parts. Studies on medical signal, image, and video processing as well as healthcare information and data analytics using AI-based tools and techniques are covered in Part 1 and Part 2, respectively. A summary of each chapter in this volume is described as follows.

Aikaterini et al. conduct a survey on the use of AI tools and methods for epilepsy patients through analysing electroencephalography (EEG) signals of brain activities. The related AI methodologies and applications are reviewed, focusing on the principles, parameters, complexity, feature selection, and classification methods for pre-ictal, ictal, post-ictal detection, seizure detection, and inter-ictal Identification. The implications pertaining to automated system integration and epileptic attributes identification are discussed.

Suresh et al. analyse EEG signals in their study on brain functions. A page ranking algorithm, which is commonly used for evaluating websites using the principle of eigenvector centrality, is leveraged for examining signals from EEG electrodes. The empirical analysis is beneficial for characterising the EEG electrodes into different categories based on cognitive activities, providing a better understanding of the cognitive behaviours of the human brain networks.

de Luise et al. present a machine learning approach to modelling the behaviours of autistic spectrum disorder (ASD) patients through recordings during therapy sessions. Audio and video information is utilised to develop a customised model for evaluation of a patient's performance during his/her interaction with other people. The results indicate the usefulness of the developed model for discriminating autistic verbal behaviours.

Remeseiro and Bolon-Cadeno investigate the use of computer vision and machine learning in ophthalmic image analysis. Case studies on retinal image quality assessment, automated computation of the arteriolar-to-venular index, as well as automated diagnosis of retinopathy of prematurity demonstrate the feasibility of the proposed method for use in daily practice, both for clinical and research purposes.

Bonechi et al. survey computer vision and machine learning methods for urine culture screening based on automatic understanding of images from Petri plates. Several segmentation techniques and some specific methods for bacterial counting and infection classification are described. A synthetic image generation approach to overcome privacy concerns and medical data paucity is presented. The generated synthetic images with annotations are beneficial for training deep learning models, leading to reliable image segmentation.

Wang and Williams outline the technical considerations of imaging pertaining to cancer biomarkers. Machine learning models are utilised for radiological data analysis in solving clinical problems. The challenges related to cancer imaging biomarkers are tackled through the development of new radiomic features.

Iwahori et al. design deep learning model for detection of lateral spreading tumour (LSP) type of polyps. Specifically, the convolutional neural networks are used to process 3D shapes obtained from endoscopic images, whereby a depth map is created under the condition of point light source illumination and perspective projection. The proposed method is able to yield high accuracy rates for LSP-type polyps detection.

Luca et al. discuss computer-aided tools to assist gastroenterologists in processing video colonoscopy and detecting colorectal cancers. In this respect, AI, machine learning and deep learning models are more useful, as compared with conventional methods. Automatic detection tools for polyps and adenomas on colonoscopy video frames are valuable for training and assisting the physicians towards objective evaluation. Deep learning is found to be useful for real-time processing of colonoscopies with very good and consistent results.

del Mar Vila et al. investigate carotid artery ultrasound images for detecting the presence of atherosclerotic plaques, in order to diagnose cardiovascular diseases. A review on the state-of-the-art methods for carotid artery segmentation, plaque classification, and risk assessment through ultrasound images with a focus on deep learning models is presented. The strengths and weaknesses are discussed. The study offers a foundation for taking advantage of the capability of deep learning, along with the associated challenges in future research.

Wang et al. examine the prediction of microvascular invasion before surgery to help doctors develop treatment plans for hepatocellular carcinoma patients. Radiomics methods are exploited to predict microvascular invasion. Specifically, a fusion model that combines clinical and radiomics magnetic resonance imaging data is devised. Random forest and support vector machines are used in the fusion model, yielding good accuracy, and area under the receiver operating characteristic curve (AUC) scores.

Qiu et al. introduce cost-effective methods for remote heart rate estimation from video images. The principle of remote photoplethysmography signal extraction through video clips is analysed, in order to facilitate heart rate estimation. In addition, mathematical models and computational algorithms for solving movement artefacts and illumination changes are developed. Deep learning methods are reviewed. A general overview on the data sets available for remote photoplethysmography learning is provided.

Nousi et al. conduct a survey on the role of data mining towards healthcare applications under pandemic environments. The survey aims to address the research questions on types of pervasive analytics involving the medical and healthcare domains, as well as the commonly used data mining methods and techniques for medical and healthcare resources.

Akbari and Unland devise a clinical decision support system for guided history and physical examination (H&P). Holonic paradigm, multi-agent system, and swarm intelligence models are exploited to develop the decision support tool. It is beneficial for managing and executing the complete H&P examination process, which include collecting the relevant data, performing the required tests, and deriving the related results.

Liu et al. present depressive severity detection using deep learning methods for automatic audio, visual, and audiovisual emotion sensing. Behavioural features such as facial expressions and speech prosody are introduced. A multi-modal behavioural data set of Chinese university students with and without depressive tendencies is formed. The experimental results indicate the usefulness of low-level features in audio-based depression detection, while deep learning-based features are effective in visual-based depression detection. Overall, behavioural features in positive-emotional speech have more potential in depressive severity identification.

Leonardi et al. study stroke management processes with deep learning models. Recurrent neural networks and their combination with convolutional models are devised for trace classification that supports quality assessment in stroke centres. The composite architecture with deep learning offers a better approach with higher accuracy scores in their study.

Bollino et al. endeavour to realise a technological platform to support the early oncological diagnosis based on an integration of an interoperable communication and clinical data management. A computer-aided detection diagnosis tool based on machine learning and deep learning is developed to assist the operator in the analysis of screening data, which include anamnestic information, blood tests, as well as instrumental and diagnostic images. The solution has great potential for physicians in developing personalised diagnostic and therapeutic strategies for cancer prevention programs.

Dykstra et al. present new insights pertaining to the implementation of AI systems in cardiovascular care. Machine learning approach is exploited to address the unique challenges faced by personalised healthcare delivery using multi-domain patient information. Insightful discussion on the solutions for data management and machine learning methods for combining the value of disparate data resources for patient-specific risk prediction modelling is provided.

The editors would like to express our gratitude to all authors and reviewers for their contributions and to the Springer editorial team for their help in this publication. The chapters presented in this volume are just a small coverage on the broad and rapidly changing AI-based methodologies in the medical and healthcare domain. Hopefully, this volume can offer readers a glimpse on the advances and applications of AI, particularly relating to signal, image, and video processing as well as information and data analytic problems, in the healthcare sector.

Waurn Ponds, Australia	Chee-Peng Lim
Adelaide, Australia	Ashlesha Vaidya
Stockton, USA	Kiran Jain
Nagpur, India	Virag U. Mahorkar
Shoreham-by-Sea, UK	Lakhmi C. Jain
May 2021	

Contents

Part I Advances in AI for Healthcare Signal, Image, and Video Processing

1 Advances in Artificial Intelligence for the Identification of Epileptiform Discharges 3
Aikaterini Karampasi, Kostakis Gkiatis, Ioannis Kakkos, Kyriakos Garganis, and George K. Matsopoulos
  1.1   Background 5
  1.2   Artificial Intelligence Tools 6
  1.3   Pre-Ictal, Ictal, Post-Ictal Detection 10
  1.4   Seizure Detection 12
  1.5   Inter-Ictal Identification 15
  1.6   Seizure Onset Zone 16
  1.7   Implications and Future Challenges 18
  References 19

2 Characterizing EEG Electrodes in Directed Functional Brain Networks Using Normalized Transfer Entropy and PageRank 27
Kaushik Suresh, Vijayalakshmi Ramasamy, Ronnie Daniel, and Sushil Chandra
  2.1   Introduction 28
  2.2   Current Approaches to Study Directional Information Flow in FBNs 30
    2.2.1   Normalized Transfer Entropy 31
    2.2.2   PageRank 32
  2.3   Materials and Methods 33
    2.3.1   Experimental Design 33
    2.3.2   EEG Data Acquisition and Pre-Processing 34
    2.3.3   Behavioral Data 35
    2.3.4   Directed Information Flow Using Normalized Transfer Entropy 35
    2.3.5   Rate of Change of Cognition 35
  2.4   Experimental Results and Discussion 36

		2.4.1	Electrode Wise Analysis	38
		2.4.2	Observation Phase	44
		2.4.3	Entire Population Group-Wise Analysis	44
	2.5	Conclusion		46
	References			47

3 Autistic Verbal Behavior Language Parameterization ... 51
Daniela López De Luise, Ben Raúl Saad, Tiago Ibacache, Christian Saliwonczyk, Pablo Pescio, and Lucas Soria

	3.1	Introduction		51
	3.2	Considerations About the Autistic Spectrum Disorder		54
		3.2.1	Degrees of Autism	55
		3.2.2	Verbal Behavior	56
	3.3	Materials and Methods		56
		3.3.1	Hardware	56
		3.3.2	Protocol	57
		3.3.3	Software	57
	3.4	Preliminary Evaluation		60
		3.4.1	Modeling the Problem with Metadata	60
		3.4.2	Advantages and Disadvantages of Using the Proposed Approach	62
	3.5	The Sounds of the Use-Case		64
	3.6	Test and Evaluation		67
		3.6.1	Pre-processing	69
		3.6.2	Variable Selection	69
		3.6.3	Automatic Timestamp Detection	74
		3.6.4	Model for Timestamp Detection	79
		3.6.5	Model Findings and Results Analysis	79
	3.7	Conclusions and Future Work		80
	References			80

4 Case Studies to Demonstrate Real-World Applications in Ophthalmic Image Analysis ... 83
Beatriz Remeseiro and Verónica Bolón-Canedo

	4.1	Introduction		84
	4.2	Related Work		85
		4.2.1	Retinal Image Quality Assessment	85
		4.2.2	Arteriolar-to-Venular Index and A/V Classification	86
		4.2.3	Retinopathy of Prematurity	88
	4.3	Case Study: Retinal Quality Assessment		90
		4.3.1	Dataset	90
		4.3.2	Methods	91
		4.3.3	Results	93
	4.4	Case Study: Arteriolar-to-Venular Index		98
		4.4.1	Datasets	99

		4.4.2	Methods	99
		4.4.3	Results	105
	4.5	Case Study: Retinopathy of Prematurity		109
		4.5.1	Datasets	110
		4.5.2	Methods	111
		4.5.3	Results	112
	4.6	Summary		117
	References			119
5	**Segmentation of Petri Plate Images for Automatic Reporting of Urine Culture Tests**			**127**
	Simone Bonechi, Monica Bianchini, Alessandro Mecocci, Franco Scarselli, and Paolo Andreini			
	5.1	Introduction		128
	5.2	Related Work		131
	5.3	Automatic Petri Plate Analysis Pipeline		134
		5.3.1	Image Acquisition	134
		5.3.2	Segmentation	135
		5.3.3	Colony Classification and Count	144
	5.4	Conclusions		148
	References			148
6	**Repurposing Routine Imaging for Cancer Biomarker Discovery Using Machine Learning**			**153**
	James W. Wang and Matt Williams			
	6.1	Introduction		153
		6.1.1	Imaging Modalities in Cancer Care	155
		6.1.2	Imaging in the Cancer Pathway	157
	6.2	Cancer Biomarker Research		159
	6.3	Machine Learning Applications in Cancer Cross-Sectional Imaging		160
		6.3.1	Lesion Detection/Classification	162
		6.3.2	Segmentation	163
		6.3.3	Cancer-Related Radiomics	164
	6.4	Preparing Radiology Data for Machine Learning		165
	6.5	Example of Biomarker Discovery: Sarcopenia in Cancer		166
		6.5.1	Defining Cancer Sarcopenia	166
		6.5.2	Scalable Solutions to Radiological Sarcopenia Assessment	168
		6.5.3	Remaining Translational Gaps	170
	6.6	Conclusion		170
	References			171

7	**Automatic Detection of LST-Type Polyp by CNN Using Depth Map**		177
	Yuji Iwahori, Shota Miyazaki, Hiroyasu Usami, M. K. Bhuyan, Boonserm Kijsirikul, Aili Wang, Naotaka Ogasawara, and Kunio Kasugai		
	7.1	Introduction	178
	7.2	Background	179
		7.2.1 Removal of Specular Reflectance Components and Generation of Lambertian Images	180
		7.2.2 Recovering 3D Shape and Creating Depth Map	181
	7.3	Construction of U-Net Using Depth Map	183
		7.3.1 Preprocessing and Construction of Dataset	183
		7.3.2 Construction of CNN Model Using U-Net Structure	185
	7.4	Experiment	188
		7.4.1 Evaluation Method	188
		7.4.2 Detection Experiment	189
	7.5	Conclusion	195
	References		195
8	**Artificial Intelligence and Deep Learning, Important Tools in Assisting Gastroenterologists**		197
	M. Luca, A. Ciobanu, T. Barbu, and V. Drug		
	8.1	Introduction	197
	8.2	Computer-Assisted Colonoscopy for CRC Early Detection	198
		8.2.1 Polyps' Semantic Segmentation	200
		8.2.2 Reviews and Meta-Analysis, Randomized Studies and AI Embedded Colonoscopy Devices	201
		8.2.3 Well Structured Labeled Databases	201
	8.3	Dealing with Video Colonoscopy Frames	202
	8.4	Deep Learning on Video Colonoscopies	204
		8.4.1 Deep Learning on Video Colonoscopies Using Nvidia Jetson Xavier	207
	8.5	Conclusions	208
	References		208
9	**Last Advances on Automatic Carotid Artery Analysis in Ultrasound Images: Towards Deep Learning**		215
	Maria del Mar Vila, Beatriz Remeseiro, Maria Grau, Roberto Elosua, and Laura Igual		
	9.1	Introduction	216
	9.2	Carotid Artery Segmentation and Intima Media Thickness Estimation in Ultrasound Images	218
		9.2.1 Deep Learning Proposal for IMT Estimation and Plaque Detection	224
	9.3	Carotid Artery Plaque Classification and Risk Assessment in 2D CA Ultrasound Images	231

		9.3.1	Data Properties: Transversal/Follow-Up, Different Devices, Image Modality, Artery Territory, Number of Samples and Ground Truth	232
		9.3.2	Work Objectives	233
		9.3.3	Image Features	237
		9.3.4	Methods and Results	239
	9.4	Discussion: Challenges in Deep Learning		240
	9.5	Conclusions and Future Perspective		241
	9.6	Appendix		241
	References			243
10	**Radiomics and Its Application in Predicting Microvascular Invasion of Hepatocellular Carcinoma**			249

Weibin Wang, Qingqing Chen, Risheng Deng, Fang Wang, Yutaro Iwamoto, Lanfen Lin, Hongjie Hu, Ruofeng Tong, and Yen-Wei Chen

	10.1	Introduction		250
		10.1.1	What is Radiomics	250
		10.1.2	What Has Been Achieved in Medical Image Analysis Using Radiomics	251
		10.1.3	Application of Radiomics in Hepatocellular Carcinoma	252
	10.2	Radiomics Signature and Prediction Model		254
		10.2.1	Medical Image Acquisition	254
		10.2.2	Calibration and Segmentation of Tumour Regions	254
		10.2.3	Feature Extraction and Quantification	256
		10.2.4	Feature Selection	257
		10.2.5	Classification and Prediction	259
		10.2.6	Material and Clinical Model	261
		10.2.7	Radiomics Model and Fusion Model for Predicting MVI	262
	10.3	Experiment		262
		10.3.1	Experimental Result	262
		10.3.2	The Direction of Future Progress	264
	10.4	Conclusion		264
	References			265
11	**Artificial Intelligence in Remote Photoplethysmography: Remote Heart Rate Estimation from Video Images**			267

Zhaolin Qiu, Lanfen Lin, Hao Sun, Jiaqing Liu, and Yen-Wei Chen

	11.1	Introduction		267
	11.2	Naive Methods		269
	11.3	Blind Signal Separation		269
		11.3.1	Independent Component Analysis	269
		11.3.2	Principal Component Analysis	270
		11.3.3	Joint Blind Signal Separation	271

11.4	Modelling	272
	11.4.1 CHROM	272
	11.4.2 Illumination Rectification	272
	11.4.3 2SR, POS	273
	11.4.4 Motion Reduction	274
11.5	Deep Learning	274
	11.5.1 Feature Extraction and Representation	275
	11.5.2 Interference Separation and Signal Enhancement	277
11.6	Popular Datasets for rPPG Learning	278
11.7	Future	279
References		281

Part II Advances in AI for Healthcare Information and Data Analytics

12 Mining Data to Deal with Epidemics: Case Studies to Demonstrate Real World AI Applications 287
Christina Nousi, Paraskevi Belogianni, Paraskevas Koukaras, and Christos Tjortjis

12.1	Introduction	288
	12.1.1 Goal and Research Questions	290
	12.1.2 Introduction to Data Mining	290
	12.1.3 Data Mining Techniques	292
	12.1.4 Chapter Overview	294
12.2	Literature Review	294
	12.2.1 Dengue Fever Analysis and Prediction with Classification and Association Rules	295
	12.2.2 Mumps Analysis with Clustering and Association Rules	296
	12.2.3 Cholera Analysis with Classification and Association Rules	296
	12.2.4 Measles Analysis with Classification	297
	12.2.5 Ebola Analysis with Clustering	298
12.3	Methodology	298
	12.3.1 Methodology Outline	298
12.4	Experiments	299
	12.4.1 Dataset	299
	12.4.2 Classification	299
	12.4.3 Clustering	303
	12.4.4 Association Rule Mining	307
12.5	Conclusion	308
	12.5.1 Discussion	309
	12.5.2 Overview of Contribution	309
	12.5.3 Future Directions	310
References		310

13 A Powerful Holonic and Multi-Agent-Based Front-End for Medical Diagnostics Systems 313
Zohreh Akbari and Rainer Unland
- 13.1 Introduction 314
- 13.2 State of the Art 318
- 13.3 Differential Diagnosis and the Holonic Medical Diagnostics System (HMDS) 323
  - 13.3.1 Differential Diagnosis as a Holonic Domain 323
  - 13.3.2 The Holonic Medical Diagnostics System 327
- 13.4 Learning in the HMDS 329
- 13.5 Simulations 335
  - 13.5.1 The Assessment of the Diagnosis Abilities 335
  - 13.5.2 The Assessment of the Self-Organization Abilities 338
- 13.6 Discussion 342
- 13.7 Conclusion 346
- References 347

14 Computer-Aided Detection of Depressive Severity Using Multimodal Behavioral Data 353
Jiaqing Liu, Yue Huang, Shurong Chai, Hao Sun, Xinyin Huang, Lanfen Lin, and Yen-Wei Chen
- 14.1 Introduction 353
- 14.2 Multimodal Behavioral Dataset of Chinese University Students with and Without Depressive Tendencies 354
  - 14.2.1 Collecting Survey Data 355
  - 14.2.2 Acquiring Behavioral Data 356
- 14.3 Computer-Aided Detection of Depressive Severity 360
  - 14.3.1 Feature Extraction 360
  - 14.3.2 Detection Model 363
- 14.4 Performance Evaluation 364
  - 14.4.1 Experimental Setup 364
  - 14.4.2 Evaluation Functions 364
  - 14.4.3 Results 365
- 14.5 Conclusions 368
- References 369

15 Classifying Process Traces for Stroke Management Quality Assessment: A Deep Learning Approach 373
Giorgio Leonardi, Stefania Montani, and Manuel Striani
- 15.1 Introduction 373
- 15.2 Background 374
  - 15.2.1 Convolutional Neural Networks 375
  - 15.2.2 Autoencoders 376
  - 15.2.3 Recurrent Neural Networks 376
- 15.3 Related Work 378

	15.4	Deep Learning Process Trace Classification for Quality Assessment	379
	15.5	Experimental Results	381
	15.6	Discussion and Conclusions	384
	References		385
16	**Synergy-Net: Artificial Intelligence at the Service of Oncological Prevention**		**389**
	Ruggiero Bollino, Giampaolo Bovenzi, Francesco Cipolletta, Ludovico Docimo, Michela Gravina, Stefano Marrone, Domenico Parmeggiani, and Carlo Sansone		
	16.1	Introduction	391
	16.2	Synergy-Net	393
		16.2.1 Medical Imaging and AI	395
		16.2.2 The Synergy-Net Architecture	397
		16.2.3 Synergy-Net: Analysed Tumours	400
	16.3	Skin Cancer	402
	16.4	Lung	407
	16.5	Colon Rectum Cancer	413
	16.6	Breast Cancer	417
	16.7	Gastric Carcinoma	418
	16.8	Thyroid Cancer	418
	16.9	Prostate Cancer	419
	16.10	Conclusions and Future Perspectives	419
	References		421
17	**New Insights on Implementing and Evaluating Artificial Intelligence in Cardiovascular Care**		**425**
	S. Dykstra, J. White, and M. L. Gavrilova		
	17.1	Introduction	425
		17.1.1 Artificial Intelligence and Machine Learning	426
		17.1.2 Relevance of Artificial Intelligence to the Future of Cardiovascular Care Delivery	427
		17.1.3 Implementing AI Within Institutional Healthcare Environments	429
	17.2	Data Capture and Management	430
		17.2.1 Data Availability	431
		17.2.2 Data Quality	433
		17.2.3 Data Generalizability	435
		17.2.4 Missing Data	436
		17.2.5 Data Permission and Privacy	438
	17.3	Model Development and Validation	440
		17.3.1 Model Development	441
		17.3.2 Model Performance Metrics May not Reflect Clinical Applicability	444
		17.3.3 Model Generalizability and Explainability	446

| | | 17.3.4 | Algorithmic Bias and Equity, Diversity and Inclusion | 447 |

17.4	Clinical Integration and Support	449
	17.4.1 Human Barriers	449
	17.4.2 Regulatory Considerations and Demonstrating Patient Value	450
17.5	Chapter Summary	452
References		453

Part I
Advances in AI for Healthcare Signal, Image, and Video Processing

Chapter 1
Advances in Artificial Intelligence for the Identification of Epileptiform Discharges

Aikaterini Karampasi, Kostakis Gkiatis, Ioannis Kakkos, Kyriakos Garganis, and George K. Matsopoulos

Abstract Epilepsy is one of the most common neurological disorders, with millions affected worldwide, disturbing the normal brain activity and causing abnormal dynamics to be initiated in various regions of the brain. In order to define the different ictal states and thus to evaluate the overall course of the patient, expert clinicians rely on Electroencephalography (EEG) denoting the differentiated events based on their experience and perception. As such, the implementation of cutting-edge Artificial Intelligence (AI) tools can not only alleviate misdetection but also provide a support bases in order to extract additional information regarding epileptic characteristics. In this chapter, AI tools and techniques that comprise distinct frameworks of epilepsy evaluation over the last decade are described while noting the performance, the methodological aspects and challenges. The related AI applications are further reviewed concerning the principles, parameters, complexity, feature selection and classification approaches and their implications in automated system integration and epileptic attributes identification.

Keywords Epilepsy · EEG · AI · Classification · Features

Table of Abbreviations

ADHD	Attention Deficit Hyperactivity Disorder
ANOVA	Analysis Of Variance
AI	Artificial Intelligence
ANN	Artificial Neural Networks
CT	Clustering Technique

A. Karampasi (✉) · K. Gkiatis · I. Kakkos · G. K. Matsopoulos
School of Electrical and Computer Engineering, National Technical University of Athens, Athens, Greece
e-mail: karampasi_k@biomig.ntua.gr

K. Gkiatis · K. Garganis
Epilepsy Monitoring Unit, St Luke's Hospital, Thessaloniki, Greece

© The Author(s), under exclusive license to Springer Nature Switzerland AG 2022
C.-P. Lim et al. (eds.), *Handbook of Artificial Intelligence in Healthcare*, Intelligent Systems Reference Library 211,
https://doi.org/10.1007/978-3-030-79161-2_1

CNN	Convolutional NN
DSS	Decision Support System
DT	Decision Trees
DTI	Diffusion Tensor Imaging
DTF	Directed Transfer Function
DWT	Discrete Wavelet Transformation
EMD	Empirical Mode Decomposition
EEG	Electroencephalogram
ED	Epileptiform Discharges
EZ	Epileptogenic Zone
FS	Feature Selection
FDA	Fisher Discriminant Analysis
FLP	Fractional Linear Prediction
FC	Functional Connectivity
fMRI	Functional Magnetic Resonance Imaging
FIS	Fuzzy Inference System
GFD	Generalized Fractal Dimensions
GP	Genetic Programming
GE	Grammatical Evolution
HFO	High Frequency Oscillations
HOS	Higher Order Spectra
IED	Inter-ictal Epileptiform Discharges
ILAE	International League Against Epilepsy
iEEG	Intracranial EEG
IMF	Intrinsic Mode Functions
kNN	K-Nearest-Neighbor
LS-SVM	Least Square SVM
LDA	Linear Discriminant Analysis
LPF	Linear Prediction Filter
LBP	Local Binary Patterns
MI	Mutual Information
NBC	Naïve Bayes Classifier
NN	Neural Network
PE	Permutation Entropy
PSR	Phase Space Representation
PCA	Principal Components Analysis
PNN	Probabilistic NN
RBF	Radial Basis Function
RF	Random Forests
RQA	Recurrence Quantification Analysis
SODP	Second Order Difference Plots
SOZ	Seizure Onset Zones
sEEG	Stereo EEG
SUDEP	Sudden Unexpected Death in Epilepsy
SVM	Support Vector Machines

WPT	Wavelet Packet Transform
WHO	World Health Organization

1.1 Background

Epilepsy is one of the most common neurological disorders, affecting more than 50 million people world-wide according to the World Health Organization (WHO) [1]. It is characterized by abnormal electrical discharges in the brain leading to various irregular phenomena (seizures), with core manifestations including alterations of consciousness and involuntary movements [2]. In this regard, scalp electroencephalogram (EEG) is considered the golden standard for diagnosing epilepsy since it provides a non-invasive approach for inspecting brain activity electrical potentials [3]. More invasive procedures such as intracranial EEG (iEEG) and stereo EEG (sEEG) describe an overall category of EEG recordings by utilizing either strips and/or grids or wires of electrodes accessing the brain directly [4]. However, the invasiveness of the iEEG (regardless of the methodology utilized) allows for sampling of a limited number of preselected brain areas only, among which, the neurologist must identify the ictal onset region, within a limited time-window, subsequently proceeding to its resection. At the same moment, iEEG investigation and subsequent brain operation encompass several dangers due to multiple surgeries [5–7]. In general, epilepsy evaluation accommodates the detection of seizure onset zones (SOZ) (i.e. describing the epileptogenic zone (EZ), which is further denoted as the cortical tissue that must be surgically resected in order for the patient to be seizure-free [8]) as well as the information regarding the state and the dynamics of the epileptic brain activity (i.e. meaning the changing rate of the signal [9]). SOZ denotes the taxonomy of the seizures categorizing them as focal (limited to a specific brain network within a single hemisphere) or generalized (referring to the involvement of bilateral hemispheric extensive networks) [10]. Since surgical removal of epileptic foci, especially in drug-resistant patients, is the adapted treatment course, identifying and marking of the exact cortical structures for extraction is of outmost importance [10].

For a robust and efficient automated detection of epileptiform discharges (ED), EEG data are usually divided and analyzed in five distinct periods, namely the non-seizure period, the pre-ictal, ictal, post-ictal and inter-ictal stages. Usually, the seizure-free interval coincides with the inter-ictal period, however, in most studies as non-seizure is considered the normal brain activity derived from healthy individuals. Specifically, the pre-ictal period has a duration of approximately 30–60 min prior to the seizure, ictal is the seizure period itself and may last from a few seconds to several minutes, whereas the post-ictal period is usually around 30 min after the ictal period [11]. Inter-ictal epileptiform discharges (IED) are identified as spikes having a duration of 20–70 ms or as sharp waves with specific characteristics lasting 70–200 ms [7]. These manifestations occur between seizures (between the post-ictal and pre-ictal period of the next seizure), yet they are pathological and they differentiate from background activity, while their EEG localization strongly corresponds to the brain regions the seizures originate from [12]. As more general definitions, one could note ictal as the seizure itself, post-ictal as an interval after the seizure and inter-ictal as a period between seizures, however this is a general rule that may be more confusing than explanatory [13, 14]. To date, identification of irregular brain activity is mostly based on visual inspection and manual annotation in order to detect all the distinct event types [15]. However, the IED are not always visible in the short time EEG recordings that are taking place rendering the SOZ identification as well as recognition of the distinct stages of the seizure ineffective [16]. What is more, most IED-detection related studies tend to use their own terminology, annotating the need for careful reading of the terms prior to interpreting the results.

Towards addressing the aforementioned concerns, the development of decision support systems (DSS) employing artificial intelligence (AI) tools can genuinely assist the expert clinicians for automatically recognizing the IED or eventually the SOZ, even in the case of the short-time iEEG or the non-invasive EEG recordings. In this direction, a variety of DSS have been implemented towards identifying the seizure onset, as well as for classifying and discriminating among the distinct EEG stages related to the ictal event (seizure). Events that would have been missed due to lack of time, experience or subjectivity issues shall be recognized with precision, leading to accurate predictions, while resolving manual annotation issues.

1.2 Artificial Intelligence Tools

Although the different studies that incorporate AI tools and techniques are comprised of distinct frameworks for epilepsy evaluation, most follow a common route namely feature extraction, feature selection and finally classification, as shown in Fig. 1.1. Notably, not all of these procedures are always employed, as they are not demanded

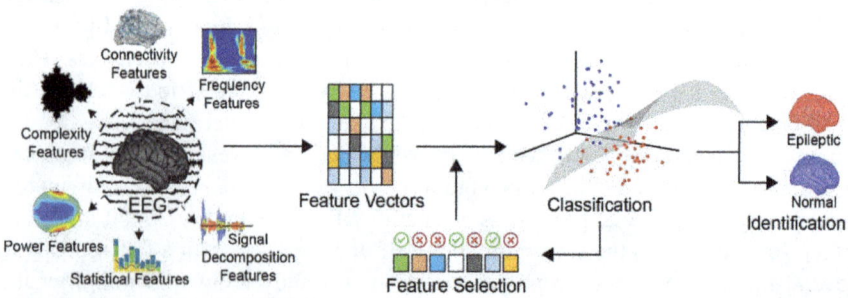

Fig. 1.1 The overall decision support system (DSS) framework is usually comprised of the feature extraction, feature selection and classification procedures. Results obtained from the classification task lead to redefining the features that will be employed

for efficacious results to be obtained. What is more, in most cases several preprocessing steps are employed (e.g. feature normalization etc.), although different in every study.

The feature extraction procedure is denoted as the calculation of various characteristics which are eventually utilized in the DSS. Those features have the potential to allow for learning of a specific pattern for discriminating stages of ED from normal EEG signal. Essentially, any metric can be used as a feature, though, the right choice of features and the significance on the final results is a subject of debate. As such, over the recent years several features have proven valuable in the effective identification of epileptic components. The most prominent include signal decomposition methods, where the initial EEG signals are decomposed into frequencies containing the representation of the initial signal in a certain range of brain wave rhythms (discrete wavelet transformation, DWT or empirical mode decomposition, EMD) or in order to further estimate a finite set of amplitude and frequency modulated components, namely the intrinsic mode functions (IMF), while utilizing the information extracted to estimate the frequency/energy content (Hilbert-Huang Transformation) [17–21]. Furthermore, signal variation and filtering methods also accommodate for the identification of distinctive epileptiform characteristics. Specifically, the calculation of the randomness of an EEG signal (entropy), the rate of variability (second order difference plots, SODP) or bispectral invariants about the formation of the brain waveforms (higher order spectra, HOS), provide appropriate measurements less prone to noise and artifacts when differentiating between the ictal-related signals and the normal ones [22–26]. In this context, statistical information can further assess the epileptic attributes by consolidating the initial signal with random noise (matched filtering), dividing it to clusters while determining common statistical properties (clustering technique, CT) and constructing histograms by calculating where EEG epochs cross a specific threshold (zero crossing interval histograms) [27–29]. Other features follow several parameters formed by the dynamic non-linear nature of the EEG (recurrence quantification analysis, RQA), the probability distribution of signal complexity (generalized fractal dimensions, GFD), image related invariant texture estimation (local binary patterns, LBP) and specific brain rhythm analysis (high frequency oscillations, HFO) [8, 30–32]. More recently, the progression of the dynamical properties of the EEG over time is employed, utilizing information for each time point (phase space representation, PSR), determining distinct signal types based on the nearby time points (Lyapunov exponents) and calculating the pairwise signal associations to form a connectivity scheme between the different brain channels (functional connectivity, FC) [5, 33–35]. It is worth mentioning that the aforementioned features may have several variations, in terms of different calculation functions and thus their exact definition may deviate among studies.

In any manner, the feature space that results from all these procedures is a high dimensional space, thus leading to the risk of overfitting and possible classification bias. In this context, feature selection (FS) frameworks are usually applied eliminating features that carry unnecessary and/or redundant information, while determining the most appropriate number of features that can lead to the optimal classification performance [36]. To alleviate overfitting or classification bias, the ratio among the instances (i.e., individuals) over the features is optimally around 3, however this is not always applicable, due to the different principles of the classification procedures incorporated in each study [37, 38]. Of note is that the vast number of FS algorithms employed for epileptiform classification procedures renders the creation of an exhaustive list impossible to make. As such, the most commonly used ictal-related FS methodologies are included in this chapter as the preceding step prior to the classification procedures. As a generalized procedure, FS takes into account each feature with regard to an objective function and ranks them accordingly. This is usually implemented on the basis of an internal classifier that discriminates features among labels either by appertaining to individual features (linear discriminant analysis, LDA), by comparing all pairs of features and retaining the most relevant ones (fisher discriminant analysis, FDA) or by discriminating instances that are close to one another (RELIEFF) [39–41]. In addition, the variance of the feature space can be utilized (principal components analysis, PCA) as well as the similarity between the feature vectors (mutual information, MI) to assess their discriminability information [10, 42]. Last but not least, evolutionary strategies can take into account the improvement of the classifier output in terms of performance eventually producing the optimal feature subset (genetic programming, GP, grammatical evolution, GE) [39, 43, 44].

The classification procedure is the main component of the DSS, with each classifier employing specific AI scripts, in terms of mathematical background, as well as statistical tools, to learn from the data provided to recognize patterns and discriminate among them. Classifiers can be distinguished into different categories with a more general taxonomy being clustering, statistical learning and rules based. Clustering classifiers divide the feature vectors into clusters (and sub-clusters) and predict the non-labeled data based on the resemblance (or feature vector proximity) of their neighbors. These classifiers include supervised and unsupervised algorithms, the most prominent of which are the k-nearest-neighbor (kNN) and k-means [41, 45–47]. Fuzzy inference system (FIS) is another clustering classification method which uses the input data based on certain parameters (such as the radius) defining the range of influence of each cluster's center on each instance [48]. Statistical learning algorithms, such as support vector machines (SVM) involve the representation of the instances in regard to the number and nature of features creating a new dimensional space onto which they will project the data [26, 49–51]. SVM, in particular, is a supervised algorithm that hypothesizes that in the new dimensional space (hyperspace), the data can be easily discriminated by calculating a finite distance between the different labels. Rules-based AI algorithms include a vast array of methodologies that range from probabilistic methods (i.e. assuming random model variables and searching thoroughly for the optimal values), best described by the extensively adopted Naïve Bayes classifier (NBC), to filtering and thresholding classifiers such as the linear prediction filter (LPF) that calculate the discrimination model by iteratively improving the coefficients of the filter depending on the repetition output and the defined threshold [32, 52]. Other algorithms like decision trees (DT) (or random forests (RF) that consist of massive numbers of DT paired with feature selection methodologies) utilize the features to construct rules that lead to the classification decision of new test data [19]. Last but not least, artificial neural networks (ANN) have gained ground over the recent years [53]. This is due to the ability of ANN to calculate and re-evaluate the cost function in a feed-forward back-propagation manner and thereby maximize their classification performance. For instance, probabilistic neural networks (PNN) are most commonly utilized in multiclass classification problems due to their distinction ability based on the Bayesian rule, while they optimize the weights of the model for the finest performance to be obtained [19, 54]. On the other hand, convolutional neural networks (CNN) are most commonly employed in 2D images, although a modified implementation for 1D signals can also be utilized, during which the features are represented after they have been convolved with a known matrix for better representation [2, 55].

All of the aforementioned AI tools are employed towards distinguishing the data in different categories. In the event of identifying a certain formation of a given signal, a binary problem exists, e.g. a new segment of signal fills the requirements or not. Nevertheless, multiclass classification problems can also arise (for instance, discriminating pre-ictal, ictal and post-ictal in an EEG recording demands three clusters/classes to be identified).

In the following sections, the AI methodologies utilized for classifying the EEG stages related to the ictal event, as well as for the identification of the seizure onset, in time, will be presented (Fig. 1.2). However, the existing literature over the last decade is exceedingly large, with many studies taking into account data from different patients, experimental designs and methods. In this context, the scope of this chapter is not to assess the efficiency of the AI tools employed, even though accuracies, where possible, are reported. For simplicity reasons other metrics are not provided, due to the differentiated metrics of each work rendering an immediate comparison among all studies not feasible. Nonetheless, in order to provide an abstract association between the different features extracted and methods that could be utilized, the studies

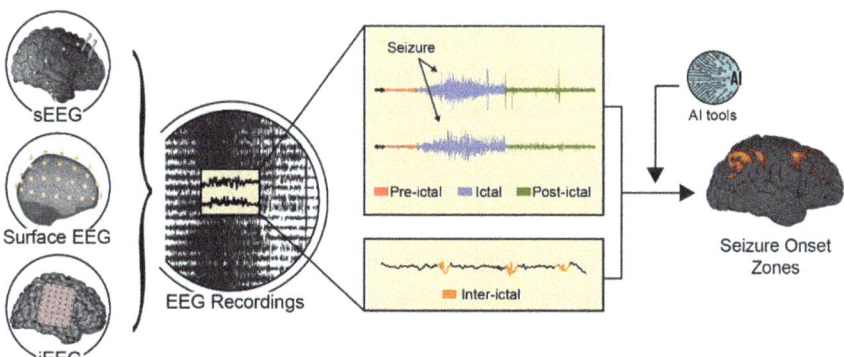

Fig. 1.2 Input data may be derived from surface or scalp EEG, stereo EEG (sEEG) using wires accessing directly the brain, or intracranial EEG (iEEG) using grids and/or strips. The distinct ictal stages are automatically determined through the AI tools using the ground truth from expert clinician, to eventually derive the seizure onset zones (SOZ)

mentioned include common or similar datasets on which each of the AI frameworks was tested.

1.3 Pre-Ictal, Ictal, Post-Ictal Detection

There are two main restrictions concerning the overall process of classifying these three distinct EEG periods: (i) the data employed for each framework and (ii) how the authors define each ictal moment. Thus, it is of great importance to demonstrate each performance along with the data that were utilized and the respective definition of the ictal stages. As such, in most scenarios, pre-ictal, ictal and post-ictal discrimination is a multiclass classification problem. Hence, a great portion of the literature that has come across this classification scheme, employ all kinds of consolidations to discriminate among them. For instance, the dataset provided by the University of Bonn contains five sets of 128-channel EEG [56]. These sets are labeled from A to E with set A and B designating surface EEG from five healthy controls with eyes open and closed respectively, while sets C, D and E accord for iEEG in the epileptogenic zone (seizure free), opposite to the epileptogenic zone (seizure free) and brain activity from the epileptogenic zone during seizure, respectively, derived from five epileptic patients. Regarding all of the abovementioned sets, in the original paper there is not a strict definition as to which interval they may refer to. As such, seizure free period in sets C and D is comprised of recordings from the EZ and opposite to the EZ brain regions. To that end, each of the studies mentioned below has defined what the implicated sets are utilized for (i.e., pre-ictal, post-ictal). Encompassing all the following pairs is a common combination for classification, facilitating analogies among the studies, although other combinations have been employed, as well.

From this standpoint, Kumar et al. [57] implemented the DWT in order to derive the approximate entropy, while utilizing SVM and neural network (NN) classifiers to discriminate between A-E, B-E, C-E, D-E, ACD-E, ABCD-E. The accuracy achieved ranged from 72.00 to 100.00% for NN, while SVM produced slightly different results ranging from 94.00 to 98.00%. In an analogous manner, another study utilized DWT followed by Hurst exponent-based feature extraction and SVM classification obtaining an accuracy of 89.00–99.00% [17]. DWT features and SVM was also employed paired with the fuzzy approximate entropy by Kumar et al. providing 93.00–100.00% accuracy between all sets' combinations, while Hsu et al. combined them with a SVM classifier with radial basis function (RBF) kernel and either GP or FDA for the feature selection procedure, trying to identify set C deriving 95.80% accuracy when employing GP and 88.00% accuracy when employing FDA [26, 39]. Other SVM implementations include least square SVM (LS-SVM) and CT features (84.90–99.90% accuracy) or histogram features deriving from calculated key-points (98.20–100.00% accuracy) [27, 51]. The robustness of DWT features was also illustrated in several other studies employing different classifiers. Lee et al. employed GP feature selection after they calculated the DWT and represented the data on a higher dimensional space (sets A-E) obtaining an accuracy of 98.20% [58]. In addition,

Guo et al. implemented DWT along with an ANN to acquire 97.75–99.60% accuracy, while Orhan et al. employed the DWT in order to calculate the centroids and probability distributions of the sub-bands, eventually, feeding them to a NN to derive their final labeling attaining 95.60–100.00% classification performance [43, 47]. In a related study, the convention of set C being the pre-ictal period, set D the post-ictal period and set E the ictal period, DWT features with a PNN achieved 83.10–99.80% classification accuracy [54]. On the other hand, Alickovic et al. employing data from [59] implemented a methodology comprised of PCA for signal pre-processing and several signal decomposition methods (IMF derived from the DWT or the wavelet packet transform, WPT) for feature calculation. Subsequently these features were fed into a RF and SVM classifier discriminating among ictal, pre-ictal and inter-ictal periods and attaining significantly high performance [19].

Alternative feature extraction approaches encompass entropy measurements as indicative characteristic of ictal-related states leading to 57.80–97.68% accuracy between the different sets with a NN technique [60]. In the same way, recurrent NN utilizing wavelet packet log energy entropy enhanced classification performance with an average of 99.85% proximity of measurement results to the true labels, while the use of permutation entropy (PE) with a SVM classifier produced an average accuracy of 86.10% [25, 61]. Moreover, LBP histogram features for 1D signals implemented along with ANN and Bayesian NN have been reported to have an attained accuracy of 93.00–99.50% and 92.80–99.50%, respectively, whereas Lyapunov exponents fed to a PNN provided multiclass classification accuracy of 98.10% [31, 34].

On this premise, it is evident that the indicative features employed in the different studies extend to an extremely large number and cannot be fully illustrated in this chapter, the same applies regarding the number of the classification methods implemented. For instance, Acharya et al. calculated several statistical measurements and classified the data by employing a variety of methods, while the FIS achieved the best performance with 98.10% accuracy in a threefold cross validation scheme [48]. In similar attempts, the utilization of the LPF provided 88.00–100.00% accuracy, while Guo et al. demonstrated that the combination of GP and a kNN classifier could lead to 93.50–99.20% accuracy accompanied by the identification of the most prominent features for discriminating ictal versus normal time periods [52, 62].

Deep learning has also been applied for the identification of ED (normal, pre-ictal, ictal and post-ictal). As such, Zhang et al. [2] utilized an enhanced CNN obtaining an accuracy of 98.90–99.90% between all sets' combinations, with the same authors also employing multiclass classification attaining a mean classification performance of 94.00–98.60%. Moreover, Xu et al. proposed a CNN which was fed with the normalized data provided by [56] to derive an accuracy of 99.39% [55]. In related studies, CNNs which were trained using EEG images rather than the signals themselves, following the rationale of a neurologist who inspects the signals, also resulted in very high classification predictions [3, 63]. Another effort was performed by employing a variety of pre-ictal lengths, number of electrodes and sampling frequencies [64]. However, although deep learning approaches in general present high-performance results, these methods diffuse the information in a way that is exceedingly difficult to decipher. In this regard, feature vectors interpretation presents several obstacles in the effort to elucidate the underlying brain processes that correspond to the epileptic moments.

In this context, AI has been implemented to detect brain activity characteristics apart from ictal states discrimination. Towards this direction, Mera-Gaona et al. [28] proposed a matched filter approach to detect whether a given spike is epileptiform or not (i.e., a normal EEG variant). This algorithm receives as its input a template spike comparing the type of spike on a given channel, by utilizing the matched filter and consequently a NN for correcting possible mistakes. Other studies utilized the GE on iEEG data from 6 patients in order to identify slow ripples versus normal brain activity, or they implemented a SVM using Lyapunov exponents to detect spike wave, sharp waves, spike and slow wave complex, sharp and slow wave complex, polyspike complex, spike rhythm [44, 65]. In order to classify spike waveforms, authors in another study implemented the DWT for both artifact removal and feature extraction purposes and, with a modified FIS, they derived 100.00% accuracy when evaluating their framework on six patients with iEEG recordings [66]. In a similar manner, Jiang et al. [67] utilized several wavelet functions to calculate the sub-bands of the signal and by composing certain rules they attained over 97.33% accuracy for detecting a certain type of spikes that were a priori noted by an expert clinician. More importantly, post-ictal detection has been referenced to as a possible biomarker for preventing sudden unexpected death in epilepsy (SUDEP) leading to the development of a linear regression model to detect the initiating and ending point of the post-ictal period [68]. In this model, probabilities of a certain time interval were determined as having exact starting and ending time-points for the post-ictal periods, subsequently thresholded in order to conclude whether the intervals would be labeled as post-ictal or not. However, no satisfying result was derived as the clinicians did not coincide on the exact starting and ending moments.

1.4 Seizure Detection

The holy grail of the neuroimaging in epilepsy studies is the identification of the seizure (i.e. ictal periods) ahead of time in order to alert the patient itself and/or the doctors and relatives to take the necessary precautions. Towards this direction, by employing data from [56], many studies utilize AI tools to discriminate dataset E from the other datasets A-D and recognize the seizure onset.

To that end, DWT was employed in binary classification schemes to discriminate set E from the other sets by Sharmila et al. [46]. They managed to achieve 100.00% accuracy when they compared normal brain waves (set A) with seizure brain waves (set E) in two classifiers, NBC and kNN. Also 100.00% accuracy was achieved for all classifiers they tested (NBC, kNN, NN, SVM) by Amin et al. when classifying seizure versus non-seizure [69]. Statistical tools, such as one-way analysis of variance (ANOVA), with combination of DWT with GFD derived features have been tested achieving high accuracy. Chen et al. [70] implemented a framework to automatically compute the optimal DWT attaining 99.33% accuracy performance. When it comes to feature selection methodologies, the LDA has proven to reach a 100.00% accuracy when employed with a SVM and the RBF kernel, while in another study, the best basis selection was utilized to keep only the most informative features in terms of discriminating the data reaching 99.45% accuracy when employing a kNN with a tenfold cross validation scheme [39, 68].

Furthermore, alternative decomposition tools, such as EMD and consecutively IMF calculation, have been extensively tested for their ability to classify ictal periods. Oweis et al. [21] has illustrated this by estimating the Hilbert-Huang frequency weights in the IMF achieving 94.00% accuracy when discriminating epileptic from normal EEG waveforms. In the same direction, Pachori et al. [18] employed the Hilbert transformation and further observed the statistical difference between EEG signal originating from seizure and normal EEG signals. The same authors have utilized this framework in iEEG data to detect seizures in focal temporal lobe epilepsy but it was only when LS-SVM classifier with the Morlet kernel was employed that they derived an accuracy of 99.50% [20, 71]. Additionally, when PSR features of the IMF were fed to a LS-SVM with the RBF kernel, a maximum accuracy of 98.33% was attained [33]. When SODP was utilized along with the EMD and the derived IMF in order to feed them to an ANN, they produced fine statistical results [22]. Statistical moments, such as mean, variance, skewness and kurtosis, in the Hilbert transformation of the IMF in the theta bands were fed to a SVM with RBF kernel by Fu et al. to achieve a 100.00% accuracy [48].

Analysis in the domain of frequency has not only been accomplished by decomposing the EEG signal in bands of frequencies, but through the spectral analysis as well, as demonstrated by Übeyli who employed it in a LS-SVM to obtain an accuracy of 99.56% [72]. Similarly, Garcés Correa et al. [7] utilized the power spectrum calculation followed by the calculation of derivatives of the signals in an attempt to locate the exact onset and offset time-points of the seizure in 21 patients that were submitted to iEEG. An alternate approach is presented in Selvakumari et al. [42], who employed the phase space as features in a PCA FS method. In this study, authors utilized a SVM to predict whether a specific segment of signal is seizure, followed by a NBC which eventually decides for the correct choice, leading to minimum errors, while the attained accuracy was 95.63%. Similarly, for dimensionality reduction purposes and the utilization of signal segments of various lengths, the RELIEFF FS algorithm was implemented to select the most informative of the features derived by the Q-Wavelet analysis, leading to 99.00% accuracy levels [40]. Wavelets were also employed by Gandhi et al. [73] by applying several levels of decomposition and selecting the approximations of level 6 and above to achieve a roughly 100.00% accuracy with the utilization of a PNN scheme.

When attempting to classify pre-ictal versus ictal periods, as to predict the incoming seizure, Rasekhi et al. [9] utilized 22 linear univariate features in a SVM classifier achieving fine results. Though, it should be noted that, in a similar attempt, Aung et al. [74] employed only one feature, namely the fuzzy entropy, achieving accuracy levels as high as 92.00%. Likewise, in such an attempt, statistical moments were calculated in Hilbert-Huang transformation following various decomposition methodologies deriving an accuracy range of 98.01–99.31% when employed in a

SVM [75]. More recently, Sharma et al. employed relative entropy, relative energy and FC measurements to predict the preictal period. They eventually attained an accuracy of 92.18% in predicting the seizure 18 min prior to it taking place [76].

Over and above the aforementioned feature extraction and classification methodological schemes, connectivity metrics have been considered for the seizure detection problems as well. A fine example that achieved 100.00% accuracy levels utilizing correlation metrics in several classifiers is the Iscan et al. study [77]. Similarly, Wang et al. demonstrated a classifier which was fed with calculations from the directed transfer function (DTF) as features using a SVM classifier with a fivefold cross validation scheme to attain an accuracy of 95.89% from 10 patients with refactory epilepsy [78]. Furthermore, it has been shown that a combination of the dynamic similarity index with the mean phase coherence can improve the seizure prediction accuracy [79].

Within this framework, a variety of machine learning methodological schemes have been employed for identifying not only the most prominent features that will result in fine performance, but also the classification scheme that will enhance this outcome. For instance, Mardini et al. implemented several classification algorithms along with GP and a variety of features achieving 100.00% accuracy when distinguishing sets A from E and sets B from E in a variety of classifiers, such as SVM, NBC, ANN or kNN, as well as in the scenario of sets AB from E when utilizing SVM, ANN, kNN [80]. kNN was also employed in a tenfold cross-validation framework using the Hurst exponent as features only to attain 100.00% accuracy [81]. In the same discrimination schemes, fractional linear prediction (FLP) (an implementation for fractal analysis similar to the GFD combined with linear prediction) was employed with a SVM and the RBF kernel to attain 95.33% accuracy [82]. A superior performance of 98.50% accuracy was obtained by Acharya et al. when utilizing an SVM, along with the HOS following the DWT [83]. Acharya et al. in a multiclass classification problem of discriminating normal, ictal and inter-ictal periods calculated the RQA parameters to feed them to several classifiers deriving the higher accuracy levels with the SVM classifier [32]. Texture features, such as the LBP, attained 99.33% accuracy when employed in a NN classifier with a tenfold cross-validation scheme [45]. The impact of the parameters used for the estimation of texture features in classification tasks have been explored by Ramanna et al. [84].

As the literature encompasses a wide range of implementations concerning either the data utilized, the AI methodologies employed as well as the framework facilitated, this chapter was restricted to limited studies in order to guide the reader through the various methodologies possible and its implication in the final results. Various extensive reviews exist that have covered the field of seizure detection in epilepsy [85].

1.5 Inter-Ictal Identification

When it comes to inter-ictal periods' identification, attention should be paid in the definition of the term each study has given as much confusion exist in this field. In contrast to the strict definition that has been given in a previous section, many studies have used different definition, such as intervals that are hours apart from seizures. As such, careful reading is necessary when interpreting the results and we do not present accuracy results in this section as direct comparison is not possible. Having this in mind, many studies have attempted to discriminate the inter-ictal waveforms from other waveforms including normal periods (i.e., compared to healthy EEG), ictal periods, pre-ictal periods.

In such manner, Kumar et al. calculated the DWT to obtain the approximation wavelet coefficients and utilize them as features to discriminate among sets C-E and D-E attaining high accuracy using a feed forward back-propagation NN [24]. Alternatively, the estimation of the IMF from the EMD were fed to a SVM classifier for distinguishing the inter-ictal from ictal intervals [50]. Notably, Bagheri et al. developed a framework to optimize the process of the identification of the IED using scalp EEG by eliminating the background activity to amplify their results. At its maximum, this methodology performed 4 times quicker utilizing a tenfold cross validation procedure where they employed wavelet, spectrogram as well as nonlinear energy operator features missing only 3% of inter-ictal periods in the EEG signal they used, which, as they mention, is not critical in an epilepsy diagnostic system [12]. Furthermore, the wavelet entropy and energy have also been estimated in an attempt to classify pre-ictal versus inter-ictal periods by manually selecting the channels that would be utilized in the overall training procedure [86].

Moreover, other features have also been utilized regarding the inter-ictal identification. For instance, Zandi et al. [29] employed zero-crossing intervals, Gaussian mixtures and similarity as well as dissimilarity indices to construct a seizure prediction system. Furthermore, in an effort to identify a relationship among inter-ictal and ictal periods, Karoly et al. [15] studied the rhythmicity of the signal's analysis in each ED. However, the authors had already observed that seizures were taking place in a certain point of time during the day, hence their results were eventually subject specific and they could not conclude whether the inter-ictal promoted or inhibited the ictal onset. For this study, 15 subjects had undergone iEEG recordings and the authors considered as pre-ictal 1 h time window preceding seizure and as the inter-ictal at least 8 h before and after seizure.

As mentioned in the previous sections of this chapter, several classification schemes have been implemented, towards the direction of identifying the most appropriate for the data in hand. In this light, Acharya et al. in an attempt of classifying normal (i.e., from healthy individuals), inter-ictal and ictal periods utilized a SVM along with the RBF kernel. HOS and texture were employed as features. However, one must notice that for the inter-ictal period, the seizure-free intervals are considered [23]. Equivalently, Lotfalinezhad et al. utilized a SVM with RBF kernel and a leave-one out cross validation scheme trying to discriminate inter-ictal from ictal periods (sets D-E) with the highest accuracy results achieved when the Hurst exponents calculation was utilized as features [87]. More recently, Truong et al. implemented a CNN in iEEG data from 21 patients, though, again defining as the pre-ictal periods at least 50 min prior to seizures and as the inter-ictal periods the seizure-free intervals [88]. Zhang et al. employed a CNN, as well, along with a leave-one-out cross-validation, fed by an extracted pattern which was created after projecting the data into a new high-dimensional space. Their overall framework was evaluated in 23 scalp EEG data from patients with different kinds of epilepsy, in order to classify pre-ictal and inter-ictal intervals [89]. Markedly, a different approach was considered from Goldstein et al. who performed an attempt to predict the length of time a video-EEG recording should take place in order for an IED to be present. What is more, they endeavored to correlate how many times an IED is present during the recording with other information, such as age, duration of epilepsy, duration of monitoring as well as with the type of the events. Their study was conducted based on data derived from 151 patients with temporal lobe epilepsy [16].

In drawing things to a close, very few studies exist to date that attempt to classify the inter-ictal spikes, i.e. IED with the strict definition of its meaning from other periods and further effort should be put into this field as it is essential for a correct epilepsy diagnosis.

1.6 Seizure Onset Zone

Classification of the distinct EEG stages, as well as the identification of the SOZ are two ostensibly irrelevant matters yet they lead to the same output, which is eventually aiding the neurologist to identify the region that produces these abnormal electrical manifestations and possibly guide the neurosurgeon as to which brain region is to be extracted. When it comes to identifying the SOZ there are two main methodologies that are employed. The leading one is by inspecting the ED and recognize the distinct events during the EEG recording, resulting to eventually identify the SOZ. The alternative technique is usually performed in invasive EEG as it consists of the calculation of the dynamics that are created before the seizure, which comprise a network representing the brain regions that initiate these abnormal electrical manifestations eventually leading to seizure. These two approaches are not distinct, considering that the latter is a consequence from the former.

Regarding the identification of the SOZ through the first approach, Geertsema et al. proposed the calculation of HFO from slow-wave-sleep segments of signal to further analyze it using the Huang-Hilbert transformation. When this framework was implemented in iEEG data from 9 individuals with a duration of at least one week, the classification accuracy varied depending on the subject [8]. More specifically, an autoregressive model was implemented towards distinguishing which electrodes are placed inside or outside the SOZ, which was further evaluated after the surgical removal of this region with the patient being seizure-free. Essentially, this algorithm detects the high residual values in the EEG data, however in some cases these spikes are being found in channels outside the SOZ, as well. Furthermore, in another work multiple statistical features were determined such as the variance, the root mean square, the difference absolute standard deviation among others, while employing a FS methodology based on MI [10]. LightGBM (a tree classifier with gradient-boosting) along with the FS procedure performed better when compared to a SVM, in almost every patient, during the identification of the channels placed in the SOZ. In a similar approach, Karthick et al. calculated the DWT-estimated statistical moments such as the mean value, variance, skewness and kurtosis for each coefficient and derived a maximum accuracy of 79.50% in an effort to identify the seizure onset on 20 patients with iEEG data [90]. As such, Random Forest outperformed other classifier implementations for the identification of the electrodes placed on the SOZ, as well as for the determination of the sparcity of the abnormal brain activity caused by the ED.

Having followed the alternate procedure, Machado et al. [91] were able to identify distinct subgroups of event types, depending on the exact location of the onset by utilizing sEEG data with a k-means algorithm, while employing the epileptogenicity index, (i.e. a quantification as to whether a specific location is implicated during the seizure or it is affected on a possible spread). Four subtypes (clusters) were eventually calculated when trying to discriminate the networks that arise during seizures in the prefrontal cortex. Similarly, Sabba et al. [92] tried to identify this network organization given that it would lead to implementing more accurate seizure detection algorithms. This course led them to recognize a pattern on the synchronization and resynchronization of the neurons firing tendency and finally to define the network dynamics during seizure. In the same direction, Kramer et al. [93] utilized depth electrodes and grids to measure the dynamic FC, while graph theory approaches derived the network that seemed to be activated during the seizure. An attempt to identify the EZ in 8 partial pharmaco-resistant epileptic patients using sEEG data was implemented in [6]. The authors employed Fourier Transformation and isolated the frequencies of interest (FOI) which were determined as having abnormal activity, when compared with other brain regions at the same time-point. When the FOIs were sorted, they were able to identify the region that was characterized as the EZ. Finally, Frusque et al. [5] employed FC in short segments of the signal that was utilized for the creation of graphs. This framework was utilized in sEEG recording from 6 patients and it managed to recognize the network relevant to each patient's SOZ.

Identifying the SOZ is of crucial importance in the study of epilepsy. As such, much attention has been given in this regard. Some studies presented here may not be the classic classification scheme, though, they are AI tools and frameworks that can accurately and reliably identify the SOZ and eventually be of help when time is critical.

1.7 Implications and Future Challenges

In this chapter, an outline of the advances of AI tools in epilepsy is presented and specifically, the employment of state of the art methods to identify the seizure onset, the distinct EEG stages (i.e., inter-ictal, pre-ictal, ictal, post-ictal) and the brain's activity re-organization during the seizure. Regarding the distinct types of epilepsy as well as the criteria based on which classification schemes may be based on in order to obtain fine performance results, the International League Against Epilepsy (ILAE) proposed an updated version of terms [94].

On this premise, several feature extraction approaches have been employed, usually combined with feature selection procedures or combinations of multiple classifiers implementations. As such, to provide an abstract indication of the AI methods efficiency, most of the epileptic studies mentioned utilize publicly available datasets. In this regard, due to the data similarity discrepancies in the performance output can be attributed to the data processing and methodologies applied.

Regarding seizure incident detection, several approaches have reported 100.00% accuracy [47, 49, 80, 95] utilizing specific sets (e.g. set A *vs* E from dataset in [46] indicated in the Pre-ictal, Ictal, Post-ictal Detection Section). Other studies that employ several combinations among the classes, which in some cases overlap each other (e.g. set C *vs* E, ABCD *vs* E), also result in very high accuracy (over 90.00%) [24, 47, 51, 61, 70, 71, 87], which is also apparent in the Inter-ictal Identification [23, 56] employing binary classification, although, expansion to multiclass classification paradigms naturally result in inferior performance [54]. Cortical characteristics such as multiple forms of epileptic spikes have also been extracted from the AI application providing an estimation of the distinct events in an individual's EEG recording and elucidating hidden epileptic substrates [64, 65].

However, one of the most prominent applications of AI in epileptic EEG signals is the detection of the distinct dynamics that initiate during the seizure, leading to the region responsible for the abnormal electrical manifestations. More specifically, the networks that are being organized prior to the seizure have proven to be of valuable information, and maybe even lead to better results, regardless of classification accuracies. For instance, functional connectivity (FC) represents a metric that estimates common brain activation among distinct brain regions and is widely utilized in a variety of studies ([5, 76, 78, 93]). However, FC is not the only tool being utilized to identify the arrangement of the brain activity, as shown in [8]. In some cases, graph theory is employed to further exploit the results of the feature extraction procedures ([5, 93]).

Especially in the field of Seizure Onset Zone identification, the results attained from the recognition of this network organization are further employed to predict the seizures, as such a tool might turn out to be of great importance. As illustrated in [76, 90] seizure onset prediction results in fine performance, however much are still to be done.

A major concern is that towards the identification of all the ictal stages one must carefully choose which time frames (from the entire EEG series) will be established as input in the AI implementation. For instance, the reported bibliography has defined several terms as the inter-ictal. However, in most cases inter-ictal moments have been labeled arbitrarily by various studies by characterizing seizure free moments as inter-ictal. This would not be of a problem, in case the pre-ictal is identified 30–60 min prior to the seizure, yet in any other instance it would present a severe issue for correct labeling. It should be noted that inter-ictal moments reflects the brain regions that are involved during the seizure while its form may vary from a spike to more complex waveforms, such as spike and wave, as it is defined [96, 97]. These abnormal manifestations may appear with lots of variations which neurologists are trained to identify, yet an automated system might miss. As such, although appropriate methodologies for identifying this form have been established, a universal approach should incorporate medical expertise apart from AI implementation [28]. In this direction, the overall procedure that takes place in following studies must provide solid data and correct labeling in order for the classification task to be unbiased. Moreover, an overall observation concerning the presented studies is that not everyone employs the same evaluation metrics (i.e., some studies only report sensitivity, specificity levels or false positive rate), thus there cannot be an immediate comparison with those which have presented accuracy performance.

To conclude, although fine results have been achieved concerning the seizure detection, as well as the classification of distinct ictal periods and the identification of the seizure onset, acquiring data with high sampling rate may determine the overall process and results. What is more, the correct initial identification and labeling of each ictal interval may also enhance the conclusions for the different AI tools implementations, providing the medical experts with automated methodologies proving a valuable and time-saving procedure. Fusion of modalities, such as the functional magnetic resonance imaging (fMRI) with concurrent EEG will also enhance such an implementation benefiting both the clinical and research community, resulting in better quality of life for the patients involved. What is more, FC is a metric of possible simultaneous activation of distinct brain regions which has been widely utilized in the field of neuroscience [98–100]. It has been proven an indicative biomarker for distinguishing among healthy individuals and patients and may be derived by several imaging methodologies, such as EEG, fMRI or even diffusion tensor imaging (DTI). Hence, an overall framework for possible disruption in either the brain activity or the physical connections (i.e. neurons) is an additional area of research, as well as the distinct mathematical tools that will be employed for its calculation. For instance, correlation metrics are usually utilized (i.e. Pearson's linear correlation, Spearman's rank correlation etc.) or even partial correlation metrics [101, 102].

References

1. Epilepsy. https://www.who.int/news-room/fact-sheets/detail/epilepsy
2. Zhang, G., et al.: MNL-network: a multi-scale non-local network for epilepsy detection from EEG signals. Front. Neurosci. **14**, (2020). https://doi.org/10.3389/fnins.2020.00870

3. Liang, W., Pei, H., Cai, Q., Wang, Y.: Scalp EEG epileptogenic zone recognition and localization based on long-term recurrent convolutional network. Neurocomputing **396**, 569–576 (2020). https://doi.org/10.1016/j.neucom.2018.10.108
4. Parvizi, J., Kastner, S.: Human intracranial EEG: promises and limitations. Nat. Neurosci. **21**(4), 474–483 (2018). https://doi.org/10.1038/s41593-018-0108-2
5. Frusque, G., Borgnat, P., Gonçalves, P., Jung, J.: Semi-automatic extraction of functional dynamic networks describing patient's epileptic seizures. Front. Neurol. **11**, (2020). https://doi.org/10.3389/fneur.2020.579725
6. Gnatkovsky, V., et al.: Identification of reproducible ictal patterns based on quantified frequency analysis of intracranial EEG signals. Epilepsia **52**(3), 477–488 (2011). https://doi.org/10.1111/j.1528-1167.2010.02931.x
7. Garcés Correa, A., Orosco, L., Diez, P., Laciar, E.: Automatic detection of epileptic seizures in long-term EEG records. Comput. Biol. Med. **57**, 66–73 (2015). https://doi.org/10.1016/j.compbiomed.2014.11.013
8. Geertsema, E.E., Visser, G.H., Velis, D.N., Claus, S.P., Zijlmans, M., Kalitzin, S.N.: Automated seizure onset zone approximation based on nonharmonic high-frequency oscillations in human interictal intracranial EEGs. Int. J. Neural Syst. (2015). https://doi.org/10.1142/S012906571550015X
9. Rasekhi, J., Mollaei, M.R.K., Bandarabadi, M., Teixeira, C.A., Dourado, A.: Preprocessing effects of 22 linear univariate features on the performance of seizure prediction methods. J. Neurosci. Methods **217**(1–2), 9–16 (2013). https://doi.org/10.1016/j.jneumeth.2013.03.019
10. Akter, M.S., et al.: Statistical features in high-frequency bands of interictal iEEG work efficiently in identifying the seizure onset zone in patients with focal epilepsy. Entropy **22**(12), (2020). Article No.: 12. https://doi.org/10.3390/e22121415
11. Parvez, M.Z., Paul, M., Antolovich, M.: Detection of pre-stage of epileptic seizure by exploiting temporal correlation of EMD decomposed EEG signals. JOMB **4**(2), 110–116 (2015). https://doi.org/10.12720/jomb.4.2.110-116
12. Bagheri, E., Jin, J., Dauwels, J., Cash, S., Westover, M.B.: A fast machine learning approach to facilitate the detection of interictal epileptiform discharges in the scalp electroencephalogram. J. Neurosci. Methods **326**, 108362 (2019). https://doi.org/10.1016/j.jneumeth.2019.108362
13. Fisher, R.S., Scharfman, H.E., de Curtis, M.: How can we identify ictal and interictal abnormal activity? Adv. Exp. Med. Biol. **813**, 3–23 (2014). https://doi.org/10.1007/978-94-017-8914-1_1
14. Fisher, R.S., Engel, J.J.: Definition of the postictal state: when does it start and end? Epilepsy Behav. **19**(2), 100–104 (2010). https://doi.org/10.1016/j.yebeh.2010.06.038
15. Karoly, P.J., et al.: Interictal spikes and epileptic seizures: their relationship and underlying rhythmicity. Brain **139**(4), 1066–1078 (2016). https://doi.org/10.1093/brain/aww019
16. Goldstein, L., Margiotta, M., Guina, M.L., Sperling, M.R., Nei, M.: Long-term video-EEG monitoring and interictal epileptiform abnormalities. Epilepsy Behav. **113**, 107523 (2020). https://doi.org/10.1016/j.yebeh.2020.107523
17. Madan, S., Srivastava, K., Sharmila, A., Mahalakshmi, P.: A case study on discrete wavelet transform based hurst exponent for epilepsy detection. J. Med. Eng. Technol. **42**(1), 9–17 (2018). https://doi.org/10.1080/03091902.2017.1394390
18. Pachori, R.B., Bajaj, V.: Analysis of normal and epileptic seizure EEG signals using empirical mode decomposition. Comput. Methods Prog. Biomed. **104**(3), 373–381 (2011). https://doi.org/10.1016/j.cmpb.2011.03.009
19. Alickovic, E., Kevric, J., Subasi, A.: Performance evaluation of empirical mode decomposition, discrete wavelet transform, and wavelet packed decomposition for automated epileptic seizure detection and prediction. Biomed. Signal Process. Control **39**, 94–102 (2018). https://doi.org/10.1016/j.bspc.2017.07.022
20. Bajaj, V., Pachori, R.B.: Epileptic seizure detection based on the instantaneous area of analytic intrinsic mode functions of EEG signals. Biomed. Eng. Lett. **3**(1), 17–21 (2013). https://doi.org/10.1007/s13534-013-0084-0

21. Oweis, R.J., Abdulhay, E.W.: Seizure classification in EEG signals utilizing Hilbert-Huang transform. Biomed. Eng. Online **10**(1), 38 (2011). https://doi.org/10.1186/1475-925X-10-38
22. Pachori, R.B., Patidar, S.: Epileptic seizure classification in EEG signals using second-order difference plot of intrinsic mode functions. Comput. Methods Prog. Biomed. **113**(2), 494–502 (2014). https://doi.org/10.1016/j.cmpb.2013.11.014
23. Acharya, U.R., et al.: Automated diagnosis of epilepsy using CWT, HOS and texture parameters. Int. J. Neural Syst. **23**(3), 1350009 (2013). https://doi.org/10.1142/S0129065713500093
24. Kumar, Y., Dewal, M.L., Anand, R.S.: Relative wavelet energy and wavelet entropy based epileptic brain signals classification. Biomed. Eng. Lett. **2**(3), 147–157 (2012). https://doi.org/10.1007/s13534-012-0066-7
25. Nicolaou, N., Georgiou, J.: Detection of epileptic electroencephalogram based on permutation entropy and support vector machines. Expert Syst. Appl. **39**(1), 202–209 (2012). https://doi.org/10.1016/j.eswa.2011.07.008
26. Kumar, Y., Dewal, M.L., Anand, R.S.: Epileptic seizure detection using DWT based fuzzy approximate entropy and support vector machine. Neurocomputing **133**, 271–279 (2014). https://doi.org/10.1016/j.neucom.2013.11.009
27. Siuly, Li, Y., (Paul) Wen, P.: Clustering technique-based least square support vector machine for EEG signal classification. Comput. Methods Prog. Biomed. **104**(3), 358–372 (2011). https://doi.org/10.1016/j.cmpb.2010.11.014
28. Mera-Gaona, M., López, D.M., Vargas-Canas, R., Miño, M.: Epileptic spikes detector in pediatric EEG based on matched filters and neural networks. Brain Inf. **7**(1), (2020). https://doi.org/10.1186/s40708-020-00106-0
29. Zandi, A.S., Tafreshi, R., Javidan, M., Dumont, G.A.: Predicting epileptic seizures in scalp EEG based on a variational Bayesian Gaussian mixture model of zero-crossing intervals. IEEE Trans. Biomed. Eng. **60**(5), 1401–1413 (2013). https://doi.org/10.1109/TBME.2012.2237399
30. Uthayakumar, R., Easwaramoorthy, D.: Epileptic seizure detection in EEG signals using multifractal analysis and wavelet transform. Fractals **21**(02), 1350011 (2013). https://doi.org/10.1142/S0218348X13500114
31. Kaya, Y., Uyar, M., Tekin, R., Yıldırım, S.: 1D-local binary pattern based feature extraction for classification of epileptic EEG signals. Appl. Math. Comput. **243**, 209–219 (2014). https://doi.org/10.1016/j.amc.2014.05.128
32. Acharya, U.R., Sree, S.V., Chattopadhyay, S., Yu, W., Ang, P.C.A.: Application of recurrence quantification analysis for the automated identification of epileptic EEG signals. Int. J. Neural Syst. **21**(3), 199–211 (2011). https://doi.org/10.1142/S0129065711002808
33. Sharma, R., Pachori, R.B.: Classification of epileptic seizures in EEG signals based on phase space representation of intrinsic mode functions. Expert Syst. Appl. **42**(3), 1106–1117 (2015). https://doi.org/10.1016/j.eswa.2014.08.030
34. Übeyli, E.D.: Lyapunov exponents/probabilistic neural networks for analysis of EEG signals. Expert Syst. Appl. **37**(2), 985–992 (2010). https://doi.org/10.1016/j.eswa.2009.05.078
35. Friston, K.J.: Functional and effective connectivity: a review. Brain Connectivity **1**(1), 13–36 (2011). https://doi.org/10.1089/brain.2011.0008
36. Ambroise, C., McLachlan, G.J.: Selection bias in gene extraction on the basis of microarray gene-expression data. PNAS **99**(10), 6562–6566 (2002). https://doi.org/10.1073/pnas.102102699
37. Foley, D.: Considerations of sample and feature size. IEEE Trans. Inf. Theory **18**(5), 618–626 (1972). https://doi.org/10.1109/TIT.1972.1054863
38. Muñoz, M.A., Villanova, L., Baatar, D., Smith-Miles, K.: Instance spaces for machine learning classification. Mach. Learn. **107**(1), 109–147 (2018). https://doi.org/10.1007/s10994-017-5629-5
39. Hsu, K.-C., Yu, S.-N.: Detection of seizures in EEG using subband nonlinear parameters and genetic algorithm. Comput. Biol. Med. **40**(10), 823–830 (2010). https://doi.org/10.1016/j.compbiomed.2010.08.005

40. Nishad, A., Pachori, R.B.: Classification of epileptic electroencephalogram signals using tunable-Q wavelet transform based filter-bank. J. Ambient Intell. Human Comput. (2020). https://doi.org/10.1007/s12652-020-01722-8
41. Wang, D., Miao, D., Xie, C.: Best basis-based wavelet packet entropy feature extraction and hierarchical EEG classification for epileptic detection. Expert Syst. Appl. **38**(11), 14314–14320 (2011). https://doi.org/10.1016/j.eswa.2011.05.096
42. Selvakumari, R.S., Mahalakshmi, M., Prashalee, P.: Patient-specific seizure detection method using hybrid classifier with optimized electrodes. J. Med. Syst. **43**(5), 121 (2019). https://doi.org/10.1007/s10916-019-1234-4
43. Guo, L., Rivero, D., Dorado, J., Rabuñal, J.R., Pazos, A.: Automatic epileptic seizure detection in EEGs based on line length feature and artificial neural networks. J. Neurosci. Methods **191**(1), 101–109 (2010). https://doi.org/10.1016/j.jneumeth.2010.05.020
44. Smart, O., Tsoulos, I.G., Gavrilis, D., Georgoulas, G.: Grammatical evolution for features of epileptic oscillations in clinical intracranial electroencephalograms. Expert Syst Appl **38**(8), 9991–9999 (2011). https://doi.org/10.1016/j.eswa.2011.02.009
45. Kumar, T.S., Kanhangad, V., Pachori, R.B.: Classification of seizure and seizure-free EEG signals using local binary patterns. Biomed. Signal Process. Control **15**, 33–40 (2015). https://doi.org/10.1016/j.bspc.2014.08.014
46. Sharmila, A., Geethanjali, P.: DWT based detection of epileptic seizure from EEG signals using Naive Bayes and k-NN classifiers. IEEE Access **4**, 7716–7727 (2016). https://doi.org/10.1109/ACCESS.2016.2585661
47. Orhan, U., Hekim, M., Ozer, M.: EEG signals classification using the K-means clustering and a multilayer perceptron neural network model. Expert Syst. Appl. **38**(10), 13475–13481 (2011). https://doi.org/10.1016/j.eswa.2011.04.149
48. Acharya, U.R., Molinari, F., Sree, S.V., Chattopadhyay, S., Ng, K.-H., Suri, J.S.: Automated diagnosis of epileptic EEG using entropies. Biomed. Signal Process. Control **7**(4), 401–408 (2012). https://doi.org/10.1016/j.bspc.2011.07.007
49. Fu, K., Qu, J., Chai, Y., Dong, Y.: Classification of seizure based on the time-frequency image of EEG signals using HHT and SVM. Biomed. Signal Process. Control **13**, 15–22 (2014). https://doi.org/10.1016/j.bspc.2014.03.007
50. Li, S., Zhou, W., Yuan, Q., Geng, S., Cai, D.: Feature extraction and recognition of ictal EEG using EMD and SVM. Comput. Biol. Med. **43**(7), 807–816 (2013). https://doi.org/10.1016/j.compbiomed.2013.04.002
51. Tiwari, A.K., Pachori, R.B., Kanhangad, V., Panigrahi, B.K.: Automated diagnosis of epilepsy using key-point-based local binary pattern of EEG signals. IEEE J. Biomed. Health Inf. **21**(4), 888–896 (2017). https://doi.org/10.1109/JBHI.2016.2589971
52. Altunay, S., Telatar, Z., Erogul, O.: Epileptic EEG detection using the linear prediction error energy. Expert Syst. Appl. **37**(8), 5661–5665 (2010). https://doi.org/10.1016/j.eswa.2010.02.045
53. Teixeira, C.A., et al.: EPILAB: A software package for studies on the prediction of epileptic seizures. J. Neurosci. Methods **200**(2), 257–271 (2011). https://doi.org/10.1016/j.jneumeth.2011.07.002
54. Gong, C., Zhang, X., Niu, Y.: Identification of epilepsy from intracranial EEG signals by using different neural network models. Comput. Biol. Chem. **87**, 107310 (2020). https://doi.org/10.1016/j.compbiolchem.2020.107310
55. Xu, G., Ren, T., Chen, Y., Che, W., A one-dimensional CNN-LSTM model for epileptic seizure recognition using EEG signal analysis. Front. Neurosci. **14**, (2020). https://doi.org/10.3389/fnins.2020.578126
56. Andrzejak, R.G., Lehnertz, K., Mormann, F., Rieke, C., David, P., Elger, C.E.: Indications of nonlinear deterministic and finite-dimensional structures in time series of brain electrical activity: dependence on recording region and brain state. Phys. Rev. E. Stat. Nonlin. Soft Matter Phys. **64**(6 Pt 1), 061907 (2001). https://doi.org/10.1103/PhysRevE.64.061907
57. Kumar, Y., Dewal, M.L., Anand, R.S.: Epileptic seizures detection in EEG using DWT-based ApEn and artificial neural network. SIViP **8**(7), 1323–1334 (2014). https://doi.org/10.1007/s11760-012-0362-9

58. Lee, S.-H., Lim, J.S., Kim, J.-K., Yang, J., Lee, Y.: Classification of normal and epileptic seizure EEG signals using wavelet transform, phase-space reconstruction, and Euclidean distance. Comput. Methods Prog. Biomed. **116**(1), 10–25 (2014). https://doi.org/10.1016/j.cmpb.2014.04.012
59. EEG Database—Seizure Prediction Project Freiburg. http://epilepsy.uni-freiburg.de/freiburg-seizure-prediction-project/eeg-database
60. Raghu, S., Sriraam, N.: Optimal configuration of multilayer perceptron neural network classifier for recognition of intracranial epileptic seizures. Expert Syst. Appl. **89**, 205–221 (2017). https://doi.org/10.1016/j.eswa.2017.07.029
61. Raghu, S., Sriraam, N., Kumar, G.P.: Classification of epileptic seizures using wavelet packet log energy and norm entropies with recurrent Elman neural network classifier. Cogn. Neurodyn. **11**(1), 51–66 (2017). https://doi.org/10.1007/s11571-016-9408-y
62. Guo, L., Rivero, D., Dorado, J., Munteanu, C.R., Pazos, A.: Automatic feature extraction using genetic programming: an application to epileptic EEG classification. Expert Syst. Appl. **38**(8), 10425–10436 (2011). https://doi.org/10.1016/j.eswa.2011.02.118
63. Goldberger, A.L., et al.: PhysioBank, PhysioToolkit, and PhysioNet: components of a new research resource for complex physiologic signals. Circulation **101**(23), E215–E220 (2000). https://doi.org/10.1161/01.cir.101.23.e215
64. Chung, Y.G., et al.: Deep convolutional neural network based interictal-preictal electroencephalography prediction: application to focal cortical dysplasia type-II. Front. Neurol. **11**, (2020). https://doi.org/10.3389/fneur.2020.594679
65. Li, Q., Gao, J., Huang, Q., Wu, Y., Xu, B.: Distinguishing epileptiform discharges from normal electroencephalograms using scale-dependent Lyapunov exponent. Front. Bioeng. Biotechnol. **8**, (2020). https://doi.org/10.3389/fbioe.2020.01006
66. Khosropanah, P., Ramli, A.R., Abbasi, M.R., Marhaban, M.H., Ahmedov, A.: A hybrid unsupervised approach toward EEG epileptic spikes detection. Neural Comput. Appl. **32**(7), 2521–2532 (2020). https://doi.org/10.1007/s00521-018-3797-2
67. Jiang, Y., Chen, W., Zhang, T., Li, M., You, Y., Zheng, X.: Developing multi-component dictionary-based sparse representation for automatic detection of epileptic EEG spikes. Biomed. Signal Process. Control **60**, 101966 (2020). https://doi.org/10.1016/j.bspc.2020.101966
68. Theeranaew, W., et al.: Automated detection of postictal generalized EEG suppression. IEEE Trans. Biomed. Eng. **65**(2), 371–377 (2018). https://doi.org/10.1109/TBME.2017.2771468
69. Amin, H.U., Yusoff, M.Z., Ahmad, R.F.: A novel approach based on wavelet analysis and arithmetic coding for automated detection and diagnosis of epileptic seizure in EEG signals using machine learning techniques. Biomed. Signal Process. Control **56**, 101707 (2020). https://doi.org/10.1016/j.bspc.2019.101707
70. Chen, D., Wan, S., Xiang, J., Bao, F.S.: A high-performance seizure detection algorithm based on discrete wavelet transform (DWT) and EEG. PLoS ONE **12**(3), (2017). https://doi.org/10.1371/journal.pone.0173138
71. Bajaj, V., Pachori, R.B.: Classification of seizure and nonseizure EEG signals using empirical mode decomposition. IEEE Trans. Inf. Technol. Biomed. **16**(6), 1135–1142 (2012). https://doi.org/10.1109/TITB.2011.2181403
72. Übeyli, E.D.: Least squares support vector machine employing model-based methods coefficients for analysis of EEG signals. Expert Syst. Appl. **37**(1), 233–239 (2010). https://doi.org/10.1016/j.eswa.2009.05.012
73. Gandhi, T., Panigrahi, B.K., Anand, S.: A comparative study of wavelet families for EEG signal classification. Neurocomputing **74**(17), 3051–3057 (2011). https://doi.org/10.1016/j.neucom.2011.04.029
74. Aung, S.T., Wongsawat, Y.: Modified-distribution entropy as the features for the detection of epileptic seizures. Front. Physiol. **11**, (2020). https://doi.org/10.3389/fphys.2020.00607
75. Mahjoub, C., Jeannès, R.L.B., Lajnef, T., Kachouri, A.: Epileptic seizure detection on EEG signals using machine learning techniques and advanced preprocessing methods. Biomed. Eng. (Biomedizinische Technik) **65**(1), 33–50 (2020). https://doi.org/10.1515/bmt-2019-0001

76. Sharma, A., Rai, J.K., Tewari, R.P.: Scalp electroencephalography (sEEG) based advanced prediction of epileptic seizure time and identification of epileptogenic region. Biomed. Eng. (Biomedizinische Technik) **65**(6), 705–720 (2020). https://doi.org/10.1515/bmt-2020-0044
77. Iscan, Z., Dokur, Z., Demiralp, T.: Classification of electroencephalogram signals with combined time and frequency features. Expert Syst. Appl. **38**(8), 10499–10505 (2011). https://doi.org/10.1016/j.eswa.2011.02.110
78. Wang, G., Ren, D., Li, K., Wang, D., Wang, M., Yan, X.: EEG-based detection of epileptic seizures through the use of a directed transfer function method. IEEE Access **6**, 47189–47198 (2018). https://doi.org/10.1109/ACCESS.2018.2867008
79. Feldwisch-Drentrup, H., Schelter, B., Jachan, M., Nawrath, J., Timmer, J., Schulze-Bonhage, A.: Joining the benefits: combining epileptic seizure prediction methods. Epilepsia **51**(8), 1598–1606 (2010). https://doi.org/10.1111/j.1528-1167.2009.02497.x
80. Mardini, W., Yassein, M.M.B., Al-Rawashdeh, R., Aljawarneh, S., Khamayseh, Y., Meqdadi, O.: Enhanced detection of epileptic seizure using EEG signals in combination with machine learning classifiers. IEEE Access **8**, 24046–24055 (2020). https://doi.org/10.1109/ACCESS.2020.2970012
81. Lahmiri, S., Shmuel, A.: Accurate classification of seizure and seizure-free intervals of intracranial EEG signals from epileptic patients. IEEE Trans. Instrum. Meas. **68**(3), 791–796 (2019). https://doi.org/10.1109/TIM.2018.2855518
82. Joshi, V., Pachori, R.B., Vijesh, A.: Classification of ictal and seizure-free EEG signals using fractional linear prediction. Biomed. Signal Process. Control **9**, 1–5 (2014). https://doi.org/10.1016/j.bspc.2013.08.006
83. Acharya, U.R., Sree, S.V., Suri, J.S.: Automatic detection of epileptic EEG signals using higher order cumulant features. Int. J. Neural Syst. **21**(05), 403–414 (2011). https://doi.org/10.1142/S0129065711002912
84. Ramanna, S., Tirunagari, S., Windridge, D.: Epileptic seizure detection using constrained singular spectrum analysis and 1D-local binary patterns. Health Technol. **10**(3), 699–709 (2020). https://doi.org/10.1007/s12553-019-00395-4
85. Siddiqui, M.K., Morales-Menendez, R., Huang, X., Hussain, A.: A review of epileptic seizure detection using machine learning classifiers. Brain Inf. **7**(1), (2020). https://doi.org/10.1186/s40708-020-00105-1
86. Gadhoumi, K., Lina, J.-M., Gotman, J.: Discriminating preictal and interictal states in patients with temporal lobe epilepsy using wavelet analysis of intracerebral EEG. Clin Neurophysiol **123**(10), 1906–1916 (2012). https://doi.org/10.1016/j.clinph.2012.03.001
87. Lotfalinezhad, H., Maleki, A.: TTA, a new approach to estimate Hurst exponent with less estimation error and computational time. Phys. A **553**, 124093 (2020). https://doi.org/10.1016/j.physa.2019.124093
88. Truong, N.D., et al.: Convolutional neural networks for seizure prediction using intracranial and scalp electroencephalogram. Neural Netw. **105**, 104–111 (2018). https://doi.org/10.1016/j.neunet.2018.04.018
89. Zhang, Y., Guo, Y., Yang, P., Chen, W., Lo, B.: Epilepsy seizure prediction on EEG using common spatial pattern and convolutional neural network. IEEE J. Biomed. Health Inform. **24**(2), 465–474 (2020). https://doi.org/10.1109/JBHI.2019.2933046
90. Karthick, P.A., Tanaka, H., Khoo, H.M., Gotman, J.: Could we have missed out the seizure onset: a study based on intracranial EEG. Clin. Neurophysiol. **131**(1), 114–126 (2020). https://doi.org/10.1016/j.clinph.2019.10.011
91. Machado, S., et al.: Prefrontal seizure classification based on stereo-EEG quantification and automatic clustering. Epilepsy Behav. **112**, 107436 (2020). https://doi.org/10.1016/j.yebeh.2020.107436
92. Cymerblit-Sabba, A., Schiller, Y.: Network dynamics during development of pharmacologically induced epileptic seizures in rats in vivo. J. Neurosci. **30**(5), 1619–1630 (2010). https://doi.org/10.1523/JNEUROSCI.5078-09.2010
93. Kramer, M.A., Eden, U.T., Kolaczyk, E.D., Zepeda, R., Eskandar, E.N., Cash, S.S.: Coalescence and fragmentation of cortical networks during focal seizures. J. Neurosci. **30**(30), 10076–10085 (2010). https://doi.org/10.1523/JNEUROSCI.6309-09.2010

94. Fisher, R.S., et al.: Operational classification of seizure types by the international league against epilepsy: position paper of the ILAE commission for classification and terminology. Epilepsia **58**(4), 522–530 (2017). https://doi.org/10.1111/epi.13670
95. Subasi, A., Ismail Gursoy, M.: EEG signal classification using PCA, ICA, LDA and support vector machines. Expert Syst. Appl. **37**(12), 8659–8666, (2010). https://doi.org/10.1016/j.eswa.2010.06.065
96. Kane, N., et al.: A revised glossary of terms most commonly used by clinical electroencephalographers and updated proposal for the report format of the EEG findings. Revision 2017. Clin. Neurophysiol. Pract. **2**, 170–185 (2017). https://doi.org/10.1016/j.cnp.2017.07.002
97. Kural, M.A., et al.: Criteria for defining interictal epileptiform discharges in EEG: a clinical validation study. Neurology **94**(20), e2139–e2147 (2020). https://doi.org/10.1212/WNL.0000000000009439
98. Woodward, N.D., Cascio, C.J.: Resting-state functional connectivity in psychiatric disorders. JAMA Psychiat. **72**(8), 743–744 (2015). https://doi.org/10.1001/jamapsychiatry.2015.0484
99. Kakkos, I., et al.: Mental workload drives different reorganizations of functional cortical connectivity between 2D and 3D simulated flight experiments. IEEE Trans. Neural Syst. Rehabil. Eng. **27**(9), 1704–1713 (2019). https://doi.org/10.1109/TNSRE.2019.2930082
100. Schumacher, J., et al.: Dynamic functional connectivity changes in dementia with Lewy bodies and Alzheimer's disease. NeuroImage: Clin. **22**, 101812, (2019). https://doi.org/10.1016/j.nicl.2019.101812
101. Dimitrakopoulos, G.N., et al.: Task-independent mental workload classification based upon common multiband EEG cortical connectivity. IEEE Trans. Neural Syst. Rehabil. Eng. **25**(11), 1940–1949 (2017). https://doi.org/10.1109/TNSRE.2017.2701002
102. Fraschini, M., Pani, S.M., Didaci, L., Marcialis, G.L.: Robustness of functional connectivity metrics for EEG-based personal identification over task-induced intra-class and inter-class variations. Pattern Recogn. Lett. **125**, 49–54 (2019). https://doi.org/10.1016/j.patrec.2019.03.025

Chapter 2
Characterizing EEG Electrodes in Directed Functional Brain Networks Using Normalized Transfer Entropy and PageRank

Kaushik Suresh, Vijayalakshmi Ramasamy, Ronnie Daniel, and Sushil Chandra

Abstract Over the years, cognitive research has been an active and evolving field, where non-invasive techniques like Electroencephalogram (EEG) play a dominant role in the study of brain functions. The electrical signals recorded from the brain using multi-channel EEG are used in a wide range of applications, making it possible to understand the concept of cognition better. It is crucial to study the non-linear and dynamic electrical signals generated from the brain in order to understand the behavior of each brain region. This study provides a better understanding of cognition by using page ranking (a widely used algorithm to rank a website in a network of sites using the principle of eigenvector centrality) of the EEG electrodes. Based on the performance in the short-term memory task called Corsi Block-tapping task (CBTT), the participants are classified into two groups, viz. good and poor performers. The directed Functional Brain Networks (FBNs) are constructed using Normalized Transfer Entropy (NTE) by considering EEG electrodes as nodes in the network, information flow between pairs of nodes as edges, and the NTE values of connectivity as edge weights. The NTE values computed during the performance of the CBTT task of the participants are compared with the baseline data for both good and poor performers. The weighted page rank algorithm is used to compute the ranks of the electrodes in terms of the cognitive load measured using NTE values of the different brain regions. The status of each electrode at the two groups is identified using the Reduction and Increase in Consistency (RIC) value. Therefore, the RIC

K. Suresh
PSG College of Technology, Coimbatore, Tamil Nadu, India

V. Ramasamy (✉)
University of Wisconsin-Parkside, Kenosha, WI, USA
e-mail: ramasamy@uwp.edu

R. Daniel
Indian Institute of Technology, Chennai, India

S. Chandra
Institute of Nuclear Medicine and Allied Sciences, DRDO, New Delhi, India

value serves as an indicator of the decrease/increase/constant in the rank of an electrode during the performance of the CBTT task compared to that during the baseline. A user-defined Observation Phase Value (OPV) number of the top-ranked electrodes is used to analyze the cognitive processes within the groups (using three different arbitrary OPV values of 10, 20, and 30). Based on the ranks of the electrodes and an OPV value of 20, the common electrodes during the baseline and CBTT task activity are classified using four different categories of occurrences (100, 81–99, 61–80 and 50–60%) for all the good and poor performers of CBTT respectively. The empirical analysis helps characterize the EEG electrodes into different categories based on cognitive activities using efficient computational techniques. The inferences made from such an analysis play a significant role in understanding the cognitive behavior of human brain networks using the directional flow of information during cognitive load-based tasks such as short-term memory CBTT task.

Keywords Directed information flow · Transfer entropy · PageRank · Electroencephalography (EEG) · Functional brain networks (FBN)

2.1 Introduction

The human brain is one of the most complex structures in the universe. Given its network with millions of neurons as it acts as the control center of the human body, it involves processing, integrating, and coordinating the information it receives from the sensory organs and making effective decisions. The non-linear and non-stationary signals generated by the human brain via its electrical communication between neurons can be observed, collected, and studied using neuroimaging (e.g., Magnetic Resonance Imaging (MRI), Positron Emission Tomography (PET), functional Magnetic Resonance Imaging (fMRI)) or neurophysiological (e.g., EEG, and Magnetoencephalography (MEG)) techniques. EEG is a non-invasive method that proves to be a valuable tool due to its significant features such as the superior temporal resolution, portability, and being completely silent during the recording of EEG. Additionally, the participants are not exposed to high-intensity magnetic fields. Identifying the hidden dynamic patterns in the underlying data from neurophysiological signals, images, social networks, and protein interaction networks poses a fundamental challenge to modeling the data as complex networks [1]. Graph-based data modeling approaches help us understand the complex nature of the networks like intranet, web, social networks, and biological networks. The complex network analysis using graph-theoretic algorithms unlocks the information that the non-stationary and non-linear signals generated by neurons can possess.

A graph/network is a mathematical representation of the brain structure consisting of nodes (vertices) and links (edges) connecting the pairs of nodes [2–4]. Researchers have studied and demonstrated the application of graph-based approaches by modeling the structural and functional connectivity of the different brain regions using statistical and network-based metrics. The different brain regions are denoted as nodes, and the association between any two regions as edges that represent the anatomical, structural and functional connections [5, 6]. The patterns of dynamic interactions obtained from the time series analysis of the EEG signals from the brain's neuronal elements can be identified using FBNs representing the distributed cognitive activity during various cognitive processes. Much of our understanding of brain connectivity depends on the way it has been measured and modeled. More research is needed to investigate the high dimensional and dynamic brain functioning data from a network perspective [7, 8]. FBNs can be constructed and visualized using linear statistical connectivity measures such as Pearson correlation and non-linear approaches such as Mutual information (MI), Granger causality, and NTE. Researchers widely use non-linear measures to characterize the behavior of the electrical signals generated from the human brain, which is itself non-linear and dynamic. An efficient algorithm called Minimum Connected Component (MCC), when applied to EEG data, extracts the significant component of a graph that distinguishes and identifies the predominant features of cognitive activity in healthy human participants. Clinical research later validated that the topological properties of networks constructed using MCC show more significant differences between Alzheimer's Disease (AD) and healthy participants better than other methods in the literature [1, 4]. Non-linear measures like MI have been used to measure the information flow between the nodes in FBNs but fail to provide details of the information flow direction. The significance of the information flow direction substantially provides a better understanding of the influence of one brain region over the other, which can be identified by measures like Granger causality and NTE. Therefore, FBNs constructed using NTE representing directed information flow within the electrodes are used in this study.

Network-based algorithms provide parameters that define the global organization of the brain and its alterations at different levels of integration [5]. PageRank, proposed by Lawrence Page and Sergey Brin, is widely used in the Google web search engine to rank websites based on relevancy and has proven to be a useful tool in a wide range of applications like medicine [9], recommendation systems [10], sports team ranking [11] and study of ecosystems [12]. We use a global ranking-based link analysis algorithm, PageRank, to rank the EEG electrodes [13]. The PageRank algorithm is used to understand the flow of information between each pair of electrodes in the FBNs. It works under the principle of eigenvector centrality, which measures a node's influence in a network. For a given set of webpages, the PageRank algorithm identifies the significant (highly ranked) webpages. A similar approach is used to rank EEG electrodes based on their cognitive activity and influence over the other electrodes in the FBNs. Based on the principle of eigenvector centrality, the PageRank algorithm ranks an electrode high if the sum of its backlink's ranks is high, which could occur when either an electrode has many backlinks, or it has fewer highly ranked backlinks [13].

In this study, the directed information flow of the EEG data is measured using the non-linear NTE metric that results in the construction of FBNs. The rate of change of cognition based on NTE values is compared between the baseline and the task data of each participant. The NTE values computed are used to rank the electrodes using the PageRank algorithm and based on the ranks of the electrodes. An extensive analysis is carried out to identify the significant electrodes based on the user-defined OPV value.

The remainder of the chapter is organized as follows. A brief review of the current approaches to identify cognitive activity, the representation of functional brain networks, applications of graphs, and information-theoretic approaches to network construction are discussed in Sect. 2.2. The experimental setup, data collection, pre-processing, and the directed information flow measure are discussed in Sect. 2.3. A detailed description of the proposed methodology of ranking the electrodes' NTE values using the PageRank algorithm to identify the electrodes that exchange more information during the CBTT task is presented in Sect. 2.4. We conclude with a summary of the finding and the contribution to complex functional brain network analysis in Sect. 2.5.

2.2 Current Approaches to Study Directional Information Flow in FBNs

While the functional interactions among the neuronal populations are highly non-linear, the amount of non-linear information transmission and its functional roles are not clear. Recent studies have explored finding measures sensitive to the directionality of information flow [2, 3]. Some of the widely used non-linear information-theoretic measures are MI, Granger Causality, and NTE [14–16]. MI tends to be one of the promising non-linear metrics. It tries to quantify the amount of information obtained about one variable through the other yet fails to identify the information flow direction. To quantify the directional coupling between variables, an approach called Granger causality was introduced with a wide range of applications in biomedicine, atmospheric sciences, fluid dynamics, finance, and neuroscience [17]. Granger causality portrays effective connectivity in the analysis of EEG/MEG data and fMRI signals. Despite its advantages, the performance is strictly restricted to the usage of structural models.

The time-directed information flow between two dynamical systems is measured using an information-theoretic statistical measurement called Transfer Entropy (TE). It overcomes the disadvantage observed in Granger causality by directly estimating the values from the data. The information flow direction changes during cognitive activity have been studied using NTE in [18, 19]. Based on the uniqueness and significance of TE, it is applied in a variety of applications in different fields such as neuroscience [18, 20], structural engineering [19, 21], complex dynamical systems [22, 23], and environmental engineering [24, 25]. TE has also been used as an essential tool to interpret the coupling in specific neuroscience papers [26–28]. The role of NTE in information flow detection and is described in the following subsection.

2.2.1 Normalized Transfer Entropy

TE, a non-linear, non-parametric, scalar measure, was proposed by Schreiber in-order to identify the magnitude and direction of the information flow [8]. Being a non-parametric method, TE tries to quantify the degree where the past values of one variable determine the future values of another variable as it is completely based on the data. Any types of models are not considered, which represents the dynamic nature of the variables.

$$p(y_{t+1}|y_t^n, x_t^m) = p(y_{t+1}|y_t^n) \tag{2.1}$$

Two-time series, $x^m = \{x_t, ..., x_{t-m+1}\}$, $y^n = \{y_t, ..., y_{t-n+1}\}$ are approximated by the Markov process with time step as t shown in Eq. 2.1 [29, 30] and the orders of the following Markov process x and y are m and n. The TE from X to Y is shown in Eq. 2.2 [26, 31].

$$TE_{X \to Y} = \sum_{y_t, y_t^n, x_t^m} p(y_{t+1}, y_t^n, x_t^m) \log\left(\frac{p(y_{t+1}|y_t^n, x_t^m)}{p(y_{t+1}|y_t^n)}\right) \tag{2.2}$$

$$NTE_{X \to Y} = \frac{TE_{X \to Y} - \langle TE_{X_{shuffle} \to Y}\rangle}{H(Y_{t+1}|Y_t)} \tag{2.3}$$

$$H(Y_{t+1}|Y_t) = -\sum_{y_{t+1}, y_t} p(y_{t+1}|y_t) \log\left(\frac{p(y_{t+1}, y_t)}{p(y_t)}\right) \tag{2.4}$$

TE is an asymmetric measure with a range of $0 < TE_{X \to Y} < \infty$ based on transition probabilities, which leads to the identification of directional and dynamic information [32]. Some noise is usually present in the TE matrices. Due to the algebraic sum of other information-theoretic quantities, many TE estimation techniques are proven to possess bias effects [17]. Therefore, removing/reducing bias is a primary task to proceed further before constructing FBN's. The TE values computed could possess considerable noise; hence, to remove the noise/bias, one efficient way is to subtract the average TE from X to Y using the shuffled version of the X denoted by ($TE_{Xshuffle \to Y}$) with the estimate of TE [33, 34]. The NTE from X to Y, which represents the amount of information transferred by X to Y is calculated, as shown in Eq. 2.3 [35].

The conditional entropy at Y at time $t + 1$ given its value at time $t(H(Y_{t+1}|Y_t))$ used in the Eq. 2.3 is calculated, as shown in Eq. 2.4. Due to the uncertainty in the TE estimations, the normalization process is carried out to increase the data redundancy and increase data integrity. NTE for two identical signals rose from 0 to a small positive value by introducing a delay factor between the two signals. NTE lies in the range $0 < NTE_{X \to Y} < 1$, where 0 indicates the no transfer of information, and the maximal transfer of information from X to Y is denoted by value 1. For each FBN constructed from the EEG data, TE for n electrodes gives nearly about $n(n-1)/2$ connections leading to an inherent overhead of exponential computations since each electrode is linked with the other n − 1 electrodes forming a fully connected weighted network.

One of the biggest challenges in decoding such huge networks is that it is complicated to characterize the nodes in the network [4]. One of the familiar techniques to reduce network size is by removing the weak/noisy/insignificant connections by using a fixed threshold value [36, 37]. The sample mean of NTE values obtained for each FBN of the respective individual is used as a threshold in this study. The threshold for each participant's FBN is different and changes from participant to participant based on their FBNs' NTE values. NTE values of connections between electrodes in the FBNs lesser than the threshold value are considered weak/insignificant electrodes and therefore removed to attain the significance of the FBNs. The following subsection describes the PageRank algorithm used on the NTE values computed in the study.

2.2.2 PageRank

PageRank was initially introduced by Google to resolve their problem encountered in the World Wide Web search engine. PageRank is a link analysis algorithm based on the principle of eigenvector centrality, which is used to rank a website in a network of sites [38]. The node's importance can be determined by the rank of the particular node among the other nodes in the network. PageRank of a node u in a directed network G with adjacency matrix A is calculated based on the incoming neighbors as shown in Eq. 2.6. A page in a network is considered to have a high rank if the sum of the ranks of its backlinks is high, which could occur based on two types of scenarios, where the page might have many backlinks or if the page has few highly ranked backlinks [13]. Calculation of the PageRank a node, as shown in Eq. 2.5 is an iterative process and continues until the convergence is met. A default damping factor of 0.85 is assumed in this study.

$$PR(u) = (1-d) + d \sum_{v \in B(u)} \frac{PR(v)}{N_v} \qquad (2.5)$$

Therefore, the PageRank used to rank the website in a network of websites is used to rank the EEG electrodes by applying the PageRank algorithm to the Directed FBNs of each participant in sets G and B constructed using NTE for both baseline and task. The information flow between the electrodes in the FBNs is treated as edge weights, which is directional. The considered edge weight is used to obtain the weighted page rank as the electrodes can be ranked according to their popularity, which indicates its number of $inlinks(w^{in}_{(v,u)}$ w) and $outlinks$ ($w^{out}_{(v,u)}$), respectively [39], as shown in Eqs. 2.6 and 2.7.

$$w^{in}_{(v,u)} = \frac{I_u}{\sum_{p \in R(v)} I_P} \tag{2.6}$$

$$w^{out}_{(v,u)} = \frac{O_u}{\sum_{p \in R(v)} O_P} \tag{2.7}$$

$w^{in}_{(v,u)} \left(w^{out}_{(v,u)} \right)$ is the weights obtained from the number of inlinks (outlinks) of page u and the number of inlinks (outlinks) of all reference pages to page v. Iu (Ip) and Ou (Op) represents the number of inlinks of page u(v) and outlinks of pages u(p). Therefore, the reference page list of page v is denoted as R(v). With the weight of the edges, the PR algorithm is modified accordingly, as shown in Eq. 2.8.

$$PR(u) = (1-d) + d \sum_{v \in B(u)} PR(v) \, w^{in}_{(v,u)} w^{out}_{(v,u)} \tag{2.8}$$

A human brain is made of billions of neurons that wire and fire together, whereas the web is one of the internet applications consisting of millions of websites. The brain works in parallel and entirely modular with some degree of specialization between the different regions. Similarly, just as the web recovers rapidly from damage, so too can the human brain through the process of plasticity. From the functionality perspective, the human brain resembles both the internet and the web. The brain carries information similar to the net and acts as an active repository of knowledge like the web. Compared with brain networks, web networks are smaller, but the fundamental structure of these two networks is the same as using simple local rules to obtain global stability. According to Krioukov, if two different real network systems possess similar structural and dynamic properties, then there exist some universal laws that could determine the dynamics of these networks [40].

2.3 Materials and Methods

This section presents detailed descriptions of the experimental setup, EEG and behavioral data collection methods used, FBN construction procedure, and the calculation of rate of change of cognition.

2.3.1 Experimental Design

Thirty healthy participants (right-handed, normal/corrected vision, normal hearing—seventeen male, thirteen female, mean age = 22.44 years; SD = 1.8) participated in the experimental study to collect EEG data while performing the visuospatial short term memory task called the Corsi-block tapping task (CBTT). The computerized

CBTT version is used for the study, which was designed using Inquisit software. The computerized version of the experiment offers several advantages, such as using two-dimensional stimuli rather than the traditional three-dimensional blocks in the wooden model, path sequences designated by color or brightness changes rather than manual pointing to the blocks [41].

The CBTT task consists of nine blocks, and the process requires the participant to observe the sequence of blocks tapped and then repeat the sequence back in the exact order. Initially, the task starts with a small number of blocks and gradually increases to nine blocks. Two trials were given per block of the same length. If this was repeated correctly, the next two trials consisted of a sequence of increasing length. Only a completely correct sequence was scored as correct; self-corrections were permitted on the computer screen as the participants had the option to correct the block sequence by clicking on them again to deselect the selected ones. The test measures the total score as the number of correct sequences identified and the longest sequence remembered, making it a reliable psychological test that assesses visuospatial short-term working memory [42].

2.3.2 EEG Data Acquisition and Pre-Processing

The data was recorded at the Department of Bio-medical engineering (BME), Defence Research and Development Organization (DRDO), Institute of Nuclear medicine and allied sciences (INMAS), Delhi, India [43]. No psychiatric disorder, neurological or physiological complications were observed among the participants. Before the commencement of the experiment, informed consent was obtained from each participant. EEG data was recorded under two different conditions, the baseline and the task (while performing the CBTT task). The baseline data was recorded for one minute (60 s) while the participants were asked to relax and focus on the screen. In the task phase, the participants were asked to undergo the CBTT task. The recording duration lengths differ from participant to participant as it is completely based on the participant's performance. Apart from the EEG data, the behavioral data consisting of the participants' performance in the CBTT task was also collected for further future analysis.

ANT-Neuro's eego™ sports system was used with 64-electrode locations, 10–20 System through Ag/AgCl electrodes to collect the EEG data from the participants. Impedance levels of the electrodes were considered below 5Ω and sampled at a rate of 1024 Hz. MATLAB R2014b was used to analyze offline the obtained EEG data. Bandpass filtering from 0.5 to 45 is done to remove the linear trends in the data. Removal of ocular artifacts was achieved using the signal projection method [44].

2.3.3 Behavioral Data

The behavioral data for the 30 participants are calculated during the recording of the EEG data while performing the CBTT task automatically. Based on the given constraints and environment of the CBTT task, the participants scored a total value based on their performance, ranging from 2 to 80. The average value of the total score range was used as a threshold value to classify the participants under two categories called the good and poor performers. Participants who scored below the average threshold value are considered poor performers, and the participants who scored above the threshold value are deemed good performers.

2.3.4 Directed Information Flow Using Normalized Transfer Entropy

Three different population sets are defined in this study to compare with the other population groups of participants. The Set E $\{P_1, ..., P_{30}\}$ denotes the entire population of participants who performed the CBTT task. The Set E is divided into two sets, G $\{P_1, ..., P_g\}$ and B $\{P_1, ..., P_b\}$ where set G denotes the good performing participants, meaning that their behavioral data total score for performing the CBTT task (referred to as "task" in the rest of the paper) is higher than the median threshold value (the median of the performance index). On the other hand, set B denotes the poor performers with lower scores. The values g and b indicate the number of good and poor performers in set G and B, respectively. It can be observed that $E = G \cup B$ and $G \cap B = \emptyset$ as a participant can be either a good or poor performer based on his total score and cannot be both a good and a poor performer.

FBNs are constructed for each participant in sets G and B using the NTE values calculated for the good performers (16) and poor performers (14) by considering the 64-channel EEG electrodes as nodes and the links between them as edges. During the initial construction of the FBNs for sets G and B, the number of edges in each FBNs is $n(n-1)/2$. The insignificant nodes in the FBNs of sets G and B were removed using a fixed threshold value of 0.02. This process drastically reduced the number of edges in each FBNs while reducing computational overheads and better interpreting the flow of information between electrodes.

2.3.5 Rate of Change of Cognition

Based on the NTE values obtained for each participant, the Rate of Change of Cognition (RCC) is calculated by finding the difference between the participant's task and baseline data, as shown in Eq. 2.9. The participants' RCC values help us understand the rate of cognition, whether the information flow increases or decreases while performing the specified task.

$$RCC(P_j) = \sum_{i=1}^{n} \text{NTE\_task}_{ij} - \text{NTE\_baseline}_{ij} \quad (2.9)$$

$$RIC_i = \begin{cases} Negative, & \text{Decrease in information flow for participant } j \\ 0, & \text{No change in information flow for participant } j \\ Positive, & \text{Increase in information flow for partifcipant } j \end{cases}$$

RCC value is determined for each participant j considered in the study, where n denotes the number of EEG electrodes used in the study. NTE_task$_{ij}$ represents the NTE value of the corresponding EEG electrode i, while the participant j is performing the specified task. NTE_baseline$_{ij}$ determines the NTE value of the electrode i during baseline for the participant j. For each participant, the RCC is the difference between NTE_task$_{ij}$ and NTE_baseline$_{ij}$. If the difference between NTE values of the task and baseline tends to be 0 (i.e., RCC$_j$ = 0), there is *no change in the information flow*. If the value is *positive* (RCC$_j$ > 0), there is an *increase in the participant's information flow* while performing the task. On the other hand, if the RCC value for a participant tends to be *negative* (RCC$_j$ < 0), it indicates a *decreased flow of information* during the task's performance compared to the baseline. Therefore, RCC helps understand the nature of cognition occurring during information flow in an individual's brain based on the baseline and task NTE values.

2.4 Experimental Results and Discussion

RCC values obtained for each participant in two different sets of population groups G and B, are shown in Table 2.1. RCC values are calculated for the groups G and B, instead of directly calculating the RCC values for the set E as E = (G ∪ B). The rate of change in cognition between the good and poor performers helps to identify the similarities or differences between the two groups, as shown in Table 2.1.

The calculations show positive RCC values for participants P_1 through P_6 categorized as good performers (i.e., NTE_task$_{ij}$ − NTE_baseline$_{ij}$ is positive). On the contrary, the RCC values for participants P_{11} through P_{16} classified as poor performers are negative (i.e., NTE_task$_{ij}$ − NTE_baseline$_{ij}$ is negative).

The line chart in Fig. 2.1 shows the respective NTE values for task, baseline, and RCC values of the participants in the two categories G (P_1 through P_6) and B (P_{11} through P_{16}) separated by the vertical dotted line.

The interesting inferences drawn from Fig. 2.1 are that the good performers (P1, P2, P3, P4, and P5) have positive RCC values compared to the poor performers (P11, P12, P13, P14, and P15) because the NTE values during the task (NTE_task) were higher than the NTE values of the baseline (NTE_baseline). It also indicates

2 Characterizing EEG Electrodes in Directed Functional Brain Networks …

Table 2.1 RCC Value of the good and poor performers[a] considered in the study

Performance	Participant	NTE_task	NTE_baseline	RCC
Good performers (G)	P1	0.1436	0.1100	0.0336
	P2	0.1485	0.1317	0.0168
	P3	0.1863	0.1145	0.0717
	P4	0.1782	0.1236	0.0547
	P5	0.2121	0.1431	0.0690
	P6	0.2283	0.1787	0.0446
Poor performers (B)	P11	0.1079	0.1411	−0.0332
	P12	0.0605	0.0850	−0.0246
	P13	0.0955	0.1602	−0.0647
	P14	0.0987	0.1014	−0.0027
	P15	0.1007	0.1081	−0.0074
	P16	0.1272	0.1495	−0.0223

[a]*Note* participants numbered based on analysis rank and not order of participation

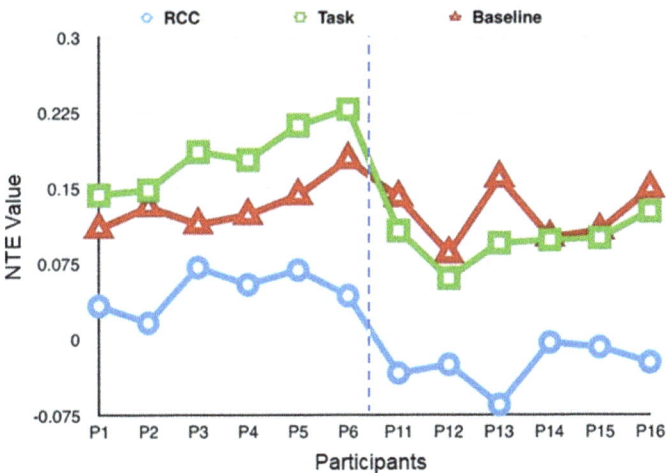

Fig. 2.1 Comparison between NTE Values (task and baseline) and the RCC values calculated for good and poor performers (separated by vertical dotted line)

the increase in the flow of information in good performers during the task performance compared to their baseline. Similarly, most of the poor performers had negative RCC values as their NTE values during baseline (NTE_Baseline) are higher than the NTE_task values showing a decrease in the flow of information during the performance of the CBTT task.

The PageRank value of each electrode among the 64-electrodes of a participant is obtained. An individual analysis of each electrode for a participant during both baseline and the task is done. An observing phase is introduced to observe the number of electrodes to be considered for future analysis based on the user-defined threshold value called the observing phase value (OPV).

2.4.1 Electrode Wise Analysis

Each electrode is individually studied to identify its behavior during the baseline and task for both good and poor performers. For instance, the rank of the electrode FP1 determined for good (P1) performer during the baseline and task are 47 and 17, respectively. Similarly, in the case of poor performers (e.g., P11), the electrode's rank in baseline and performing tasks are 58 and 1, respectively, as shown in Table 2.2. Based on the electrode ranks during baseline and task, an effective measure to identify the change of rank among electrodes is determined using the RIC approach. RIC computed as a difference in rank of a particular electrode during the task (Rank_task$_i$, i = 1 to 64) and baseline (Rank_baseline$_i$, i = 1 to 64) is shown in Eq. 2.10. It helps in understanding the electrode's behavior while the participant is not doing any cognitive activity and during the performance of the CBTT task.

$$RIC_i = Rank\_task_i - Rank\_baseline_i \quad (2.10)$$

$$RIC_i = \begin{cases} Negative, & Status = RIR, \text{ Reduction in the rank of electrode } i \\ 0, & Status = CIR, \text{ Consistency in the rank of electrode } i \\ Positive, & Status = IIR, \text{ Increase in the rank of electrode } i \end{cases}$$

Based on the RICi value, the status of the electrode i is identified. Suppose the RIC value of an electrode is negative (RIC < 0), the status is considered as *Reduction in Rank* (RIR) as an increase in the information flow of that electrode during the task compared to the baseline is observed. If RIC = 0, then the electrode's status is *Consistent in Rank* (CIR) as there are no changes in the electrode's baseline and task ranks. An electrode receives a status of an *Increase in Rank* (IIR) when the RIC is positive (RIC > 0), and it denotes a decrease in the information flow of an electrode during the task compared to the baseline. An example of the rank of electrodes calculated using page rank for good (P2) and poor performer (P13) and the RIC values are shown in Table 2.2.

The distribution percentages of RIC values calculated for good (P2) and poor performer (P13) presented in Table 2.2 are shown in Table 2.3.

It can be observed that ~60 and ~50% of the electrodes have shown an increase in rank for good performer and poor performer. On the contrary, many electrodes have reduced in rank in the poor performer than the good performer. Electrodes like F3, FCZ, and FC4 (FT8 and P5) are consistent in rank among the good performer (poor performer). All the electrodes from the temporal lobe were reduced in rank

2 Characterizing EEG Electrodes in Directed Functional Brain Networks ...

Table 2.2 Ranks of the EEG electrodes along with their RIC status

Lobe	Electrode	Good performer (P2)						Electrode	Poor performer (P13)					
		Baseline		Task		RIC			Baseline		Task		RIC	
		Rank	Wt	Rank	Wt	Val	Status		Rank	Wt	Rank	Wt	Val	Status
Central	C2	46	0.0092	18	0.0187	−28	RIR	CP2	51	0.0118	34	0.0139	−17	RIR
	C3	22	0.016	8	0.0236	−14	RIR	C3	63	0.0105	57	0.0089	−6	RIR
	CP6	29	0.0139	20	0.0177	−9	RIR	C4	49	0.0122	44	0.0118	−5	RIR
	C5	61	0.0038	59	0.0077	−2	RIR	C2	8	0.0227	5	0.0258	−3	RIR
	C6	40	0.0103	47	0.0102	7	*IIR*	CP4	13	0.0195	19	0.0163	6	*IIR*
	Cz	4	0.0485	12	0.0212	8	*IIR*	CP5	37	0.0128	49	0.0101	12	*IIR*
	CP4	17	0.0173	26	0.016	9	*IIR*	C1	26	0.0147	43	0.0118	17	*IIR*
	C1	39	0.0107	53	0.0087	14	*IIR*	CP1	28	0.0142	47	0.0104	19	*IIR*
	CP3	20	0.0168	42	0.0117	22	*IIR*	CP6	40	0.0126	59	0.0089	19	*IIR*
	C4	10	0.0265	35	0.0136	25	*IIR*	CP3	16	0.0178	41	0.0121	25	*IIR*
	CP5	2	0.0502	37	0.013	35	*IIR*	Cz	34	0.0129	61	0.0087	27	*IIR*
	CP1	14	0.0189	50	0.0089	36	*IIR*	C5	18	0.0169	56	0.0093	38	*IIR*
	CP2	1	0.0542	54	0.0086	53	*IIR*	C6	15	0.018	54	0.0095	39	*IIR*
Frontal	F3	63	0.0032	17	0.0189	−46	RIR	FT8	58	0.0105	1	0.0399	−57	RIR
	AF8	58	0.005	14	0.0197	−44	RIR	FP1	60	0.0105	18	0.0177	−42	RIR
	FP2	50	0.008	6	0.024	−44	RIR	Fz	44	0.0124	3	0.0291	−41	RIR
	F1	62	0.0036	25	0.0166	−37	RIR	AF8	61	0.0105	29	0.0144	−32	RIR
	F5	47	0.0091	11	0.0219	−36	RIR	FC6	59	0.0105	28	0.0146	−31	RIR
	FP1	41	0.0102	7	0.0238	−34	RIR	FPz	36	0.0128	8	0.0243	−28	RIR

(continued)

Table 2.2 (continued)

Lobe	Electrode	Good performer (P2)							Electrode	Poor performer (P13)						
		Baseline		Task		RIC				Baseline		Task		RIC		
		Rank	Wt	Rank	Wt	Val	Status			Rank	Wt	Rank	Wt	Val	Status	
	FC2	57	0.0058	23	0.017	−34	RIR		F7	55	0.0115	32	0.014	−23	RIR	
	AF4	59	0.0045	34	0.014	−25	RIR		AF7	33	0.0129	16	0.0201	−17	RIR	
	Fz	42	0.0101	21	0.0176	−21	RIR		AF4	23	0.0148	7	0.0248	−16	RIR	
	F8	24	0.0156	3	0.0284	−21	RIR		FP2	38	0.0127	25	0.0152	−13	RIR	
	FC6	60	0.0041	46	0.0103	−14	RIR		F3	25	0.0148	13	0.0213	−12	RIR	
	F4	52	0.0073	40	0.012	−12	RIR		F5	35	0.0128	24	0.0152	−11	RIR	
	FT8	38	0.0112	38	0.0126	0	*CIR*		F6	31	0.013	20	0.0162	−10	RIR	
	FCZ	64	0.0031	64	0.0054	0	*CIR*		FC3	52	0.0117	42	0.012	−10	RIR	
	FC4	56	0.006	56	0.0082	0	*CIR*		AF3	21	0.0153	11	0.0221	−10	RIR	
	FT7	18	0.0172	19	0.0178	1	*IIR*		F1	39	0.0127	39	0.0124	0	*CIR*	
	AF7	28	0.0144	30	0.0152	2	*IIR*		FC2	54	0.0116	58	0.0089	4	*IIR*	
	F7	54	0.0068	57	0.0082	3	*IIR*		FC4	19	0.0168	23	0.0156	4	*IIR*	
	F2	53	0.007	58	0.0079	5	*IIR*		FCZ	27	0.0143	37	0.0129	10	*IIR*	
	FC3	55	0.0061	62	0.0063	7	*IIR*		F4	50	0.0119	63	0.0082	13	*IIR*	
	F6	45	0.0092	55	0.0084	10	*IIR*		FT7	3	0.0299	17	0.0196	14	*IIR*	
	AF3	51	0.0074	63	0.0061	12	*IIR*		FC1	43	0.0125	60	0.0088	17	*IIR*	
	FC5	27	0.0146	43	0.0116	16	*IIR*		F2	11	0.0196	36	0.0131	25	*IIR*	

(continued)

Table 2.2 (continued)

Lobe	Electrode	Good performer (P2)						Electrode	Poor performer (P13)						
		Baseline		Task		RIC			Baseline		Task		RIC		
		Rank	Wt	Rank	Wt	Val	Status		Rank	Wt	Rank	Wt	Val	Status
	FPz	43	0.0098	60	0.0073	17	IIR	FC5	20	0.0157	46	0.0104	26	IIR
	FC1	12	0.0222	29	0.0158	17	IIR	F8	12	0.0195	53	0.0096	41	IIR
Mastoid	M1	8	0.0268	24	0.0169	16	IIR	M1	62	0.0105	4	0.0262	−58	RIR
	M2	13	0.0205	31	0.0152	18	IIR	M2	64	0.0105	38	0.0129	−26	RIR
Occipital	O1	3	0.0502	1	0.0653	−2	RIR	O1	53	0.0116	12	0.0221	−41	RIR
	Oz	32	0.0135	49	0.0091	17	IIR	O2	1	0.0395	2	0.0399	1	IIR
	O2	9	0.0267	61	0.0068	52	IIR	Oz	6	0.0237	64	0.0082	58	IIR
Parietal	P7	31	0.0136	10	0.0225	−21	RIR	P5	42	0.0125	15	0.0202	−27	RIR
	P8	34	0.0127	15	0.0196	−19	RIR	P6	24	0.0148	10	0.0235	−14	RIR
	PO7	25	0.0154	16	0.0192	−9	RIR	P3	45	0.0123	33	0.014	−12	RIR
	PO8	19	0.0168	13	0.0199	−6	RIR	PO4	56	0.0112	45	0.0112	−11	RIR
	PO6	23	0.016	22	0.0174	−1	RIR	P4	47	0.0123	40	0.0121	−7	RIR
	P3	26	0.0153	28	0.0159	2	IIR	PO3	29	0.0141	27	0.0148	−2	RIR
	PO5	30	0.0136	33	0.0143	3	IIR	P2	9	0.0205	9	0.0239	0	CIR
	PO4	5	0.0302	9	0.0233	4	IIR	P7	41	0.0125	52	0.0097	11	IIR
	Pz	33	0.013	44	0.0115	11	IIR	PO7	14	0.0193	26	0.0149	12	IIR
	POz	36	0.012	48	0.0092	12	IIR	POz	22	0.0149	35	0.0135	13	IIR

(continued)

Table 2.2 (continued)

Lobe	Electrode	Good performer (P2)							Electrode	Poor performer (P13)						
		Baseline		Task			RIC			Baseline		Task			RIC	
		Rank	Wt	Rank	Wt		Val	Status		Rank	Wt	Rank	Wt		Val	Status
	P5	15	0.0185	27	0.0159		12	*IIR*	P8	32	0.013	48	0.0103		16	*IIR*
	PO3	16	0.0175	32	0.0144		16	*IIR*	PO6	4	0.0287	21	0.016		17	*IIR*
	P6	35	0.0126	52	0.0088		17	*IIR*	P1	5	0.0249	30	0.0142		25	*IIR*
	P1	11	0.0252	39	0.0125		28	*IIR*	PO5	30	0.0136	55	0.0093		25	*IIR*
	P4	6	0.0292	36	0.0131		30	*IIR*	Pz	17	0.0169	50	0.01		33	*IIR*
	P2	7	0.0284	45	0.0107		38	*IIR*	PO8	10	0.0197	62	0.0087		52	*IIR*
Temporal	T7	44	0.0092	2	0.032		−42	RIR	TP7	48	0.0122	6	0.0254		−42	RIR
	T8	37	0.0118	5	0.0251		−32	RIR	T7	57	0.0111	31	0.014		−26	RIR
	TP8	21	0.0161	4	0.0259		−17	RIR	T8	46	0.0123	22	0.0159		−24	RIR
	TP7	49	0.0082	41	0.0118		−8	RIR	TP8	7	0.0235	14	0.0212		7	*IIR*

Table 2.3 Distribution (%) of RIC status of the EEG electrodes in different lobes

Lobe	#Electrode	Good performer (P2)			Poor performer (P13)		
		CIR	IIR	RIR	CIR	IIR	RIR
Frontal	39.68	12.00	40.00	48.00	4.00	36.00	60.00
Parietal	25.40	–	68.75	31.25	6.25	56.25	37.50
Central	20.63	–	69.23	30.77	–	69.23	30.77
Temporal	6.35	–	–	100.00	–	50.00	50.00
Occipital	4.76	–	66.67	33.33	–	66.67	33.33
Mastoid	3.17	–	100.00	0.00	–	0.00	100.00
Total %	100.00	4.76	53.97	41.27	3.17	49.21	47.62

for the good performer. Similarly, the distribution of electrodes from good and poor performer has increased and reduced in rank in the Central and Occipital lobe.

The ranks of the top 20 electrodes for performers P2 (good) and P13 (poor) are visualized using a bump plot (Rank plot) for baseline and task, as shown in Fig. 2.2.

The variables poor_base and poor_task represent the electrode ranks during the baseline and task of the poor performer (P13), respectively, and good_baseline and

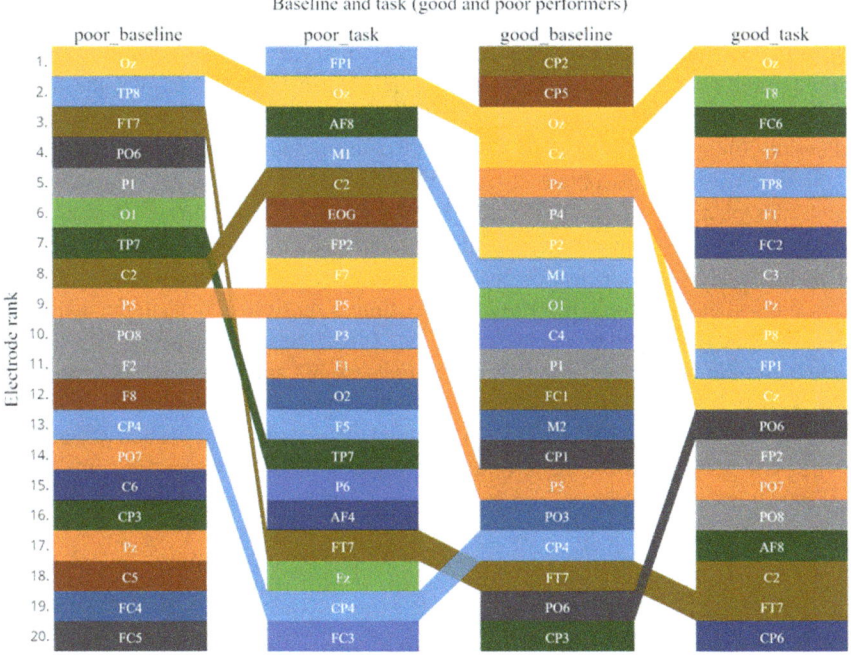

Fig. 2.2 PageRank of the top 20 EEG electrodes for baseline and task using rank plot for good (P2) and poor (P13) performers

good_task represent the ranks of the electrode during baseline and task of the good performer (P2), respectively.

2.4.2 Observation Phase

The user-defined OPV value determines the number of electrodes to be chosen for further analysis. In this study, OPV values were assumed as 10, 20, and 30 (Regions A, B, and C), respectively. The analysis is carried out under three categories: good versus good performers, poor versus poor performers, and good versus poor performers. OPV set of each performer consists of the top OPV number of highly ranked electrodes, the occurrence of each electrode e_i, i = 1 to 64 in all the performers' OPV set belonging to a group (good, poor) is calculated. The common electrodes for each group for three different OPV values, such as 10, 20, and 30, are identified based on the occurrence value. Figure 2.3 represents the common electrodes between two good performers (P2 and P3) and two poor performers (P12 and P20) during baseline and task.

Figure 2.3a and b represent the common electrodes of two good performers (P2 & P3) during baseline and task. The common electrodes of poor performers (P12 & P20) during baseline and task are visualized in Fig. 2.3c and d. It is apparent from Fig. 2.3 that electrode Oz plays a significant role among both groups (good, poor) performers. The common set of electrodes obtained for each performer during the baseline and task is different from each other. It can be observed that the highly ranked common electrodes in region A with the OPV value of 10 is a subset of the electrodes obtained using OPV value 20 in Region B and 30 in Region C.

Similarly, electrodes obtained using OPV value 20 (Region B) is a subset of electrodes obtained using OPV value 30 (Region C). The Observation phase and OPV values are used to identify the highly ranked electrodes by easing the process of analyzing all the 64 electrodes. It also helps visualize the dominant and significant electrodes in each group's performers, providing a feasible way to understand and infer the behavior of the respective electrode. The electrode Oz tends to be a highly ranked common electrode among good performers (P2 and P3) during baseline and task. The electrodes Oz and PO7 tend to be the highest-ranked common electrode among poor performers (P12 and P20). It may be concluded that the activity at PO7 in the poor performers is related to a P300 wave. It could represent, at some level, that poor performers "recognize" a mistake (or rather a mismatch or odd-ball) but can't consciously correct that error [45].

2.4.3 Entire Population Group-Wise Analysis

After analyzing the electrodes' rank using page rank, a generalized approach is considered for the study based on the OPV values. For all the performers in both

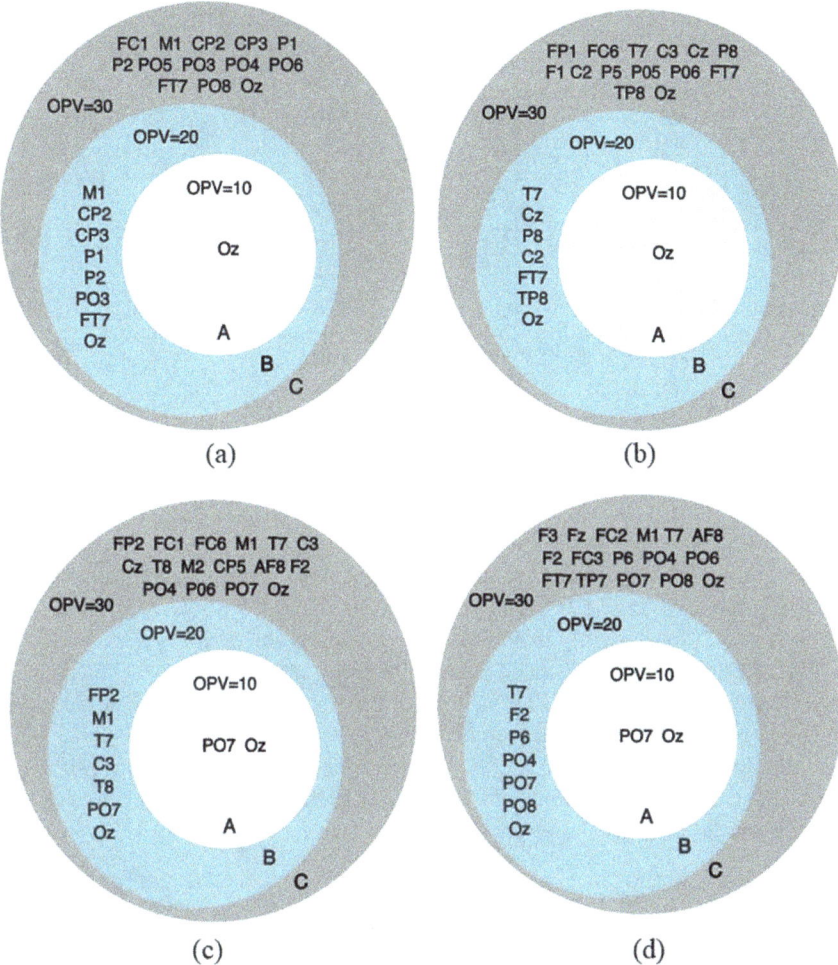

Fig. 2.3 Common electrodes of good performers and poor performers during baseline and task with three different OPV levels. Common electrodes between two good performers P2 and P3 during **a** baseline, and **b** CBTT task, and Common electrodes between poor performers P12 and P20 during **c** baseline, and **d** CBTT task

groups, the common electrodes in terms of the percentage of occurrence of a specific electrode with an OPV value of 20 for good and poor performers are shown in Table 2.4.

The set of common electrodes obtained from the highly ranked OPV set is initially identified in the user-defined OPV value. The common electrodes that occur in the entire population (100%) of a specific group are the *Constantly Highly Ranked Electrodes* (CHRE). Therefore, CHRE electrodes identified for the poor performers

Table 2.4 Percentage of common electrodes occurring during baseline and task for good and poor performers with OPV value 20

Percentage of common electrodes (%)	Poor performers		Good performers	
	Baseline	Task	Baseline	Task
100	PO7, Oz	Oz	Oz, P1	Oz
81–99	C2	P6	FT7	–
61–80	T7, F2, P1, PO6, TP8	FP1, FP2, AF8, F1, FC3, FT7	CP2, F5, CP3, CP4, P2, PO8	Pz, P6, PO5, PO4
50–60	C3, C4, T8, Pz, FC4, C5, C6, CP3, CP4, P5, PO8	P3, O2, F5, F2, CP3, CP4, P5, TP7, PO7	CP5, CP1, P4, C2, P5, P6, PO5, TP7, TP8, PO7	FC5, T7, Cz, P8, POz, AF8, P2, TP7, TP8

during baseline are PO7 and Oz. The common electrode that occurs in nearly 80–99% of the entire poor performer population is electrode C2 during baseline and electrode P6 during the task. CHRE electrodes among good performers are Oz and P1 during the CBTT task and Oz during baseline as they occur in common to all the good performers. It may be noted that the electrodes like FC5, T7, CZ, P8, POz, AF8, P2, TP7, and TP8 occur only in 50–60% of the entire good performer's population.

The experimental analysis intends to initially provide a novel way of ranking the EEG electrodes based on the NTE values, identify the rate of change of cognition in different groups of performers, then classify the electrodes based on the change of rank into three different categories (viz. IIR, RIR, and CIR) during baseline and task using RIC approach, and finally identify the (dis)similaritites of the electrodes during baseline and task for good and poor performers with a user-defined OPV value of 20.

2.5 Conclusion

This state-of-the-art research study includes measuring the electrodes' behavior using page ranking of the 64 EEG electrodes during the performance of the CBTT task. Directed FBNs are constructed using NTE depicting the directed information flow, and the insignificant edges are removed from the network using the sample mean as a threshold. The RCC values obtained suggested that the rate of change in cognition in good performers in CBTT task is higher than that in the poor performers. Applying the page rank algorithm over the directed FBNs helped to understand better the subtle changes in cognition in each electrode during the baseline and CBTT task by each participant. Reduction, increase, and consistency in rank for each electrode during its baseline and CBTT task were calculated. All the electrodes from the temporal lobe showed reduced rank for good performers. One possible reason might be that the good performers can better encode information (while not their primary function, the temporal lobes have also been associated with some memory encoding).

Similarly, most of the electrodes in poor performers followed an increase in rank as the amount of information flow during task performance was less compared to the baseline. The percentage of commonly occurring electrodes for 50–100% performers of the respective group are identified. It can be noted that electrodes like C2, PO7, Oz, and P6 are 81% common in most poor performers, followed by electrodes like FT7, Oz, P1, which are 81% common in most of the good performers. The empirical results reveal that Oz is the only CHRE electrode since it occurs commonly among all the good and poor performers. This is far from unexpected given the visual nature of the task and that the Oz electrode records activity from the primary visual cortex. The experiments will be repeated on more participants to determine the best OPV values, which helps automate the process. The future direction of the research is to apply a combination of advanced computational techniques on the directed information flow data in FBNs to gather detailed insights about the cognitive changes in different brain regions during multiple levels of cognitive tasks.

References

1. Vijayalakshmi, R., Nandagopal, D., Tran, M., Abeynayake, C.: A novel feature extraction algorithm for IED detection from 2-D images using minimum connected components. Procedia Comput. Sci. **114**, 507–514 (2017)
2. Shovon, M.H.I., Nandagopal, D., Vijayalakshmi, R., Du, J., Cocks, B.: Cognitive load driven directed information flow in functional brain networks. In: Neural Information Processing, ICONIP 2015. Lecture Notes in Computer Science, vol. 9492, pp. 332–340. Springer (2015)
3. Shovon, M.H.I., Nandagopal, D., Cocks, B., Vijayalakshmi, R.: Capturing cognition via EEG-based functional brain networks. In: Emerging Trends in Neuro Engineering and Neural Computation, Series in BioEngineering, pp. 147–172. Springer, Singapore (2017)
4. Vijayalakshmi, R., Nandagopal, D., Dasari, N., Cocks, B., Dahal, N., Thilaga, M.: Minimum connected component—a novel approach to detection of cognitive load-induced changes in functional brain networks. Neurocomputing **170**, 15–31 (2015)
5. Vecchio, F., Miraglia, F., Rossini, P.M.: Connectome: graph theory application in functional brain network architecture. Clin. Neurophysiol. Pract. **2**, 206–213 (2017)
6. Thilaga, M., Vijayalakshmi, R., Nadarajan, R., Nandagopal, D.: Shortest path-based network analysis to characterize different cognitive load states of human brain using EEG based functional brain networks. J. Integr. Neurosci. 1–23 (2018)
7. Bullmore, E., Sporns, O.: Complex brain networks: Graph theoretical analysis of structural and functional systems. Nat. Rev. Neurosci. **10**(3), 186–198 (2009)
8. Wig, G.S., Schlaggar, B.L., Petersen, S.E.: Concepts and principles in the analysis of brain networks. Ann. N.Y. Acad. Sci. **1224**, 126–146 (2011)
9. Newton, P.K., Mason, J., Behtel, K., Bazhenova, L.A., Nieva, J., Kuhn, P.: A stochastic Markov chain model to describe lung cancer growth and metastasis. PLoS ONE **7**(4), (2012)
10. Wang, J., Liu, Z., Zhao, H.: Group recommendation based on the PageRank. J. Netw. **7**(12), 2019–2024 (2012)
11. Lazova, V., Barskanov, L.: PageRank approach to ranking national football teams. In: 12th International Conference on Informatics and Information Technologies Correspondence, CIIT (2015)

12. Allesina, S., Pascual, M.: Googling food webs: can an eigenvector measure species' importance for coextinctions? PLOS Comput. Biol. **5**(9), e1000494 (2009)
13. Brin, S., Page, L.: The anatomy of a large-scale hypertextual web search engine. Comput. Netw. ISDN Syst. **30**(1–7), 107–117 (1998)
14. Marinazzo, D., Liao, W., Chen, H., Stramaglia, S.: Nonlinear connectivity by Granger causality. Neuroimage **58**(2), 330–338 (2011)
15. Nandagopal, D., Vijayalakshmi, R., Cocks, B., Dahal, N., Dasari, N., Thilaga, M., Shamshu Dharwez, S.: Computational techniques for characterizing cognition using EEG data—new approaches. Procedia Comput. Sci. **22**, 699–708 (2013)
16. Shovon, M.H.I., Nandagopal, D., Vijayalakshmi, R., Du, J.T., Cocks, B.: Directed connectivity analysis of functional brain networks during cognitive activity using transfer entropy. Neural Process. Lett. **45**(3), 807–824 (2015)
17. Gencaga, D.: Transfer Entropy. Entropy **20**(288), 1–4 (2018)
18. Gourévitch, B., Eggermont, J.J.: Evaluating information transfer between auditory cortical neurons. Neurophysiology **97**, 2533–2543 (2007)
19. Overbey, L.A., Todd, M.D.: Dynamic system change detection using a modification of the transfer entropy. J. Sound Vib. **322**(1), 438–453 (2009)
20. Sabesan, S., Narayanan, K., Prasad, A., Iasemidis, L.D., Spanias, A., Tsakalis, K.: Information flow in coupled non-linear systems: application to the epileptic human brain. Data Mining Biomed. **7**, 483–503 (2007)
21. Overbey, L.A., Todd, M.D.: Effects of noise on transfer entropy estimation for damage detection. Mech. Syst. Signal Process. **23**, 2178–2191 (2009)
22. Majda, A.J., Harlim, J.: Information flow between subspaces of complex dynamical systems. Proc. Natl. Acad. Sci. **104**(23), 9558–9562 (2007)
23. Liang, X.S., Kleeman, R.: Information transfer between dynamical system components. Phys. Rev. Lett. **95**(24), (2005)
24. Ruddell, B.L., Kumar, P.: Ecohydrologic process networks: 1. Identification. Water Resour. Res. **45**(W03419), (2009)
25. Ruddell, B.L., Kumar, P.: Ecohydrologic process networks: 2. Analysis and characterization. Water Resour. Res. **45**(W03420), (2009)
26. Vicente, R., Wibral, M., Lindner, M., Pipa, G.: Transfer entropy-a model-free measure of effective connectivity for the neurosciences. J. Comput. Neurosci. **30**(1), 45–67 (2001)
27. Wibral, M., Rahm, B., Rieder, M., Lindner, M., Vicente, R., Kaiser, J.: Transfer entropy in magnetoencephalographic data: quantifying information flow in cortical and cerebellar networks. Prog. Biophys. Mol. Biol. **105**(1–2), 80–97 (2011)
28. Vakorin, V.A., Krakovska, O.A., McIntosh, A.R.: Confounding effects of indirect connections on causality estimation. J. Neurosci. Methods **184**, 152–160 (2009)
29. Schreiber, T.: Measuring information transfer. Phys. Rev. Lett. **85**(2), 461–464 (2000)
30. Lindner, M., Vicente, R., Priesemann, V., Wibral, M.: TRENTOOL: a Matlab open-source toolbox to analyze information flow in time series data with transfer entropy. BMC Neurosci. **12**(119), (2011)
31. Kaiser, A., Schreiber, T.: Information transfer in continuous processes. Physica D **166**, 43–62 (2002)
32. Vicente, R., Wibral, M., Lindner, M., Pipa, G.: Transfer entropy-a model-free measure of effective connectivity for the neurosciences. J. Comput. Neurosci. **30**(1), 45–67 (2011)
33. Sabesan, S., Narayanan, K., Prasad, A., Iasemidis, L., Spanias, A., Tsakalis, K.: Information flow in coupled non-linear systems: application to the epileptic human brain. Springer Optim. Appl. **7**, 483–502 (2007)
34. Neymotin, S.A., Jacobs, K.M., Fenton, A.A., Lytton, W.W.: Synaptic information transfer in computer models of neocortical columns. J. Comput. Neurosci. **30**, 69–84 (2011)
35. Gourévitch, B., Eggermont, J.J.: Evaluating information transfer between auditory cortical neurons. J. Neurophysiol. **97**, 2533–2543 (2007)
36. Zalesky, A., Fornito, A., Bullmore, E.T.: Network-based statistic: identifying differences in brain networks. Neuroimage **53**, 1197–1207 (2010)

37. Telesford, Q.K., Simpson, S.L., Burdette, J.H., Hayasaka, S., Laurienti, P.J.: The brain as a complex system: using network science as a tool for understanding the brain. Brain Connectivity **1**(4), 295–308 (2011)
38. Gleich, D.F.: PageRank beyond the Web (2014). ArXiv, abs/1407.5107
39. Xing, W., Ghorbani, A.: Weighted PageRank algorithm. In: Proceedings of the Second Annual Conference on Communication Networks and Services Research, pp.305–314. IEEE (2004)
40. Krioukov, D., Kitsak, M., Sinkovits, R.S., Rideout, D., Meyer, D., Boguñá, M.: Network cosmology. Sci. Rep. **2**(793), 1–6 (2012)
41. Berch, D.B., Krikorian, R., Huha, E.M.: The corsi block-tapping task: methodological and theoretical considerations. Brain Cogn. **38**(3), 317–338 (1998)
42. Kessels, R.P.C., van Zandvoort, M.J.E., Postma, A., Kappelle, L.J., de Haan, E.H.F.: The corsi block-tapping task: standardization and normative data. Appl. Neuropsychol. **7**(4), 252–258 (2000)
43. Daniel, R., Pandey, V., Bhat, K.R., Rao, A.K., Singh, R., Chandra, S.: An empirical evaluation of short-term memory retention using different high-density EEG based brain connectivity measures. In: 2018 26th European Signal Processing Conference (EUSIPCO), pp. 1387–1391. Rome (2018). https://doi.org/10.23919/EUSIPCO.2018.8553587
44. Uusitalo, M.A., Ilmoniemi, R.J.: Signal-space projection method for separating MEG or EEG into components. Med. Biol. Eng. Comput. **35**, 135–140 (1997)
45. Picton, T.W.: The P300 wave of the human event-related potential. J. Clin. Neurophysiol. **9**(4), 456–479 (1992). https://doi.org/10.1097/00004691-199210000-00002. PMID: 1464675

Chapter 3
Autistic Verbal Behavior Language Parameterization

Daniela López De Luise, Ben Raúl Saad, Tiago Ibacache, Christian Saliwonczyk, Pablo Pescio, and Lucas Soria

Abstract In severe degrees of ASD (Autistic Spectrum Disorder), patients are not able to produce or understand natural language, and they also have social disorders that make it difficult the communication with other people. Their natural language presents different degrees of alteration, reaching in some cases the impossibility of speaking. This chapter presents an approach to model the patient's behavior by processing recordings during the therapy. Video and audio data provide certain hidden patterns as we already presented in previous work. By using Machine Learning, it is possible to obtain a customized model that makes it possible to evaluate the individual's performance during his interaction with other people. The model inputs a specific set of stereotyped responses collected in a systematic way, labeled as patterns. Those movements and sounds, represents how patterns in audio and video relate to stimuli from the environment. Findings allow to discriminate when and how there is a reaction, an autistic verbal behavior.

Keywords Autistic spectrum disorder · Natural language processing · Linguistics · Sound processing

3.1 Introduction

Autism is a neuron-developmental disorder characterized by a triad of symptoms that can be observed since the first years of life. They mainly consist of impaired language development, stereotyped behaviors associated with restricted interests, and social interaction disorder [1]. About 1 in 54 children born in 2008 have been identified with

---

D. L. De Luise (✉)
CI2S Lab, Buenos Aires, Argentina
e-mail: mdldl@ci2s.com.ar

T. Ibacache · P. Pescio · L. Soria
IDTI Lab—Facultad de Ciencia y Tecnología—UADER, Concepción del Uruguay, Argentina

B. R. Saad · C. Saliwonczyk
CAETI—Universidad Abierta Interamericana, Buenos Aires, Argentina

Autistic Spectrum Disorder (ASD) according to estimates from Centers for Disease Control and Prevention, CDC's Autism and Developmental Disabilities Monitoring (ADDM) Network [2]. ASD is more than 4 times more common among boys than among girls [3]. About 1 in 6 (17%) children aged 3–17 years were diagnosed with a developmental disability, as reported by parents, during a study period of 2009–2017. These included autism, attention-deficit/hyperactivity disorder, blindness, and cerebral palsy, among others [4]. The World Health Organization changes those numbers to one in 160 children, but based on a study of Mayada et al. in 2012, that use a survey instead of statistical inference of patients' records [5]. In recent years there have been plenty of studies providing data about how many people in the world are being affected by ASD. Nowadays results are yet not conclusive due to various reasons, among others samples used are from different records, diagnostic procedures, experimental designs, ages ranges, etc. Despite all, it can be said that at least 60–70 people in 10,000 are diagnosed with traditional autism. Many others remain in a borderline, not diagnosed or even misdiagnosed. Despite the imprecision with the numbers, the community agrees in its increasing rate in countries where autism were tracked.

Children with autistic disorders can have significant social, communication, and behavioral problems. The Diagnostic and Statistical Manual of Mental Disorders (DSM), is the most relevant diagnostic classification system. The World Health Organization (WHO) considers autism as pervasive developmental disorders, characterized by a wide variety of clinical and behavioral expressions that are the result of multiple factors related to developmental dysfunctions of the central nervous system [2].

On the other hand, children with these types of disorders show significant cognitive deficits in different areas [7]. Many of the characteristics of children with Generalized Developmental Disorder (PDD) and autism could present alterations in their attention processes [8]. Autistic people have particular difficulties in interpreting socially relevant information, since socially significant stimuli are physically complex. Problems with social interaction, are combined with cognitive and physical symptoms, but their timings, severity, and nature may be quite different [9].

The alteration of verbal language can reach the complete impossibility of speech [10]. It is associated with Sensory processing disorder (SPD), a condition in which a person does not respond normally to sounds, smells, textures, and other stimuli. Many times autistic is associated to both hearing loss or hyperacusis, that can be general or focused on a certain sound. Other typical manifestation is the "stimming", a short for self-stimulatory behavior, sometimes also called "stereotypical" behavior. In a person with autism, stimming usually refers to specific behaviors that include hand-flapping, rocking, spinning, or repetition of words and phrases.

It is important to note that subtler forms of stimming are also a part of most people's behavior patterns. The main differences between autistic and typical stimming are the type, quantity, and obviousness of the behavior. In general, behaviors are described as "stims" when they go beyond what is culturally tolerated. Sometimes they can be quite extreme and are legitimately upsetting or even frightening to typical people. There are cases where autistic people stim by making loud noises that can sound threatening or scary [11]. In other cases they hit themselves with their hands, or bang their heads against the wall. Those manifestations that go beyond certain limits, are problematic for a variety of reasons [12].

People with ASD, find it difficult to stop stimming. Stim appears when the individual is excited, happy, anxious, overwhelmed, or because it feels comforting. It helps the patient to handle overwhelming sensory input (too much noise, light, heat, etc.) [13].

It's not fully understood why stimming usually goes along with autism. Many experts believe it is a tool for self-regulation and self-calming. It could be an outgrowth of the sensory processing dysfunction that often goes along with autism [14].

In this project it is important, since the autistic stim relates to feelings of anxiety, fear, anger, excitement, anticipation, and other strong emotions [15]. They also stim to help themselves handle overwhelming sensory input (too much noise, light, heat, etc.). Therefore, the external manifestations could serve as a clue to understand the individual's status and thoughts.

In certain cases, stimming are with certain behaviors that are a sort of rudimentary communications but are understood as a distraction. The distinction in those cases is very hard. The parameterization of verbal behavior, proposed in this work is useful to do that discrimination.

There are some extra features in the body expression of people suffering autism. For example "echolalia". It consists of the precise repetition, or echoing, of words and sounds. Echolalia can be a symptom of various disorders, but it is most often associated with autism. It is one of the first ways in which children with ASD uses to communicate, and represents a relevant tool for speech-language therapy [16].

But it is important to note that echolalia has no communicative meaning at all in severe cases of autism. It may simply be a self-calming tool working as good as any other like hand-flapping or rocking. In those cases it is an imitation of human speech without grasping the meaning behind those sounds. So, it can be another way to calm themselves when they're anxious or cope with overwhelming sensory challenges. Thus, echolalia may work as a form of self-stimulation or stimming.

Other people on the autism spectrum use "prefabricated" phrases and scripts to communicate ideas when it is too difficult for them to formulate their own novel speech patterns. From this perspective, echolalia is an important first step toward more typical forms of spoken communication.

Any case, autistic verbal behavior can provide very useful information to understand what is happening inside the mind of the patient. As every individual has its own set of stimmings, phrases and scripts, a model can work as a dual translator machine to and from the environment.

This article follows this approach, certain studies that process utterances to determine whether a patient has ASD or not, and combine them with own findings on stimming and audio processing.

Authors started using five different musical notes are composed which are described by: pitch, intensity and features of timbre: frequency, amplitude, harmonic composition or waveform [17]. Different tests were carried out with autism spectrum patients using those notes as stimuli. Experiences were filmed and the reactions they had to each note (movements of hands, arms, head, feet, sounds, etc.). The protocol included filming, and hand-made descriptions on sheets. All the information was used to perform statistics and develop a set of main features. It should be noted that this type of evaluation contrasts with the proposal, where the patient's sound production is analyzed.

In the next stage, simple visual information is added. To do that, the study performed by Cheol-Hong and Ahmed [18] was considered. It presents a new method for automatic detection of stereotyped behavior patterns using data from an accelerometer. Orthogonal subspaces are extracted from the sensor data, which are used to generate a clustering of the dictionary and in turn for the representation of signals. The algorithm was improved for the detection of new events that were unknown. In [19] a study carried out at the University of Southern California (USA) of the design of an emotionally directed interactive agent for boys with autism, called Rachel, is presented. In it, an incorporated conversation agent (RCT) was developed to achieve the interaction of patients, previously diagnosed with autism, who participated together with their parents, interacting with the RCT. The agent produces different scenarios that represent emotions such as angry, sad, happy and scared; with the aim of allowing a controlled evaluation of the communication skills of children with ASD. Although this work is extensive, it lacks of statistics and result validations.

The current work, takes some of the above approach. Instead of a specific interaction, the current therapies are considered. This is because the routines are very important for this type of patients. Changing the activities and/or the therapist affects the study. The processing is also different: the audio and video recordings are processed in parallel, with statistical evaluation and an automated model that serves as a tool for later evaluation of the activity. Both models (audio and video) will be afterwards related using the timestamp. Previous publications introduced some preliminary findings [20]. In this work, only audio processing is considered.

The rest of this paper organizes as follows: Sect. 3.2 presents some of the main working considerations about ASD, Sect. 3.3 introduces the proposal, materials and methods, Sect. 3.4 describes a testing protocol and preliminary considerations of the use case, Sect. 3.5 is the test for audio recordings of the use case, and Sect. 3.7 has conclusions and future work.

3.2 Considerations About the Autistic Spectrum Disorder

This section presents main aspects of the project. First, it introduces main definitions of ASD, starting with the three degrees of autism, and their stims. They are important since the article focuses in the severe conditions, which is the third degree. Then it introduces Skinner's verbal behavior, definition that is used to determine the model's variables.

3.2.1 Degrees of Autism

The DSM-V [21] of the American Psychiatric Association, establishes a classification guide, a coding used by much of the scientific community to diagnose different mental disorders. According to the authors [22] those who suffer from ASD experience a series of symptoms based on Wing's triad, these disorders refer to social interaction, communication and lack of flexibility in reasoning and behavior. In turn, there are classifications of different degrees in the guides and manuals, which leads specialists [22] to affirm that despite Wing's classification, no person suffering from ASD is similar to another in terms of their observable characteristics.

People who are diagnosed with Autism Spectrum Disorder ASD have deficiencies in communication and social interaction. The DSM-V guide determines the level of ASD on a three-grade scale, detailed below.

- **Grade 1**. Need Help

In this stage, there is still social communication. The patient can be without on-site help, but presents deficiencies in social communication causing major problems. Typically has difficulty initiating social interactions and there are clear examples of atypical or unsatisfactory responses to the social openness of other people. May appear to have little interest in social interactions. For example, a person who is able to speak in complete sentences and who establishes communication but whose extensive conversation with other people fails and whose attempts to make friends are eccentric and usually unsuccessful.

Typically have restricted and repetitive behaviors. The behavioral inflexibility causes significant interference with performance in one or more contexts, with difficulty alternating activities. The organizational and planning problems make autonomy difficult.

- **Grade 2**. Needs Notable Help

Patient has very reduced social communication, but with notable deficiencies in verbal and non-verbal social communication skills; apparent social problems even with on-site help; limited initiation of social interactions; and reduced response or abnormal responses to the social openness of other people. For example, a person who emits simple sentences, whose interaction is limited to very specific special interests, and who has very eccentric non-verbal communication.

As in grade 1, presents restricted and repetitive behaviors, with behavioral inflexibility, difficulty coping with changes, or other restricted/repetitive behaviors often appear clearly to the casual observer and interfere with functioning in various contexts. Also presents anxiety and/or difficulty in changing the focus of action.

- **Grade 3**. Needs Very Notable Help

This degree is the most severe condition with almost none social communication. Presents severe deficits in verbal and nonverbal social communication skills cause severe functional impairment, very limited initiation of social interactions, and minimal response to other people's social openness. For example, a person with few intelligible words who rarely initiates interaction and who, when he does, performs unusual strategies only to meet needs and only responds to very direct social approaches. Behaviors are restricted and repetitive, with inflexibility, extreme difficulty coping with changes, or other restricted/repetitive behaviors significantly interfere with functioning across the board. Intense anxiety/difficulty in changing focus of action.

3.2.2 Verbal Behavior

In DSM-V there is a mention of verbal and non-verbal social communication, when indicating one of the problems that patients with ASD present. Skinner [23] carried out studies on verbal behavior, indicating that vocal language is only a part or subset, arguing that the emission of sounds or certain actions such as gestures are verbal even though they are not part of an organized language, since they provoke a reaction in the listener or observer similar to the emission of vocal language and therefore must be part of the verbal behavior.

Repetitive and stereotyped behaviors are considered an important symptom of autism spectrum disorders (ASD). Jumping, turning, and other rhythmic body movements were described in the first patients originally described in Kanner's series [24, 25].

Leo Kanner conducted an evaluation in the case study with 8 boys and 3 girls, describing various repetitive movements such as: rhythmic jumping, clapping, sucking sounds, walking on tiptoe, not looking directly at the face, continuous repetition of words and/or phrases. Later, in 1979, Wing and Gould [25] determined that people with Autism Spectrum Disorder have problems in three areas: (a) They cannot develop skills in reciprocal social interaction. (b) They have difficulties in their verbal and non-verbal communication and (c) they have restricted patterns of behavior and interests. These symptoms are known as the Wing Triad.

3.3 Materials and Methods

This section describes how the use case is being designed, the hardware and software used for data collection, and certain preliminary considerations for the testing.

3.3.1 Hardware

For the use case, a therapy session with a patient diagnosed with severe ASD (degree 3) is considered. The patient's age is 13 years old, native from Argentina, with parents authorization. The activity analyzed cover several typical tasks: identification, concentration, pointing, etc. The interaction was registered in a video recording, with a Sony Handycam HDR-CX250, with 5 sound channels.

3.3.2 Protocol

The video has a total duration of stimmings, phrases and scripts 22:00 min. As the scope of this article covers only audio, it was extracted as a wav file.

All the procedure was also registered in printed forms. The use case consists of a set of sounds and movements of the original video, that are part of the patient's verbal behavior and allows to identify the different actions. From them it is expected to derive the audio and visual stimmings, phrases and scripts, as introduced in Sect. 3.1. The initial set of clues was manually registered in an online Google spreadsheet.

The worksheet was divided into the following columns: Time, Action, Characteristics, Comments. That original worksheet was extended to add two new columns with the timestamp before the starting of the visual/audio clue, of a possible stimulus, and a similar column with the duration of the behavior. The Action column, which is the stim observed (a body movements, or certain noise or sound produced by the patient). A short description of these movements is recorded in the Characteristics column; and finally, in the Comments column, there are the actions and expressions that the therapist performs at each opportunity.

The next step to prepare the use case is to convert this sheet into a list of stims with every repetition during the recorded session, and relevant information for its automatic detection. Part of the resulting document is in Table 3.1.

While the registration has been traditionally performed manually according to the actions of the patient and the indications of the therapist, the actions are those that were described in the introduction section. There are many papers explaining them, and for the aim of this project, they were added to the protocol. An excerpt of that long list of detectable movements and sounds are in Table 3.2 and is based on the work of Riviere [26].

The last step to prepare the use case is to adapt Table 3.1 to use the listing in Table 3.2. This way, any clue detected represents a stimming, or specific utterance.

3.3.3 Software

For processing, five versions of a prototype were written in Python, and five versions in Octave. Both languages are frequently used for signal processing, statistical analysis and certain mining procedures [27–33].

The final version of the prototype, consists of a python module with several functions. The visual and audio signals required the Python and Octave library LTFAT,

Table 3.1 Time-sheet of Stimulus upon every sound slice detected

Reference	Time$_1$	Time$_2$	Time$_3$	Time$_4$	Time$_5$	Time$_6$	Time$_7$
Time slice 1	0:00:00	2:31:00	3:58:00	4:18:00	5:17:00	6:52:00	7:25:00
Label: iuuu		He moved or was someone in the room, before he had lost focus on the therapist	The book is given	The therapist stood up	Most of the time she is standing behind him hace uuuuu	A vehicle is heard in the background while passing the pages of his book	He got bored reading the book a second time and turning the pages seemed
Time slice 2	1:57:00	2:07:00	2:19:00	2:52:00	3:18:00	7:03:00	8:20:00
Label: aaaa	You won the token (Buenisimoooooo) + timer beep + eye contact to therapist + gives him yellow toy	Token arrangement	Points to card and the therapist congratulates him + gives him red toy	Buenisimoooooo (good)	He gives him yellow ball, (Bienmm Excellentee)	Wait for the stimulation of the therapist to turn the page	Look at the floor, he gets bored of waiting
...							
...							
Time slice 4	3:40:00	10:30:00	16:25:00	16:30:00	18:10	19:09:00	
Clapping Sound 4	Given the lack of attention to him, the therapist takes a long time in his notes	He asks for silence, takes him a glass and plate and touches his mouth. Seems eager to play and win the lollipop	Sneezing and health	Sneezing and health	They clean his nose	He's bored now, he makes many new movements, he stretches, he wants to finish now	

Table 3.2 ASD typical behavior

Movement/sound	Description
Rhythmic jumps	The body sitting/standing, the patient facing the front, performs vertical stentorian movements with/without arm movements
Clapping	It is the action of clapping the palms of the hands together repeatedly as a sign of both approval (joy) and, sometimes, rejection
Sucking sounds	It is the effect of producing a sound similar to the sucking of the bottle or the mother's breast when drinking milk
Walk on tiptoe	It is the action of walking on the balls of the feet without contact between the heels and the ground. It hits both feet at the same time
Do not look to the face directly	The patient, seen from the front, does not direct his gaze towards us but appears skewed, to the right (more frequently) or to the left

The list continues...

and Octave libraries Signal and Control. LTFAT provides signal processing algorithms for use with Octave and Python software. The other two completes some basic processing that are part of the current testing, like FFT, modulus of a complex signal, mean, covariance and Fast Walsh-Hadamard Transform (FWHT), wavelets, design of FIR and IIR filters, spectral analysis, etc.

The use of the Fourier transform does not solve the problem of a better localization of a signal. In addition, we will have problems if the events are presented very close to each other since it will be very difficult to differentiate behaviors within the same window width.

The mathematical tool that helps solve these problems is the Wavelet Transform. This transform can detect high frequency phenomena. Once we choose the window size, the frequencies are analyzed with the same time and frequency resolutions, different from what happens in the Wavelet Transform which has a window size adapted to the frequencies.

This work, based on the BIOTECH project, applies also Morphosyntactic Linguistic Wavelets (MLW). An intelligent system capable of providing in-depth information on the reasoning process related to linguistic expressions [34]. It has been applied in the past to interpret WEB content, automatic summarization, dialogue profiles, texts and author profiles, bilingualism effects in young children, etc. [35, 36].

To be able to process with MLW it is mandatory to have linguistic expressions made by the patients. To overcome the lack of language articulations, the project is based on the concept of verbal behavior [37], replacing language production with specific audio and video clues.

Verbal behavior is becoming widely accepted as a crucial perspective for autism spectrum disorder in therapies; Greer [38] expresses that there is more and more evidence on onto-genetics, the sources of language and its development that leads to a renewed interest in the theory that verbal ability in humans is the result of evolution and onto-genetics of development.

Another important aspect to consider is the particularity of each individual. Experts claim [9] that skills training should be intensive, but also personalized for best results. This article does not cover the MLW production, or the traditional wavelets (like Daubechis 7 or 8), as they are out of the scope of this work.

3.4 Preliminary Evaluation

For this activity the data-set is the audio, obtained according to the steps described in the protocol (see Sect. 3.3). The main goal here is to identify the timestamps corresponding to stimming sounds or any audible activity of the patient, that could be related to any stimulus from the environment.

During the exhaustive revision, 88 instances of interactions were identified. Each one was labeled and then clustered by similarity. For instance, sounds similar to the expression "iuuu" were called Sound 1; the expressions like "aaaa" are Sound 2; "brrrr" is Sound 3, the clapping is Sound 4, and so on. It is important to note that certain sounds, such as the expression of joy, are very complex for a precise identification and not considered in the list.

On several occasions, each background sound is accompanied by a sound or movement of the patient, for example in the order number 4, 5, 14, 21, 28, 29, 33, 36, 43, 46, 47, 57, 58, 59, 74, 77, 79, 80, 81. On other occasions, the patient performs the clapping movement accompanied by one of the sounds registered, for example in the order number 1, 2, 22, 24, 44, 75, 78, 82. In addition, slice of sound 1 is associated with a movement and expression as if it were angry as recorded in the order 15, 61, 69, 83.

3.4.1 Modeling the Problem with Metadata

The model consists of a set of clues, and the variables that best describe them. In this process it is important to find out which is the specific set of clues used by the patient of the use case, taken from Table 3.2. To avoid any biasing in the detection and parameterization of the clues, a sliding windows algorithm on the entire data-set is used to detect when every sound slice is being repeated. Then the modeling needs to determine a very important subset of parameters: the similarity threshold of every variable comparison.

Four main variables were used, A and B, which would be the variables to store the sound file used; AA and AB whose function is to store the number of seconds that each loaded sound consists of.

Also, it uses two for loops from 1 to AA/AB whose main objective is to divide and compare both sounds for every second (The graph will vary based on this). An

3 Autistic Verbal Behavior Language Parameterization

if conditional where it is stated that, if both sounds are equal in a given second, they are stored in a variable C. The pseudo-code of the mentioned algorithm is in Fig. 3.1.

Regarding the graphical part, it consists of LTFAT functions, where it is plotted from the scale on the X and Y axes, and the variation of sound with the previously mentioned variable C is displayed (Fig. 3.2 and a zoom-in in Fig. 3.3).

Every sound has 4 sub-slices labeled SS1 to SS4, in order from the first second to the last. Figures have the following color code:

Fig. 3.1 Sliding Windows for matching the pattern slice

```
function retval = SlidingWindows4 ()
B="TherapyVideo.wav"
A = "Slice.wav"
N = 1e3;
AA = size(A); #Matrix size to make the for in the comparison
AB = size(B);
#Sliding Windows comparison
for i = 1 : AA,
  for j = 1 : AB,
    if metaDataComparison (A(i), B(j))  #meta data are simmilar
      C(i) = A(i)
    endif
  endfor
endfor
endfunction
x = SlidingWindows4()
save salidasw.csv x(1:100)
```

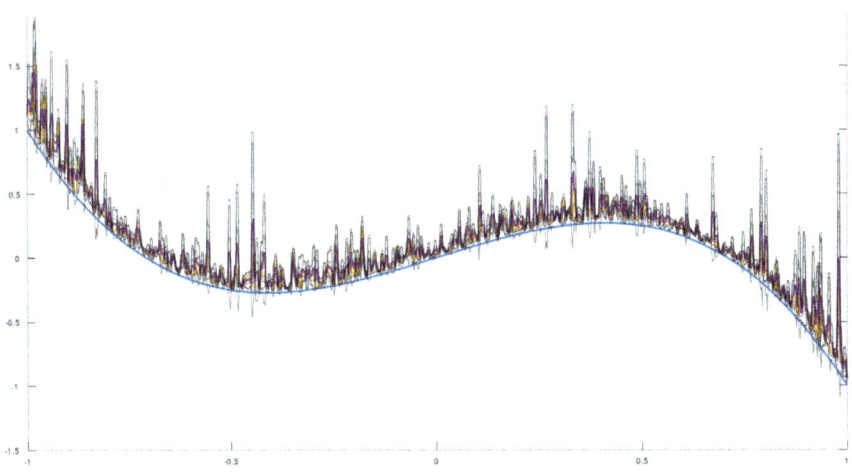

Fig. 3.2 Sliding Windows graphical output

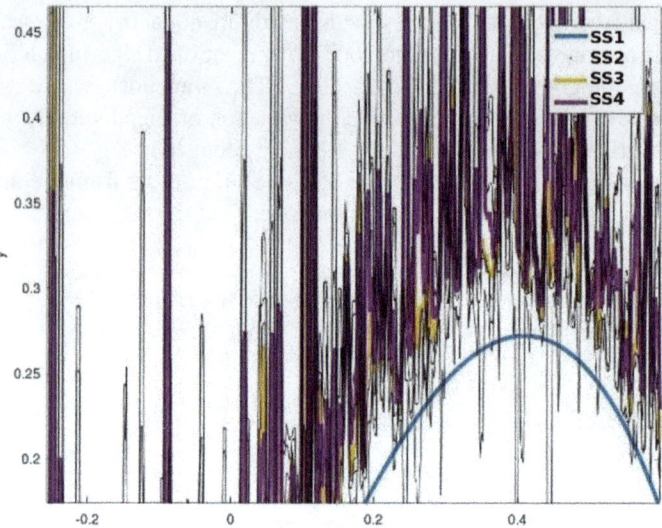

Fig. 3.3 Sliding Windows graphical output with zoom in

- **Blue** - SS1
- **Red dot** - SS2.
- **Yellow** - SS3.
- **Violet** - SS4.
- **Black** − $_i$ SS$_i$.

The plot shows the metadata corresponding to each Sub Slice of a pattern.

The plot shows the differences between metadata values for the video sub parts, as being processed for sound pattern. Running the algorithm using the Sliding Windows with two cut pointers algorithm [39] on sounds results in Fig. 3.4.

The plot represents the main curve representing the variations between the current slice and slice 1 is now bi-modal. This is because the comparison is second by second and not the entire slice. Since the sensibility is bigger, the plot shows that behind the global behavior shown in Fig. 3.2, there are moments where metadata representing the sound matches better in some parts.

3.4.2 Advantages and Disadvantages of Using the Proposed Approach

The Sliding Windows technique, was implemented in several versions, with certain pros and odds each one. The first version was created in Python, after an investigation

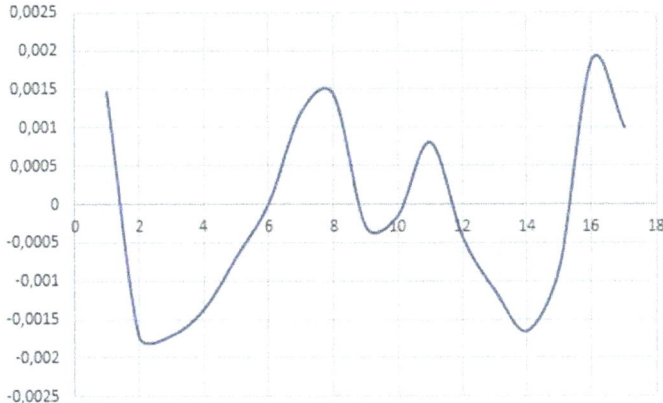

Fig. 3.4 Sliding Windows with 2 cut-points

of the case, the frequency, duration and comparison of similarities were obtained. The biggest downside is that it requires different libraries for it to work.

Then the first version was made in Octave, the result of investigating the operation of the software thoroughly, it is possible to pass an audio strip and that it reflects a graph detailing the different sounds that were detected. The disadvantage is that it is not possible to load more than one audio strip at a time and it is also very impractical to compare different graphics.

The second version was made also in Octave, can pass two different audio strips, obtaining a graph in which it is analyzed in which points there are coincidences.

The remaining versions are in Python, but based on the algorithm in Fig. 3.5, and is able to read a selected audio strip, a number of coefficients, the wavelet's

```
function retval = AplicoWvlet (zPatron, zInput, tipoWavelet, canal, numCoefWv)
f=input1;
[f,fs] = audioread (input1);
J = input2; % number of coefficients
wvNom = input3; % the wavelet to apply
%reduce input to one channel
[c,info] = fwt(f(:,canal),wvNom,J,1); % apply the wavelet and return coefficients
plotwavelets (c, info,fs,'dynrange',90);
## Frequency bands of the transform with x-axis in a long scale and band
## peaks normalized to 1. Only positive frequency band is shown
[g,a] = wfbt2filterbank({wvNom,J,'dwt'});
filterbankfreq(g,a,20*1024,'linabs','posfreq','plot','inf','flog');
% show the information structure of the signal
info
%return coefficients
retval=c;
endfunction
```

Fig. 3.5 Wavelets algorithm

parameters, and the type and number of audio channel. The last version can show analytical graphs and output a file with timestamps, and parameters in csv format.

3.5 The Sounds of the Use-Case

The analysis of every slice provides information on how often certain pattern is being repeated during the interaction with the patient. This type of information intends to make it relevant how every slice acts as a vocabulary for the individual. Following this conception Table 3.2 becomes a reference of that to expect when there is a stimulus, to confirm where is the focus at any moment.

All the selected sound patterns were made to compare each one of them and draw more precise conclusions about the behavior of the data. The comparison of the sound clippings, despite being different in their specific content, apparently have a very similar result between them.

Table 3.3 show the most relevant clippings, the echoic sound (Label), the internal ID (IDU), the order of first instance (FI), the timestamp of the first instance (Time), the threshold defined to determine is the cumulative distances between a metadata in the pattern is similar to metadata in some part of the video (MetaDtThreshold), the threshold defined to determine is the distance between certain metadata in the pattern is similar to metadata in some part of the video (PatternThreshold) and the number of sub-slices of the pattern (NumSubSlices).

Table 3.4 summarizes a selection of the first eight selected clippings considered to be the most repetitive in the recording. The plots show the wavelet description in every case. They are so frequent in the original interaction with the patient that are used as patterns of reactions.

The table makes it clear that every pattern has its own set of values. Something interesting arises when the numeric values of the ten first wavelets are compared. They have exact the same value for half of the code values, for all the patterns (see Table 3.5).

Table 3.3 Summary of patterns detected in the interaction

Label	IDU	FI	Time	MetaDtThreshold	PatternThreshold	NumSubSlices
iuiuiuui.wav	1	1	10:10	0.5	0.4	4
iuiuiuu.wav	2	2	14:22	0.5	0.4	4
iuiuiuiu.wav	3	3	13:30	0.5	0.4	4
iuiuiuiu.wav	4	3	13:30	0.5	0.4	4
iuiuiui.wav	5	1	7:23	0.5	0.4	4
iuiuiu.wav	6	0	0:00	0.5	0.4	4
iuuu.wav	7	4	2:53	0.5	0.4	4
iuiuiu.wav	8	0	10:17	0.5	0.4	4

3 Autistic Verbal Behavior Language Parameterization

Table 3.4 Plots of the pattern's wavelet encoding

Wavelets 1–10 of patterns		
IDU 1	IDU 2	IDU 3
IDU 4	IDU 5	IDU 6
IDU 7	IDU 8	

Table 3.5 Shared WV-coefficient in patterns

MetaData<x>SubSlice<y>	Pattern IDU	Coefficient
MtDt1SS1	[1…8]	0.0010946527865457112
MtDt3SS1	[1…8]	1321.678276643991
MtDt1SS2	[1…8]	5.6848702944657583e−05
MtDt3SS2	[1…8]	1320.678276643991
MtDt1SS3	[1…8]	−0.00099214605055142672
MtDt3SS3	[1…8]	1319.678276643991
MtSt1SS4	[1…8]	−0.00034117011565242596
MtDt2SS4	[1…8]	1318.678276643991

In the first column **MetaData<x>SubSlice<y>**, represents the meta-data number x of the sub-slice y. For instance MtDt1SS1 is the first meta-data of the first sub-slice. Being the meta-data, the slice selected. Table 3.6 shows the differences between wavelets.

Table 3.6 Peculiar WV-coefficient in patterns

IDU	MtDt2SS1	MtDt2SS2	MtDt2SS3	MtDt2SS4
1	−0.0020528575776779	0.000258812900079	−0.000245072739345	−0.001520474883871 44
2	0.002197774753675 1	−0.003481925534852	0.002276476081460 1	0.000693833371500096
3	−0.000973553361635 4	−0.000102468070003	0.000113669083227 6	−0.001303448825948 86
4	0.003132295832909 5	−0.004955072342362	−0.000232883456961 8	0.003182710319363 32
5	−0.000163574328507 2	−0.002160975862761	0.001170077212972 7	0.000922812954996 67
6	0.000777712413649 74	−0.000633479491237	0.001768172638893 2	−0.001159264358836 96
7	0.001260975846586	0.004033220214 35	−0.001881736903387 5	0.004830114072217 03
8	0.002785511914547	0.000599980364665 99	0.003198385519591 4	4.368454103618233 8

3 Autistic Verbal Behavior Language Parameterization

Table 3.7 WV-coefficient in patterns

IDU1	IDU2	IDU3	IDU4	IDU5	IDU6	IDU7	IDU8
−0.00036	−0.00052	−0.00005	−0.00015	−0.00159	0.00645	−0.00019	−0.00015
0.00037	0.00032	−0.00001	−0.00005	0.00118	−0.00702	−0.00005	−0.00005
−0.0009	−0.00073	−0.00005	0.00004	−0.00063	0.00566	−0.00019	−0.00005
0.00119	0.00096	−0.00004	0.00034	−0.00005	−0.00209	−0.00001	−0.00012
−0.0009	−0.00088	−0.00008	0.00042	0.00069	−0.00144	−0.00019	0.00001
0.00006	0.00065	0.00048	−0.00081	−0.00116	0.00222	0.00009	−0.00023
0.00045	−0.00062	−0.00048	0.00094	0.00064	−0.00065	−0.0002	0.00023
−0.00096	0.0004	0.0005	−0.00108	0.00035	−0.00256	0.00022	−0.00006
0.99973	0.0002	−0.00032	0.00093	−0.00151	0.00447	−0.00014	0
−0.0004	−0.00078	0.00016	−0.00122	0.00193	−0.00502	0.00005	0.00008

Finally, Table 3.7 has the wavelet decomposition of the eight patterns as a whole (without Sub-slicing and metadata).

3.6 Test and Evaluation

The previous section describes the main features that allow to determine that the entire audio has only eight sound patterns that may represent a kind of stimming, as they have identical parameters and repeat several times. This section, is the statistical evaluation and validation of the previous findings.

The variables considered for the lightweight version of the detection and their parameters are in Table 3.8.

In order to study how the model works for a single pattern, Pattern4 is considered from the entire list (see Table 3.9).

Sound recording was extracted from the original video into a.wav file. The sampling rate is fs = 44,100. Audio stream has every instances sampled as a tuple of 2 values, here named as X and Y.

The files obtained after Octave processing are labeled SalPattern1.Rami<x>.csv, with x = [1.0.3].

Patterns 9 and 10 are slices that seem to be a distorted version of one of the previous patterns. They were kept since there is still possibility that they are new patterns.

In the table **SalPattern1.Rami<x>.csv** stands for the output file of input **Rami<x>**, with <x> being the sequential ID of the input wav. There are up to 3 files, that is x = [1.0.3], since the original video had to be partitioned to adequate it to the computational availability of the project.

This section focuses on Pattern4, selected at random to show the case study. Table 3.10 describes the case of Pattern4.

Table 3.8 Fast detection variables and parameters

Variable	Description	Parameters
AVG-DifX, AVG-DifY	Average difference between first and second coordinate of the wave sample	Coordinate = {1, 2}
minX, minY	Minimum value of the first coordinate	Coordinate = 1
maxX, maxY	Maximum value of the second coordinate	Coordinate = 2
AvgCovX, AvgCovX	Average xcov, which is Compute covariance at various lags [=correlation(x-mean(x), y-mean(y))]	Coordinate = {1, 2}
MaxDifWalsh-HadamardX, MaxDifWalsh-HadamardY	Maximum of the differences in Fast Walsh-Hadamard Transform (FWHT) of every slice against the window of the video	*order = Hadamard, number of elements = 64*
R-CoefFFT	Coefficient R of covariance of FFT harmonics	numCoefFFT = 30
difCoefFFT	Difference between FFT coefficients of the slice versus the window	NumCoefFFT = 30
Threshold for FFT comparison		uFFT = 0.0005
Threshold for accumulated differences		Utot = 3

Table 3.9 Set of patterns detected in the video

Pattern	ID
iu iu iu iu 12,47	Pattern1
iu iuiuiu 3,20	Pattern2
iuiuiu 10,17	Pattern3
iuiuiu min 0	Pattern4
iuiuiui 7,23	Pattern5
iuiuiuiu 8,34	Pattern6
iuiuiuiu 13,30	Pattern7
iuiuiuu 14,22	Pattern8
iuiuiuui 10,10	Pattern9
iuiuuiiu 4,15	Pattern10
iuuu 2,53	Pattern11

3   Autistic Verbal Behavior Language Parameterization

Table 3.10 Data processed for Pattern 4

File	Records	Time	Pre-processed file
SalPattern4.Rami1.csv	1,048,576	441"	SalPattern4.set1.csv
SalPattern4.Rami2.csv	1,048,576	441"	SalPattern4.set2.csv
SalPattern4.Rami3.csv	1,046,199	440"	SalPattern4.set3.csv
Total	3,143,351		

The file length corresponds to a rate of 2.378 samples per second, in order to reduce the computational power required. The sampling change is performed after reading in Octave with 44,100 as a sampling rate. The last column is the name after certain pre-processing required for the exploratory analysis with WEKA 3.8.4

3.6.1 Pre-processing

From the previous considerations, the new version of the data-set has to be processed with WEKA to determine the most reduced set of variables to be used for the model of Pattern4. To do that there is the following pre-processing:

Step 1. Files SalPattern4.set<n>.csv, needs to change the regional setting in Octave to the one in LibreOffice Calc:. A script in Octave changes "," to ";" and "." to ",".
Step 2. With LibreOffice Calc every numeric column is changed to numeric format with leading sign, and 8 decimals. When needed until 20 decimals are defined. The file is then exported to CSV format.
Step 3. A script in Octave changes "," to "." and ";" to ","
Step 4. Import data in WEKA (c).

It is important to note that all the processing is being made with open source, standard in the field: Octave and WEKA. Both of them very used by its compatibility with other tools (like python and Java), its flexibility, cross platform installation, and deep Learning abilities. Furthermore, every graphic in this paper was performed in these tools.

3.6.2 Variable Selection

This section explains the variable selection procedure and justification. Some are based on practical criteria, others required more sophisticated approaches like Subset Evaluation algorithms based on information provided of the variables and PCA.

Variables *hit*, and *tira* are discarded, since in this version of the project, *hit* depends only on *ScoreTotal*; and *tira* is the name of the pattern's use case, which is the same for every instance under the scope of present study. For this process there is not wavelet or any other extra feature considered, so *ScoreTotal* and *ScoreParcial* are equal (the accumulated scoring and the scoring due to basic features), thus *ScoreTotal* is also discarded. Features considered as basic features are in Table 3.11.

The data-set presents no missing values by construction, and all (except *tira*, which is the pattern name) are numbers. The distribution of *ScoreParcial* (see Fig. 3.6) shows that a few instances are close to 0.1, the value of the highest approximation of the current slice to the pattern. Figures 3.7, 3.8 and 3.9 show similar behavior.

Zones with highest R are the ones candidates to be the pattern, since coefficients trend to follow a similar sequence. It is important to note that peaks are not located in

Table 3.11 Features considered for processing

Feature	Description
AVG-DifX	Average of the difference in value X between Pattern and current slice of the audio
AVG-DifY	Average of the difference in value y between Pattern and current slice of the audio
AvgCovX	Average of the covariance in value X between Pattern and current slice of the audio
AvgCovY	Average of the covariance in value Y between Pattern and current slice of the audio
minX, minY	Minimum of difference in value X and Y respectively
maxX, maxY	Maximum of difference in value X and Y respectively
MaxDifWalsh-HadamardX	Maximum of difference in Walsh-Hadamard transform coefficients in value X
MaxDifWalsh-HadamardY	Maximum of difference in Walsh-Hadamard transform coefficients in value Y
difCoefFFT-1 ... 30	Difference between coefficients FFT1... FFT30 between pattern and slice
R-CoefFFT'	Coefficient R of FFT covariance between pattern and Slice

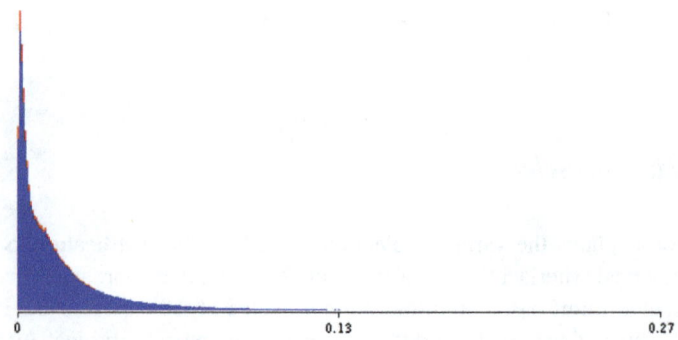

Fig. 3.6 Dispersion of *ScoreParcial*

3 Autistic Verbal Behavior Language Parameterization

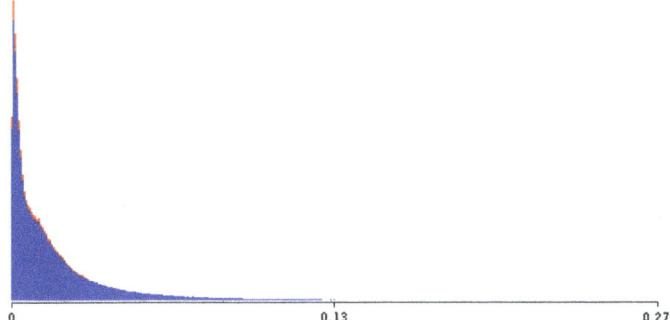

Fig. 3.7 Dispersion *MaxDifWalsh-HadamardX*

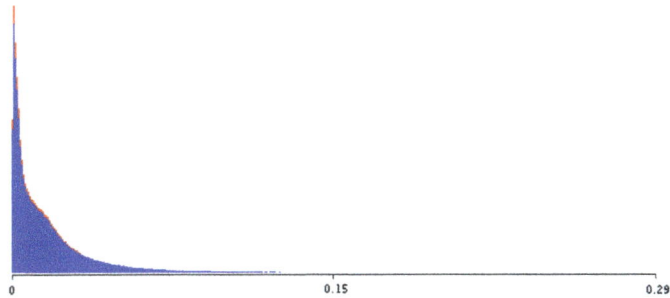

Fig. 3.8 Dispersion *MaxDifWalsh-HadamardY*

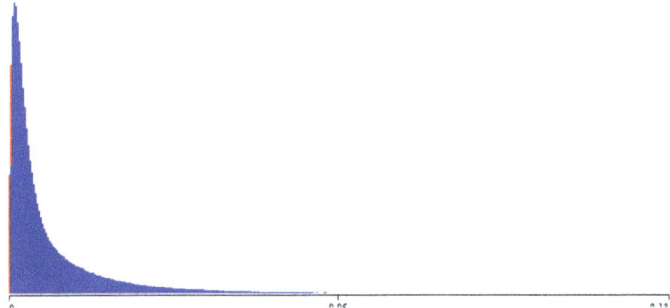

Fig. 3.9 Dispersion Pattern4 *RcoefFFT*

a single timestamp starting the pattern, because of the sampling rate—A good model will be able to determine if this corresponds to the Pattern4 or a similar sound.

The next step in WEKA, for attribute selection process starts with all attributes except those discarded previously.

(i) **Subset considering class *ScoreParcial***

The algorithm for attribute selection requires an Attribute selector and a search method. As an standard approach the ***selector*** recommended by WEKA by default is ***CfsSubsetEval***, that evaluates the worth of a subset of attributes by considering the individual predictive ability of each feature along with the degree of redundancy between them.

The *Search* method selected is ***BestFirst***. This way, the algorithm Searches the space of attribute subsets by greedy hill-climbing augmented with a backtracking facility. Setting the number of consecutive non-improving nodes allowed controls the level of backtracking done. Best first may start with the empty set of attributes and search forward, or start with the full set of attributes and search backward, or start at any point and search in both directions (by considering all possible single attribute additions and deletions at a given point).

The test runs with 39 attributes and 100,000 records. The evaluation mode is "evaluate on all training data". The attribute Subset Evaluator runs supervised, considering the *class* of type numeric ***ScoreParcial***. The CFS Subset Evaluator includes locally predictive attributes.

The selected attribute with 9: 1 scoring is ***R-CoefFFT***.

The result can be explained as currently, scoring depends on FFT differences between FFT in X and Y, so the algorithm is detecting the deep relationship between both measures and not information dependency with the entire set of features.

The same test is performed with *Selector CfsSubsetEval* and *Search* method ***Greedy Stepwise***, a greedy forward (or backward) search through the space of attribute subsets. May start with no/all attributes or from an arbitrary point in the space. Stops when the addition/deletion of any remaining attributes results in a decrease in evaluation. Can also produce a ranked list of attributes by traversing the space from one side to the other and recording the order that attributes are selected. The parameters selected are for forward search, starting with no attribute.

As in the previous test, the selected attribute with 9:1 scoring is ***R-CoefFFT***, Merit of best subset found: 0.159 also identical to ***BestFirst***.

From all this analysis, the *ScoreTotal* depends mainly on the covariance coefficient of the FFT values of the patterns. The rest of the thresholds determined for closeness between pattern and slice features contribute less to it.

The next section evaluates, beyond *ScoreTotal*, how features contribute to ***R-CoefFFT***.

(ii) **Subset considering class *R-CoefFFT***

In order to explore how features contribute to values of FTT covariance, *ScoreTotal* y ignored and the algorithm runs with *Evaluator CfsSubsetEval* and *Search BestFirst*. Class is ***R-CoefFFT***.

Results Merit of the best subset found rises up to 0.44 selecting only ***AVG-DifX*** attribute, as relevant. Scoring depends on FFT differences between FFT in X and Y, so the algorithm shows the deep relation between both measures. The same Evaluator with ***GreedyStepwise*** results in the same variable and merit (see Table 3.12).

3 Autistic Verbal Behavior Language Parameterization

Table 3.12 Ranked attributes with GreedyStepwise

Order	ID	Attribute	Order	ID	Attribute
1	19	DifCoefFFT-11	17	31	DifCoefFFT-23
2	16	DifCoefFFT-8	18	32	DifCoefFFT-24
3	17	DifCoefFFT-9	19	34	DifCoefFFT-26
4	11	DifCoefFFT-3	20	21	DifCoefFFT-13
5	10	DifCoefFFT-2	21	35	DifCoefFFT-27
6	9	DifCoefFFT-1	22	36	DifCoefFFT-28
7	7	MaxDifWalsh-HadamardY	23	30	DifCoefFFT-22
8	2	AVG-DifX	24	29	DifCoefFFT-21
9	3	AVG-DifY	25	28	DifCoefFFT-20
10	4	AvgCovX	26	27	DifCoefFFT-19
11	5	AvgCovY	27	22	DifCoefFFT-14
12	6	MaxDifWalsh-HadamardX	28	23	DifCoefFFT-15
13	18	DifCoefFFT-10	29	24	DifCoefFFT-16
14	20	DifCoefFFT-12	30	25	DifCoefFFT-17
15	37	DifCoefFFT-29	31	26	DifCoefFFT-18
16	33	DifCoefFFT-25	32	1	Timespamp

The *Evaluator* **ClassifierAttributeEval** evaluates the worth of an attribute by using a user-specified classifier. This time a simple ZEROR is selected (a tree with just one node). The Search method is leaded by a *RANKER*, that ranks attributes by their individual evaluations. Works in conjunction with attribute evaluators (ReliefF, GainRatio, Entropy etc.). In the case of *ZeroR*, it is GainRatio. Table 3.13 shows the ranking.

Relevance of attributes are: 38, 14, 12, 13, 15, 19, 16, 17, 11, 10, 9, 7, 2, 3, 4, 5, 6, 18, 20, 37, 33, 31, 32, 34, 21, 35, 36, 30, 29, 28, 27, 22, 23, 24, 25, 26, 1. A few FFT coefficients characterize the shape of the sound wave of Pattern4. Also the difference in fast transform Walsh Hadamard. They can be used to perform a fast testing in real time instead of all the 39 features.

(iii) **PCA**

Since all nominal attributes were removed in pre-processing, Principal Components Analysis (PCA) can be useful to identify and avoid inter-dependencies among features. Ir works in conjunction with a Ranker search. Dimension reduction is accomplished by choosing enough eigenvectors to account for some percentage of the variance in the original data-default 0.95 (95%). Attribute noise can be filtered by transforming to the PC space, eliminating some of the worst eigenvectors, and then transforming back to the original space. But it is not considered for obtaining a new rotated set of axis but to evaluate the information provided by the attributes.

Table 3.13 Ranked attributes **ClassifierAttributeEval** for R-coefFFT

Order	Score	Attribute	Order	Score	Attribute
1	38	DifCoefFFT-30	19	20	DifCoefFFT-12
2	14	DifCoefFFT-6	20	37	DifCoefFFT-29
3	12	DifCoefFFT-4	21	33	DifCoefFFT-25
4	13	DifCoefFFT-5	22	31	DifCoefFFT-23
5	15	DifCoefFFT-7	23	32	DifCoefFFT-24
6	19	DifCoefFFT-11	24	34	DifCoefFFT-26
7	16	DifCoefFFT-8	25	21	DifCoefFFT-13
8	17	DifCoefFFT-9	26	35	DifCoefFFT-27
9	11	DifCoefFFT-3	27	36	DifCoefFFT-28
10	10	DifCoefFFT-2	28	30	DifCoefFFT-22
11	9	DifCoefFFT-1	29	29	DifCoefFFT-21
12	7	MaxDifWalsh-HadamardY	30	28	DifCoefFFT-20
13	2	AVG-DifX	31	27	DifCoefFFT-19
14	3	AVG-DifY	32	22	DifCoefFFT-14
15	4	AvgCovX	33	23	DifCoefFFT-15
16	5	AvgCovY	34	24	DifCoefFFT-16
17	6	MaxDifWalsh-HadamardX	35	25	DifCoefFFT-17
18	18	DifCoefFFT-10	36	26	DifCoefFFT-18
			37	1	Timespamp

As *ScoreParcial* is a derived formula provided it depends mainly on *R-CoefFFT*, it is not considered for this analysis. Table 3.12 shows the output of PCA, denoting that every variable and the 25 first FFT coefficients are relevant.

Selected attributes are 1, 2, 3, 4, 5, 6, 7, 8, 9, 10, 11, 12, 13, 14, 15, 16, 17, 18, 19, 20, 21, 22, 23, 24, 25: a total of 25 of 38. Although just *R-cofFFT* describes properly the pattern detection criteria, the entire set of features until *coefFFT-18* provide relevant information about the signal, and therefore must be kept in the data-set analysis. The rest of the FFT coefficients are not relevant.

3.6.3 Automatic Timestamp Detection

To validate the timestamp of the automatically processed slices, a comparison against hand made table of occurrences is performed. Since the previous analysis detected that there are "hit ranges" of timestamps instead of single matches, a clustering is performed to find the scope of the regions. The same clustering with the entire set, serves to evaluate the matching performance. Hit ranges are in the reduced set

3   Autistic Verbal Behavior Language Parameterization   75

Table 3.14 Timestamp for hand made matching of Pattern4

Time (min)	Time (s)	Timestamp	Test set	Stimulus
4.16	256	608,697	1	4.14'
7.23	443	1,053,331	2	2.22'
10.10	610	1,450,412	2	10.08'
14.10	850	2,021,065	2	14.09'
16.35	995	2,365,835	3	6.33'

Table 3.15 Matching of Pattern4

Timestamp	Time	MaxDifWalsh-HadamardX	MaxDifWalsh-HadamardY	R-coefFFT
621,804	4' 20''	0.000655651	0.000399113	0.320047
729,992	5' 7''	0.000473976	0.00031662	0.449992

containing only registers marked with highest ***ScoreTotal*** (or ***R-coefFFT***, as shown previously, works a the metric corresponding to the ***ScoreParcial*** indicator).

(i)   **Validation with hand made registering**

Table 3.1 shows part of a hand made Time-sheet of Stimulus—sound detected. For Pattern 4, the corresponding entry details are in Table 3.14.

Every entry has a stimulus associated. In the case of Pattern 4, the stimulus is in the background sound: birdsong. The conversion to timestamp is using the reduced sampling rate determined during pre-processing.

Table 3.15 shows the corresponding timestamps of hits detected in the first test set (from timestamp 1 to 1,048,576), representing the first portion of the video, with a length of 7' 21''.

It can be seen that there is one more matching not detected previously, as those timestamps correspond to a fast and loud aggregation of sounds. In both cases MaxDifWalsh-HadamardX, MaxDifWalsh-HadamardY and R-coefFFT have values different from the rest. The converted timestamp to minutes also has certain differences probably due to the ability of the evaluator to calculate the time. Figures 3.10 and 3.11 shows the dispersion of MaxDifWalsh-HadamardX and R-coefFFT, highlighted the timestamps with best matching of Pattern4. As the case of the rest of the figures, they are plots from WEKA.

Figure 3.10 shows detected matchings as minimal values of the MaxDifWalsh-HadamardX (maximum of the difference for Walsh Hadamard coefficients in X range).

For R-CoefFFT (Fig. 3.11), there are some extra values around the optimum of the selected timestamp, due to the sampling rate, the granularity is big. In the following analysis (clustering with the entire set) there are two timestamps ranges of hits (that also have ScoreParcial, ScoreTotal, and R-coefFFT hight) instead of one (see portions in red of Fig. 3.12). Despite this is an improvement to the hand-made registration

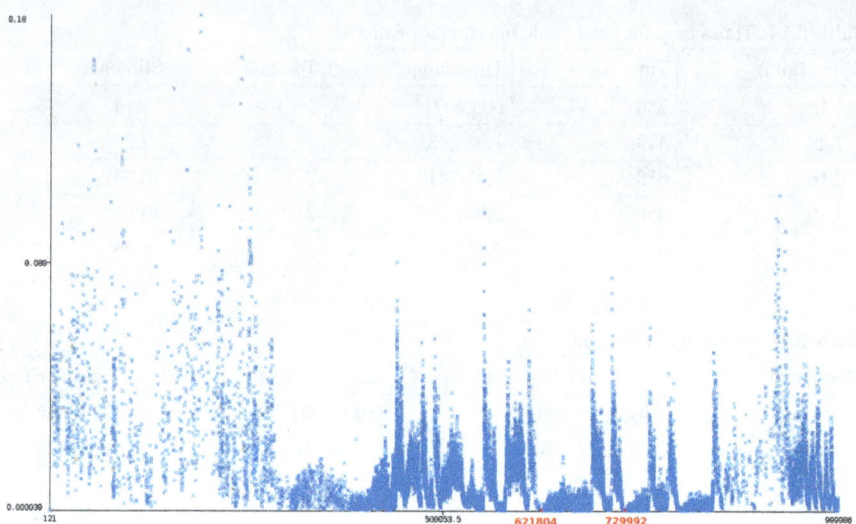

Fig. 3.10 Timestamp versus MaxDifWalsh-HadamardX

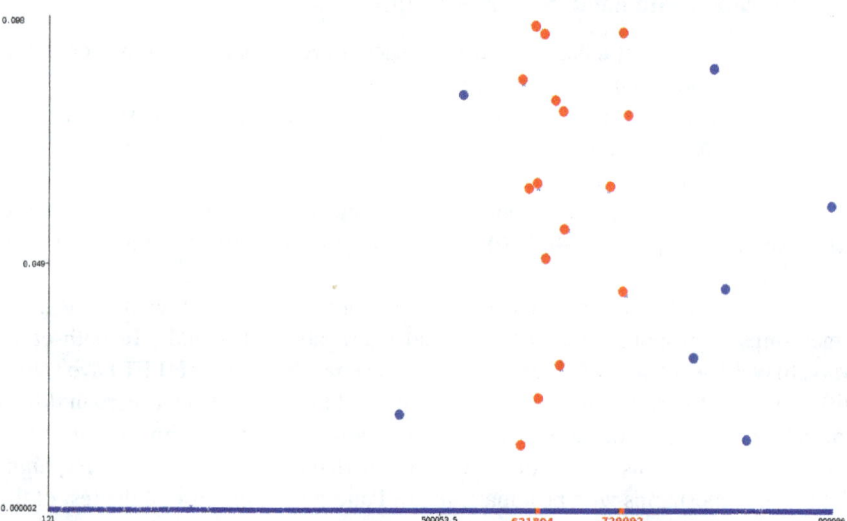

Fig. 3.11 Timestamp versus R-CoefFFT

(with only one match), it is not good enough to precise when the pattern starts. The model with NN fixes this problem (see section "Model for timestamp detection").

(ii) **Clustering with the entire set**

To cluster instances Simple K-Means is the fastest algorithm to process the set 1. Parameter $K = 2$ clusters, for detecting if the model is able to split features related

3 Autistic Verbal Behavior Language Parameterization

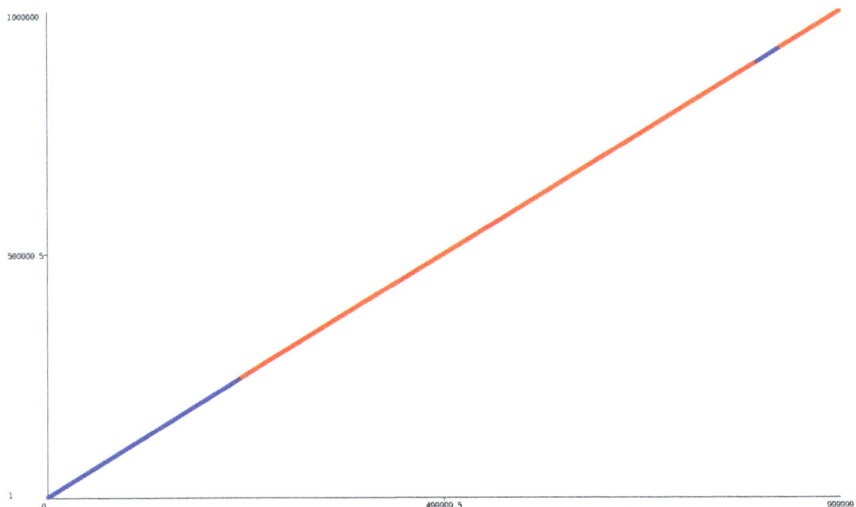

Fig. 3.12 Matching of Pattern4: Timestamp versus instance number

to Pattern4, all the features selected in the previous section are used. Other parameters are: distance function Euclidean Distance, maxIterations (maximum number of iterations) 500, numExecutionSlots (number of execution threads to use. Must be equal to the number of available cpu/cores) 1, dontReplaceMissingValues (Replace missing values globally with mean/mode) false, preserveInstancesOrder (Preserve order of instances) false, InitializationMethod (The initialization method to use) Random, fastDistanceCalc (Use cut-off values for speeding up distance calculation, but suppressing the calculation and output of the within cluster sum of squared errors/sum of distances) false, and Seed value of 10. It takes 9 s to build the clusters for 1,000,000 records, Within cluster sum of squared errors: 271,479.03. Table 3.16 has the final cluster centroids.

It detects that there are 2 clusters one with low R-CoefFFT and the other with high values. It corresponds to MaxDifWalsh values. A total of 272,799 Clustered Instances (27%) belong to cluster 1 (lower differences) and 727,201 (73%) are in cluster 0. Values of difCoedFFT-1 to difCoedFFT-18 are fewer in cluster 1 than in cluster 0, due to the proximity of those instances to the pattern. Several sounds that aren't Pattern 4 are in the cluster. This implies that K-means is not good enough to detect with precision where the pattern matches. Figure 3.12 shows the cluster distribution of Pattern4.

The cluster detects the two main time periods when the pattern is present (portions in red), but the model lacks of enough specificity.

(iii) **Clustering with reduced set**

The reduced set of attributes are 25 (the original data-set has 39 attributes), and 42,682 registers (drifted from the starting 1,048,576 instances). The clustering process now takes only 0.81 s and clustered instances are organized as follows: cluster 1 with

Table 3.16 Clustering details

Attribute	Full data	Cluster# 0	1
	(1,000,000.0)	(727,201.0)	(272,799.0)
AVG-DifX	0.0387	0.0131	0.0482
AVG-DifY	0.0338	0.0114	0.0422
MaxDifWalsh-HadamardX	0.0173	0.0374	0.0097
MaxDifWalsh-HadamardY	0.0166	0.0353	0.0096
R-CoeffFFT	0.0075	0.0047	0.015
difCoefFFT-1	2.95	3.5736	2.7161
difCoefFFT-2	2.5176	3.35	2.2054
difCoefFFT-3	2.1955	2.9226	1.9227
difCoefFFT-4	2.6231	3.6645	2.2324
difCoefFFT-5	2.4688	3.5241	2.0729
difCoefFFT-6	2.595	3.4923	2.2584
difCoefFFT-7	4.8701	5.4453	4.6543
difCoefFFT-8	3.6354	4.3074	3.3834
difCoefFFT-9	2.529	3.3567	2.2185
difCoefFFT-10	2.0781	3.1077	1.6918
difCoefFFT-11	4.0816	4.8391	3.7975
difCoefFFT-12	3.3608	4.2408	3.0307
difCoefFFT-13	3.0082	3.9483	2.6555
difCoefFFT-14	2.0709	3.7964	1.4237
difCoefFFT-15	2.1553	3.0641	1.8144
difCoefFFT-16	2.0514	3.1202	1.6505
difCoefFFT-17	2.4121	3.4797	2.0117
difCoefFFT-18	2.1623	3.1289	1.7998

8272 (19%), and cluster 0 with 34,410 (81%). Although there are fewer timestamps classified as matching zone, the precision is still poor.

The hit found by using the main features have matching ranges, because the sampling rate is high (44,100 samples per second) compared to the time granularity for speech instances in language processing (seconds).

The initial hit rate, just considering R-Coeff reduced set 1 from 1,000,000 to 42,682 records. (The adjusted hit with a combination of MaxDifWalsh-Hadamard, AVG-Dif, AVG-Cov and difCoefFFT-1 to difCoefFFT-18 improved fitness but it needs to be even better. I the following sections Neural Model is able to perform a better classification of the true matching.

3   Autistic Verbal Behavior Language Parameterization   79

Table 3.17 NN model with test sets

Set	instances	Correctly classified instances (%)	Incorrectly classified instances
1	1,048,576	98.62	1
2	1,048,576	91.98	5
3	1,046,199	99.14	2

3.6.4 Model for Timestamp Detection

This section describes the simple neural model for timestamp detection of Pattern4. As precision of AvgCovX and have scientific notation, AvgCovXe15 instead which is 10^{15} times smaller. data-sets are considered in a reduced version with only relevant attributes in the previous analysis: Timespamp, AVG-DifX, AVG-DifY, MaxDifWalsh-HadamardX, MaxDifWalsh-HadamardY, R-CoefFFT, AvgCovXe15, AvgCovYe15 and HIT.

Table 3.17 is the summary of the models obtained, using Multilayer Perceptron of 9 input nodes, one hidden layer of 5 units and one output unit. In all cases Test mode is split using 66.0% for training and remainder for testing.

Kappa statistics (0.98) and classification results suggest that the model is good for detecting Pattern4.

3.6.5 Model Findings and Results Analysis

Table 3.18 is Table 3.14 extended with the NN model findings: timestamp found with the Perceptron network, and the number of records representing the hit (column Length derived).

There are two new rows with extra matchings detected automatically: timestamp 1,224,527 and 1,930,712. From these results it can be said that matching timestamp is more accurate when the model finds a matching, and that the number is higher than in hand-made evaluation of the recording.

Table 3.18 Timestamp for hand made matching of Pattern4

Time (min)	Time (s)	Timestamp	Test set	Timestamp derived	Length derived	Stimulus
4.16	256	608,697	1	608,697	2	4.14'
7.23	443	1,053,331	2	1,053,332	5	2.22'
8.35	515	1,224,527	2	1,224,504	2	8.34'
10.10	610	1,450,412	2	1,449,996	3	10.08'
13.32	812	1,930,712	2	1,928,767	2	13.29'
14.10	850	2,021,065	2	1,998,262	1	14.09'
16.35	995	2,365,835	3	2,365,876	4	16.33'

3.7 Conclusions and Future Work

This paper presents an introduction of main characteristics of patients suffering Autistic spectrum Disorder. Those that has not preserved verbal behavior have severe problems to communicate. They can't articulate any language in the sense that has been traditionally defined. After analyzing the recording of a patient's interaction, it is possible to determine several repetitive movements and sounds, that are present upon certain stimuli. The sounds can be considered as part of a pattern to evaluate when it is a verbal behavior during the interaction. All the patterns have certain basic characteristics. FFT coefficients are not enough to detect similarities between a pattern and the sound track. Considering the covariance of the difference between pattern and wav file, of coefficients in fast transform Walsh Hadamard and FFT are the best option. They can be used to perform a fast testing in real time. Several parameters and coefficients were considered but are not relevant. The model derived in this chapter is a neural Network, using as parameters the covariance of differences between FFT coefficients and Walsh Hadamard. The test made with the use case is able to detect one matching not detected previously, and more accurate timestamps. The findings in this paper might be considered as a first step to evaluate other patient's interactions and their features. Other pending activities are: implement a prototype that makes it simpler to drift off sound patterns and evaluate them automatically, apply similar considerations to video recordings, track the evolution in time of the communication of the individual.

References

1. Filipek, P.A., Accardo, P.J., y Ashwal, S.: Parameter practice: detection and autistic diagnose. Neurology **55**, 468479 (2000)
2. Maenner, M.J., Shaw, K.A., Baio, J., et al.: Prevalence of autism spectrum disorder among children aged 8 years—autism and developmental disabilities monitoring network, 11 Sites, United States. In: MMWR Surveillance Summaries 2020, vol. 69(No. SS-4), pp. 1–12 (2016)
3. Zablotsky, B., Black, L.I., Maenner, M.J., Schieve, L.A., Danielson, M.L., Bitsko, R.H., Blumberg, S.J., Kogan, M.D., Boyle, C.A.: Prevalence and trends of developmental disabilities among children in the United States: 2009–2017. Pediatrics **144**(4), e20190811 (2019)
4. Mayada, et al.: Global prevalence of autism and other pervasive developmental disorders. Autism Res. **5**(3), 160–179 (2012)
5. Sevilla, M.d.S.F., Bermúdez, M.O.E., Sánchez, J.J.C.: How many people have autism? Theor. Rev. Int. J. Dev. Educ. Psychol. INFAD. N1 V1, 769–786 (2013). ISSN 0241-9877
6. Greer, R.D.: The wide application of behavior analysis to schooling behavior (CABAS®). Behav. Soc. Matter
7. Krans, B.: Small humanoid robot helps children with ASD. Healthline News (2013). Obtained from http://www.healthline.com/healthnews
8. Greer, R.D.: The comprehensive application of behavior analysis to schooling. (CABAS®). Behav. Soc. Issues **7**(1) (1997)
9. Bustamante, P., Lafalla, A., Coria, N., Agüero, M., López de Luise, D., Parra, C., Azor, R., Moya, J., Cuesta, J.: Protocol for evaluation of somatic and oral behavior to sound stimuli in patients with autism spectrum. CI2S Lab. Pringles 10- P2. University of Burgos (2016)

10. Kuiper, M.W., Verhoeven, E.W., Geurts, H.M.: Stop making noise! auditory sensitivity in adults with an autism spectrum disorder diagnosis: physiological habituation and subjective detection thresholds. J. Autism Dev. Disord. **49**(5), 2116–2128 (2019). https://doi.org/10.1007/s10803-019-03890-9
11. Summers, J., Shahrami, A., Cali, S., et al.: Self-injury in autism spectrum disorder and intellectual disability: exploring the role of reactivity to pain and sensory input. Brain Sci. **7**(11), 140 (2017). Published 26 Oct 2017. https://doi.org/10.3390/brainsci7110140
12. Marsh, K.L, Isenhower, R.W., Richardson, M.J., et al.: Autism and social disconnection in interpersonal rocking. Front. Integr. Neurosci. **7**, 4 (2013). Published 18 Feb 2013. https://doi.org/10.3389/fnint.2013.00004
13. Mazefsky, C.A., Herrington, J., Siegel, M., et al.: The role of emotion regulation in autism spectrum disorder. J. Am. Acad. Child. Adolesc. Psychiatry. **52**(7), 679–688 (2013). https://doi.org/10.1016/j.jaac.2013.05.006
14. Mazefsky, C.A., White, S.W.: Emotion regulation: concepts & practice in autism spectrum disorder. Child. Adolesc. Psychiatr. Clin. N. Am. **23**(1), 15–24 (2014). https://doi.org/10.1016/j.chc.2013.07.002
15. van Santen, J.P., Sproat, R.W., Hill, A.P.: Quantifying repetitive speech in autism spectrum disorders and language impairment. Autism Res. Off. J. Int. Soc. Autism Res. **6**(5), 372–383 (2013). https://doi.org/10.1002/aur.1301
16. De Luise, D.L., Azor, R., Párraga, C.: Autistic verbal behavior. Automated model of the patient profile—audio. Edit. Académica Española (2015). ISBN 978-3-659-07183-6
17. Cheol-Hong, N., Ahmed, H.: Novel pattern detection in children with autism spectrum disorder using iterative subspace identification. Department of Electrical and Computer Engineering University of Minnesota, USA (2010). 978-1-4244-4296-6/10 ©2010 IEEE ICASSP 2010. PPS 2266/2269
18. Mower, E., Black, M.P., Flores, E., Williams, M., Narayanan, S.: Design of an emotionally targeted interactive agent for children with autism. University of Southern California (USC), 2011. IEEE (2011). 978-1-61284-350-6/11
19. De Luise, D.L.: Autistic verbal behavior parameters. Paper presented in: 9th International Workshop on Soft Computing Applications (SOFA 2020). Arad-Romania, 27–29 November 2020. Hosted by "Aurel Vlaicu" University of Arad (2020)
20. DSM-V Encoding update®. Supplement to the Diagnostic and Statistical Manual of Mental Disorders, 5th edn. American Psychiatric Association (2014)
21. Ministry of Science and Innovation Spain. Clinical practice guide for the management of patients with autism spectrum disorders in primary care. Nipo: 477-09-052-8. ISBN: 978-84-451-3244-9: Estilo Estugraf Impresores, S.L. Pol. Ind. Los Huertecillos, Nave 13 - 28350 Ciempozuelos (Madrid) (2009)
22. Skinner, B.F.: Verbal Conduct (Trans.: R. Ardila, Edit. T. Mexico) (1981) ISBN 968-24-0987-X
23. Kanner, L. (1943). Autistic disturbances of affective contact. Nervous Child. N2, (217250) (Trans: T.S. Vicario). Published in the Spanish Journal of Intellectual Disability Siglo Cero. www.feaps.org
24. Wing, L.: The definition and prevalence of autism: a review. Eur. Child Adolesc. Psychiatry **2**, 61–74 (1993)
25. Riviere, A.M.: The little boy with autism (2000). ISBN: 9788460702610
26. Python in practice: create better programs using concurrency, libraries, and patterns (Developer's Library), 1st Edición. Mark Summerfield. ISBN-13: 978-0-321-90563-5
27. Fluent Python: Clear, concise, and effective. Ramalho, Luciano. ISBN-13: 978-1491946008
28. Beazley, D., Jones, B., Jones, K.: Python Cookbook, 3rd edn. O'Reilly Media, Inc. ISBN: 9781449340377
29. Automate the Boring Stuff with Python. Al Sweigart. Free to read under a Creative Commons License. ISBN-13: 9781593279929
30. Summerfield, M.: Python 3. Editorial: ANAYA MULTIMEDIA. (INFORMATICA). Año de edición: 2009 (2009). ISBN: 978-84-415-2613-6

31. Baghai-Ravary, L., Beet, S.: Automatic speech signal analysis for clinical diagnosis and assessment of speech disorders (2013). ISBN 978-1-4614-4574-6
32. Biing-Hwang, J., Rabiner, L., Wilpon, J.: On the use of bandpass liftering in speech recognition. IEEE Trans. Acoust. Speech Sig. Process. **35**(7), 947–954 (1987). https://doi.org/10.1109/TASSP.1987.1165237
33. De Luise, D.L., Hisgen, D., Cabrera, A., y Morales Rins, M.: Modeling dialogs with linguistic wavelets. Theory Pract. Mod. Comput. **1**, 11–13 (2012)
34. De Luise, D.L.: Morphosyntactic linguistic wavelets for knowledge management. InTechOpen **8**, 167–189 (2012). https://doi.org/10.5772/35438
35. De Luise, D.L., Hisgen, D.: MLW and bilingualism: case study and definition of basic techniques. IGI global: Advanced Research and Trends in New Technologies, Software, Human-Computer Interaction, and Communicability, pp. 568–600 (2013)
36. Sundberg, M.L.: A brief overview of a behavioral approach to language assessment and intervention for children with autism association for behavior analysis newsletter, 30(3) (2007)
37. Greer, D.: The ontogenetic selection of verbal capabilities: contributions of skinner's verbal behavior theory to a more comprehensive understanding of language. Int. J. Psychol. Psychol. Ther. **8**(3), 363–386 (2008)
38. Two Pointer with Sliding Window Algorithm to Compute the Longest Substring with at most K Distinct Characters (2020) Taken from https://helloacm.com/
39. Fumarola, F., Ciampi, A., Annalisa, A., Malerba, D.: A sliding window algorithm for relational frequent patterns mining from data streams. In: 12th International Conference on Discovery Science (2009). http://dx.doi.org/10.1007/978-3-642-04747-3_30

Chapter 4
Case Studies to Demonstrate Real-World Applications in Ophthalmic Image Analysis

Beatriz Remeseiro and Verónica Bolón-Canedo

Abstract In the digital era we live in, people are able to generate and store data at an unprecedented rate. This explosion in available data for further analysis is as evident in medicine as it is elsewhere. Numerous artificial intelligence techniques been applied to different medical problems with the aim of automating time-consuming, and often subjective, manual tasks implemented by practitioners in diverse specialties. This chapter focuses on several real-world applications in ophthalmic image analysis. In this context, the objective quality assessment of retinal images plays an important role to guarantee the success of any computer-aided system. For this reason, we first present a case study on retinal image quality assessment, which uses computer vision and machine learning techniques. Additionally, we introduce two other case studies: the automatic computation of the arteriolar-to-venular index, a predictive biomarker of cerebral atrophy and cardiovascular events; and the automatic diagnosis of retinopathy of prematurity, a disease affecting low birth weight infants that shows a high amount of disagreement among experts. The experimental results presented were obtained on several datasets, both public and private, and demonstrate their suitability to be used in daily practice, both for clinical and research purposes.

Keywords Image analysis · Artificial intelligence · Ophthalmology · Retinal image · Machine learning

---

Part of the content of this chapter was previously published in *Computer Methods and Programs in Biomedicine* (https://doi.org/10.1016/j.cmpb.2013.04.007, https://doi.org/10.1016/j.cmpb.2015.06.004), *IEEE Proceedings* (https://doi.org/10.1109/IJCNN.2017.7966429), and *The Visual Computer* (https://doi.org/10.1007/s00371-020-01863-z)

B. Remeseiro (✉)
Department of Computer Science, Universidad de Oviedo,
Campus de Gijón s/n, 33203 Gijón, Spain
e-mail: bremeseiro@uniovi.es

V. Bolón-Canedo (✉)
Centro de Investigación CITIC, Department of Computer Science, Universidade da Coruña,
Campus de Elviña s/n, 15071 A Coruña, Spain
e-mail: veronica.bolon@udc.es

© The Author(s), under exclusive license to Springer Nature Switzerland AG 2022
C.-P. Lim et al. (eds.), *Handbook of Artificial Intelligence in Healthcare*,
Intelligent Systems Reference Library 211,
https://doi.org/10.1007/978-3-030-79161-2_4

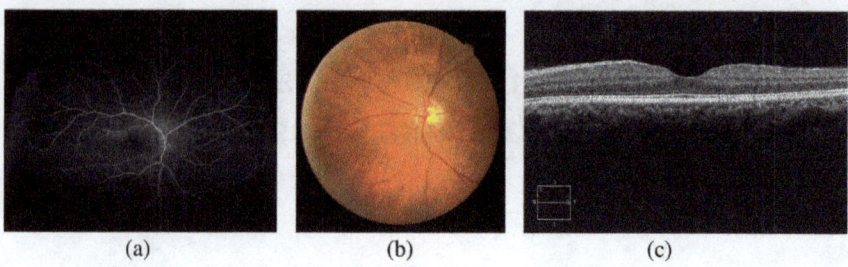

Fig. 4.1 Examples of different eye imaging modalities: **a** fluorescein angiography [6], **b** retinography [7], and **c** optical coherence tomography [8]

4.1 Introduction

Ophthalmology is an area of medicine and surgery that deals with the prevention, diagnosis, and treatment of eye diseases and other problems related to vision. In order to diagnose any possible eye disorder, ophthalmologists perform different techniques for eye examination, such as visual acuity [1] or ocular tonometry [2]. Moreover, there are several eye imaging modalities used by practitioners in their clinical and research routines. Some examples are following detailed:

- Fluorescein angiography [3] is a simple technique that involves injecting a dye and was adopted by early pioneers in medical retina research to study the retinal vasculature (see Fig. 4.1a).
- Retinography [4] is a technique that shows the optic fundus of the retina allowing to observe the retinal vessels and other structures, such as the optic disc (see Fig. 4.1b).
- Optical coherence tomography (Optical coherence tomography) [5] is a non-invasive method that provides a cross-sectional image of the retina and its structures in real-time (see Fig. 4.1c).

As for the most common eye diseases [9], they can be grouped in those related to the retina, such as glaucoma or macular degeneration; and those related to the eye surface, such as dry eye or conjunctivitis. Artificial intelligence techniques have been used in the last decades to automatize the analysis of ophthalmic images, thus supporting practitioners in the diagnosis and/or monitoring a great variety of eye diseases [10, 11]. Additionally, there are other diseases and several vascular disorders that can be also diagnosed and monitored by examining the eyes and their structure through ophthalmic images.

Human blood circulation can be observed in-vivo in the eye, allowing to diagnose several systemic diseases that affect the retinal vessels in such a way that they become thicker or narrower [12, 13]. Some of these diseases include diabetes, with a 8.5% of global prevalence among adults according to the WHO[1]; raised blood pressure,

---

[1] World Health Organization: http://www.who.int/en/.

which is estimated to cause about the 12.8% of the total of all deaths worldwide as reported by WHO; and different vascular disorders. More specifically, diabetic retinopathy frequently causes vessel diameter alterations [14], whilst dilatation and elongation of main arteries and veins are often associated with hypertension and other cardiovascular pathologies [15].

In this context, retinography images are one of the most widely used imaging modalities. For this reason, retinographies have been commonly used as input data in many screening tools and computer-aided diagnosis systems for glaucoma [16, 17], macular degeneration [18, 19], or diabetic retinopathy [20, 21], among other diseases. The success of these systems is highly dependent on the quality of the retinal images. For this reason, the field of retinal image quality assessment has increased its interest in recent years, as we analyze in the first case study of this chapter. The other two cases studies are focused on two specific topics: the automatic estimation of the arteriolar-to-venular index, correlated with cardiovascular diseases such as stroke or atherosclerosis [22]; and the understanding of the causes of inter-expert variability in the diagnosis of retinopathy of prematurity.

4.2 Related Work

The human eye is one of the most important organs of our body. Abnormalities can cause changes in the anatomy of the eye that are difficult and time consuming to detect. For this reason, artificial intelligence and image processing have had a huge impact on the detection and treatment of eye diseases. We can find several books that delve into this topic [23, 24]. Some reviews are devoted to specific diseases, such as diabetic retinopathy [25–27], while the most recent ones study the application of deep learning to this topic [28–30]. The remainder of this section explores the related work on the topics of the three case studies that will be then described: retinal image quality assessment, arteriolar-to-venular index, and retinopathy of prematurity diagnosis.

4.2.1 Retinal Image Quality Assessment

The goal of image quality assessment is to provide quantitative metrics which can automatically predict perceived image quality. The simplest metrics are the mean squared error and the peak signal-to-noise ratio, which quantify global distortions and so they cannot reflect local spatial variations in the image. This problem has motivated a new philosophy with the structural similarity (Structural Similarity Index) index [31], a well-known metric in the current state-of-art. It presents a change in the fundamental assumption from the intensity error based image quality assessment by suggesting that the structural information is the key component of visual quality. Some of its variants are multi-scale SSIM (MS-SSIM) [32], three-component weighted SSIM (3-SSIM) [33], and information weighted SSIM (IW-SSIM) [34].

Although image quality assessment has been a topic of intense research over the last decades and the development of general purpose algorithms is growing tremendously, its application to retinal imaging is still immature and some fundamental challenges remain unsolved. However, there is no doubt that it plays a crucial role to guarantee the appropriate behavior of the computer-aided systems developed for the prevention and diagnosis of diseases such as diabetes [35] or hypertension [36]. In this context, retinal image quality assessment has to be performed in such a way that it simulates clinicians' criteria. One of the first works on this topic was proposed by Lee et al. [37], who analyzed the correlation between histogram similarity and image quality, while some years later Fleming et al. [38] focused on the correlation between image blurring and blood vessels visibility.

Other works are based on the eye structures that should be observed in a retinal image of good quality [39]. In this sense, Giancarlo et al. [40] proposed to measure the quality of retinal images from the performance achieved by vessel segmentation algorithms, whilst Welikala et al. [41] suggested to use the segmented vessel maps in a similar way.

Different image properties were also used for retinal image quality assessment. For example, Davis et al. [42] used features such as color, luminance and contrast, Dias et al. [43] focused on the color and the contrast, and Remeseiro et al. [44] proposed an approach based on color and texture properties. For their part, Paulus et al. [45] combined global clustering with local sharpness and texture features. Statistical and structural measures have also proven useful in this context, as reported in [46]. More recently, Abdel-Hamid [47] proposed a non-reference quality index based on the sharpness and the wavelet decomposition of retinal images.

Other noteworthy works include the adaptation of structural indexes, such as the MS-SSIM, to the visual system [48]; and the proposal of explainable methods to detect low quality images [49].

4.2.2 Arteriolar-to-Venular Index and A/V Classification

The arteriolar-to-venular ratio (Arteriolar-to-Venular Ratio) has been shown to be associated with several risk factors such as cardiovascular or inflammatory biomarkers [50], and correlated with different diseases including stroke or atherosclerosis [22]. The Arteriolar-to-Venular Ratio represents the relationship between the calibers of both arteries and vein, measured within a standard ring area around the optical disc. Consequently, the automatic calculation of the Arteriolar-to-Venular Ratio requires an accurate classification of blood vessels into arteries and veins, also known as A/V classification, which has become a leading topic in retinal image analysis over the last years [51].

Arteries are brighter and thinner than veins, and the central reflex at the inner part is more obvious in arteries. This difference between arteries and veins has been used in many A/V classification approaches to assign A/V labels to vessel pixels. In this sense, Montoro et al. [52] analyzed the appearance of the retinal tree in different color spaces, including RGB and HSV, to extract relevant features such as the hue mean, the variance of the red contrast and the mean of the saturation contrast. Irshad et al. [53] presented an automatic method for A/V classification based on intensity and gradient features. Using only four color features, Relan et al. [54] proposed a squared-loss mutual information clustering to perform the retinal vessel classification. An early diagnostic tool for various diseases was presented by Xu et al. [55], using not only color features extracted from the CIE xyY color space, but also texture features based on both first- and seconder-order statistics. With the final target of detecting hypertensive retinopathy, Akbar et al. [56] proposed the used of a hybrid set of features that includes both color and statistical based texture features for A/V classification. Huang et al. [57] proposed a wide set of features and then applied a feature selection method based on genetic-search. In this manner, they obtained a subset of features that were fed to a linear discriminant analysis for the final A/V classification.

In addition to image properties, the structural information of both arteries and veins in the retinal tree has also been considered for A/V classification. For example, Mirsharif et al. [58] presented a structural method for blood vessel classification in which intersection and bifurcation points were processed, after computing features such as vessel widths or pixel intensities in different color spaces (RGB, HSL, and LAB). In the field of structural information, graph-based approaches are also commonly found in the literature. Graph search was used in [59] as part of an automatic method for retinal vessel identification, in which features such as orientation, width, and intensity of each vessel segment were used to find the optimal graph. A different approach for A/V classification was presented in [60], whose authors used the graph extracted from the retinal vasculature combined with a set of intensity features. Estrada et al. [61] proposed a graph-theoretic framework using the vessel tree topology along with domain-specific features. On the other hand, a more global framework was proposed by Hu et al. [62], who generated a vessel network composed of vessel segments and their potential connectivity, and made use of a graph-based meta-heuristic algorithm for the final A/V classification. In this context, although applied to ultra-wide-field-of-view retinal images, Pellegrini et al. [63] proposed a graph cut approach for A/V classification by using hand-crafted features, which include local vessel intensity and vascular morphology. More recently, Zhao et al. [64] adapted the concept of dominant set clustering to estimate the vascular network of the retinal blood vessels, and used intensity and morphology features to finally classify its pixels.

Deep learning techniques started to be applied to the A/V classification problem. Meyer et al. [65] proposed a novel approach based on convolutional neural networks (Convolutional Neural Networks) to classify the pixels belonging to the retinal vasculature tree into arteries and veins. Some popular datasets include vessels pixels manually labeled not only as artery or vein, but also as uncertain. This uncertainty is due to the difficulty found by the specialists to label some vessel pixels in retinal images, mainly because of the limitations of acquisition devices. In this context,

Galdran et al. [66] proposed a Convolutional Neural Networks trained to classify the pixels into one of four classes (background, artery, vein, and uncertain), thus providing an automatic segmentation of the vasculature tree.

Regarding the computation of the Arteriolar-to-Venular Ratio, Niemeijer et al. [67] presented an automatic method for Arteriolar-to-Venular Ratio estimation where arteries and veins were classified by means of an iterative algorithm that used centerline pixel features and crossing/bifurcation points of the vascular tree. In [68], an Arteriolar-to-Venular Ratio monitoring system was presented, which analyzed different images from the same patient using a registration approach to measure the vessel widths at the same points in all the images. Three automatic approaches for the estimation of the Arteriolar-to-Venular Ratio were compared in [69], defined as different methodologies for optic disc and vessel segmentation, vessel caliber estimation, and A/V classification. More recently, Mendonça et al. [70] proposed two new methods for Arteriolar-to-Venular Ratio estimation, both based on the retinal vasculature: one fully automatic and the other one that allows user interaction through the RetinaCAD system [60]. This method was further improved in [71], with an automatic method for A/V classification and Arteriolar-to-Venular Ratio estimation based on the local contrast between arteries and veins, combined with a graph propagation strategy.

Improving the illumination properties of retinal images for a more accurate A/V classification was also the focus of attention in several recent works. Mustafa et al. [72] proposed a new approach, based on low pass and Gaussian filters, to correct the illumination. Varnousfaderani et al. [73] presented a method for non-uniform illumination removal, by normalizing the luminance using the LUV color space; and for contrast enhancement, by histogram shifting. Huang et al. [74] presented a new normalization technique that allows to compute four new features related to the lightness reflection of vessels, adequate for A/V classification.

4.2.3 Retinopathy of Prematurity

Retinopathy of prematurity (Retinopathy of Prematurity) is a disease affecting low-birth weight infants, in which blood vessels in the retina of the eye develop abnormally and cause potential blindness. Retinopathy of Prematurity is diagnosed from dilated retinal examination by an ophthalmologist, and may be successfully treated by laser photocoagulation if detected appropriately [75]. Despite these advances, Retinopathy of Prematurity continues to be a major cause of childhood blindness throughout the world [76]. This is becoming increasingly significant in middle-income countries in Latin America, Eastern Europe and Asia because these countries are expanding neonatal care, yet have limited expertise in Retinopathy of Prematurity. In addition, the number of infants at risk for Retinopathy of Prematurity throughout the world is increasing dramatically because of improved survival rates for premature infants [77], while the availability of adequately-trained ophthalmologists to perform Retinopathy of Prematurity screening and treatment is decreasing [78].

An international classification system was developed during the 1980 s, and revised in 2005, to standardize clinical Retinopathy of Prematurity diagnosis [79]. One key parameter of this classification system is called "plus disease", and is characterized by tortuosity of the arteries and dilation of the veins in the posterior retina. Plus disease is a boolean parameter (present or absent), and is the most critical parameter for identifying severe Retinopathy of Prematurity. Numerous clinical studies have shown that infants with Retinopathy of Prematurity who have plus disease require treatment to prevent blindness, whereas those without plus disease may be monitored without treatment. Therefore, it is essential to diagnose plus disease accurately and consistently.

Ataer-Cansizoglu et al. [80], proposed a method to investigate whether there are groups of observers who decide consistently with each other and if there exist important features these experts mainly focus on. Their approach involved a hierarchical clustering of the experts using a pairwise similarity based on mutual information between the diagnostic decisions. They also performed an analysis to see the dependence between experts' decisions and image-based features, which enabled to qualitatively assess whether there are popular features for the group of observers obtained through clustering.

However, high levels of inconsistency among experts when diagnosing Retinopathy of Prematurity have been demonstrated [81, 82]. Inter-expert variability in clinical decision making is an important problem which has been widely studied in the literature for several decades [83]. Much of this previous work has examined inter-expert variability in the interpretation of ophthalmic images [81, 84]. There are also studies which focus on the variability in diagnosis of acute diseases such as prostate cancer [85], breast cancer [86], melanoma [87], papillary carcinoma [88], and polycystic ovary disease [89]. Although there is a broad range of studies on analysis of inter-expert variability, few of them focus on investigating its underlying causes [80, 90–92].

Understanding the causes of disagreement among experts is a challenging problem. In the cognitive process during clinical diagnosis, some features may be considered more important by certain experts than by others. If two experts consider different sets of features during diagnosis, then we might expect to see a strong disagreement between them. Hence, such a feature-observer analysis enables us to understand the underlying causes of inter-expert variability.

Determining expert agreement on relative Retinopathy of Prematurity disease severity has been studied in the last few years. Bolón-Canedo et al. [93] proposed a methodology to identify important features for experts and check whether the selected features reflect the pairwise agreements/disagreements. Kalpathy-Kramer et al. [94] demonstrated that although experts showed poor absolute agreement, they had relative agreement on disease severity, suggesting that the use of pairwise rankings and a continuous severity score could improve agreement. Ghergherehchi et al. [95] pointed out in their study that, apart from popular potential explanations for the disagreement (focus on narrower or wider field of view, unfamiliarity with digital images, magnification and apparent severity of the standard photograph, etc.), there are also differences in diagnostic consistency among groups of experts separated both geographically and chronologically. These findings have implications for clinical care, research, and education, and highlight the need for a more precise definition of plus disease and objective diagnostic methods for Retinopathy of Prematurity.

The irruption of deep learning techniques has led to performance comparable to those of expert physicians, but has brought the drawback that it is not possible to ensure that the same clinical factors are learned in the deep representations. Graziani et al. [96] investigated the relationship between the handcrafted and the deep learning features in the context of Retinopathy of Prematurity diagnosis, showing that the curvature, diameter and tortuosity of the segmented vessels are indeed relevant to the classification.

4.3 Case Study: Retinal Quality Assessment

Different image analysis techniques have demonstrated its adequacy in the ophthalmic field in order to diagnose several diseases, such as diabetes [12, 14] or hypertension [13, 15]. The performance of these techniques depends, among other factors, on the quality of the input images. For this reason, retinal quality assessment should be considered as a preliminary step that precedes the use of any computer-aided system focused on retinal imaging.

This case study presents a reliable method that addresses the objective quality assessment of retinal images by means of a binary classification task [44, 70]. It is based on the characterization of the retinal images by color and texture properties, and uses feature selection techniques to select the final feature vector. This vector is finally classified into one of the two target categories (good quality, poor quality) by means of different supervised learning algorithms. This four-step methodology provides satisfactory results thanks to its ability to identify relevant components (texture analysis), as well as color spots and illumination problems (color analysis).

4.3.1 Dataset

The experimentation was carried out on a dataset composed of 330 images with the following distribution [44]: 183 images of good quality and 147 of poor quality. The images were acquired and labeled by experts of the Portuguese Regional Administration of Health—North (ARSN). The dataset presents a high level of variability, including normal and pathological cases, two acquisition devices (Canon Inc, Carl Zeiss Meditec AG), and five spatial resolutions (1444×1444, 1728×2592,

4 Case Studies to Demonstrate Real-World Applications …

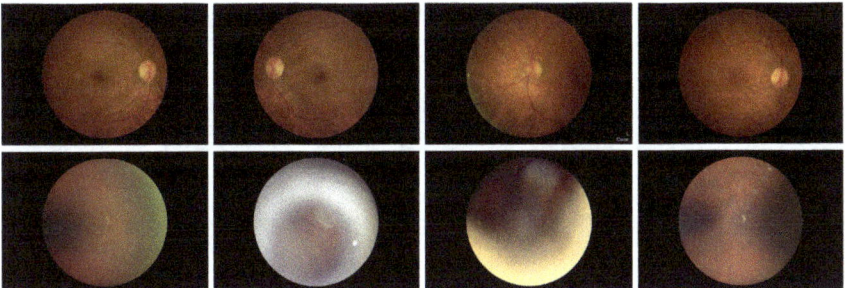

Fig. 4.2 Representative retinal images: (top) good quality images, and (bottom) poor quality images

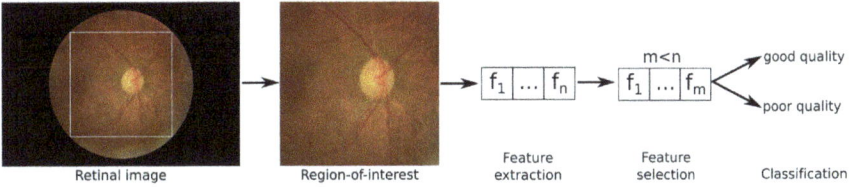

Fig. 4.3 Steps of the methodology for retinal image quality assessment

1958×2196 2056×2124, and 2304×3456). Figure 4.2 depicts some representative retinal images of the dataset, corresponding to the two categories considered (good quality, poor quality).

4.3.2 Methods

The objective assessment of retinal image quality consists of four main steps, as illustrated in Fig. 4.3. The first stage entails the extraction of the region of interest that will be subsequently processed. The second stage involves the analysis of the underlying color and texture properties, thus obtaining a feature vector per input image. In the third step, feature selection techniques are applied to select a representative subset of image features. Finally, in the last stage, input images are classified into of the two target categories: good quality, poor quality.

4.3.2.1 Region of Interest

Retinal images, as depicted in Fig. 4.4a, are in the RGB color space [97] and include a black background that does not contain relevant information for the classification. Experts who manually analyze these images focus their attention on the central part

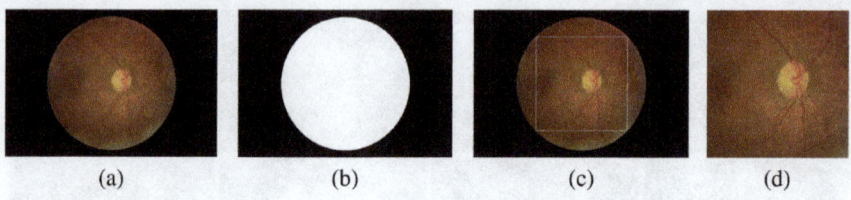

Fig. 4.4 Extraction of the region of interest: **a** input image, **b** circular mask, **c** square of maximum area inside the mask, and **d** ROI

that corresponds to the retina, including relevant landmarks such as the optic disc and the blood vessels.

Based on that, input images are firstly preprocessed to detect their region of interest (Region of Interest). For this purpose, the following steps are applied:

1. Obtain a circular mask to detect the retina, using the histogram of the red component of the RGB input images and a threshold computed from its mode (see Fig. 4.4b).
2. Locate the Region of Interest by calculating the square with the maximum area that fits within the circular mask previously obtained (see Fig. 4.4c, d).

4.3.2.2 Feature Extraction

This step consists in computing a set of discriminative features from the ROIs previously computed. Analyzing the retinal images depicted in Fig. 3.1, several differences can be highlighted between good quality and poor quality images: (1) good quality images have a similar appearance in terms of color, compared to the color differences observed in poor quality images, which may also present lighting anomalies and color spots; and (2) relevant eye landmarks (e.g., the optic disc, the blood vessels) can be observed in good quality images, while they are generally occluded or barely observable in poor quality images.

Based on this information, the features extracted from retinal images are based on color and texture properties. On the one hand, three color modalities are used to take into account the differences related to color and illumination conditions. The following options are considered for color analysis [44]:

- **Grayscale**. Region of Interest images are transformed from RGB to grayscale, obtaining a single component (G_r).
- **RGB** [97]. The three color components (R, G, B) of Region of Interest images are considered without any transformation.
- **CIELAB** [98]. Region of Interest images are transformed from RGB to CIELAB, obtaining three color components (L, a, b).

On the other hand, several texture descriptors are used to detect eye structures and other components useful for discrimination among the two classes. For this purpose, the different color components previously obtained are analyzed in terms of texture using the following descriptors [44]:

- **Butterworth filters** [99]. The feature vector is obtained by computing a uniform histogram [100] of 16 bins from the filtered image. Vector size: 16 features per color component.
- **Gabor filters** [101]. As in the previous case, a 16-bin uniform histogram is computed to define the feature vector. Vector size: 16 features per color component.
- **Discrete wavelet transform** [102]. The feature vector is defined by three statistic measures computed from the original image and the four sub-images obtained after wavelet decomposition, applied once or twice. Vector size: (one scale) 7 features per color component, and (two scales) 12 features per color component.
- **Gaussian Markov random fields** [103]. The feature vector is obtained by computing the directional variances [104] of the texture model parameters, generated with a Chebyshev distance d. Vector size: $4 \times d$ features per color component.
- **Co-occurrence features** [105]. The feature vector is defined by the mean and the range of 14 statistics computed from the gray level co-occurrence matrices, generated with a Chebyshev distance. Vector size: 28 features per color component.

4.3.2.3 Feature Selection

Feature selection is a machine learning technique employed to detect the most important features for a given classification task [106]. Thus, in this stage we apply different feature selection methods to select a set of relevant features from the ones previously obtained, thus removing those that are irrelevant and/or redundant. Among the different methods found in the literature, three popular techniques were employed: correlation-based feature selection [107], consistency-based filter [108], and INTERACT [109].

4.3.2.4 Classification

The last step consists in classifying the input image into one of the two categories considered: good quality or poor quality. In order to solve this binary classification task, five different machine learning algorithms were applied: naive Bayes [110], C4.5 [111], random forest [112], and support vector machine (Support Vector Machine) [113].

4.3.3 Results

This section reports the results achieved by applying the methodology previously described to the dataset acquired by the ARSN [44] (see Sect. 4.3.1), including a

Table 4.1 Butterworth filters: accuracy (%) of the four classifiers for each band of frequency (in increasing order)

Classifiers	Bank of nine filters								
	1	2	3	4	5	6	7	8	9
Naive Bayes	93.64	93.03	92.73	90.00	85.15	80.30	73.33	62.12	60.91
	93.64	93.03	91.52	89.70	86.97	80.61	73.03	63.03	61.21
	95.45	95.15	93.03	91.82	86.97	82.12	77.27	76.97	73.03
C4.5	92.73	95.15	93.33	90.30	82.12	76.67	72.42	72.73	77.58
	92.73	93.94	91.82	90.00	89.09	80.91	73.33	72.42	74.85
	94.85	94.85	93.64	92.73	86.06	82.12	80.61	81.21	79.39
Random forest	92.42	94.55	92.73	90.00	84.24	78.36	71.82	67.58	74.24
	93.33	94.24	95.45	92.73	89.39	84.24	77.58	72.12	77.88
	94.85	95.15	93.03	94.85	89.70	83.03	84.24	83.64	83.03
Support vector machine	96.06	96.36	96.06	95.15	91.52	82.42	76.67	80.91	78.48
	97.58	96.97	96.67	96.36	95.15	89.70	80.30	81.82	85.45
	96.06	96.67	96.06	95.45	93.33	88.18	87.27	89.39	89.39

From top to bottom, each cell includes the results for grayscale, RGB and CIELAB. Best result is in bold face

deep analysis of the different techniques and algorithms considered. In particular, the adequacy of the different methods for texture and color analysis were first analyzed, using the four classifiers considered (naive Bayes, C4.5, random forest, and Support Vector Machine).

Table 4.1 shows the results obtained by a bank of nine Butterworth filters, each one with a different bandpass to cover the whole frequency spectrum. As can be observed, the lowest frequency bands are more discriminative than the intermediate and highest ones, in the same way that the use of color information outperforms grayscale images. Moreover, the results are quite competitive for the first three bandpass filters, exceeding a 90% of accuracy regardless the color space and the classifier. The best result was achieved when applying the Support Vector Machine to the features obtained with the first band of frequency and the three RGB channels, with an accuracy of 97.58%.

Table 4.2 includes the results obtained by a bank of 16 Gabor filters, defined by the combination of four orientations and four spatial frequencies (filters from 1 to 4 correspond to the lowest frequency, whilst the highest one is represented by filters from 13 to 16). Analyzing the results, it can be seen how the two highest frequencies (filters from 9 to 16) outperform the two lowest ones, with a clear benefit of using color information compared to grayscale. Regarding the learning algorithms, the Support Vector Machine was again the most competitive classifier, achieving a maximum accuracy of 90.61% in several configurations.

Table 4.3 reports the results obtained by four different mother wavelets based on the well-known Haar and Daubechies [114]. As can be seen, both Haar and Daubechies provide similar performance. Regarding the number of scales, the addi-

Table 4.2 Gabor filters: accuracy (%) of the four classifiers for each pair orientation-frequency (in increasing order)

Classifiers	Bank of 16 filters															
	1	2	3	4	5	6	7	8	9	10	11	12	13	14	15	16
Naive Bayes	68.48	68.79	69.39	68.79	70.91	71.52	71.82	71.21	72.12	72.73	73.03	73.03	72.12	71.82	74.24	71.82
	73.03	73.33	73.03	73.03	75.15	75.76	75.76	76.36	74.55	75.15	74.85	75.76	76.36	76.97	76.67	75.15
	75.45	75.45	76.06	75.15	74.85	75.45	74.85	75.15	76.06	75.15	76.36	75.45	76.06	77.88	78.18	76.67
C4.5	73.94	69.70	69.70	71.82	72.12	73.94	71.82	71.82	74.55	76.36	79.09	76.06	77.88	77.58	79.39	74.55
	76.67	75.76	75.15	79.09	72.42	75.45	73.64	75.45	78.79	77.88	82.73	74.55	74.85	79.09	76.36	80.00
	76.67	78.48	76.06	78.18	69.70	76.67	73.64	76.97	76.67	80.61	78.48	77.58	85.15	81.52	80.30	83.94
Random forest	75.76	75.45	76.06	80.91	76.36	75.15	76.67	74.24	80.30	80.00	77.88	81.21	82.42	79.70	85.45	79.70
	82.12	81.82	81.82	81.52	76.36	81.82	81.52	81.21	83.33	81.21	82.12	80.91	80.61	83.64	84.55	84.55
	82.12	80.61	82.73	81.52	77.27	79.70	79.70	78.79	80.61	79.70	79.09	81.52	85.15	86.06	84.85	85.45
Support vector machine	79.09	79.39	80.00	79.39	79.70	79.70	79.39	79.39	84.24	85.76	85.45	84.55	84.24	86.67	84.85	86.06
	85.45	87.58	86.06	86.36	86.67	86.06	86.36	85.45	86.36	87.58	87.88	87.58	88.48	90.61	90.61	90.00
	87.27	86.67	86.97	86.67	88.79	88.18	88.48	88.48	**90.61**	89.09	89.39	89.70	**90.61**	89.09	89.70	89.39

From top to bottom, each cell includes the results for grayscale, RGB and CIELAB. Best result is in bold face

Table 4.3 Discrete wavelet transform: accuracy (%) of the four classifiers for each mother wavelet, using one and two scales

Classifiers	Four mother wavelets with two scales							
	Haar		Daub4		Daub6		Daub8	
	1	2	1	2	1	2	1	2
Naive Bayes	74.85	75.15	73.94	73.94	74.55	73.03	74.85	72.12
	78.48	76.06	80.00	75.45	80.00	77.27	79.70	76.36
	83.03	72.73	83.33	73.33	84.55	75.45	84.24	74.55
C4.5	73.64	83.94	72.12	83.03	70.91	76.36	70.61	80.61
	81.21	89.39	84.24	83.94	86.06	81.82	82.42	83.94
	84.24	86.67	85.76	83.03	84.85	81.52	85.45	84.85
Random forest	79.39	88.18	79.09	83.64	78.48	80.61	82.12	81.21
	88.48	93.33	87.58	88.18	87.27	86.97	86.67	87.58
	87.58	90.00	87.88	85.15	87.58	84.55	86.67	85.76
Support vector machine	82.42	93.33	82.12	84.55	80.00	84.24	83.64	79.09
	91.21	**95.45**	91.21	90.00	90.91	90.61	90.30	90.30
	89.39	93.94	88.48	90.00	89.09	90.61	89.09	88.48

From top to bottom, each cell includes the results for grayscale, RGB and CIELAB. Best result is in bold face

tional features obtained with two iterations seems to be useful for the problem at hand. The best result obtained in this case is 95.45% of accuracy with the Support Vector Machine, and corresponds to the Haar mother wavelet with two scales applied to RGB images.

Table 4.4 shows the results obtained by Gaussian Markov fields, using seven Chebhyshev distances to define the concept of neighborhood. As can be observed, the intermediate distances are the most discriminative for the classification task. Once again, the use of color information seems to be adequate for the characterization of the quality image properties. The highest accuracy (98.48%) is here obtained by the Support Vector Machine classifier when using the fifth distance applied to the three components of the CIELAB color space.

Table 4.5 includes the results obtained by co-occurrences features, also using seven Chebhyshev distances to define the concept of neighborhood. Unlike the previous method, the highest distance is the more adequate in this case. However, the same conclusion can be extracted regarding the competitiveness of the two color spaces compared to the grayscale images. It is worth mentioning that the co-occurrence features combined with the CIELAB color space and the Support Vector Machine classifier outperform any other configuration previously analyzed, with an accuracy of 99.09%.

After analyzing the different methods for color and texture analysis, the two best configurations were considered for further experimentation: Gaussian Markov random fields (distance $d = 5$) and co-occurrence features (distance $d = 7$), both combined with the CIELAB color space and the Support Vector Machine. Table 4.6

4 Case Studies to Demonstrate Real-World Applications ...

Table 4.4 Gaussian Markov random fields: accuracy (%) of the four classifiers for each distance

Classifiers	Neighborhoods defined by seven distances						
	1	2	3	4	5	6	7
Naive Bayes	67.88	67.27	67.27	67.58	67.58	67.58	67.27
	70.30	70.30	70.00	70.00	69.70	69.70	69.70
	84.55	81.52	87.58	83.03	86.36	83.33	84.85
C4.5	67.58	71.52	86.36	86.06	84.85	84.24	83.64
	83.33	87.58	91.21	89.09	88.48	87.88	89.70
	87.88	88.48	91.21	92.73	94.24	94.24	93.64
Random forest	76.36	75.45	87.58	86.97	86.36	86.67	84.55
	87.27	87.88	88.79	91.82	89.39	90.30	87.88
	90.00	88.79	90.91	93.03	95.76	94.55	94.24
Support vector machine	77.88	83.94	95.76	96.67	96.97	97.27	94.85
	87.88	92.73	97.27	98.18	97.58	97.58	96.36
	94.55	97.58	98.18	98.18	**98.48**	98.18	97.88

From top to bottom, each cell includes the results for grayscale, RGB and CIELAB. Best result is in bold face

Table 4.5 Co-occurrence features using the 14 statistics: accuracy (%) of the four classifiers for each distance

Classifiers	Neighborhoods defined by seven distances						
	1	2	3	4	5	6	7
Naive Bayes	76.67	81.21	91.52	93.94	93.33	91.21	91.52
	78.18	79.39	86.36	89.09	91.52	90.61	91.52
	80.61	84.55	90.00	93.33	95.15	96.06	96.97
C4.5	81.52	90.00	92.12	94.55	92.12	92.73	92.42
	86.67	93.64	92.73	94.85	94.85	93.33	94.24
	90.00	90.91	93.03	93.33	93.03	95.15	93.33
Random forest	88.48	92.12	93.94	94.24	95.15	95.15	94.55
	92.73	93.03	94.55	94.55	95.76	95.15	95.76
	92.73	94.24	96.36	95.45	96.36	97.58	97.27
Support Vector Machine	93.73	96.36	96.36	97.27	97.27	96.97	96.97
	94.55	96.36	96.67	97.58	97.58	97.88	96.97
	96.06	96.67	97.58	98.18	98.48	98.48	**99.09**

From top to bottom, each cell includes the results for grayscale, RGB and CIELAB. Best result is in bold face

Table 4.6 Feature selection: support vector machine accuracy (%) and number of features (in brackets) for the most competitive texture extraction methods using the CIELAB color space

Texture features	Filter methods			
	No feature selection	Correlation-based feature selection	Cons	INT
Gaussian Markov random fields (Distance 5)	94.48 (60)	97.88 (8)	96.67 (9)	96.97 (10)
Co-occurrence features (Distance 7)	99.09 (84)	**99.09** (**17**)	96.67 (5)	98.48 (14)

No feature selection means that no feature selection was performed, whilst the other columns are the filters applied: correlation-based feature selection (Correlation-based feature selection), consistency-based filter (Cons), and INTERACT (INT). Best result is in bold face

shows the figures obtained when applying different feature selection methods to the feature vectors computed with each method. As can be seen, the three feature selection techniques select a subset of features considerable smaller than the original one, with a slight degradation in terms of performance in the majority of configurations. Among all the results, it is noteworthy the one achieved by the co-occurrence features method (distance $d = 7$) combined with the Correlation-based Feature Selection method. Note that this combination is able to reach the maximum accuracy (99.09%) despite its aggressive reduction in the number of features, from 84 to only 17.

4.4 Case Study: Arteriolar-to-Venular Index

Several systemic diseases affect the structure of the retinal vascular network, causing different changes in the retinal blood vessels (e.g., diameter alterations, elongation, etc.). In this context, the arteriolar-to-venular ratio (Arteriolar-to-Venular Ratio) plays an important role since it has been shown to be associated with several risk factors such as cardiovascular or inflammatory biomarkers [50], and correlated with different diseases including stroke or atherosclerosis [22]. The Arteriolar-to-Venular Ratio represents the relationship between the calibers of both arteries and veins, measured within a standard ring area around the optical disc. Consequently, the automatic calculation of the Arteriolar-to-Venular Ratio requires an accurate classification of blood vessels into arteries and veins, also known as A/V classification, which has become a leading topic in retinal image analysis over the last years [51].

This case study presents an automatic, unsupervised method for A/V classification and Arteriolar-to-Venular Ratio estimation [71]. It uses the local contrast as a simple, yet powerful image feature to distinguish between arteries and veins, along with multilevel thresholding and graph propagation. Notice that the graph propagation procedure combines the labels obtained by applying multilevel thresholding to the local contrast feature with the graph structure. The combination of both steps implies a competitive advantage, due to the reduction in the number of cases in which errors in only one of the two steps imply an increase in terms of the misclassification rate.

4.4.1 Datasets

The experiments performed in this case study used two different public datasets. The INSPIRE dataset [115] is composed of 40 eye fundus images with a spatial resolution of 2392 × 2048 pixels, which are optic disc-centered. It includes two Arteriolar-to-Venular Ratio measures for each image computed by two ophthalmologists using a semi-automated computer program developed at the University of Wisconsin. Additionally, a manual classification of the arteriolar-to-venular tree has been considered as the ground truth for the A/V classification. It was obtained by labeling each vessel pixel with one of the following labels: artery, vein, and uncertain.

The DRIVE dataset [7] is composed of 40 retinal images, which are fovea-centered and were captured with a resolution of 565 × 584 pixels. It includes manual segmented images for validation purposes and, based on them, the RITE dataset was created in [116] to provide an A/V reference standard, which has been considered in this research. Note that this standard was generated by labeling each vessel pixel with one of the following options: artery, vein, overlap, and uncertain.

4.4.2 Methods

The automatic classification of retinal blood vessels requires the detection of several landmarks, allowing the A/V classification and the final computation of the Arteriolar-to-Venular Ratio. Figure 4.5 illustrates the whole procedure, where the main steps are highlighted with a blue background. First, a retinal image is segmented to obtain the optic disc and the blood vessels. Next, the feature extraction step is carried out to calculate the local contrast of vessel pixels and, in parallel, the vasculature graph is computed. Using both of them, a multilevel thresholding is applied to obtain two A/V classified images: a robust initial classification that includes the uncertain label, and a total classification used for achieving a full coverage rate. Next, the artery/vein labels of the initial classification are propagated to those segments classified as uncertain, using the graph structure. Finally, the region of interest is defined and the Arteriolar-to-Venular Ratio is estimated.

4.4.2.1 Optic Disc Segmentation

The optic disc (Optic Disc) is the entry point for the major retinal blood vessels. Its segmentation is an important step in the automatic calculation of the Arteriolar-

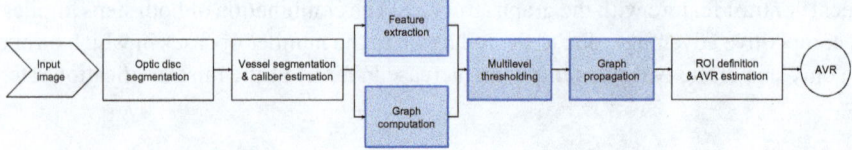

Fig. 4.5 Steps of the methodology for A/V classification and AVR estimation

to-Venular Ratio index, as the measuring region is centered in the Optic Disc and depends on the Optic Disc diameter. Optic Disc segmentation is carried out following the method proposed in [117], a robust algorithm based on multi-resolution sliding band filters.

4.4.2.2 Vessel Segmentation and Caliber Estimation

Since the Arteriolar-to-Venular Ratio index is calculated from the vessel calibers, another important step is to segment the retinal blood vessels and estimate their calibers. For the vessel segmentation, the method originally presented in [118] is considered, including the further improvements proposed in [119], which add an increased adaptation to image size and field-of-view and a decreased sensitivity to parameter settings. To estimate the vessel calibers, the Euclidean distance is calculated from the central pixel of the segmented vessels and its closest background pixel.

4.4.2.3 Feature Extraction

On color retinal images, arteries are often brighter than veins since their blood contains, respectively, oxygenated and deoxygenated hemoglobin. However, the background of retinal images is not homogeneous and it affects the visual appearance of vessel pixels. For this reason, this approach uses a simple and single feature for artery-vein discrimination: the local contrast. Note that this feature represents the local variation measured as the difference between vessel pixel intensities and the background tissue intensities that surrounds them in a local neighborhood.

Due to the discrimination power of the red channel to distinguish arteries from veins [120], it was extracted from the RGB input image and subsequently normalized [121]. For each vessel pixel (i, j), the local contrast C is calculated as:

$$C[i, j] = |I[i, j] - B[i, j]|, \qquad (4.1)$$

where I is the normalized red channel of the original image [120], and B is the average of the background pixels in a neighborhood determined by a $(2k + 1)$ square window centered at (i, j) calculated as:

$$B[i, j] = \frac{1}{N_{i,j}} \sum_{u=-k}^{k} \sum_{v=-k}^{k} I[i+u, j+v]M[i+u, j+v], \qquad (4.2)$$

where $N_{i,j}$ is the number of background pixels in the neighborhood:

$$N_{i,j} = \sum_{u=-k}^{k} \sum_{v=-k}^{k} M[i+u, j+v], \qquad (4.3)$$

and M is the mask corresponding to the vessel segmented images:

$$M[i', j'] = \begin{cases} 0 & \text{if } (i', j') \text{ is a vessel pixel} \\ 1 & \text{if } (i', j') \text{ is a background pixel.} \end{cases} \qquad (4.4)$$

4.4.2.4 Graph Computation

The graph extracted from the segmented retinal vasculature proved to be adequate for A/V classification [60, 61]. The original procedure is summarized as follows [60]:

1. **Graph extraction.** The vessel center-lines are firstly obtained from the segmented image to finally generate a vascular network composed of nodes and links. Nodes represent the intersection points in the vascular tree, whilst links represent vessel segments between intersection points.
2. **Graph modification.** The graph is modified to avoid the following common errors: node splitting, missing link, and false link. Next, all vessels around the optic disc are removed since, in this area, the vessels are not relevant for the Arteriolar-to-Venular Ratio estimation and the graph may not be reliable.
3. **Node type decision.** The nodes are classified into different categories: connecting point, meeting point, bifurcation point, and crossing point. For this purpose, the degree of a node (i.e., the number of adjacent nodes) and other characteristics (e.g., the angle between the connected links) are used. The possible node types for each degree are summarized as follows: a) nodes of degree 2 are a connecting point or a meeting point; b) nodes of degree 3 are a meeting point or a bifurcation point; c) nodes of degree 4 are a meeting point, a bifurcation point, or a crossing point; and d) nodes of degree 5 are a crossing point.

The graph originally obtained may include some errors regarding the node types. Aiming at avoiding them and reducing the number of unknown points, the following improvements are applied:

- **Nodes of degree 2 and 3**. The concept of almost parallel vessels is introduced with a condition to check if the angle between links is $\leq 15°$. If this condition is met, the node is classified as a meeting point in order to distinguish between the artery link and the vein link.

- **Nodes of degree 2.** The concept of link convergence is introduced with a condition to the check if the angle between links is ≤ 90° and is oriented to the optic disc. If this condition is met, the node is classified as meeting point in order to distinguish between the artery link and the vein link.

4.4.2.5 Multilevel Thresholding

After computing the local contrast and the graph, the average contrast of each graph link (segment) is computed as:

$$C_s = \frac{1}{N} \sum_{(i,j) \in s} C[i,j] \qquad (4.5)$$

where N is the number of pixels (i, j) that belongs to the segment s, and $C[i, j]$ refers to the local contrast (Eq. 4.1).

Given that the local contrast on the veins is higher than the local contrast on the arteries, this feature is used to classify the graph segments into arteries and veins. The idea is to consider the local contrast of the graph segments, and compute the histogram of each contrast level. Then, a multilevel thresholding based the Otsu's algorithm [122] is applied to search the two thresholds (th_1 and th_2) that minimize the intra-class contrast variance. Based on them, a partial classification with three target classes is computed for each segment s:

$$PC = \begin{cases} \text{artery} & \text{if } C_s \leq th_1 \\ \text{vein} & \text{if } C_s \geq th_2 \\ \text{uncertain} & \text{otherwise.} \end{cases} \qquad (4.6)$$

In parallel, an average threshold is computed as $th_\mu = \frac{th_1 + th_2}{2}$, to avoid any unclassified segment and guarantee a full coverage rate at some point in the process. In this case, a total classification is computed for each segment s:

$$TC = \begin{cases} \text{artery} & \text{if } C_s \leq th_\mu \\ \text{vein} & \text{otherwise.} \end{cases} \qquad (4.7)$$

As stated before, the background brightness varies along the retinal image due to light reflection changes from the spherical-shaped eye surface. This affects the local brightness and contrast of the vessel pixels, and can be easily confirmed by inspecting the image mean intensity on the four quadrants centered at the Optic Disc, or by observing the decreasing intensity when moving away from the Optic Disc. For these reasons, the multilevel thresholding is applied to the segments located at different regions of interest. In particular, we consider two different regions of interest (see Fig. 4.6): four quadrants Q centered at the Optic Disc, and three bands B with different distances to the Optic Disc. Combining these two regions of interest with the two approaches for segment classification, four A/V classified images were obtained:

Fig. 4.6 Regions of interest: **a** four quadrants centered at the optic disc, and **b** three bands with different distances to the optic disc

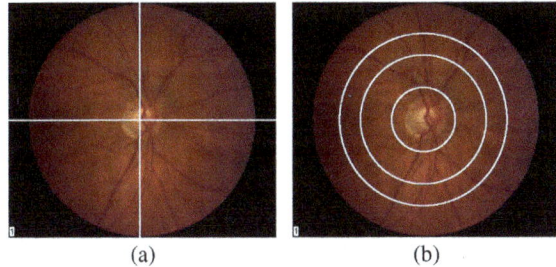

(a) (b)

Partial Classification for Quadrants and Partial Classification for Bands as partial classifications for quadrants and bands, respectively; and, equivalently, Total Classification for Quadrants and Partial Classification for Bands as total classifications.

With the main aim of benefiting from both approaches, and given the heterogeneity of images and datasets, the four A/V classified images are combined as detailed in Algorithm 1. In this manner, two final classifications are obtained: a partial classification (Partial classification) that includes three categories (artery, vein, and uncertain), and a total classification (Partial Classification for Bands) that only includes the two main categories (artery and vein). The first one can be defined as an initial, robust A/V classification that is further completed by means of graph propagation. Given that in the graph propagation step not all the uncertain segments of the Partial classification can be finally classified, Partial Classification for Bands is here defined to be used in case of uncertainty, thus allowing to achieve a fully coverage rate in A/V classification. Note that in this case, and according to some preliminary experiments, the Total Classification for Quadrants is used in case of disagreements between both total classifications (Total Classification for Quadrants and Partial Classification for Bands).

4.4.2.6 Graph Propagation

A graph propagation algorithm is used to obtain the final A/V classification. It consists in combining the information obtained in the previous steps: the node types of the graph (graph computation step), and the classified segments (multilevel thresholding step).

Given an initial classification for the graph segments, the algorithm for graph propagation is detailed as follows:

1. For each *uncertain* segment, get the classes of its two nodes using the following rules defined for the different node types:

    - *Connecting point*: There is only one connected link, so the class of the node is the class of the connected link.
    - *Bifurcation point*: There are two connected links, so the class of the node depends on their classes: (1) if one link is labeled as *uncertain*, then the class

Algorithm 1: Combination of the four A/V classified images.

Data: graph G, A/V classified images for quadrants Q and bands B: partial classifications Partial Classification for Quadrants and Partial Classification for Bands, and total classifications Total Classification for Quadrants and Partial Classification for Bands

Result: final A/V classified images: partial classification Partial classification, total classification Partial Classification for Bands

1 initialize partial classification $PCF := 0$
2 **for** *each segment $s \in G$* **do**
3   **if** $PCQ_s = PCB_s$ **then**
4          $PCF_s := PCQ_s$
5   **else if** $PCQ_s = uncertain$ **then**
6          $PCF_s := PCB_s$
7   **else if** $PCB_s = uncertain$ **then**
8          $PCF_s := PCQ_s$
    else
9          $PCF_s := uncertain$
    end
end
10 initialize total classification $TCF := PCF$
11 **for** *each segment $s \in G$* **do**
12   **if** $TCF_s = uncertain$ **then**
13         $TCF_s := TCQ_s$
end

of the node is the class of the other link; (2) if both links are labeled equally, then the class of the node is their class; (3) otherwise, the class of the node is *uncertain*.
- *Meeting point with two adjacent links*: There is only one connected link, so the class of the node is the opposite of the connected link.
- *Meeting point with three adjacent links*: The meeting link is determined using angles and distances between the adjacent links. Next, the rules for connecting and meeting points with two adjacent links are applied, as appropriate.
- *Crossing point*: The connecting link is determined using angles and distances between the adjacent links. Next, the rules for connecting and bifurcation points are applied, as appropriate.

2. For each *uncertain* segment, if both node classes are the same, then apply the propagation by labeling the segment with the corresponding class.
3. Repeat 1 and 2 until no more graph segments are re-labeled as artery or vein.

Finally, the partial and total classifications previously obtained are used to apply the graph propagation algorithm as detailed in the following:

1. Use the partial classification (Partial classification) to initially label all the segments as artery, vein or uncertain.
2. Apply the algorithm for graph propagation.

3. Use the total classification (Partial Classification for Bands) to label the fully *uncertain* segments (i.e., those segments with the two nodes labeled as *uncertain*).
4. Apply the algorithm for graph propagation.
5. Apply the algorithm for graph propagation but also spreading to the partially *uncertain* segments (i.e., those segments with one of the two nodes labeled as *uncertain*), using the label of the *known* node.
6. Use the total classification (TFC) to label all the remaining *uncertain* segments.

4.4.2.7 Region of Interest Definition and AVR Estimation

Arteriolar-to-Venular Ratio is computed from the vessel calibers inside a standard region of interest (Region of Interest), a ring-shaped area within 0.5 to 1.0 Optic Disc diameter from the Optic Disc boundaries [123]. The Arteriolar-to-Venular Ratio index is defined as the quotient between two values, which are calculated using the Knudtson's revised formula [123]: the central retinal artery equivalent (Central Retinal Artery Equivalent) and the central retinal vein equivalent (Central Retinal Vein Equivalent). For Arteriolar-to-Venular Ratio measurement, an approach similar to the one proposed by Niemeijer et al. [67] is applied: (1) six regions are considered to obtain distinct Arteriolar-to-Venular Ratio regional values, based on the six largest arteries and veins of each region; and (2) the Arteriolar-to-Venular Ratio index for the whole image is computed as the average of the six regional values.

4.4.3 Results

This section reports the results obtained by applying the method presented in this case study to two different datasets, INSPIRE and DRIVE. Additionally, a comparison with other state-of-the-art approaches is analyzed in depth.

4.4.3.1 INSPIRE Dataset

The comparative analysis performed for this dataset includes the method presented here [71] and seven state-of-the-art approaches [57, 60, 61, 64, 67, 120, 124]. The performance metrics used in the evaluation process are [71]: accuracy, both centerline accuracy (Centerline Accuracy) and pixel-wise accuracy (Pixel-wise Accuracy); sensitivity (Sens.), with veins as positive samples; specificity (Spec.), with arteries as negative samples; and vessel caliber (vc), which makes reference to the caliber of the vessel pixels considered in the evaluation ($vc > 0$ means all vessel pixels).

Table 4.7 shows the results achieved with the different methods considered, some of them supervised and others unsupervised. Analyzing the individual results in terms of the different vessel calibers, it can be observed that, in general, the pixel-wise accuracy (Pixel-wise Accuracy) is greater than the centerline accuracy (Centerline

Accuracy). This fact shows that the three automatic methods that provide the accuracy rates in this manner tend to classify correctly the largest vessels. Therefore, there is an increase in the accuracy rates when all the vessel pixels are considered instead of just those on the centerline. Two of these methods [60, 120] are quite similar in terms of image features, with the main difference in terms of the learning process: the first one is an unsupervised method, whilst the second one is supervised. If they are compared, it can be observed that the supervised method slightly outperforms the unsupervised one for all vessel calibers, except the largest one ($vc > 20$ pixels). However, the unsupervised approach has the main benefit of be independent of a previous image labeling since no training phase is needed. Including the method proposed by Remeseiro et al. [71] in the comparative, we can see that it outperforms the unsupervised approach in most cases ($vc > 5, 10, 15$ and 20 pixels). Besides, it also outperforms the supervised approach when considering the three largest vessel calibers and provides accuracy rates over 96% in the best case. Note that these results are particularly relevant because a key requirement for Arteriolar-to-Venular Ratio calculation is the correct classification of the main (largest) vessels. Furthermore, this method has the same advantage of the unsupervised one: it does not require any training, which means stability and independence of the image dataset. With respect to the other methods, they do not provide results in terms of vessel calibers, limiting the comparative analysis. Huang et al. [57] provides the highest accuracy rate in terms of Centerline Accuracy, but at the expense of 100 features and a supervised classifier, thus limiting the generalization to new datasets. In terms of sensitivity and specificity, the most competitive results were achieved with the method proposed by Zhao et al. [64]. However, the authors do not analyze how their algorithm behaves with the largest vessels, since they do not estimate the Arteriolar-to-Venular Ratio index.

Figure 4.7 illustrates the qualitative results of two sample images from the INSPIRE dataset. The results of the A/V classification method presented in this chapter can be visually compared with the manual labeling (ground truth images). As can be observed, the partial classification provides a robust, preliminary categorization of the blood vessels into arteries (blue), veins (red), and uncertain (green). These initial labels are next spread trough the graph by means of the different propagation stages, in order to achieve the final classification into arteries and veins.

Table 4.8 summarizes some Arteriolar-to-Venular Ratio statistics for the complete INSPIRE dataset, including the two human observers and three different approaches [67, 69, 71]. As can be seen, the mean errors generated by comparing the automatic results to the reference ones are very similar, regardless the approach considered. In order to statistically analyze them, the Friedman test [125] was applied using two different error sets: the errors of the observer 2 and the three automatic methods compared to the observer 1, and the errors of the observer 1 and the three automatic methods compared to the observer 2. According to the results obtained, there are no significant differences among the three automatic approaches and the two observers, thus demonstrating the adequacy of the method presented in this case study.

Table 4.7 INSPIRE dataset: results of different approaches for A/V classification

Method	S/U	Num. feats.	Vessel caliber	Acc. CA	Acc. PA	Sens.	Spec.
Huang et al. [57]	S	100	vc > 0 px	0.92	–	0.90	0.91
Niemeijer et al. [67]	S	27	vc > 0 px	–	–	0.78	0.78
Dashtbozorg et al. [60]	S	30	vc > 0 px	0.85	0.88	0.91	0.86
			vc > 5 px	0.87	0.89	–	–
			vc > 10 px	0.90	0.91	–	–
			vc > 15 px	0.93	0.93	–	–
			vc > 20 px	0.93	0.93	–	–
Estrada et al. [61]	U	3	vc > 0 px	0.91	–	0.92	0.90
Zhao et al. [64]	U	23	vc > 0 px	–	–	0.96	0.97
Lyu et al. [124]	U	–	vc > 0 px	0.85	–	0.79	0.90
Dashtbozorg [120]	U	30	vc > 0 px	0.82	0.86	0.85	0.80
			vc > 5 px	0.83	0.86	–	–
			vc > 10 px	0.87	0.89	–	–
			vc > 15 px	0.90	0.91	–	–
			vc > 20 px	0.94	0.95	–	–
Remeseiro et al. [71]	U	1	vc > 0 px	0.79	0.84	0.91	0.79
			vc > 5 px	0.84	0.88	–	–
			vc > 10 px	0.91	0.92	–	–
			vc > 15 px	0.93	0.94	–	–
			vc > 20 px	0.96	0.96	–	–

S/U stands for supervised and unsupervised methods, respectively; and Num. feats. refers to the number of image features used for classification

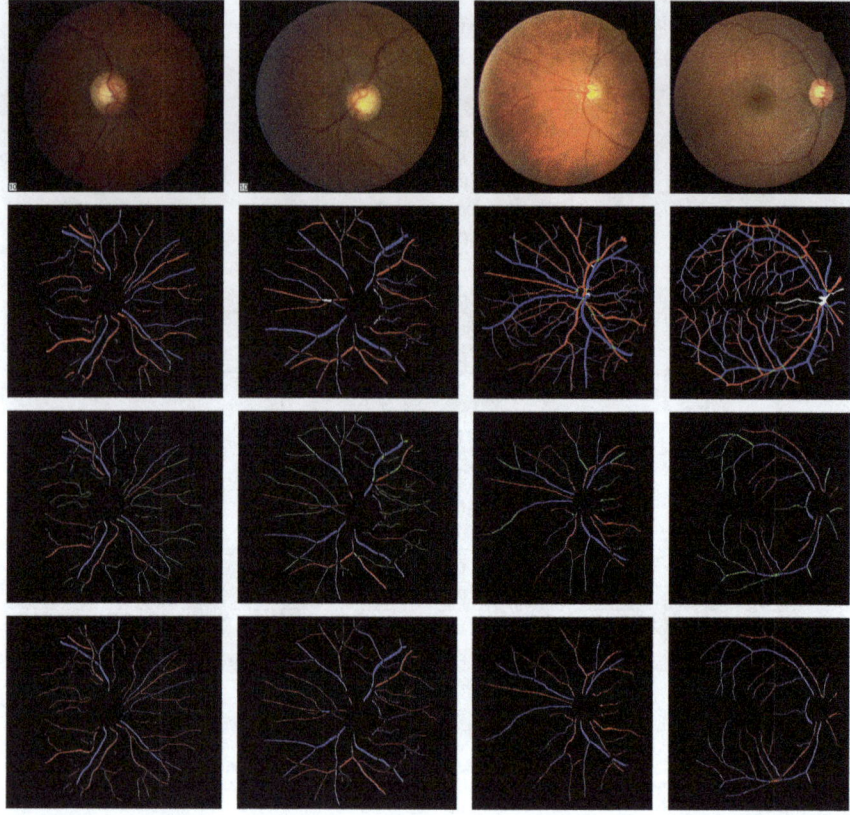

Fig. 4.7 From left to right: two INSPIRE images, and two DRIVE images. From top to bottom: original images, ground truth for A/V classification, partial classification (PCF), and final classification after graph propagation

4.4.3.2 DRIVE Dataset

As with the INSPIRE dataset, a comparative analysis with several A/V classification methods applied to the DRIVE dataset was carried out. In this case, the method presented here [71] was compared with eight state-of-the-art approaches [57, 60–62, 64, 67, 120, 124]. All the methods were evaluated using the following performance measures: centerline accuracy (Centerline Accuracy), pixel-wise accuracy (Pixel-wise Accuracy), sensitivity (Sens.), and specificity (Spec). Two additional metrics suggested by Hu et al. [62] were also considered: coverage rate (Coverage Rate), which represents the ratio of vessel pixels classified as *arteries* and *veins* over all the vessel pixels labeled in the ground truth, except the ones labeled as *uncertain*; and overall accuracy (Overall Accuracy), which represents the pixel-wise accuracy but also includes the *overlapping* pixels of the ground truth.

Table 4.8 INSPIRE dataset: arteriolar-to-venular ratios (AVR) and errors (E), considering two human observers

Method	Measure	Mean	St. deviation	Maximum	Minimum
Observer 1	AVR	0.67	0.08	0.93	0.52
Observer 2	AVR	0.66	0.08	0.85	0.45
	E	0.05	0.05	0.29	0.00
Niemeijer et al. [67]	AVR	0.67	0.07	0.81	0.55
	E1	0.06	0.04	0.15	0.01
	E2	0.06	0.06	0.28	0.00
Dashtbozorg et al. [69]	AVR	0.65	0.07	0.82	0.49
	E1	0.05	0.04	0.16	0.00
	E2	0.05	0.05	0.22	0.00
Remeseiro et al. [71]	AVR	0.64	0.08	0.91	0.53
	E1	0.06	0.07	0.28	0.00
	E2	0.06	0.05	0.23	0.00

Note that E1 and E2 refer to the errors with respect to the observers 1 and 2, respectively

Table 4.9 depicts the results obtained with the different methods considered. The results achieved with the method presented here [71] demonstrate its robustness, with competitive performance values and a 100% of coverage rate. In addition, these results are also comparable with the ones obtained for the INSPIRE dataset, demonstrating the adequacy of this method to the problem at hand, regardless of the dataset. In this sense, it is worth noting the poor performance of the approach proposed by Huang et al. [57], with an accuracy of 0.72 compared with the 0.92 achieved with INSPIRE. The rest of the methods present similar performances with a full coverage rate (100%), except the approach proposed by Hu et al. [62] that achieves a 0.86 of overall accuracy with a coverage rate of 83.55%.

Figure 4.7 depicts the qualitative results of two sample images from the DRIVE dataset. The ground truth images can be visually compared with the partial classifications, which include some uncertain segments (green), and the outcomes obtained after applying the propagation step that guarantees a full coverage rate.

4.5 Case Study: Retinopathy of Prematurity

As mentioned in Sect. 4.2.3, Retinopathy of Prematurity is a disease that affects low-birth weight infants, which can potentially cause blindness. It is usually diagnosed following an international classification system [79] that searches for the presence of "plus disease", defined as presenting tortuosity of the arteries and dilation of the veins in the posterior retina. One of the main problems in diagnosing this disease is the

Table 4.9 DRIVE dataset: results of different approaches for A/V classification

Method	S/U	Num. feats.	Coverage rate (%)	Acc. CA	Acc. PA	Acc. OA	Sens.	Spec.
Huang et al. [57]	S	100	100	0.72	–	–	0.71	0.74
Dashtbozorg et al. [60]	S	30	100	0.87	–	–	0.90	0.84
Hu et al. [62]	S	31	83.55	–	–	0.86	–	–
Niemeijer et al. [67]	S	27	–	–	–	–	0.80	0.80
Estrada et al. [61]	U	3	100	0.92	–	–	0.92	0.92
Zhao et al. [64]	U	23	100	–	–	–	0.93	0.94
Dashtbozorg [120]	U	30	100	–	–	–	0.87	0.84
Lyu et al. [124]	U	–	100	0.83	–	–	0.87	0.78
Remeseiro et al. [71]	U	1	100	0.79	0.82	0.82	0.88	0.79

S/U stands for supervised and unsupervised methods, respectively; and Num. feats. refers to the number of images features used for classification

high level of disagreement among experts [81, 82], so understanding the underlying causes of inter-expert variability is a key issue.

In this case study, we present a methodology for investigating the important features for the experts when diagnosing Retinopathy of Prematurity [93], using feature selection techniques. After selecting the useful features for each expert, a similarity analysis is carried out to see if the selected features can reflect the disagreement among experts. Finally, some classifiers are trained to check the accuracy of the prediction using the results of the feature selection process.

4.5.1 Datasets

The experiments were performed on a dataset of 34 images that had been previously rated by 22 experts [81, 126]. These experts, utilizing a secure website to review a set of retinal images, were asked to classify each of the 34 retinal posterior pole images as either "plus", "pre- plus", "neither", or "cannot determine". A total of 66 features have been extracted, some of which were curve-based and others of which were tree-based. For data analysis, "cannot determine" decisions were excluded since there were few observers who decided "cannot determine" for at least one sample.

Figure 4.8 shows the different diagnoses given by the different experts for each image. Note that there are some images in which all the 19 experts agreed (such as images 6, 10, 11, or 34) while there are other images in which the experts did not coincide in their diagnoses (such as images 5, 14, 16, or 25).

4 Case Studies to Demonstrate Real-World Applications ...

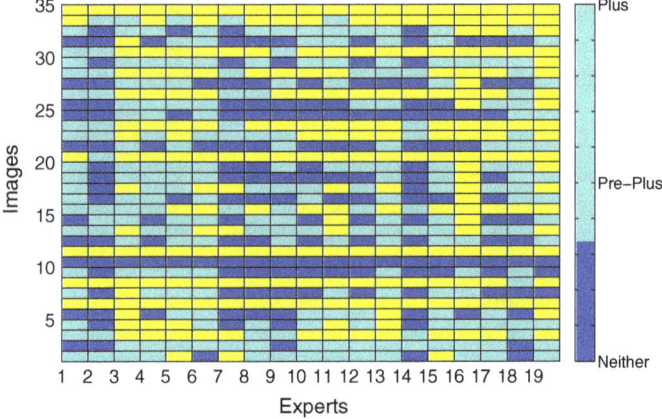

Fig. 4.8 Labels given by experts

4.5.2 Methods

A four-step methodology is applied to understand the causes of inter-expert variability in Retinopathy of Prematurity diagnosis, as illustrated in Fig. 4.9. First, the problem needs to be analyzed to check if disagreement among experts exists. Second, several feature selection methods are applied to discover which features are the most important to each individual expert. Third, a similarity analysis is performed to check if, for experts with a high ratio of agreement, the feature selection methods also select similar features. Finally, the classification performance is calculated in order to see whether the selected features are sufficient for a correct classification of the given samples.

1. **Assessment of experts' agreement**. Bearing in mind that the main objective of this case study is to evaluate the causes of disagreement among experts, it is necessary to use measures that are able to calculate the amount of disagreement. These measures can be divided into two main groups: pairs' tests and group tests. The former involve a comparison between two reference criteria (e.g., a pair of experts, or a human expert and a computer-aided diagnosis system). Pairs' tests include contingency tables, percentage agreement methods and the Kappa statistic. Group tests, on the other hand, offer an overall view of the set of experts by locating each expert in relation to the others. Examples of group tests include the Williams' index.

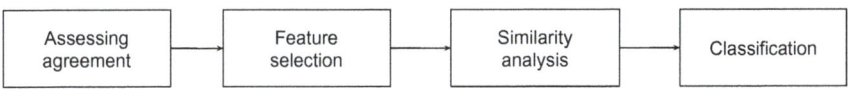

Fig. 4.9 Steps of the research methodology for ROP

2. **Feature selection**. The second step involves the use of feature selection methods trying to find out the important features for each expert. Feature selection is a well-known machine learning technique which aims to identify the relevant features for a problem and discarding the irrelevant ones, in some cases even achieving an improvement in the performance of automatic classifiers compared to classification systems using all features [106]. Among the broad suite of feature selection methods available in the literature, we employ correlation-based feature selection (Correlation-based Feature Selection) [107], consistency-based filter [108], INTERACT [109], Information Gain [127], ReliefF [128] and Recursive Feature Elimination for Support Vector Machines (Support Vector Machine—Recursive Feature Elimination) [129], since they are widely used and based on different metrics ensuring some variability in our comparative analysis. It has to be noted that three of these methods return a subset of optimal features (Correlation-based Feature Selection, INTERACT, and Consistency-based) whilst the remaining three return a ranking of all the features (Information Gain, ReliefF, and Support Vector Machine—Recursive Feature Elimination).
3. **Similarity analysis**. After determining the degree of variability among experts and the important features for each expert, it is interesting to study if, for those experts with a high degree of agreement among them, the selected features are also similar. Thus, similarity measures are used, which evaluate the sensitivity of the result given by a feature selection algorithm to variations in the training set (in this case, to variations in the class label). It is expected that, for those experts who show a reasonable amount of agreement in their labels, the features returned by the feature selection methods would be similar. Three different measures are employed: Jaccard index, Spearman correlation coefficient, and Kendall Index. While using these measures, we consider whether the feature selection method returns a subset of optimal features (Jaccard) or a ranking of features (Spearman).
4. **Classification**. The last step of the methodology is devoted to checking if the features selected as relevant for each expert are enough for building an automatic system able to classify new images in "plus", "pre-plus" or "neither". In addition to this, entrusting the task of distinguishing between class labels to an automatic classification system can be helpful to solve the problem of the high variability among experts, since this type of systems are objective and rely on the characteristics of the data. In this case, four popular classifiers are used: C4.5 [111], naive Bayes [110], k-nearest neighbors [130], and support vector machine (Support Vector Machine) [113].

4.5.3 Results

To assess the experts agreement, Fig. 4.10 shows the percentage of agreement and the Kappa statistic between each pair of experts. As can be seen, the Kappa statistic is more conservative than the percentage agreement. In any case, the maximum agreement between experts is reported between experts 12 and 17, and there are

4 Case Studies to Demonstrate Real-World Applications ...   113

four pairs of experts who show high level of agreement. In general, the experts who obtained the highest percentage agreement and Kappa statistic with other experts were 8, 10, 12, and 17. On the contrary, the experts who achieved the lowest ratios of agreement with the remaining experts were 2, 7, and 11.

Moving to the second step of the methodology, Fig. 4.11 shows the number of times that a feature was selected for the label given by each expert according to the selection obtained by Correlation-based Feature Selection, INTERACT, and consistency-based. As can be seen, there are some features that are mostly selected by these filters, which are the mean of the tortuosity index in veins, followed by the same feature in arteries, mean acceleration and CM2 of tortuosity index in veins, and maximum of MBLF in arteries.

In the case of ranker methods (Information Gain, ReliefF and Support Vector Machine—Recursive Feature Elimination), we calculated a combination of all the rankings for each method, using the SVM-Rank technique [131]. In Table 4.10 we can see the top 10 features ranked by Information Gain, ReliefF and Support Vector Machine—Recursive Feature Elimination, respectively (after combining the 19 rankings with SVM-rank). It is interesting to note that the feature that is ranked in the first position for the three ranker methods is, again, the mean of the tortuosity index in veins, confirming its crucial importance.

Next we checked if, for experts with a high ratio of agreement, the feature selection methods also selected similar features. For the subset filters (Correlation-based Feature Selection, Consistency-based and INTERACT) we calculated the Jaccard-index for each pair of experts and the subsets of features selected by these methods, as seen in Fig. 4.12. Notice that the higher the value, the higher the similarity. In general, the similarity between subsets is low, as it is expected because feature selection methods tend to be very sensible to variations in the data. It is interesting to note that, for the three subset methods, some of the experts with a low ratio of agreement (see Fig. 4.10) also obtained low similarities regarding their optimal subsets of features. For example, this happens with experts 2 and 11. On the other hand, the similarity between the features selected by experts 12 and 17 (who obtained high percentage agreement and Kappa statistic) and the remaining experts is quite high.

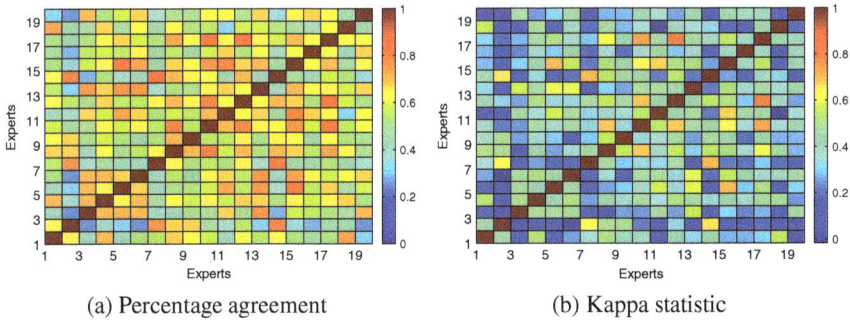

(a) Percentage agreement   (b) Kappa statistic

Fig. 4.10 Agreement among experts considering three classes: plus, pre-plus, neither

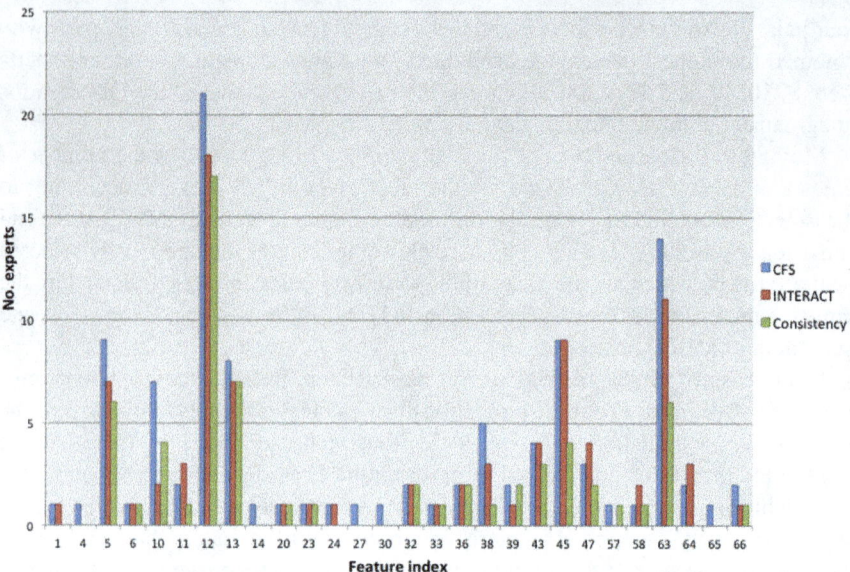

Fig. 4.11 Features selected by correlation-based feature selection, INTERACT and consistency-based feature selection methods

Table 4.10 Top 10 features ranked by information gain, ReliefF and support vector machine—recursive feature elimination

Index	description	Index	description	Index	description
12	Mean TI (v)	12	Mean TI (v)	12	Mean TI (v)
13	CM2 TI (v)	5	Mean Acc (v)	63	Max MBLF (a)
63	Max MBLF (a)	63	Max MBLF (a)	5	Mean Acc (v)
5	Mean Acc (v)	45	Mean TI (a)	23	2nd Min DCC (v)
21	CM3 diameter (v)	6	CM2 Acc (v)	25	Max DDC (v)
22	Min DDC (v)	13	CM2 TI (v)	24	2nd Max DDC (v)
27	CM2 DDC (v)	37	Max Acc (a)	29	Min MBLF (v)
20	CM2 diameter (v)	46	CM2 TI (a)	20	CM2 diameter (v)
19	Mean diameter (v)	10	2nd Max TI (v)	32	CM2 MBLF (v)
23	2nd Min DCC (v)	36	2nd Min Acc (v)	21	CM3 diameter (v)
(a) Information Gain		(b) ReliefF		(c) SVM-RFE	

It is indicated if features belong to a vein (v) or to an artery (a)

Figure 4.13 shows the Spearman correlation coefficient for each pair of experts for the rankings of features obtained by Information Gain, ReliefF and Support Vector Machine—Recursive Feature Elimination, where, again, the higher the value, the higher the similarity between rankings. It is easy to see that the rankings obtained by Information Gain are much more similar to the percentage agreement than those obtained by ReliefF and Support Vector Machine—Recursive Feature Elimination. This happens because Information Gain is a univariate method (each feature is considered independently) whereas ReliefF and Support Vector Machine—Recursive

4 Case Studies to Demonstrate Real-World Applications ...

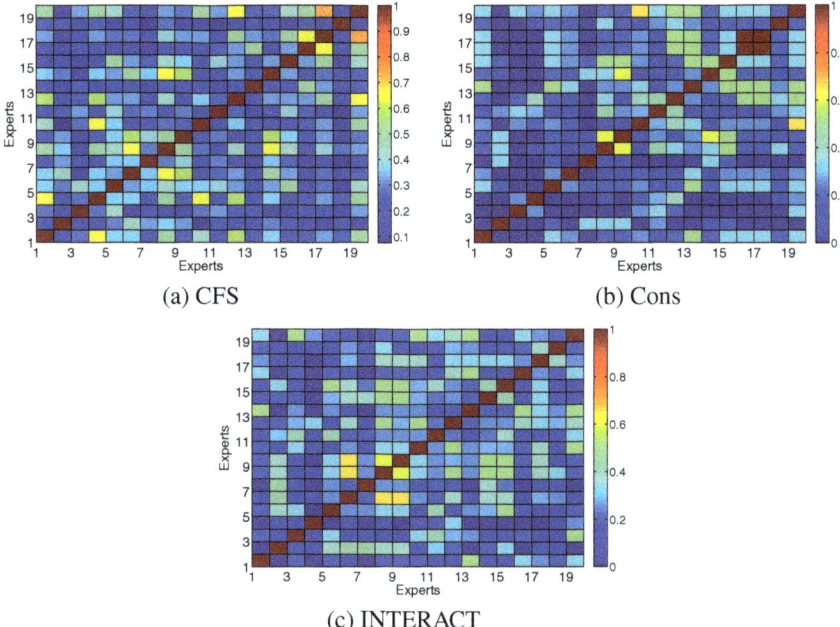

Fig. 4.12 Jaccard-index for subset filters

Feature Elimination are multivariate methods (they consider relationships between features). So, univariate filters such as Information Gain tend to obtain more stable rankings than multivariate methods. Focusing on the results achieved by the filter Information Gain, one can see that the rankings for the experts 2, 7 and 11 are very dissimilar compared with the rankings obtained by the remaining experts, since these experts had not achieved high rates of agreement with other experts. On the contrary, the similarities between the rankings achieved by experts 12 and 17 are again fairly high.

Finally, and in order to check if the features selected by the different methods are sufficient for a correct classification of the data, we performed some classification experiments. Since we have the data labeled by 19 different experts, we opted for determining the class label by majority vote. For the subset filters (Correlation-based Feature Selection, consistency-based and INTERACT) we have used the union of all the subsets of features selected for all the experts. For the ranker methods (Information Gain, ReliefF and Support Vector Machine—Recursive Feature Elimination) we used the ranking obtained by SVM-rank after combining the rankings for all the experts. Since for ranker methods we need to establish a threshold, we opted for classifying with top 50% of the ranked features.

In Table 4.11 we can see the average test classification results (using leave-one-out cross-validation) for all classifiers and feature selection methods. We also trained a classifier using all features (i.e., without feature selection (No Feature Selection))

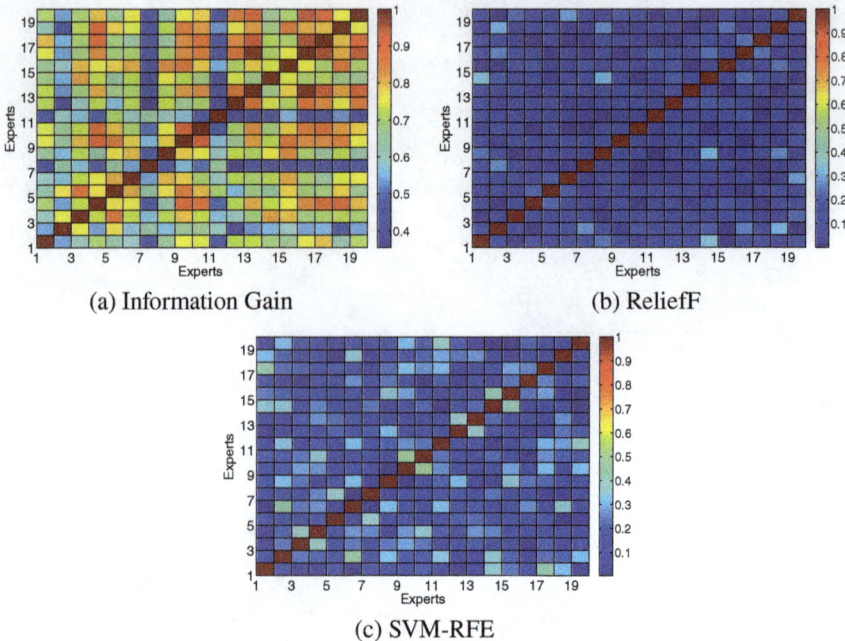

Fig. 4.13 Spearman correlation coefficient for rankings feature selection methods

Table 4.11 Average classification error (%) using leave-one-out cross-validation

Method	C4.5	Naive Bayes	k-NN	SVM
No feature selection	58.82	38.24	64.71	44.12
Correlation-based feature selection	52.94	35.29	44.11	38.24
Consistency-based filter	70.59	32.35	44.12	38.24
INTERACT	70.59	32.35	44.11	38.24
Information GAIN	41.18	41.18	50.00	35.29
ReliefF	70.59	35.29	58.82	41.18
Support vector machine—recursive feature elimination	52.94	**20.59**	47.06	32.35

Best result is in bold face

as displayed in the first row of the table. Notice that the best result was achieved using feature selection (Support Vector Machine—Recursive Feature Elimination + Naive Bayes) and that, for all classifiers, feature selection is able to improve the classification error, which demonstrates that this problem contains irrelevant features that can hinder the process of classification.

To assess the automatic system globally, group tests were applied to the results obtained from the complete analysis of the 19 experts plus the system (in this case, the best option was Support Vector Machine - Recursive Feature Elimination + Naive Bayes in Table 4.11). Figure 4.14 shows the Williams' indices obtained using both

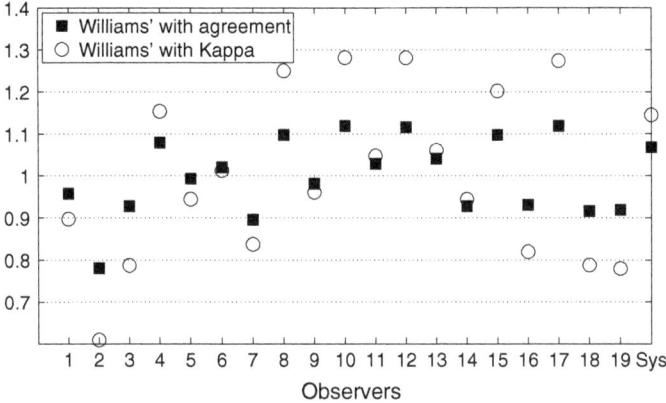

Fig. 4.14 Williams' index calculated utilizing percentage agreement and the Kappa statistic as agreement measurements

the percentage agreement and the Kappa value measures. From among the Williams' indices obtained, the highest indices correspond to expert 10, which means that this expert exhibits the highest agreement with the remaining experts. For the system, the indices obtained are greater than 1, from which it can be deduced that (a) the agreement between the system and the group of experts is greater than the agreement among experts, and (b) the influence of chance is practically null, as is to be expected from an automatic computer-based system. Therefore, results indicate that the system can be asserted to behave in a similar manner to the experienced experts.

4.6 Summary

This chapter presents three real world applications in ophthalmic image analysis, an area in which retinographies are one of the most widely used imaging modalities. In this context, the objective assessment of the quality in retinal images plays an important role to guarantee the success of any computer-aided system. First, we presented a case study on retinal image quality assessment, consisting of a four-step method that localizes the region of interest in which some relevant image properties are computed, including color and texture features. Next, feature selection is applied to select the most relevant properties and, finally, supervised classification is performed to determine if the input image is of poor or good quality. The second case study was related to the automatic computation of the arteriolar-to-venular ratio (Arteriolar-to-Venular Ratio), a predictive biomarker of cerebral atrophy and cardiovascular events in adults. Different image processing techniques and unsupervised methods have been demonstrated to be useful for Arteriolar-to-Venular Ratio estimation. In particular, our case study uses the local contrast between blood vessels and their surrounding background to compute the vascular structure of the retina, and then applies multilevel thresholding and graph propagation to classify the blood vessels into arteries and veins, allowing to finally compute the Arteriolar-to-Venular Ratio. Finally, the third case study is devoted to the automatic diagnosis of retinopathy of prematurity, a disease affecting low birth weight infants that shows a high amount of disagreement among experts. Discrepancies in the sets of important features considered by different experts have been identified as a possible cause of variability in the diagnosis of Retinopathy of Prematurity. Our case study uses feature selection techniques to discover the most important features considered by a given expert. Finally, an automated diagnosis system using machine learning methods is built in order to check if this approach can be helpful to diagnose Retinopathy of Prematurity and understand high inter-rater variability. The experimental results presented in this chapter were obtained by applying the different methods of the case studies to several datasets, both public and private, proving to be useful for daily practice.

Glossary

AVR	Arteriolar-to-Venular Ratio
CRAE	Central Retinal Artery Equivalent
CRVE	Central Retinal Vein Equivalent
CA	Centerline Accuracy
CR	Coverage Rate
CNN	Convolutional Neural Networks
CFS	Correlation-based Feature Selection
FS	FS Feature Selection
NB	Naive Bayes
OA	Overall Accuracy
oct	Optical coherence tomography
OD	Optic Disc
PCQ	Partial Classification for Quadrants
PCB	Partial Classification for Bands
PCF	Partial classification
PA	Pixel-wise Accuracy
ROP	Retinopathy of Prematurity
ROI	Region of Interest
SVM	Support Vector Machine
SSIM	Structural Similarity Index
SVM-RFE	SVM-RFE Support Vector Machine—Recursive Feature Elimination
TCQ	Total Classification for Quadrants
TCB	Total Classification for Bands
TCF	Total classification

References

1. Holladay, J.T.: Visual acuity measurements. J. Cataract Refract. Surg. **30**(2), 287–290 (2004)
2. Kutzscher, A.E., Kumar, R.S., Ramgopal, B., Rackenchath, M.V., Devi, S., Nagaraj, S., Moe, C.A., Fry, D.M., Stamper, R.L., Keenan, J.D.: Reproducibility of 5 methods of ocular tonometry. Ophthalmol. Glaucoma **2**(6), 429–434 (2019)
3. Spaide, R.F., Klancnik, J.M., Cooney, M.J.: Retinal vascular layers imaged by fluorescein angiography and optical coherence tomography angiography. JAMA Ophthalmol. **133**(1), 45–50 (2015)
4. Quintí Foguet, VAMPAHICA Study Group, Rodríguez, A., VAMPAHICA Study Group, Marc Saez, VAMPAHICA Study Group, Ubieto, A., VAMPAHICA Study Group, Beltrán, M., VAMPAHICA Study Group, et al.: Usefulness of optic fundus examination with retinography in initial evaluation of hypertensive patients. Am. J. Hypertension **21**(4), 400–405 (2008)
5. Puzyeyeva, O., Lam, W.C., Flanagan, J.G., Brent, M.H., Devenyi, R.G., Mandelcorn, M.S., Wong, T., Hudson, C.: High-resolution optical coherence tomography retinal imaging: a case series illustrating potential and limitations. J. Ophthalmol. (2011)
6. Ding, L., Bawany, M.H., Kuriyan, A.E., Ramchandran, R.S., Wykoff, C.C., Sharma, G.: RECOVERY-FA19: Ultra-Widefield Fluorescein Angiography Vessel Detection Dataset. IEEE Dataport (2019) https://dx.doi.org/10.21227/m9yw-xs04
7. Niemeijer, M., Staal, J.J., van Ginneken, B., Loog, M., Abramoff, M.D.: DRIVE: Digital Retinal Images for Vessel Extraction (2004). http://www.isi.uu.nl/Research/Databases/DRIVE
8. Gholami, P., Lakshminarayanan, V.: Optical coherence tomography image retinal database. Inter-university Consortium for Political and Social Research (2019)
9. Galloway, N.R.: Kwaku Amoaku. Common Eye Diseases and their Management. Springer, W.M., Galloway, P.H., Browning, A.C., Galloway, N.R. (2006)
10. Nayak, J., Acharya, R., Subbanna Bhat, P., Shetty, N., Lim, T.-C.: Automated diagnosis of glaucoma using digital fundus images. J. Med. Syst. **33**(5), 337 (2009)
11. Remeseiro, B., Barreira, N., García-Resúa, C., Lira, M., Giráldez, M.J., Yebra-Pimentel, E., Penedo, M.G.: iDEAS: a web-based system for dry eye assessment. Comput. Methods Progr. Biomed. **130**, 186–197 (2016)
12. Yimlui Cheung, C., Kamran Ikram, M., Klein, R., Wong, T.Y.: The clinical implications of recent studies on the structure and function of the retinal microvasculature in diabetes. Diabetologia **58**(5), 871–885 (2015)
13. Yuki, M., Akitaka, T., Kyoko, K., Masahiro, A., Ken, O., Tomoaki, M., Yumiko, A.-K., Kazuaki, M., Nagahisa, Y.: Age-and hypertension-dependent changes in retinal vessel diameter and wall thickness: an optical coherence tomography study. Am. J. Ophthalmol. **156**(4), 706–714 (2013)
14. Heitmar, R., Lip, G.Y.P., Ryder, R.E., Blann, A.D.: Retinal vessel diameters and reactivity in diabetes mellitus and/or cardiovascular disease. Cardiovasc. Diabetol. **16**(1), 56 (2017)
15. Ding, J., Lay Wai, K., McGeechan, K., et al.: Retinal vascular caliber and the development of hypertension: a meta-analysis of individual participant data. J. Hypertension **32**(2), 207 (2014)
16. Hagiwara, Y., Wei Koh, J.N., Hong Tan, J., Bhandary, S.V., Laude, A., Ciaccio, E.J., Tong, L., Rajendra Acharya, U.: Computer-aided diagnosis of glaucoma using fundus images: a review. Comput. Methods Progr. Biomed. **165**, 1–12 (2018)
17. Raghavendra, U., Fujita, H., Bhandary, S.V., Gudigar, A., Hong Tan, J., Rajendra Acharya, U.: Deep convolution neural network for accurate diagnosis of glaucoma using digital fundus images. Inf. Sci. **441**, 41–49 (2018)
18. Rajendra Acharya, U., Hagiwara, Y., Koh, J.E.W., Hong Tan, J., Bhandary, S.V., Krishna Rao, A., Raghavendra, U.: Automated screening tool for dry and wet age-related macular degeneration (ARMD) using pyramid of histogram of oriented gradients (PHOG) and nonlinear features. J. Comput. Sci. **20**, 41–51 (2017)

19. Burlina, P.M., Joshi, N., Pekala, M., Pacheco, K.D., Freund, D.E., Bressler, N.M.: Automated grading of age-related macular degeneration from color fundus images using deep convolutional neural networks. JAMA Ophthalmol. **135**(11), 1170–1176 (2017)
20. Niemeijer, M., Abramoff, M.D., Ginneken, B.V.: Information fusion for diabetic retinopathy CAD in digital color fundus photographs. IEEE Trans. Med. Imaging **28**(5), 775–785 (2009)
21. Abràmoff, M.D., Reinhardt, J.M., Russell, S.R., Folk, J.C., Mahajan, V.B., Niemeijer, M., Quellec, G.: Automated early detection of diabetic retinopathy. Ophthalmology **117**(6), 1147–1154 (2010)
22. Bretschger Seidelmann, S., Claggett, B., Bravo, P., Gupta, A., Farhad, H., Carli, M.D., Solomon, S.: Retina vessel caliber in atherosclerotic cardiovascular event prediction: the atherosclerosis in communities study. J. Am. Coll. Cardiol. **67**(13), 1893 (2016)
23. Ng, E.Y.K., Rajendra Acharya, U., Rangayyan, R.M., Suri, I.S.: Ophthalmological Imaging and Applications. CRC Press (2014)
24. Robert, K.: Image Analysis for Ophthalmological Diagnosis. Springer (2016)
25. Teng, T., Lefley, M., Claremont, D.: Progress towards automated diabetic ocular screening: a review of image analysis and intelligent systems for diabetic retinopathy. Med. Biol. Eng. Comput. **40**(1), 2–13 (2002)
26. Fonager Nørgaard, M., Grauslund, J.: Automated screening for diabetic retinopathy-a systematic review. Ophthal. Res. **60**(1), 9–17 (2018)
27. Kawaguchi, A., Sharafeldin, N., Sundaram, A., Campbell, S., Tennant, M., Rudnisky, C., Weis, E., Damji, K.F.: Tele-ophthalmology for age-related macular degeneration and diabetic retinopathy screening: a systematic review and meta-analysis. Telemed. e-Health **24**(4), 301–308 (2018)
28. Grewal, P.S., Oloumi, F., Rubin, U., Tennant, M.T.S.: Deep learning in ophthalmology: a review. Can. J. Ophthalmol. **53**(4), 309–313 (2018)
29. Wei Ting, D.S., Pasquale, L.R., Peng, L., Campbell, J.P., Lee, A.Y., Raman, R., Siew, G., Tan, W., Schmetterer, L., Keane, P.A., Yin Wong, T.: Artificial intelligence and deep learning in ophthalmology. Br. J. Ophthalmol. **103**(2), 167–175 (2019)
30. Maryam, B., Muhammad, H., Anam, F.: Application of deep learning for retinal image analysis: a review. Comput. Sci. Rev. **35** (2020)
31. Wang, Z., Bovik, A.C., Sheikh, H.R., Simoncelli, E.P.: Image quality assessment: from error visibility to structural similarity. IEEE Trans. Image Process. **13**(4), 600–612 (2004)
32. Wang, Z., Simoncelli, E.P., Bovik, A.C.: Multiscale structural similarity for image quality assessment. Conference Record of the Thirty-Seventh Asilomar Conference on Signals, Systems and Computers **2**, 1398–1402 (2003)
33. Li, C., Bovik, A.C.: Three-component weighted structural similarity index. In: IS&T/SPIE Electronic Imaging, pages 72420Q–72420Q (2009)
34. Zhou, W., Qiang, L.: Information content weighting for perceptual image quality assessment. IEEE Trans. Image Process. **20**(5), 1185–1198 (2011)
35. Tan Nguyen, T., Lin Wang, L., Yin Wong, T.: Retinal vascular changes in pre-diabetes and prehypertension new findings and their research and clinical implications. Diab. Care **30**(10), 2708–2715 (2007)
36. Coll-de Tuero, G., González-Vázquez, S., Rodríguez-Poncelas, A., Antònia Barceló, M., Barrot-de-la Puente, J., Penedo, M.G., Pose-Reino, A., Pena-Seijo, M., Saez, M.: Retinal arteriole-to-venule ratio changes and target organ disease evolution in newly diagnosed hypertensive patients at 1-year follow-up. J. Am. Soc. Hypertension **8**(2), 83–93 (2014)
37. Lee, S.C., Wang, Y.: Automatic retinal image quality assessment and enhancement. In: Medical Imaging, pages 1581–1590 (1999)
38. Fleming, A.D., Philip, S., Goatman, K.A., Olson, J.A., Sharp, P.F.: Automated assessment of diabetic retinal image quality based on clarity and field definition. Investig. Ophthalmol. Vis. Sci. **47**(3), 1120–1125 (2006)
39. Niemeijer, M., Abramoff, M.D., van Ginneken, B.: Image structure clustering for image quality verification of color retina images in diabetic retinopathy screening. Med. Image Anal. **10**(6), 888–898 (2006)

40. Giancardo, L., Abràmoff, M.D., Chaum, E., Karnowski, T.P., Meriaudeau, F., Tobin, K.W.: Elliptical local vessel density: a fast and robust quality metric for retinal images. In: 30th Annual International Conference of the IEEE Engineering in Medicine and Biology Society, pages 3534–3537 (2008)
41. Alex Welikala, R., Foster, P., Hynes Whincup, P., Regina Rudnicka, A., Owen, C.G., Strachan, D.P., Barman, S.A., et al.: Automated retinal image quality assessment on the UK Biobank dataset for epidemiological studies. Comput. Biol. Med. **71**, 67–76 (2016)
42. Davis, H., Russell, S., Barriga, E., Abramoff, M., Soliz, P.: Vision-based, real-time retinal image quality assessment. In: 22nd IEEE International Symposium on Computer-Based Medical Systems, pages 1–6 (2009)
43. Pires Dias, J.M., Manta Oliveira, C., da Silva Cruz, L.: Retinal image quality assessment using generic image quality indicators. Inf. Fusion **19**, 73–90 (2014)
44. Remeseiro, B., Maria Mendonça, A., Campilho, A.: Objective quality assessment of retinal images based on texture features. In: International Joint Conference on Neural Networks, pages 4520–4527 (2017)
45. Jan, P., Jörg, M., Rüdiger, B., Joachim, H., Georg, M.: Automated quality assessment of retinal fundus photos. Int. J. Comput. Assist. Radiol. Surg. **5**(6), 557–564 (2010)
46. Fleming, A.D., Philip, S., Goatman, K.A., Sharp, P.F., Olson, J.A.: Automated clarity assessment of retinal images using regionally based structural and statistical measures. Med. Eng. Phys. **34**(7), 849–859 (2012)
47. Lamiaa, A.-H., Ahmed, E.-R., Georg, M.: No-reference quality index for color retinal images. Comput. Biol. Med. **90**, 68–75 (2017)
48. Jorge, P., Julián, E., Carmen, V., David, M.: Retinal image quality assessment through a visual similarity index. J. Mod. Opt. **60**(7), 544–550 (2013)
49. Costa, P., Campilho, A., Hooi, B., Smailagic, A., Kitani, K., Liu, S., Faloutsos, C., Galdran, A.: EyeQual: accurate, explainable, retinal image quality assessment. In: 16th IEEE International Conference on Machine Learning and Applications, pages 323–330 (2017)
50. Vincent, D., Isabelle, C., Ryo, K., Jean-Paul, C., Max, V., Pierre, F., Karen, R., Cecile, D.: Retinal vascular caliber is associated with cardiovascular biomarkers of oxidative stress and inflammation: the POLA study. PloS One **8**(7) (2013)
51. Moazam Fraz, M., Remagnino, P., Hoppe, A., Uyyanonvara, B., Rudnicka, A.R., Owen, C.G., Barman, S.A.: Blood vessel segmentation methodologies in retinal images–a survey. Comput. Methods Progr. Biomed. **108**(1), 407–433 (2012)
52. Montoro, A., Morales, S., Naranjo, V., Lopez-Mir, F., Alcaniz, M.: Feature extraction for retinal vascular network classification. In: IEEE-EMBS International Conference on Biomedical and Health Informatics, pages 404–407 (2014)
53. Irshad, S., Usman Akram, M., Ayub, S., Ayaz, A.: Retinal blood vessels differentiation for calculation of arterio-venous ratio. In: International Conference Image Analysis and Recognition, pages 411–418 (2015)
54. Relan, D., Ballerini, L., Trucco, E., MacGillivray, T.: Retinal vessel classification based on maximization of squared-loss mutual information. In: Machine Intelligence and Signal Processing, pages 77–84. Springer (2016)
55. Xu, X., Ding, W., Abràmoff, M.D., Cao, R.: An improved arteriovenous classification method for the early diagnostics of various diseases in retinal image. Comput. Methods Progr. Biomed. **141**, 3–9 (2017)
56. Akbar, S., Usman Akram, M., Sharif, M., Tariq, A., Khan, S.A.: Decision support system for detection of hypertensive retinopathy using arteriovenous ratio. Artif. Intell. Med. **90**, 15–24 (2018)
57. Huang, F., Dashtbozorg, B., Tan, T., ter Haar Romeny, B.M.: Retinal artery/vein classification using genetic-search feature selection. Comput. Methods Progr. Biomed. **161**, 197–207 (2018)
58. Qazaleh, M., Farshad, T., Hamidreza, P.: Automated characterization of blood vessels as arteries and veins in retinal images. Comput. Med. Imaging Graph. **37**(7), 607–617 (2013)
59. Joshi, V.S., Reinhardt, J.M., Garvin, M.K., Abramoff, M.D.: Automated method for identification and artery-venous classification of vessel trees in retinal vessel networks. PloS One **9**(2), (2014)

60. Dashtbozorg, B., Maria Mendonça, A., Campilho, A.: An automatic graph-based approach for artery/vein classification in retinal images. IEEE Trans. Image Process. **23**(3), 1073–1083 (2014)
61. Estrada, R., Allingham, M.J., Mettu, P.S., Cousins, S.W., Tomasi, C., Farsiu, S.: Retinal artery-vein classification via topology estimation. IEEE Trans. Med. Imaging **34**(12), 2518–2534 (2015)
62. Hu, Q., Abràmoff, M.D., Garvin, M.K.: Automated construction of arterial and venous trees in retinal images. J. Med. Imaging **2**(4), (2015)
63. Enrico, P., Gavin, R., Tom, M., van Hemert, J., Graeme, H., Emanuele, T.: A graph cut approach to artery/vein classification in ultra-widefield scanning laser ophthalmoscopy. IEEE Trans. Med. Imaging **37**(2), 516–526 (2017)
64. Zhao, Y., Xie, J., Zhang, H., Zheng, Y., Zhao, Y., Qi, H., Zhao, Y., Su, P., Liu, J., Liu, Y.: Retinal vascular network topology reconstruction and artery/vein classification via dominant set clustering. IEEE Trans. Med, Imaging (2019)
65. Ines Meyer, M., Galdran, A., Costa, P., Maria Mendonça, A., Campilho, A.: Deep convolutional artery/vein classification of retinal vessels. In: International Conference Image Analysis and Recognition, pages 622–630 (2018)
66. Galdran, A., Meyer, M.I., Costa, P., Mendonça, A.M., Campilho, A.: Uncertainty-Aware Artery/Vein Classification on Retinal Images. In: IEEE International Symposium on Biomedical Imaging, pages 556–560 (2019)
67. Niemeijer, M., Xu, X., Dumitrescu, A.V., Gupta, P., van Ginneken, B., Folk, J.C., Abràmoff, M.D.: Automated measurement of the arteriolar-to-venular width ratio in digital color fundus photographs. IEEE Trans. Med. Imaging **30**(11), 1941–1950 (2011)
68. Vázquez, Sonia G., Barreira, Noelia, Penedo, Manuel G., Rodríguez-Blanco, Maria: Reliable monitoring system for arteriovenous ratio computation. Comput. Med. Imaging Graph. **37**(5), 337–345 (2013)
69. Dashtbozorg, B., Maria Mendonça, A., Campilho, A.: Assessment of retinal vascular changes through arteriolar-to-venular ratio calculation. In: International Conference Image Analysis and Recognition, pages 335–343 (2015)
70. Maria Mendonça, A., Remeseiro, B., Dashtbozorg, B., Campilho, A.: Automatic and semi-automatic approaches for arteriolar-to-venular computation in retinal photographs. In: Medical Imaging 2017: Computer-Aided Diagnosis, volume 10134, page 101341L (2017)
71. Remeseiro, B., Maria Mendonça, A., Campilho, A.: Automatic classification of retinal blood vessels based on multilevel thresholding and graph propagation. Vis. Comput. **1–15** (2020)
72. Azani Mustafa, W., Yazid, H., Bin Yaacob, S.: Illumination correction of retinal images using superimpose low pass and gaussian filtering. In: International Conference on Biomedical Engineering, pages 1–4 (2015)
73. Varnousfaderani, E.S., Yousefi, S., Belghith, A., Goldbaum, M.H.: Luminosity and contrast normalization in color retinal images based on standard reference image. In: Medical Imaging 2016: Image Processing, volume 9784, page 97843N (2016)
74. Huang, F., Dashtbozorg, B., ter Haar Romeny, B.M.: Artery/vein classification using reflection features in retina fundus images. Mach. Vis. Appl. **29**(1), 23–34 (2018)
75. Early Treatment for Retinopathy of Prematurity Cooperative Group et al.: Revised indications for the treatment of retinopathy of prematurity: results of the early treatment for retinopathy of prematurity randomized trial. Arch. Ophthalmol. **121**(12), 1684 (2003)
76. Clare, G., Allen, F.: Childhood blindness in the context of VISION 2020: the right to sight. Bull. World Health Organ. **79**(3), 227–232 (2001)
77. Clare, G., Alistair, F., Luz, G., Graham, Q., Renato, S., Patricia, V., Andrea, Z., et al.: Characteristics of infants with severe retinopathy of prematurity in countries with low, moderate, and high levels of development: implications for screening programs. Pediatrics **115**(5), e518–e525 (2005)
78. Kemper, A.R., Wallace, D.K.: Neonatologists' practices and experiences in arranging retinopathy of prematurity screening services. Pediatrics **120**(3), 527–531 (2007)

79. International Committee for the Classification of Retinopathy of Prematurity et al.: The international classification of retinopathy of prematurity revisited. Arch. Ophthalmol. **123**(7), 991 (2005)
80. Ataer-Cansizoglu, E., Kalpathy-Cramer, J., You, S., Keck, K.M., Erdogmus, D., Chiang, M.F.: Application of machine learning principles to analysis of underlying causes of inter-expert disagreement in retinopathy of prematurity diagnosis. Methods Inf, Med (2014)
81. Chiang, M.F., Jiang, L., Gelman, R., Du, Y.E., Flynn, J.T.: Interexpert agreement of plus disease diagnosis in retinopathy of prematurity. Arch. Ophthalmol. **125**(7), 875–880 (2007)
82. Wallace, D.K., Quinn, G.E., Freedman, S.F., Chiang, M.F.: Agreement among pediatric ophthalmologists in diagnosing plus and pre-plus disease in retinopathy of prematurity. J. Am. Assoc. Pediatr. Ophthalmol. Strabismus **12**(4), 352–356 (2008)
83. Feinstein, A.R.: A bibliography of publications on observer variability. J. Chron. Diseas. **38**(8), 619–632 (1985)
84. Azuara-Blanco, A., Jay Katz, L., Spaeth, G.L., Vernon, S.A., Spencer, F., Lanzl, I.M.: Clinical agreement among glaucoma experts in the detection of glaucomatous changes of the optic disk using simultaneous stereoscopic photographs. Am. J. Ophthalmol. **136**(5), 949–950 (2003)
85. Evans, A.J., Henry, P.C., Van der Kwast, T.H., Tkachuk, D.C., Watson, K., Lockwood, G.A., Fleshner, N.E., Cheung, C., Belanger, E.C., Amin, M.B., et al.: Interobserver variability between expert urologic pathologists for extraprostatic extension and surgical margin status in radical prostatectomy specimens. Am. J. Surg. Pathol. **32**(10), 1503–1512 (2008)
86. Garibaldi, J.M., Zhou, S.M., Wang, X.-Y., John, R.I., Ellis, I.O.: Incorporation of expert variability into breast cancer treatment recommendation in designing clinical protocol guided fuzzy rule system models. J. Biomed. Inform. **45**(3), 447–459 (2012)
87. Farmer, E.R., Gonin, R., Hanna, M.P.: Discordance in the histopathologic diagnosis of melanoma and melanocytic nevi between expert pathologists. Hum. Pathol. **27**(6), 528–531 (1996)
88. Elsheikh, T.M., Asa, S.L., Chan, J.K.C., DeLellis, R.A., Heffess, C.S., LiVolsi, V.A., Wenig, B.M.: Interobserver and intraobserver variation among experts in the diagnosis of thyroid follicular lesions with borderline nuclear features of papillary carcinoma. Am. J. Clin. Pathol. **130**(5), 736–744 (2008)
89. Amer, S., Li, T.C., Bygrave, C., Sprigg, A., Saravelos, H., Cooke, I.D.: An evaluation of the inter-observer and intra-observer variability of the ultrasound diagnosis of polycystic ovaries. Hum. Reproduct. **17**(6), 1616–1622 (2002)
90. Taylor, G.A., Voss, S.D., Melvin, P.R., Graham, D.A.: Diagnostic errors in pediatric radiology. Pediatr. Radiol. **41**(3), 327–334 (2011)
91. Senapati, G., Levine, D., Smith, C., Estroff, J.A., Barnewolt, C.E., Robertson, R.L., Poussaint, T.Y., Mehta, T.S., Werdich, X.Q., Pier, D., et al.: Frequency and cause of disagreements in imaging diagnosis in children with ventriculomegaly diagnosed prenatally. Ultrasound Obstetr. Gynecol. **36**(5), 582–595 (2010)
92. Ataer-Cansizoglu, E., You, S., Kalpathy-Cramer, J., Keck, K., Chiang, M.F., Erdogmus, D.: Observer and feature analysis on diagnosis of retinopathy of prematurity. In: IEEE International Workshop on Machine Learning for Signal Processing, pages 1–6. IEEE (2012)
93. Bolón-Canedo, V., Ataer-Cansizoglu, E., Erdogmus, D., Kalpathy-Cramer, J., Fontenla-Romero, O., Alonso-Betanzos, A., Chiang, M.F.: Dealing with inter-expert variability in retinopathy of prematurity: a machine learning approach. Comput. Methods and Progr. Biomed. **122**(1), 1–15 (2015)
94. Kalpathy-Cramer, J., Peter Campbell, J., Erdogmus, D., Tian, P., Kedarisetti, D., Moleta, C., Reynolds, J.D., Hutcheson, K., Shapiro, M.J., Repka, M.X., et al.: Plus disease in retinopathy of prematurity: improving diagnosis by ranking disease severity and using quantitative image analysis. Ophthalmology **123**(11), 2345–2351 (2016)
95. Ghergherehchi, L., Jin Kim, S., Campbell, P.J., Ostmo, S., Chan, P.R.V., Chiang, M.F.: Plus disease in retinopathy of prematurity: more than meets the icrop? Asia-Pac. J. Ophthalmol. **7**(3), 152–155 (2018)

96. Graziani, M., Brown, J.M., Andrearczyk, V., Yildiz, V., Peter Campbell, J., Erdogmus, D., Ioannidis, S., Chiang, M.F., Kalpathy-Cramer, J., Müller, H.: Improved interpretability for computer-aided severity assessment of retinopathy of prematurity. In: Medical Imaging 2019: Computer-Aided Diagnosis, volume 10950, page 109501R. International Society for Optics and Photonics (2019)
97. Sangwine, S.J., Horne, R.E.N.: The Colour Image Processing Handbook. Springer Science & Business Media (2012)
98. McLaren, K.: The development of the CIE 1976 (L*a*b) uniform colour-space and colour-difference formula. J. Soc. Dyers Colour. **92**(9), 338–341 (1976)
99. Rafael, C.: Gonzalez, Woods. Digital Image Processing. Pearson/Prentice Hall, R.E. (2008)
100. Ramos, L., Penas, M., Remeseiro, B., Mosquera, A., Barreira, N., Yebra-Pimentel, E.: Texture and color analysis for the automatic classification of the eye lipid layer. In: International Work-Conference on Artificial Neural Networks, pages 66–73 (2011)
101. Grigorescu, S.E., Petkov, N., Kruizinga, P.: Comparison of texture features based on Gabor filters. IEEE Trans. Image Process. **11**(10), 1160–1167 (2002)
102. Jensen, A., Cour-Harbo, A.L.: Ripples in Mathematics: The Discrete Wavelet Transform. Springer Science & Business Media (2001)
103. Havard, R., Leonhard, H.: Gaussian Markov Random Fields: Theory and Applications. CRC Press (2005)
104. Erdogan, C., DeLiang, W.: Texture segmentation using gaussian-markov random fields and neural oscillator networks. IEEE Trans. Neural Netw. **12** (2001)
105. Haralick, R.M., Shanmugam, K., Dinstein, I.: Texture features for image classification. IEEE Trans. Syst. Man Cybernet. **3**, 610–621 (1973)
106. Guyon, I., Elisseeff, A.: An introduction to variable and feature selection. J. Mach. Learn. Res. **3**, 1157–1182 (2003)
107. Hall, M.A.: Correlation-Based Feature Selection for Machine Learning. Ph.D. thesis, The University of Waikato (1999)
108. Manoranjan, D., Huan, L.: Consistency-based search in feature selection. Artif. Intell. **151**(1), 155–176 (2003)
109. Zheng, Z., Huan, L.: Searching for interacting features. Int. Joint Conf. Artif. Intell. **7**, 1156–1161 (2007)
110. Irina, R.: An empirical study of the naive bayes classifier. IJCAI Workshop Emp. Methods Artif. Intell. **3**(22), 41–46 (2001)
111. Quinlan, J.R.: C4.5: Programs for Machine Learning. Elsevier (2014)
112. Leo, B.: Random forests. Mach. Learn. **45**(1), 5–32 (2001)
113. Vapnik, V.N.: Statistical Learning Theory. Wiley (1998)
114. Ingrid, D.: Ten Lectures on Wavelets, vol. 61. SIAM (1992)
115. Niemeijer, M., Xu, X., Dumitrescu, A.V., Gupta, P., van Ginneken, B., Folk, J.C., Abramoff, M.D.: INSPIRE-AVR: Iowa Normative Set for Processing Images of the Retina—Artery Vein Ratio (2011). http://www.medicine.uiowa.edu/eye/inspire-datasets/
116. Hu, Q., Garvin, M.K., Abramoff, M.D.: RITE: Retinal Images vessel Tree Extraction (2015). https://medicine.uiowa.edu/eye/rite-dataset
117. Dashtbozorg, B., Maria Mendonça, A., Campilho, A.: Optic disc segmentation using the sliding band filter. Comput. Biol. Med. **56**, 1–12 (2015)
118. Maria Mendonca, A., Campilho, A.: Segmentation of retinal blood vessels by combining the detection of centerlines and morphological reconstruction. IEEE Trans. Med. Imaging **25**(9), 1200–1213 (2006)
119. Maria Mendonça, A., Remeseiro, B., Dashtbozorg, B., Campilho, A.: Automatic and semi-automatic approaches for arteriolar-to-venular computation in retinal photographs. In: SPIE Medical Imaging 2017: Computer-Aided Diagnosis, volume 10134, page 101341L (2017)
120. Dashtbozorg, B.: Advanced Image Analysis for the Assessment of Retinal Vascular Changes, Ph.D thesis, Universidade do Porto (2015). https://repositorio-aberto.up.pt/handle/10216/78851?locale=en

121. Marco, F., Enrico, G., Alfredo, R.: Luminosity and contrast normalization in retinal images. Med. Image Anal. **9**(3), 179–190 (2005)
122. Nobuyuki, O.: A threshold selection method from gray-level histograms. IEEE Trans. Syst. Man Cybern. **9**(1), 62–66 (1979)
123. Knudtson, M.D., Lee, K.E., Hubbard, L.D., Yin Wong, T., Klein, R., Klein, B.E.: Revised formulas for summarizing retinal vessel diameters. Curr. Eye Res. **27**(3), 143–149 (2003)
124. Lyu, X., Yang, Q., Xia, S., Zhang, S.: Construction of retinal vascular trees via curvature orientation prior. In: IEEE International Conference on Bioinformatics and Biomedicine, pages 375–382 (2016)
125. Demšar, J.: Statistical comparisons of classifiers over multiple data sets. J. Mach. Learn. Res. **7**, 1–30 (2006)
126. Gelman, R., Jiang, L., Du, Y.E., Elena Martinez-Perez, M., Flynn, J.T., Chiang, M.F.: Plus disease in retinopathy of prematurity: pilot study of computer-based and expert diagnosis. J. Am. Assoc. Pediatr. Ophthalmol. Strabismus **11**(6), 532–540 (2007)
127. Ross Quinlan, J.: Induction of decision trees. Mach. Learn. **1**(1), 81–106 (1986)
128. Kononenko, I.: Estimating attributes: analysis and extensions of RELIEF. In: Machine Learning: ECML-94, pages 171–182. Springer (1994)
129. Isabelle, G., Jason, W., Stephen, B., Vladimir, V.: Gene selection for cancer classification using support vector machines. Mach. Learn. **46**(1–3), 389–422 (2002)
130. Aha, D.W., Kibler, D., Albert, M.K.: Instance-based learning algorithms. Mach. Learn. **6**(1), 37–66 (1991)
131. Joachims, T.: Training linear SVMs in linear time. In: 12th ACM SIGKDD International Conference on Knowledge Discovery and Data Mining, pages 217–226. ACM (2006)

Chapter 5
Segmentation of Petri Plate Images for Automatic Reporting of Urine Culture Tests

Simone Bonechi, Monica Bianchini, Alessandro Mecocci, Franco Scarselli, and Paolo Andreini

Abstract Recently, significant improvements in biological and medical decision support systems have been obtained by using hybrid methods, based on a combination of advanced image processing techniques, artificial intelligence tools, fuzzy logic, genetic algorithms, and Bayesian modeling. In particular, the development of intelligent tools for the automatic reporting of medical analyses (screening systems) has attracted increasing research interest, due to their higher reliability, accuracy, reduced staff time, and lower costs. In this chapter, we propose a survey of computer vision and machine learning methods employed for the urine culture screening based on Petri plate automatic image understanding. Petri plates are used for bacterial cultures, which are employed in a wide variety of microbiological tests, from food and beverage safety assessments to environmental control, and to many specific clinical analyses (f.i. urine culture). Several segmentation techniques and some specific approaches to perform bacterial counting and infection classification are described below, along with a synthetic image generation approach required to overcome privacy concerns and medical data paucity. Indeed, during the last decade, deep learning has had a devastating impact on image processing, achieving exceptional results. Nonetheless, most of these improvements rely on fully annotated data, being the annotation procedure inherently difficult and expensive. The generated synthetic annotated images can be profitably used to train deep architectures, enabling reliable image segmentation.

S. Bonechi
Department of Computer Science, University of Pisa, Pisa, Italy
e-mail: simone.bonechi@unisi.it

S. Bonechi · M. Bianchini (✉) · A. Mecocci · F. Scarselli · P. Andreini
Department of Information Engineering and Mathematics, University of Siena, Siena, Italy
e-mail: monica.bianchini@unisi.it

A. Mecocci
e-mail: alessandro.mecocci@unisi.it

F. Scarselli
e-mail: franco.scarselli@unisi.it

P. Andreini
e-mail: paolo.andreini@unisi.it

© The Author(s), under exclusive license to Springer Nature Switzerland AG 2022
C.-P. Lim et al. (eds.), *Handbook of Artificial Intelligence in Healthcare*,
Intelligent Systems Reference Library 211,
https://doi.org/10.1007/978-3-030-79161-2_5

Keywords Automatic urine culture screening · Deep learning · Image analysis

5.1 Introduction

Bacteria are a group of microscopic prokaryotic single-cell organisms belonging to the Monera kingdom. They live in almost every environment on the earth and grow very rapidly. Bacterial reproduction is asexual and mostly occurs by binary cell fission, so that the process of bacterial growth is constituted basically by the gradual increase in the quantity of cell components. Bacterial cells are cultured in microbiological laboratories, in predetermined media and under controlled conditions. Microbial cultures are used for the identification of microorganisms and of their abundance in a sample, and they represent one of the primary diagnostic methods for the recognition of causative agents of infectious diseases. Bacteria and other microorganisms grow in specially prepared Petri plates containing nutrient rich media. The solid medium used for the cultivation of bacterial cells is known as agar. The colonies of bacteria that form in the agar can be analyzed to recover the type of microorganisms and their abundance.

Among bacterial diseases, Urinary Tract Infections (UTIs), together with those of the respiratory tract, are of great clinical relevance for the high frequency with which they are found in common medical practice and because of the complications arising therefrom. UTIs can target the urethra, bladder or kidneys and they are mainly caused by Gram-negative microorganisms, with a high prevalence of *Escherichia coli* (*E. coli*, 70%)—which usually lives in the digestive system and in the bowel—even if clinical cases frequently occur where complicated infections are caused by Gram-positive or multi-resistant germs, on which the common antimicrobial agents are ineffective, leading to therapeutic failures. The occurrence of UTIs varies in dependence of age and gender, as well as based on the socioeconomic background of the patients. Moreover, specific sub-populations at increased risk of UTIs include infants, pregnant women, elderly people, persons with urological abnormalities, patients with spinal cord injuries and/or catheters, with diabetes, multiple sclerosis, and AIDS. Particularly for women, the lifetime risk of having a UTI is greater than 50%. Pregnant women seem no more prone to UTIs than other women. Yet, when the UTI occurs during pregnancy, it is more likely that the infection extends to the kidneys, giving rise to more serious pathologies. For this reason, health care providers routinely screen pregnant women for UTIs during the first three months of pregnancy. On the other hand, nosocomial urinary tract infections account for up to 40% of all hospital-acquired infections and, most importantly, nosocomial pathogens causing UTIs tend to have a higher antibiotic resistance than simple UTIs [1].

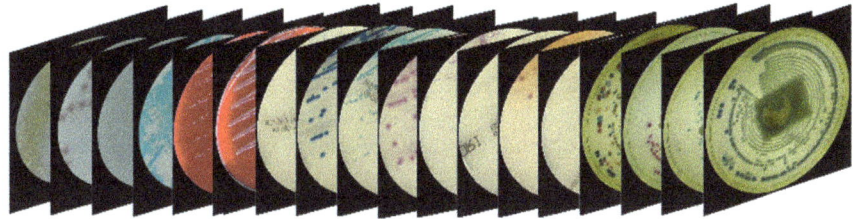

Fig. 5.1 Some examples of different culture grounds and streaking procedures

Therefore, the urine culture is a screening test[1] in the case of hospitalized patients and pregnant women. In the standard protocol, the urine sample is seeded on a Petri dish that holds a culture substrate, used to artificially recreate the environment required for the bacterial growth. There exists a variety of culture media (Fig. 5.1), which allow to perform different kinds of analysis, from isolating specific types of bacteria, to promoting a wide range of microbial growth.

The seeding procedure (streaking) consists on spreading the urine sample over the whole plate and can be performed both manually or automatically, with an *ad hoc* device. Then, the plate is incubated in a controlled environment for a fixed time period (16–24 h). After the incubation phase, each plate is examined by a microbiologist with the aim of recognizing the possible presence of bacterial colonies—and to establish their species and number—adding some more time to the medical report emission. This common situation deviates significantly from clinicians' needs for rapid results, targeted therapy, avoiding the use of broad-spectrum antibiotics and improving patient management.[2] Moreover, the traditional analysis procedure suffers from possible errors arising in the visual, qualitative, inspection of the dishes—due to the skills and the expertise of the operator—whereas difficulties also arise in the traceability of samples and results [11]. Automated urine analysis devices improve the ability of labs to screen more samples, producing results in less time than manual screening. Additionally, the redeployment and lower grading of staff, with the increased turnover and speed of urine screening, can provide economic benefits of automated over manual screening.

Indeed, an area where Artificial Intelligence (AI) has the potential to achieve some highly beneficial advantages for everyone—especially patients and medical professionals, but also clinical management staff—is the healthcare. In this field, many medical applications have been developed based on AI, ranging from pneumonia risk prediction [17], to diagnosis of prostate cancer based on NMRs [51] and skin lesion prognostic classification [13, 22, 53]. Moreover, AI and machine learning are

---

[1] The term *screening* is used here in its common meaning of a routine test performed on a large population to identify those who are likely to develop a specified disease. Instead, in in vitro diagnostics it stands for preventive analyses aimed at establishing if a sample is positive or not.

[2] Rapid reporting is crucial, especially when pediatric patients are involved, since, in this case, the infection symptoms are not always specific, while it is urgent to decide if an antibiotic therapy is necessary or not and when to start it.

providing tools to enable medical practitioners and researchers to make sense of the flood of medical data. AI and other technical innovations are helping to ensure that data are appropriately cleaned, managed, and shared in the healthcare ecosystem. Specifically, the analysis of medical images—which can be captured by many different analysis tools, from simple cameras (for example, in the case of Petri dish images) to specialized machinery for MRI, ultrasound and radiography—have also benefited significantly from the introduction of deep learning in computer vision. In this chapter, we intend to draw a brief history of the rapid evolution that has occurred in the last decade in medical image processing—specifically in semantic segmentation techniques—using the automatic analysis of images of Petri dishes as a case study [36]. In fact, semantic segmentation is a fundamental step in image analysis and understanding, since it provides a pixel-level characterization of the scene. Moreover, in this chapter, we use semantic segmentation to perform background subtraction, which allows us to isolate the informative content of the image to be employed in subsequent analyses. Starting from classical computer vision techniques, which involve choosing an *ad hoc* color space to represent the images and employing filtering and statistical approaches to characterize different type of data contained therein, we finally describe very recent semantic segmentation approaches based on deep learning. Indeed, this chapter reflects the transition occurred in the last decade in computer vision, in which deep learning has progressively superseded traditional image processing techniques. In fact, recently, deep learning has pushed the state of the art in many visual recognition tasks, achieving outstanding results [35, 40, 40]. Beside, most of these improvements rely on fully annotated data, being the annotation procedure inherently difficult and costly. This is especially true for semantic segmentation, which requires pixel-wise annotations. Moreover, in biological and medical applications, the problem of collecting large set of annotated samples is even more crucial, due to privacy issues and data shortage, while dealing with a reduced number of fully annotated data, without significantly affecting the recognition performance, is one of the most active research field in computer vision. Such problem has a particularly relevant impact in the automatic Petri plate analysis, where the data distribution is unbalanced—with a small number of bacterial species found with high frequency and a lot of very rare infections; hence, it is usually necessary to deal with under-represented classes with a reduced number of available samples—while the bacterial growth is supported by a variety of different substrates, used either to isolate a specific strain or a multitude of different bacteria (i.e., for screening tests). Thus, the complete characterization of the whole variability of substrates, species and also sowing techniques would require a considerable amount of resources.

To face these problems and foster the use of deep learning tools in the automatic analysis of agar plates, we also present a novel method for generating synthetic images of Petri dishes, which naturally blend bacterial colonies in existing images of empty dishes. A simple heuristic also allows us to deal with the natural differences in reflectance within the colonies. The generated images are then used to train fully-Convolutional Networks, with state-of-the-art performance for semantic segmentation.

After the segmentation, detected bacterial colonies can then be classified based on machine learning techniques which are also briefly described in this chapter. Finally, besides the infection identification and classification, also the bacterial count can be automatically performed, giving an estimate of the number of microorganisms per milliliter of urine.

Automatic reporting of urine culture plates can guarantee a substantial speedup of the whole analysis procedure, also avoiding the continuous transition between sterile and external environments which is typical in the standard protocol. The final outcomes can be stored, along with the related analysis records (i.e. the image, the infection type and the colony count). An overview of the literature related to this work is given in Sect. 5.2, while the whole processing pipeline is described in Sect. 5.3. More precisely, Sect. 5.3.1 describes how images can be acquired, based on a low cost device that is able to capture the image and, in the meanwhile, to extract only the part related to the plate, which must be saved for later processing. Section 5.3.2 reports on the evolution of segmentation methods to separate bacterial colonies from the growing seed, also defining an automatic engine for synthetic Petri plate generation. Instead, Sect. 5.3.3 accounts for the classification and the estimation of the infection severity (bacterial count). All the proposed techniques, along the pipeline, are supported by experimental results assessing their viability and performance. Finally, some conclusions and future perspectives are drawn in Sect. 5.4.

5.2 Related Work

The image processing pipeline described in this chapter is mainly related to three research topics, i.e. automatic agar plate analysis, synthetic data generation and image segmentation, whose literature is examined below.

Automatic agar plate analysis
The automatic analysis of agar plates has a long history. Specialized recording and processing systems for automatic bacterial counting were originally proposed in the late 1950s [2, 42]. Subsequently, bacterial colony counting systems were realized using particular transforms, like the distance transform on binarized images [45], or the watershed transform on grayscale images [15, 54]. A grayscale morphological analysis was also proposed in [39]. A particular lighting technique was presented in [19], with the aim of producing salient points on the colonies to simplify their counting. In [44], a method based on segment classification has been proposed for the segmentation of images, while the free software OpenCFU [26] uses a multiple-threshold segmentation method and a watershed transformation for the separation of confluent segments. More recently, a bacterial counting and classification approach, based on a custom background subtraction procedure and on shallow feedforward neural networks, has been proposed in [5–7], while a background subtraction technique based on a mixture of Gaussians (MOG) is used in [4]. Moreover, based on

bag of visual words (BOVWs), an image may be represented as a set of features [20, 34]. Features consist of keypoints and descriptors. Keypoints are the salient points in the image and, no matter the image is rotated, shrunk, or expanded, its keypoints will remain the same, whereas descriptors are labels associated to the keypoints. Keypoints and descriptors can be used to construct vocabularies and to represent each image as a frequency histogram of features [20]. A bag-of-word approach for infected plate detection and colony classification was used in [3]. Finally, [24] exploits a proprietary image processing method for the colony segmentation of blood agar plates, employing Convolutional Neural Networks (CNNs) on the obtained segments for the bacterial count. Indeed, to the best of our knowledge, the approaches presented in [8, 9] are the first to propose the use of convolutional neural networks for the bacterial colony semantic segmentation problem.

Synthetic data generation
Synthetic datasets are an economic and scalable alternative to the human ground-truth supervision in machine learning. In recent years, several computer vision researches have used synthetic data to face a variety of different problems. For instance, in [30, 43], virtual environments have been exploited for the pedestrian detection problem faced by neural networks. Synthetic data were also used for text detection [28, 32], and pose estimation [16, 46]. Furthermore, also in the field of semantic segmentation, some approaches have recently been proposed. Large collections of synthetic images of driving scenes in urban environments were generated in [48, 50], while synthetic indoor scenes were exploited by [29]. Indeed, despite the widespread production of synthetic data for real-world images, their use for medical imaging applications has been relatively scarce. In fact, unlike conventional real-world images—that may show a limited range of object diversity—medical images capture information of biological tissues, organs, or may be the result of laboratory analysis, and can contain unique patient-specific or instrument-specific textures that are difficult to model. An interesting contribution can be found in [41], where adversarial training is used to make real medical images more like synthetic images, hypothesizing that clinically-relevant features can be preserved via self-regularization. Moreover, in [10], Generative Adversarial Networks (GANs) were employed for synthesizing high quality retinal images, along with the corresponding semantic label-maps, to be used instead of real images during the training process of a semantic segmentation network.

Image segmentation
Image segmentation is an important research field in image processing and pattern recognition. It is the process of partitioning a digital image into many segments (composed by sets of pixels). The goal of segmentation is to change the representation of an image into something that is more meaningful and easier to analyze. Among many other possible examples, a traditional approach to image segmentation is given by the use of a Gaussian Mixture Model (GMM). In particular, in this framework, a color image is considered as the result of a GMM to which several Gaussian random variables contribute. Based on this assumption, segmentation can be viewed as a maximum likelihood parameter estimation problem, that can be solved by the expectation-maximization (EM) algorithm [25]. In the vast literature

addressing image segmentation via GMMs (f.i., [33, 47]), a comprehensive survey on classic computer vision approaches, also including GMMs, can be found in [52]. The goal of segmentation is to partition an image into several coherent parts, but without giving any specific meaning to each part. On the other hand, the semantic segmentation goal is to partition the image into semantically meaningful parts, and to classify each part into one of a set of pre-determined classes. Recently, much effort has been spent on semantic image segmentation because it can provide a meaningful overall description of the content of an image. Semantic segmentation can be also formulated as the process of making dense predictions by inferring the class of objects represented by each pixel of an image [18, 40, 55]. Relatively large datasets, with fully pixel-wise annotated natural images, have been created with this purpose: for example, PASCAL_VOC 2012 [23] and MS-COCO [38] for object segmentation and COCO_TS [12] and MLT_S [14] for scene text segmentation. Conversely, in medical imaging, the number of available samples is generally smaller, making small networks, with a reduced number of parameters, the only viable approach that can be usually employed. Indeed, one of the most successful deep learning model in medical image analysis is the U-net architecture [49], which uses a standard convolutional network, followed by an upsampling part of up-convolutions combined with skip-connections. In this chapter, we advocate the use of synthetically generated images to train more complex architectures, such as the Pyramid Scene Parsing Network [55].

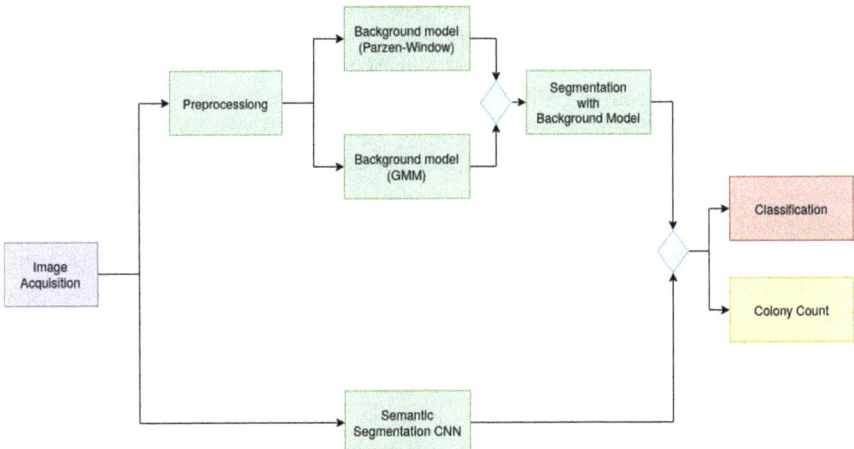

Fig. 5.2 Petri plate analysis pipeline

5.3 Automatic Petri Plate Analysis Pipeline

The following sections describe the whole image processing pipeline, based on the workflow depicted in Fig. 5.2. In particular, after the data acquisition (Sect. 5.3.1), how segmentation of Petri plate images can be carried out is illustrated (Sect. 5.3.2), employing both classical computer vision techniques and Convolutional Neural Networks (CNNs). In fact, CNNs are able to directly process the original image—without the need for preprocessing, aimed at cleaning it of non-informative contents—automatically extracting the foreground information used in the next steps for the classification and count of bacterial infections. Based on standard techniques, instead, three different phases can be distinguished, aimed at removing noise from the image, clustering uniform areas therein, and constructing a background model through which segmentation can start. The next step in the pipeline consists in representing segmented images in a suitable form to be used in conjunction with machine learning tools, which means applying *ad hoc* feature extraction techniques. Finally, connectionist models for the automatic reporting of the urine culture analysis are described in Sect. 5.3.3.

5.3.1 Image Acquisition

Most of the experiments reported in this chapter are based on various image sets both publicly available (as the MicrobIA Dataset, released by the University of Brescia, Italy) or, mainly, collected by the Copan WASPLab specimen processor at the Microbiology and Virology Laboratory of the Careggi Hospital in Florence, Italy—the reference center for microbiological and virological tests in the Tuscany region that processes more than 250 urine cultures per day. Copan WaspLab is designed to seed the plate and acquire the image at the end of the incubation phase. During the years, we have also processed other sets of data (f.i. inoculated with the bioMérieux Previ Isola system or manually seeded) for which an acquisition system is not available. In fact, in order to realize a whole processing pipeline, a low-cost device was developed to provide also small peripheral laboratories with an instrument for easy and reliable digital data acquisition. Indeed, to recognize the type of infection and accurately estimate the bacterial load, it is fundamental to avoid imperfections due to manual plate handling and to acquire a good quality image of the Petri dish. Therefore, images are captured by the automatic camera setup shown in Fig. 5.3. After the acquisition, a suitable preprocessing step is applied to locate the region of interest (the Petri dish), and to guarantee it occupies the appropriate position inside the field of view. At this point the image can be saved along with auxiliary clinical information.

In detail, the automatic acquisition is performed as follows: a simple and fast algorithm, based on change detection and morphological filtering, is applied and the image is acquired only when the dish is correctly positioned, the scene is well

5   Segmentation of Petri Plate Images for Automatic …

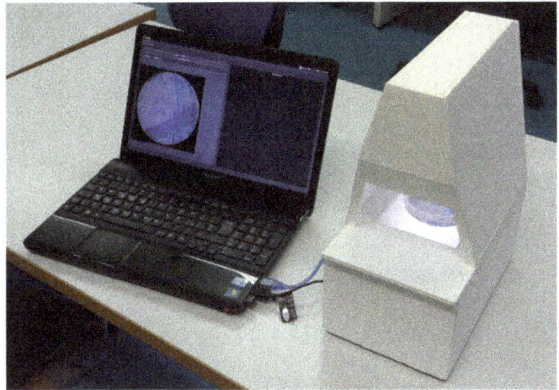

Fig. 5.3 The automatic acquisition setup

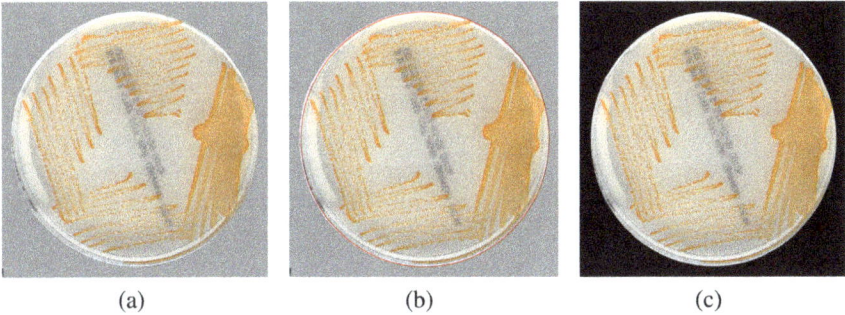

(a)   (b)   (c)

Fig. 5.4 In **a**, the Petri dish on the acquisition device; in **b**, the RoI selected by the Hough transform and, in **c**, the stored image

illuminated, and no movements are observed. Before saving the image, the Petri dish is isolated from the rest of the scene, using an Hough circle transform [4], to detect the circular Region of Interest (RoI) (Fig. 5.4).

5.3.2 Segmentation

This section is the core of this chapter and shows the evolution that has occurred over the past decade from standard computer vision techniques to convolutional neural networks. In particular, we describe the Petri plate segmentation stage showing how convolutional neural networks improve the results.

Segmentation with standard computer vision techniques

Based on the schema depicted in the top part of Fig. 5.2, the segmentation stage

Fig. 5.5 Example of a Petri plate with noisy elements (written text and label) highlighted in red. Instead, the blue rectangles represent the regions that contain the patients' data (blurred for privacy issues)

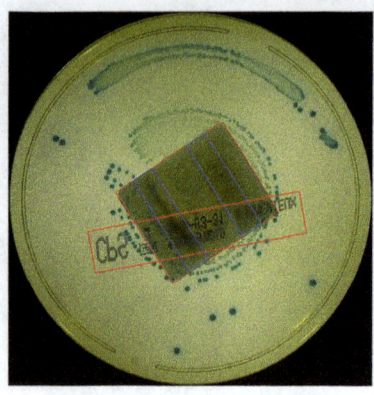

can be divided into three main phases (preprocessing, background segmentation, foreground segmentation), which will be deepened in the following.

Image preprocessing
In general, the plate-handling process requires some ancillary data that are added on the plate before or after the urine culture seeding procedure (for instance, a written text with the manufacturer name, a label for the patient traceability, etc.). In this paragraph, to describe a particular case study, the plates shown in Fig. 5.5 have been employed. The text they contain identifies the type of culture medium (Agar chromID CPS) and the manufacturer's brand. Moreover, a label is pasted underneath with the patient name and an identification bar code (see Fig. 5.5). These elements have a fixed shape and dimension, but their position can change from image to image [4]. They negatively affect the classification process and must be removed.

Written text removal—The text must be localized and removed from the image. To this aim, a template matching approach has been employed, based on a written text sample, manually extracted from an empty plate. Being the text almost the same for all the plates, the manual operation needs to be performed only once, at the very beginning of the preprocessing phase (thereafter it is stored in the system). Gradient variations (based on the Sobel filtering procedure) were later evaluated to gain independence from light alterations. Then, the Normalized Cross Correlation (NCC) has been used to detect the text position. While the text appearance is almost fixed (and can be stored), its rotation is not, and must be compensated. To this end, different rotated versions of the acquired template are applied to the image, selecting the best match. To speed up the process, the template search area is limited to a sub-part of the whole image. In fact, the text printing process grants some tolerance limits to positional variability (for example, the distance between the text position and the center of the image cannot exceed a given threshold).

Label removal—Another element that can be present on the image and that must be removed is the label, which is attached under the plate and contains the patient's name. The image acquisition device uses the backlight, so that the light passes through both the semitransparent culture medium and the label, being mostly absorbed by the last one. As a result, the label area is always darker than the surroundings. To segregate the label, an adaptive threshold is used, obtained by applying the Otsu's method to the image luminance. The binary mask gained after thresholding contains the darkest regions in the plate (some colonies and the label). A morphological opening is then employed to regularize the mask shape, based on a circular structuring element, with a diameter slightly smaller than the shortest label side. In this way, bacterial colonies and other artifacts, smaller than the label, are removed. Finally, the Minimum Perimeter Enclosing Rectangle of the largest connected component is computed, recovering the label position. Pixels belonging to this rectangle are disregarded during further processing steps. To save the images without worrying about privacy issues, the patient's name is also blurred by applying a severe smoothing on some fixed positions of the detected label (Fig. 5.5).

Background models
In order to separate the colonies from the background, a background-removal process based on chromatic information should be employed. Therefore, as a preliminary step, a color space analysis has been performed by studying the distribution of background colors in different color spaces. To analyze the chromogenic medium ground, used in the experiment described in this section, the CIE-Lab color space appeared to be the most suitable and, for this reason, it is used during the modeling of the background. The chromatic background model can be defined based on supervised training techniques, during which a human expert is required to select a set of different regions belonging to the background from some training images. In the following, two different techniques are described, respectively based on Parzen-window and Gaussian mixtures, to model the background of a Petri dish image.

Model based on Parzen–window—The chromatic components $((a,b)$ in the CIE-Lab color space) of the pixels belonging to the background regions are extracted and a median filter is applied on these values to reduce the effect of noisy samples. Then, the color histogram distribution is estimated by a Parzen–window with a Gaussian shape, according to Eq. (5.1):

$$p_B(\vec{c}) = \frac{1}{N} \sum_{i=1}^{N} \frac{1}{h_N^2} \phi\left(\frac{\vec{c}-\vec{c}_i}{h_N}\right) \quad (5.1)$$

where $p_B(\vec{c})$ represents the estimated probability density function of the the background, N is the number of observations, $\phi()$ is a Gaussian kernel function, h_N is a selected scale factor, and $\vec{c}_i$ is the chromatic vector of the i-th background sample.

Model based on Gaussian mixtures—Although the acquisition device uses a controlled illumination system, the effect of agar inhomogeneities, and of light disturbances from the external environment, produces relevant brightness variations in the background. Moreover, the presence of some particular type of infections (e.g. Proteus Mirabilis) significantly changes the culture ground appearance (see Fig. 5.6).

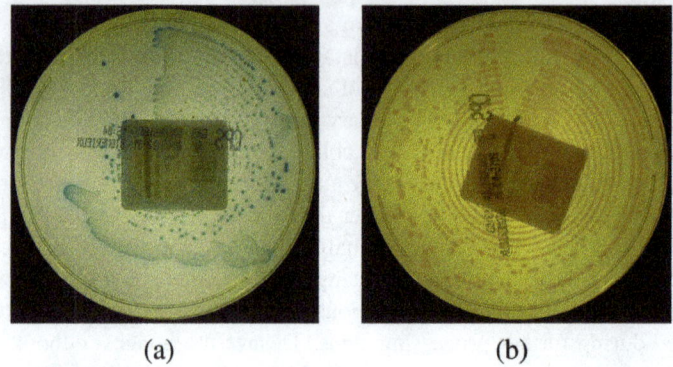

Fig. 5.6 In **a**, the typical background color and, in **b**, the background appearance changed by the Proteus Mirabilis infection

By analyzing the background color samples by means of the Mardia and Henze–Zirkler normality tests [4], it has become evident that a simple Gaussian model is unsuitable for modeling the two background clusters. For this reason, a Gaussian Mixture Model (GMM) has been adopted to describe the corresponding multimodal density function:

$$p(\theta) = \sum_{i=1}^{K} \Phi_i N(\mu_i, \Sigma_i)$$

where $\theta = (\vec{\mu}, \vec{\Sigma})$ collects the mixture parameters, and the i-th vector component is characterized by a normal distribution with weight Φ_i, mean μ_i and covariance matrix Σ_i. The number of mixture components has been empirically chosen by observing the data contour lines, while the Expectation-Maximization (EM) algorithm has been used to estimate the mixture parameters.

Background removal Once the background model has been defined, a Mean-Shift segmentation algorithm is used to compensate for local background inhomogeneities. For each segment, the (*a,b*) modal values are compared with the background model and, if the posterior probability of the background is greater, the corresponding segment is considered to be part of the culture ground. Some specific type of infections (as the *Candida bacterium*) cannot be classified by using chromatic information only, because their color is very similar to the background. In this case, spatial features (i.e., obtained with edge detection techniques) must be used to get a suitable segmentation performance. In Fig. 5.7, some results are reported.

Foreground segmentation
Similar approaches employed for the background can be used also to model the foreground that contains the colonies. Again a supervisor must select a set of regions

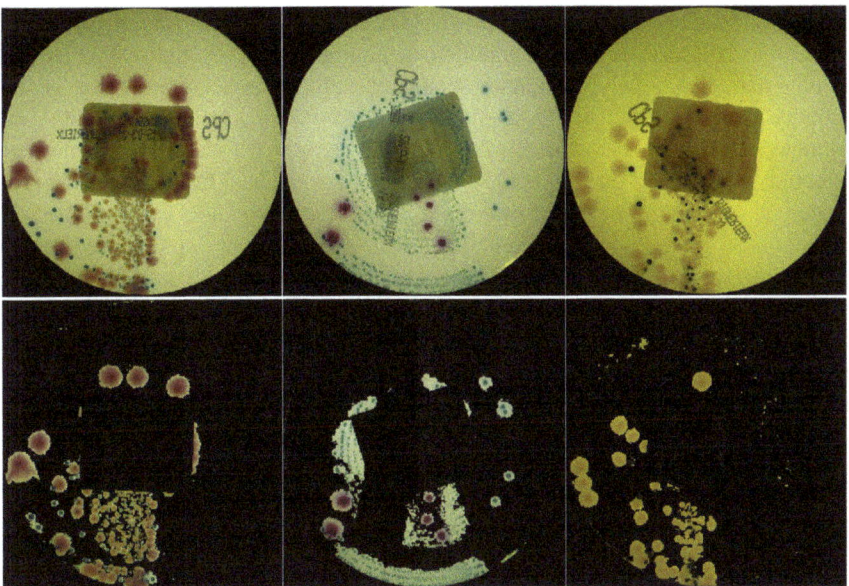

Fig. 5.7 Original images (in the top row) with the results of the background subtraction procedure at the bottom (the background and all noisy elements are in black)

belonging to seven different infection classes,[3] coming from the training set images. Therefore, seven models are created and used to estimate the conditional probability density function relative to each possible infection ($p_k(\vec{c})$; $k = 1, 2, \ldots, N_c$, where $N_c = 7$). These functions are then compared with the background probability density function to define the chromatic regions that can give rise to classification uncertainty [5]. Normally, these regions are detected in the pixels surrounding the colonies because their boundaries are not always sharp, especially for some types of infections.

Uncertain region disambiguation—The background near a colony slightly changes its colors according to the type of bacterium grown on the dish. To solve this problem, those pixels that cannot be assigned with reasonable certainty to a particular class are marked as *uncertain*. A specific postprocessing step is realized for these pixels, taking into account also local spatial properties like discontinuities (edges), that are typically present between the colonies and the background. Furthermore, by comparing the histograms of the uncertain region and the segments close to it, the classification of these ambiguous pixels is refined [5].

Segmentation with Convolutional Neural Networks and Synthetic Data
The use of a convolutional neural network to segment Petri dish images avoids the preprocessing and postprocessing steps by performing segmentation directly on the

---

[3] *E. coli*, KES (Klebsiella, Enterobacter, Serratia), *Enterococcus faecalis*, *Streptococcus agalactiae*, Pseudomonas, *Proteus mirabilis*, and *Staphylococcus aureus*.

original image. The main issue in adopting this approach is that training deep networks, which contain millions of parameters, requires a significant amount of labeled training data. Semantic segmentation requires pixel-level annotations whose generation by a human expert is very costly in term of both time and money. Therefore, segmentation datasets are generally quite smaller compared with the large scale classification collections, such as ImageNet [21]. In the medical field, this problem is exacerbated by the presence of rare diseases and privacy issues, which makes the collection of a large number of annotated data even more difficult. Indeed, in the case of the Petri plate analysis, to the best of our knowledge, only one public dataset is available (MicrobIA Dataset[4]), released by the University of Brescia (Italy). Such dataset only contains a segmentation ground-truth for a small set of blood agar plates, being barely enough to train a large CNN and inadequate to represent the huge variety of different growing media and species that can be found on Petri plates. For this reason, a synthetic image generator is presented, which can be used to cheaply produce large datasets of fully annotated images of Petri plates.

Synthetic Petri plate generation

The proposed generation engine is able to produce a huge variety of realistic images that can be used to train a deep neural network capable of generalizing to real data. Some examples of synthetic images are shown in Fig. 5.8. The generator pipeline (see Fig. 5.9) can be described as follows:

- A suitable set of background images and colony prototypes is collected;
- For each colony prototype, a generation model is built;
- A seeding procedure is simulated;
- Randomly selected patches are blended onto the background images, following the seeding simulation.

Background and token collection—From the MicrobIA image dataset, we extracted a set of single bacterial colony prototypes (tokens). Each token includes a small image crop which contains the colony and a background/foreground mask that allows to recognize if a pixel belongs to the culture ground or to the colony. We also gathered a small set of images of empty plates, representing Petri dishes free of infections, on which the colonies are blended. A set of 16 different background images and 30 tokens are used in our simulations, augmented using different scale, rotations and lightness to increase variability.

Colony models—The generation of the colony model consists of two steps. First, each token is analyzed to generate a model of the background that will be used as a reference. Then, this reference is exploited to produce a generative model of the colony that is independent from the background. The procedure is summarized in the steps below.

- Background model generation—the background colors of each token are quantized in a fixed number of **k** clusters through k-means, to speed-up the algorithm and

---

[4] http://www.microbia.org/index.php/resources.

5 Segmentation of Petri Plate Images for Automatic ...

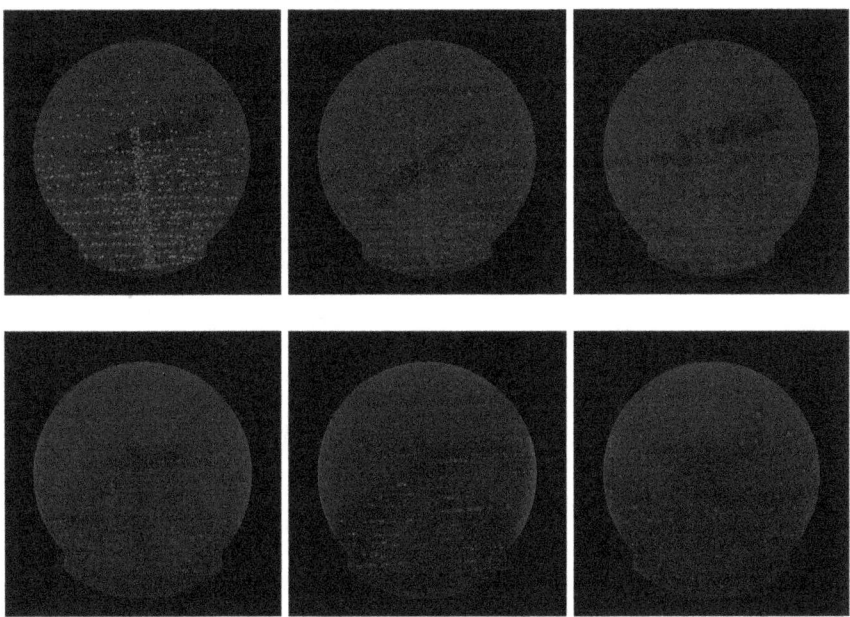

Fig. 5.8 Some examples of synthetically generated blood agar plate images (top row); images taken from the MicrobIA Haemolysis dataset (bottom row)

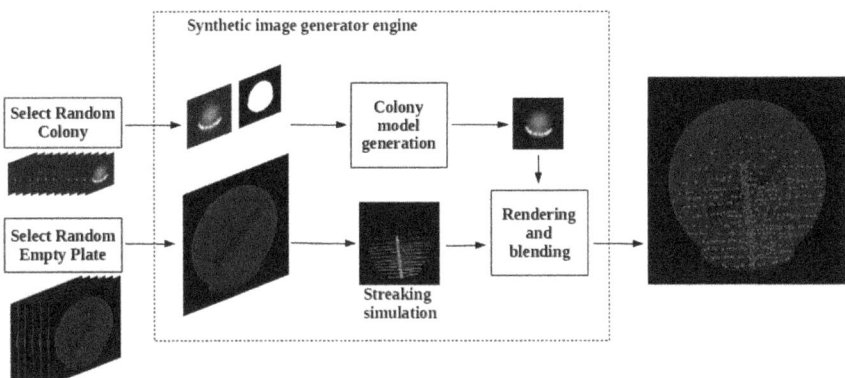

Fig. 5.9 Scheme of the synthetic agar plate image generation procedure

smooth the model, removing small changes in the appearance of the substrate. Then, for each pixel $\mathbf{p}_{x,y}$ belonging to a colony, the centroid $\mathbf{r}_k$ with the minimum L_2 distance in the CIE-Lab space is chosen, to represent the background reference for the current pixel.
- Colony model—the generative model of the colony, which will be used during the blending procedure, is calculated, subtracting from each colony pixel $\mathbf{p}_{x,y}$ the corresponding reference value:

$$\mathbf{m}_{x,y} = \mathbf{p}_{x,y} - \mathrm{argmin}_{\mathbf{r}_k}(||\mathbf{p}_{x,y} - \mathbf{r}_k||) \qquad (5.2)$$

Streaking simulation—In microbiology, several methods are available to plate out cells. The plate streaking process consists in inoculating the surface of an agar plate with a high dilution of a biological sample. The sample streaking can be manual or automatic and it can follow different patterns, leading to a variety of topologies for the distribution of the bacterial colonies over the agar plates. In this experiment, we have simulated the streaking procedure of the WASPLab automation system[5] used in the MicrobIA Dataset. Still, the same approach can be applied to any kind of streaking method. The distribution is modeled by a Wasserstein GAN with Gradient Penalty (WGAN–GP) [27], which is trained with the segmentation labels extracted from the training set of the MicrobIA Haemolysis Dataset. In our setup, starting from a noisy vector, we generate a set of label-maps representing realistic bacterial growth distributions [9].

Rendering and blending procedure—The rendering procedure takes a set of colony models as input and blends them on a background image (i.e. an agar plate without any bacterial growth), following the topology provided by the seeding simulator. Our proposed method is also devised to tackle the following problem: a colony is a conglomerate of bacterial cells with a three-dimensional structure and with the most inner part which is generally more voluminous than the outer. Hence, from an optical point of view, the center of the colony is much more opaque (i.e. there is a greater concentration of molecules absorbing the light radiation). The following approach is used to simulate this behavior. A specific blurring is applied to the background image in the regions where the colony models will be attached. In particular, for such regions, every pixel color $\mathbf{b}'_{x,y}$ is replaced with a weighted sum of $\overline{\mathbf{b}}$ and $\mathbf{b}_{x,y}$, where $\overline{\mathbf{b}}$ is the average color of background pixels inside the region, and $\mathbf{b}_{x,y}$ is the actual pixel value (see Eq. 5.3). The weighting factor $\alpha_{x,y}$ follows a normal distribution, enhancing the blurring effect in the innermost part of the patch. Formally:

$$\mathbf{b}'_{x,y} = \alpha_{x,y}(\overline{\mathbf{b}}) + (1 - \alpha_{x,y})\mathbf{b}_{x,y} \text{ with } \alpha_{x,y} = \frac{1}{2\pi\sigma^2}e^{-\frac{(x-x_0)^2+(y-y_0)^2}{2\sigma^2}} \qquad (5.3)$$

---

[5] http://www.copanusa.com/products/automation/wasplab//%7Bpath=.

5 Segmentation of Petri Plate Images for Automatic ...

Table 5.1 Segmentation results, obtained using the three different experimental setups

Experimental setup	Pixel accuracy (%)	Mean IoU (%)
Synthetic images	98.29	82.79
Real images	99.19	85.30
Synthetic and real images	99.26	86.33

where (x, y) are the spatial coordinates of the patch and (x_0, y_0) are the coordinates of its center. The colony models are then added to the blurred background image, producing the final result. A dedicated procedure also accounts for the overlapping of different colonies. Indeed, in the overlapping regions, each pixel is associated with the colony with the nearest centroid, and the area near the contours is Gaussian-smoothed to avoid a crisp visual separation. Finally, to obtain a photorealistic effect, the style transfer algorithm proposed in [37] is employed to further improve the quality of the generated images.

Semantic segmentation with the Pyramid Scene Parsing network
In this chapter, the Pyramid Scene Parsing (PSP) network [55] is used to perform the semantic segmentation of the bacterial colonies. The experiments described in this section were conducted on the MicrobIA Haemolysis dataset, collecting 324 images of blood agar plates. However, thanks to the synthetic plate generator, a deep convolutional neural network could potentially be used to segment other types of Petri dish images as well.

The PSP is a deep fully-convolutional neural network, built on the ResNet model [31] for image classification. To enlarge the receptive field of the neural network, a set of dilated convolutions [18] replaces standard convolutions in the ResNet part of the network. Then, a pyramid pooling module is used to gather context information, followed by both an upsampling and a concatenation layer, to form the final feature representation. This representation is then fed into a convolutional layer, to get the expected per-pixel prediction.

To establish the contribution of the injection of synthetic data during training, we proceeded with the following experimental setup:

- Synthetic images—training on synthetic data only;
- Real images—training on real data from the MicrobIA dataset only;
- Synthetic and real images—training on synthetic data and fine-tuning on real data from the MicrobIA dataset.

The obtained results are reported in Table 5.1.

The segmentation model, trained on real images from the MicrobIA Dataset, produces a mean intersection over union (IoU) of 85.30%, which can be considered as a baseline. When the network is pre-trained on artificial examples and fine-tuned on real data, an improvement of 1.03% in the mean IoU is obtained on the test set. Instead, when only synthetic data are used during training, the mean IoU drops down by 2.51%. Both these results prove the importance of the injection of synthetic data

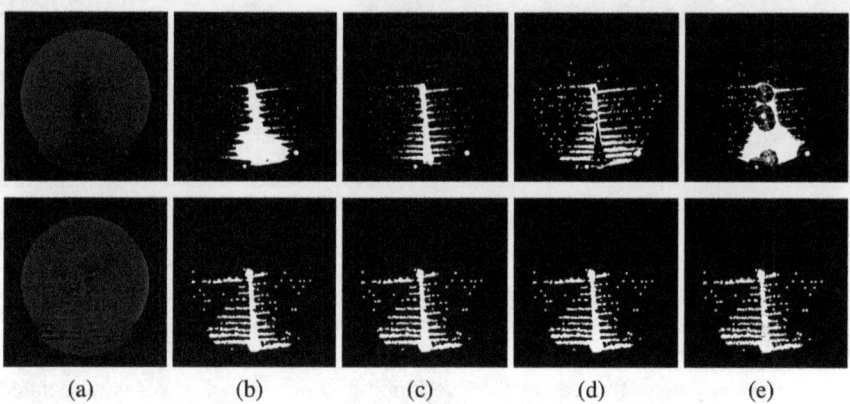

Fig. 5.10 Original images. **a** Results obtained with synthetic images, real images and both real and synthetic images, respectively, in **b–d**. Ground-Truth images (**e**)

during training. In particular, the small difference in performance obtained using only real or only synthetic data is an interesting result. This suggests that, when real agar plate images are not available (with respect to different culture grounds or bacterial species), a deep segmentation network can be used anyway, trained on synthetic data only.

In Fig. 5.10, a qualitative comparison of the results is shown. In the first row, we can observe that, using only synthetic images, the network learns to segment the isolated colonies but fails to identify the confluent growth. This behavior can be observed in almost all the images in the test set. We can also note that the network is able to recognize the colony shape more accurately when trained on both real and synthetic data, although it is not clear if this is due to the augmented number of available examples or to the rough annotation often provided in the MicrobIA Dataset [see (e) in the first row of Fig. 5.10]. Instead, in the second row, an example in which synthetic images suffice to obtain the correct result is depicted.

5.3.3 Colony Classification and Count

The main focus of this chapter is the semantic segmentation of Petri dish images, using both standard computer vision and deep learning techniques. However, segmentation is only the first step towards implementing an automated urine culture test reporting tool. The automatic examination of the image of a Petri dish consists of defining what types of infections have grown on the plate and in what quantity, i.e. carrying out the classification and counting of the colonies, which will be explained in the following.

Colony classification

The classification of the bacterial species grown on a Petri dish is a very difficult task and, actually, biologists are able to perform this operation using their a priori knowledge of the problem and thanks to the extraordinary ability of the human visual system.

Some culture grounds are studied to produce, in the grown colonies, specific features that allow to distinguish among different species of bacteria. An example of a widely used culture ground with this characteristic is the UriSelect 4, a chromogenic, milky, and opaque medium, used to isolate and enumerate microorganisms of the urinary tract. UriSelect 4 is specifically designed to identify infections by color. It incorporates two chromogenic substrates for the detection of β-galactosidase and β-glucosidase enzymes. Strains that produce β-glucosidase, such as enterococci and the KES group, form colonies that generate a turquoise/purplish blue coloration. Instead, *Escherichia coli* evidences red–pink colonies, because of the β-galactosidase production. Finally, Uriselect 4 also contains tryptophan, in order to detect members of the Proteae group (Proteus-Providencia-Morganella), that appear as brown-orange colonies, due to tryptophane désaminase.

However, distinguishing different types of infections within these macro-classes is a very difficult task, at least if the classification is based on color information only. To face this problem, a multi-stage procedure was settled, aimed at partitioning, at first, among infections which share similar chromatic features, producing a sort of pre-classification. After that, different classifiers, trained on both chromatic features and class-specific auxiliary information, are implemented to distinguish within each group. Actually, the pre-classification phase reveals the (expected) existence of three main groups, which can be identified by their color: red for *E. coli*, blue for Enterococcus Faecalis, KES and *Streptococcus agalactiae*, and yellow for Pseudomonas, Proteus and *Staphylococcus aureus*.[6] Among the seven diverse types of UTIs, only *E. coli* is characterized by red colonies, so that it can be recognized as a result of this step. Considering the other two classes, instead, the pre-classification phase allows only an infected/not-infected response, with further, specific, information needed to identify each particular type of infection. For instance, in the blue class, the colony diameter is useful for discriminating between *Enterococcus faecalis* (small colonies, 0.5–1.5 mm) and KES (2–3 mm), whereas, in the yellow class, Proteus infections can be distinguished from the others by the presence of a halo surrounding the colonies.

To collect the data for the pre-classification module, the (a, b) color components of the colony in the CIE-Lab space can be considered. Based on these two color features a simple MLP architecture or a multi-class SVM with a Gaussian kernel can be trained. In the last case, to face the multi-class problem at hand, our approach consisted in training three classifiers able to recognize one category out of three, in a one-vs-all framework. In both cases, an accuracy above 99.7% can be reached.

---

[6] By the way, according to the manufacturer specification, UriSelect 4 can be used for the direct identification of *E. coli* (pink–red colony), Enterococcus (blue colony), and Proteus (yellow–brown colony), as well as for the presumptive identification of other species.

Considering the classification of blue colonies (*Enterococcus faecalis*, KES, *Streptococcus agalactiae*), a fundamental issue still arises, since unpredictable chromatic variations may be revealed when multiple infections are present and overlap on the same Petri dish. To address this problem, isolated colonies must be recognized first, then this information is used to forecast the kind of UTI possibly present in the overlapping regions. A relevant example is related to the contemporary presence of *E. coli* and *E. faecalis*, which produce overlapping regions very similar, in color, to a KES infection. This is a well-known situation and, therefore, such an a priori knowledge may be used during the classification stage. When isolated colonies of *E. coli* and *E. faecalis* are detected, if a KES region is also detected on the same dish, the latter is classified as a possible Coli/Faecalis overlapping region, which is also statistically more likely than having the simultaneous presence of *E. coli*, *E. faecalis* and KES.[7] Based on the experiments, such an assumption significantly improves the classification accuracy. Indeed, results obtained again by using an MLP and an SVM allow to get comparable performance, with about 82.6% of accuracy. Lastly, the same training approach was applied for discriminating within the yellow class (Pseudomonas, Proteus and *Staphylococcus aureus*), with comparable performance. However, for the yellow class, the significance of the obtained results, from the statistical point of view, is very low, due to the very small number of available examples. Since the three types of infections that produce yellow/brown colony are quite distinguishable from a visual inspection, it is likely that a greater number of examples will actually guarantee a performance boost. Finally, it is worth noting that about 70% of the urinary tract infections are due to *E. coli* bacterium, which can be classified during the first step of the procedure, with an accuracy of about 100%.

Colony count

The second fundamental step in automatic reporting of urine culture tests based on images of Petri dishes is the evaluation of the infection severity, which corresponds to counting the number of colonies grown on the substrate after the incubation phase. The severity is expressed in CFU/ml (Colony-Forming Units per ml) by using a logarithmic evaluation scale. Usually, a plate can be considered positive if the number of microorganisms per milliliter of urine exceeds 10^5. Actually, the bacterial load is obtained by multiplying the number of colonies counted on the dish by the inverse of the seeding dilution rate. Colony counting is a repetitive and time demanding task, inherently prone to human error. Moreover, it should be observed that calculating the microbial density from the colony count have some intrinsic limitations, due to the fact that the colony-forming units can be a single cell, a chain of cells or a whole clump of cells.

To face these problems, we propose an automatic procedure aimed at estimating the infection severity. An automated system is not affected by fatigue and can produce quickly accurate results. For this reason, if used as a support system, it can be highly beneficial in reducing the cost and efforts of the colony counting procedure. Our approach consists in a multi-stage algorithm, based on a prior search of individual,

---

[7] Actually, Petri dishes on which many different infections are simultaneously present are considered to be contaminated and are of little interest to biologists.

5 Segmentation of Petri Plate Images for Automatic ...

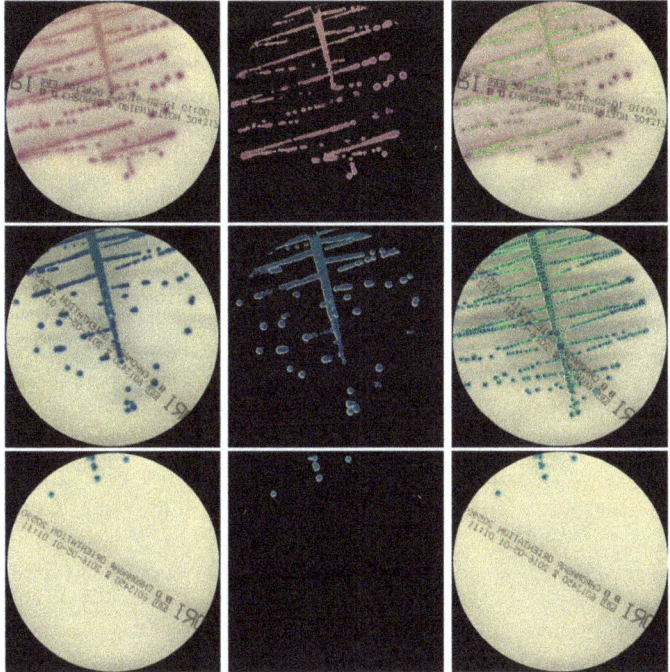

Fig. 5.11 In the first column, the original images, in the second, the output of the background removal procedure, and, in the last one, the extracted colonies, ready to be counted

not overlapping, colonies which are used to enucleate colonies belonging to slightly overlapping regions. After the ground seed identification phase, a binary image is constructed, where the background is represented by the substrate and the foreground by the colonies. Single colonies normally show a roughly circular shape and can be easily identified according to this feature. In particular, the smallest enclosing circle is evaluated for each connected component and, if the ratio between the circular area and the area of the component is less than a fixed threshold (chosen via a trial-and-error procedure), it is considered to be a colony. This simple approach is not effective in significantly overlapping regions. In this case, the convexity of each colony contour is calculated, also highlighting sub-contours with a convex shape. Then, the best ellipse (in the least square sense), that fits each sub-contour, is selected, and used to build a score matrix, that takes into account both the axes rate and the ellipse points belonging (or not) to the contour. Finally, the score matrix is used to remove all the non-relevant ellipses. Some results obtained with the proposed processing pipeline are reported in Fig. 5.11.

The colonies discovered in this way are counted to estimate the infection severity. Following this procedure, the obtained responses of the automated system coincide with those of the biologists (who represent our ground truth) with an accuracy of 92.1%.

5.4 Conclusions

Urinary tract infections (UTIs) can be originated by diverse microbes, including fungi, viruses, and bacteria, being bacteria the most common cause. Normally, bacteria that enter the urinary tract are rapidly removed by the body before they produce symptoms. However, sometimes, bacteria overcome the body's natural defences, with UTIs currently affecting more than 150 million people annually. In this chapter, with the aim of providing the description of a whole software pipeline to automatically analyse Petri plates coming from urine culture exams, we have described, in a historical perspective, some techniques useful to preprocess images of Petri dishes. In particular, we have focused our attention on segmentation techniques—starting from classical computer vision approaches to modern CNN-based models—able to enucleate bacterial colonies from the culture ground, for the successive steps of infection classification and colony count. From a broader perspective, this work describes the evolutionary parable of computer vision in the last decade, with the progressive transition from classical image processing techniques to the intensive use of deep learning. The main limitation of deep learning methods, at least for medical image processing, remains the need for a large number of examples—a topic addressed in the chapter through the generation of synthetic data. However, the creation of support tools for the automatic analysis of screening tests remains of fundamental importance, due to their ability to relieve doctors of heavy and repetitive tasks, without ignoring their invaluable experience.

References

1. National institute of diabetes and digestive and kidney diseases, urinary tract infections in adults. URL https://www.niddk.nih.gov/health-information/health-topics/urologic-disease/bladder-infection-uti-in-adults
2. Alexander, N., Glick, D.: Automatic counting of bacterial cultures–a new machine. IRE Trans. Med. Electron., 89–92 (1958)
3. Andreini, P., Bonechi, S., Bianchini, M., Baghini, A., Bianchi, G., Guerri, F., Galano, A., Mecocci, A., Vaggelli, G.: Extraction of high level visual features for the automatic recognition of UTIs. In: International Workshop on Fuzzy Logic and Applications, pp. 249–259. Springer (2016)
4. Andreini, P., Bonechi, S., Bianchini, M., Garzelli, A., Mecocci, A.: ABLE: An automated bacterial load estimator for the urinoculture screening. In: Proceedings of the 5th International Conference on Pattern Recognition Applications and Methods, pp. 573–580. SCITEPRESS–Science and Technology Publications, Lda (2016)
5. Andreini, P., Bonechi, S., Bianchini, M., Garzelli, A., Mecocci, A.: Automatic image classification for the urinoculture screening. Comput. Biol. Med. **70**, 12–22 (2016)
6. Andreini, P., Bonechi, S., Bianchini, M., Mecocci, A., Di Massa, V.: Automatic image analysis and classification for urinary bacteria infection screening. In: Murino, V., Puppo, E. (eds.) Image Analysis and Processing–ICIAP 2015, pp. 635–646. Springer International Publishing, Cham (2015)

7. Andreini, P., Bonechi, S., Bianchini, M., Mecocci, A., Di Massa, V.: Automatic image classification for the urinoculture screening. In: Intelligent Decision Technologies, pp. 31–42. Springer (2015)
8. Andreini, P., Bonechi, S., Bianchini, M., Mecocci, A., Scarselli, F.: A deep learning approach to bacterial colony segmentation. In: International Conference on Artificial Neural Networks, pp. 522–533. Springer (2018)
9. Andreini, P., Bonechi, S., Bianchini, M., Mecocci, A., Scarselli, F.: Image generation by GAN and style transfer for agar plate image segmentation. Comput. Methods Prog. Biomed. **184** (2020)
10. Andreini, P., Bonechi, S., Bianchini, M., Mecocci, A., Scarselli, F., Sodi, A.: A two stage GAN for high resolution retinal image generation and segmentation. arXiv preprint, arXiv:1907.12296 (2019)
11. Ballabio, C., Venturi, N., Scala, M.R., Mocarelli, P., Brambilla, P.: Evaluation of an automated method for urinoculture screening. Microbiol. Med. **5**(3), 178–180 (2010)
12. Bonechi, S., Andreini, P., Bianchini, M., Scarselli, F.: COCO_TS dataset: pixel–level annotations based on weak supervision for scene text segmentation. In: International Conference on Artificial Neural Networks, pp. 238–250. Springer (2019)
13. Bonechi, S., Bianchini, M., Bongini, P., Ciano, G., Giacomini, G., Rosai, R., Tognetti, L., Rossi, A., Andreini, P.: Fusion of visual and anamnestic data for the classification of skin lesions with deep learning. In: International Conference on Image Analysis and Processing, pp. 211–219. Springer (2019)
14. Bonechi, S., Bianchini, M., Scarselli, F., Andreini, P.: Weak supervision for generating pixel-level annotations in scene text segmentation. Pattern Recogn. Lett. **138**, 1–7 (2020)
15. Brugger, S.D., Baumberger, C., Jost, M., Jenni, W., Brugger, U., Mühlemann, K.: Automated counting of bacterial colony forming units on agar plates. PloS one **7**(3) (2012)
16. Busto, P.P., Liebelt, J., Gall, J.: Adaptation of synthetic data for coarse-to-fine viewpoint refinement. In: BMVC, pp. 14.1–14.12 (2015)
17. Caruana, R., Lou, Y., Gehrke, J., Koch, P., Sturm, M., Elhadad, N.: Intelligible models for healthcare: Predicting pneumonia risk and hospital 30–day readmission. In: Proceedings of the 21th ACM SIGKDD International Conference on Knowledge Discovery and Data Mining, pp. 1721–1730 (2015)
18. Chen, L.C., Papandreou, G., Kokkinos, I., Murphy, K., Yuille, A.L.: Deeplab: Semantic image segmentation with deep convolutional nets, atrous convolution, and fully connected CRFs. IEEE Trans. Pattern Anal. Mach. Intell. **40**(4), 834–848 (2017)
19. Corkidi, G., Diaz-Uribe, R., Folch-Mallol, J., Nieto-Sotelo, J.: COVASIAM: An image analysis method that allows detection of confluent microbial colonies and colonies of various sizes for automated counting. Appl. Environ. Microbiol. **64**(4), 1400–1404 (1998)
20. Csurka, G., Dance, C.R., Fan, L., Willamowski, J., Bray, C.: Visual categorization with bags of keypoints. Proc. ECCV **1**, 1–2 (2004)
21. Deng, J., Dong, W., Socher, R., Li, L.J., Li, K., Fei-Fei, L.: Imagenet: A large–scale hierarchical image database. In: IEEE Conference on Computer Vision and Pattern Recognition, 2009. CVPR 2009, pp. 248–255. IEEE (2009)
22. Esteva, A., Kuprel, B., Novoa, R.A., Ko, J., Swetter, S.M., Blau, H.M., Thrun, S.: Dermatologist-level classification of skin cancer with deep neural networks. Nature **542**(7639), 115–118 (2017)
23. Everingham, M., Eslami, S.A., Van Gool, L., Williams, C.K., Winn, J., Zisserman, A.: The Pascal visual object classes challenge: a retrospective. Int. J. Comput. Vision **111**(1), 98–136 (2015)
24. Ferrari, A., Lombardi, S., Signoroni, A.: Bacterial colony counting with convolutional neural networks in digital microbiology imaging. Pattern Recognit. **61**, 629–640 (2017)
25. Fu, Z., Wang, L.: Color image segmentation using Gaussian mixture model and EM algorithm. In: Communications in Computer and Information Science, vol. 346, pp. 61–66. Springer (2012)

26. Geissmann, Q.: OpenCFU, a new free and open-source software to count cell colonies and other circular objects. PloS one **8**(2) (2013)
27. Gulrajani, I., Ahmed, F., Arjovsky, M., Dumoulin, V., Courville, A.: Improved training of Wasserstein GANs. arXiv preprint arXiv:1704.00028 (2017)
28. Gupta, A., Vedaldi, A., Zisserman, A.: Synthetic data for text localisation in natural images. In: IEEE Conference on Computer Vision and Pattern Recognition (2016)
29. Handa, A., Patraucean, V., Badrinarayanan, V., Stent, S., Cipolla, R.: Synthcam3d: Semantic understanding with synthetic indoor scenes. arXiv preprint arXiv:1505.00171 (2015)
30. Hattori, H., Naresh Boddeti, V., Kitani, K.M., Kanade, T.: Learning scene–specific pedestrian detectors without real data. In: Proceedings of the IEEE Conference on Computer Vision and Pattern Recognition, pp. 3819–3827 (2015)
31. He, K., Zhang, X., Ren, S., Sun, J.: Deep residual learning for image recognition. In: Proceedings of the IEEE Conference on Computer Vision and Pattern Recognition, pp. 770–778 (2016)
32. Jaderberg, M., Simonyan, K., Vedaldi, A., Zisserman, A.: Reading text in the wild with convolutional neural networks. Int. J. Comput. Vis. **116**(1), 1–20 (2016)
33. Ji, Z., Huang, Y., Sun, Q., Cao, G.: A spatially constrained generative asymmetric Gaussian mixture model for image segmentation. J. Vis. Commun. Image Represent. **40**(B), 611–626 (2016)
34. Koniusz, P., Yan, F., Mikolajczyk, K.: Comparison of mid-level feature coding approaches and pooling strategies in visual concept detection. Comput. Vis. Image Underst. **117**(5), 479–492 (2013)
35. Krizhevsky, A., Sutskever, I., Hinton, G.E.: Imagenet classification with deep convolutional neural networks. In: Advances in Neural Information Processing Systems, pp. 1097–1105 (2012)
36. Kulwa, F., Li, C., Zhao, X., Cai, B., Xu, N., Qi, S., Chen, S., Teng, Y.: A state-of-the-art survey for microorganism image segmentation methods and future potential. IEEE Access **7**, 100243–100269 (2019)
37. Li, Y., Fang, C., Yang, J., Wang, Z., Lu, X., Yang, M.H.: Universal style transfer via feature transforms. Adv. Neural. Inf. Process. Syst. **2017**, 386–396 (2017)
38. Lin, T.Y., Maire, M., Belongie, S., Hays, J., Perona, P., Ramanan, D., Dollár, P., Zitnick, C.L.: Microsoft COCO: Common objects in context. In: European Conference on Computer Vision, pp. 740–755. Springer (2014)
39. Liu, A., Liu, Z., Song, L., Han, D.: Adaptive ideal image reconstruction for bacteria colony detection. In: Information Technology and Agricultural Engineering, pp. 353–360. Springer (2012)
40. Long, J., Shelhamer, E., Darrell, T.: Fully convolutional networks for semantic segmentation. In: Proceedings of the IEEE Conference on Computer Vision and Pattern Recognition, pp. 3431–3440 (2015)
41. Mahmood, F., Chen, R., Durr, N.J.: Unsupervised reverse domain adaptation for synthetic medical images via adversarial training. IEEE Trans. Med. Imaging **37**(12), 2572–2581 (2018)
42. Mansberg, H.: Automatic particle and bacterial colony counter. Science **126**(3278), 823–827 (1957)
43. Marin, J., Vázquez, D., Gerónimo, D., López, A.M.: Learning appearance in virtual scenarios for pedestrian detection. In: 2010 IEEE Conference on Computer Vision and Pattern Recognition (CVPR), pp. 137–144. IEEE (2010)
44. Masala, G.L., Bottigli, U., Brunetti, A., Carpinelli, M., Diaz, N., Fiori, P.L., Golosio, B., Oliva, P., Stegel, G.: Automatic cell colony counting by region-growing approach. Nuovo Cimento-C **30**(6), 633–646 (2007)
45. Mukherjee, D.P., Pal, A., Sarma, S.E., Majumder, D.D.: Bacterial colony counting using distance transform. Int. J. Biomed. Comput. **38**(2), 131–140 (1995)
46. Papon, J., Schoeler, M.: Semantic pose using deep networks trained on synthetic RGB–D. In: Proceedings of the IEEE International Conference on Computer Vision, pp. 774–782 (2015)
47. Reynolds, D.A.: Encyclopedia of Biometrics, chap. Gaussian Mixture Models (2009)

48. Richter, S.R., Vineet, V., Roth, S., Koltun, V.: Playing for data: ground truth from computer games. In: European Conference on Computer Vision, pp. 102–118. Springer (2016)
49. Ronneberger, O., Fischer, P., Brox, T.: U-net: Convolutional networks for biomedical image segmentation. In: International Conference on Medical Image Computing and Computer-Assisted Intervention, pp. 234–241. Springer (2015)
50. Ros, G., Sellart, L., Materzynska, J., Vazquez, D., Lopez, A.M.: The SYNTHIA dataset: A large collection of synthetic images for semantic segmentation of urban scenes. In: Proceedings of the IEEE Conference on Computer Vision and Pattern Recognition, pp. 3234–3243 (2016)
51. Rossi, A., Hosseinzadeh, M., Bianchini, M., Scarselli, F., Huisman, H.: Multi-modal Siamese networks for diagnostically similar lesion retrieval in prostate MRI. IEEE Trans. Med. Imaging **40**(3), 986–995 (2021)
52. Roy, K.K., Phadikar, A.: Automated medical image segmentation: A survey. In: Proceedings of International Conference on Computing, Communication & Manufacturing (2014)
53. Tognetti, L., Bonechi, S., Andreini, P., Bianchini, M., Scarselli, F., Cevenini, G., Moscarella, E., Farnetani, F., Longo, C., Lallas, A., et al.: A new deep learning approach integrated with clinical data for the dermoscopic differentiation of early melanomas from atypical nevi. J. Dermatol, Sci (2020)
54. Zhang, C., Chen, W.B., Liu, W.L., Chen, C.B.: An automated bacterial colony counting system. In: IEEE International Conference on Sensor Networks, Ubiquitous and Trustworthy Computing, 2008. SUTC'08, pp. 233–240. IEEE (2008)
55. Zhao, H., Shi, J., Qi, X., Wang, X., Jia, J.: Pyramid scene parsing network. In: 2017 IEEE Conference on Computer Vision and Pattern Recognition (CVPR), pp. 6230–6239 (2017)

Chapter 6
Repurposing Routine Imaging for Cancer Biomarker Discovery Using Machine Learning

James W. Wang and Matt Williams

Abstract Cancer care generates large quantities of medical imaging data during diagnosis, treatment and follow-up. This chapter presents an overview on the clinical background and setting for the opportunistic development of cancer imaging biomarkers from such routine imaging. The chapter is aimed at the clinicians with a data science interest as well as data scientists with a clinical interest, and touches on computational approaches on radiological data to solve clinical problems. The chapter outlines the technical considerations of imaging, where it occurs in the cancer pathway, and challenges to overcome in order to develop new radiomic features.

Keywords Cancer biomarker · Cancer radiomics · Convoluted neural networks · Medical image processing · Sarcopenia

6.1 Introduction

Biomedical imaging is a cornerstone of clinical practice, and forms a key part of diagnosis, together with clinical review and biological investigations. Routine clinical practice generates a wealth of radiological data, often in response to a specific clinical query at a single time point (e.g. looking for pneumonia on a chest radiograph). It is uncommon for this data to be used beyond its immediate purpose or as a historical reference. Yet scans contain additional information beyond that needed to answer the original question they were requested for, with incidental clinical findings present in a quarter of all scans [1]. Incidental findings can be both beneficial and harmful. At times, they lead to unnecessary investigation and treatment of benign pathology. At other times, 64% of cancers found in a screening programme for asymptomatic colorectal cancers were in other organs allowing their early detection and treatment [2]. These findings represent some of the imaging by-products that can be harnessed for additional clinical utility.

J. W. Wang (✉) · M. Williams
Computational Oncology Lab, Institute for Global Health Innovation, Imperial College London & Radiotherapy Department, Charing Cross Hospital, London, UK
e-mail: james.wang04@imperial.ac.uk

Medical imaging visualises tissues and organs through electromagnetic radiation, magnetic resonance and ultrasonography. Each is a technologically unique modality, and therefore a universal approach at harvesting meaningful incidental data is not feasible. Methods need to be tailored against the clinical context, patient, as well as the imaging modality. Both normal and pathological scan findings that specifically link to human physiological processes are categorised as biomarkers, which are measurable findings of a physiological state. Biomarker research has the potential to change how we view and treat diseases, and is continuously being updated with new understanding of existing imaging features and emergence of new imaging technology. However, new technology carries financial risks and time investment, and when layered onto existing standards of practice adds to both scanning time and training requirements ultimately impacting existing bottlenecks within radiology, that of scanner (and staff) time and patient time.

The scale of imaging data being generated annually is massive. 42.1 million imaging tests were reported in England alone in 2017, with the most common investigation being plain radiography (22.9 million), followed by ultrasonography (9.37 million) and Computerized Tomography (CT—4.82 million) [3]. The demand for imaging increases annually, increasing by 3.6% in England in 2017. Cancer care (oncology) is heavily reliant on imaging, as it is a disease that has the propensity to spread throughout the body. Cancer cells can acquire the ability to travel through bloodstream and lymphatics and lodge in distant organs in a process known as metastases. The detection of these metastases has a drastic impact on the treatment goal (cure versus palliation), and the response of the cancer to an ongoing treatment. Atypical surveillance schedule in a metastatic patient usually consists of scans every three months, accruing dozens of scans in their patient journey. Oncology is therefore a clinical speciality with a radiology rich component ripe for biomarker exploration. All medical imaging is stored digitally, representing an ever-increasing dataset that can be tapped for biomarker research. Current medical imaging is interpreted radiologists, human specialists trained via pattern recognition to recognize pathology. The limited pool of domain expertise is already rationed within clinical services, and thus represents an obstacle of scale in the face of ever-increasing workload, and limits the amount of time that can be dedicated to the generation and screening of new radiological biomarkers.

With advances in processor speeds in computer chips, computational power has become cheaper and easier to access. This has allowed renewed interest in computationally taxing methods such as machine learning (ML). Machine learning is the use of algorithms to can learn complex patterns in vast amounts of data order to predict outcomes. Machine learning is particularly suited to high-dimensional data, where data points per sample exceed sample size by many orders of magnitude. One example of high dimensional data is medical imaging, where each set of images contains thousands of voxel datapoints, their spatial relationship and meta-data such as time and age of the patient. High dimensionality combined with availability of large digitalised datasets has therefore made radiology a fertile ground for machine learning applications, where studies have demonstrated diagnostic equivalence between a machine learning and a radiologist for specific tasks such as breast cancer screening

[4]. Although imaging data will vary depending on modality and acquisition, the formatting remains reasonably structured in the form of voxel-coordinate pairings and accompanying meta-data, as opposed to unstructured free text records. The goal of this chapter is threefold: (i) to introduce the clinical environment in which cancer imaging occurs; (ii) to navigate the opportunities and challenges for computational research in this space; (iii) provide an example as one of the starting points for both clinicians and computer scientists on applying machine learning to cancer imaging.

6.1.1 Imaging Modalities in Cancer Care

To understand where we can generate additional clinical utility from cancer imaging, we have to cover the imaging modalities and how they apply to cancer care. Cancer is a disease born of accumulated DNA mutations within a cell which have escaped the body's natural efforts of repair and containment. Thus, pro-proliferative signals are amplified and anti-proliferative signals are dampened, leading to growth and the eventual potential to invade locally and spread to seed distally. One cancer cell can multiply into generations of clones, growing large enough to be eventually visualised on medical imaging. Cancer cell quantity is a function of tumour volume, meaning that a 0.5 cm lesion typically contains 10 million cells and a 1 cm lesion will contain 100 million cells [6]. These are the minimum thresholds for radiological detection but typically still too small to be symptomatic, which is why tumours are often detected after they have grown large enough to produce symptoms.

A summary of common imaging technologies are outlined in Table 6.1. There are well established protocols dictating the use of specific modalities for specific cancers. These are picked on the balance of accessibility and anatomical definition in relation to organs being investigated. Diagnostic radiology interrogates anatomy using these modalities to evaluate structure and function. Interventional radiology combines

Table 6.1 Summary of common medical imaging technologies

Imaging modality	Radiograph	Ultrasound	Computed tomography	Magnetic resonance imaging
Technology	Ionising radiation	Sound waves	Ionising radiation	Magnet
Result	2D	Dynamic 2D	3D	3D
Deployability	Quick, cheap	Quick, cheap	Quick	Long, expensive
Indication	Bone, lung pathology, mammograms	(Superficial) Soft tissue, perinatal	Internal structures	Internal structures

diagnostics with procedural elements to e.g., obtain biopsy or better target an intervention. Nuclear medicine combines radioisotopes with diagnostics and intervention to better visualise and target cancer tissues.

The most prevalent radiological examination is the plain radiograph, a two-dimensional snapshot of select anatomy onto radiosensitive film via the projection of X-rays. Radiographs are quick to acquire and form the majority of first line imaging investigations done in acute and primary care, and can be the first visualisation of cancer e.g., in the lungs of someone presenting with a persistent cough. X-rays are a form of ionizing radiation, meaning that they have the potential to interact with and disrupt cellular DNA they pass through. Given that cancer is a disease of DNA mutation, one of the main risks with investigations producing ionizing radiation is secondary cancer risk.

Ultrasonography (US) is portable, flexible, does not require ionizing radiation, but is the most operator dependent. This leads to large variations in sensitivity dependent on equipment, clinical indication, patient morphology, reference standards and operator experience. Scan results are displayed as a two-dimensional acoustic impedance map from the reflection of ultrasound waves generated by the probe. Because US has limited efficacy at depth and does not work with air-filled cavities, it is better suited to superficial anatomy such as in the breast or neck area. Scan interpretation is done in real time, supported by a digital set of images captured during scanning which are contextual to the immediate operator and therefore difficult for others to interpret.

Ionizing radiation is also used in computed tomography (CT) scanning, which is capable of quickly reconstructing three-dimensional anatomy for the entire body after passing through a circumferential scanner. Compared to a plain radiograph, CT requires more advanced hardware and longer scanning sequences. CT plays a key part in detecting and measuring solid malignancy burden in the body and is usually paired with tools such as the Response Evaluation Criteria in Solid Tumours (RECIST), but incurs a higher dose of ionizing radiation compared to radiographs [5]. A single chest radiograph is the equivalent of five days of background radiation whilst an abdominal CT is the equivalent of 80 chest radiographs [6]. Excess radiation can be harmful by inducing cardiovascular disease and tumour development thus limiting the frequency of CT use, especially outside the field of cancer care or in the curative setting. This restriction is relaxed when the benefits of image visualisation outweigh the radiation dose, such as response assessment in an individual who has established incurable cancer. CT can be combined with radioisotope scans, which use radioactively labelled glucose to demonstrate metabolic active tissues such as cancer.

Magnetic Resonance Imaging (MRI) interrogates the behaviour of hydrogen atoms abundant water and fat tissues within the body through applied strong magnetic field. The scanner requirements are the highest in both hardware, staff and time. MRI is particularly beneficial in distinguishing soft tissue pathology and has a range of acquisition settings allowing for suppression and enhancement of specific tissues. Like US, MRI does not utilise ionizing radiation, and is therefore free of the concerns of secondary cancer. MRI is used in the evaluation of brain lesions and in assessing the detail of pelvic organs (such in the case of rectal cancers). Example slices of

6 Repurposing Routine Imaging for Cancer Biomarker ...

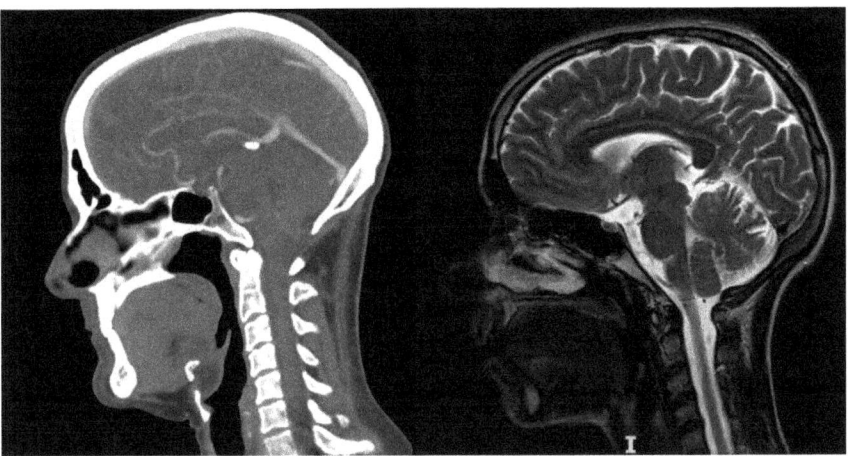

Fig. 6.1 Reconstructed CT (left) and MRI (right) images. Bone shows as white on CT, while soft tissue is better captured on MRI

reconstructed MRI and CT images of the head in normal individuals are shown in Fig. 6.1 for comparison.

Ultrasonography aside, clinical interpretation is usually divorced from the scanning process. The separation of image capture and reporting prevents any post-hoc manipulation once exported from the image acquisition equipment, but allows radiologists flexibility in reporting. A goal at this point may be to replace the human element with AI that automatically interprets a scan. AI is capable of performing a singular task well, but lacks the flexibility to interact with complex human biology and is therefore unlikely to replace human radiologists in the near future [4]. For example, in a patient with symptoms suggestive of cancer, an AI might be able to exclude cancer without correctly diagnosing the underlying illness. Furthermore, much AI work relies on an established "ground truth", which can be diagnostic labels against which the algorithm can train. Medicine remains an evolving science, and not all of it is understood, hence if new pathologies (e.g. COVID-19 infective changes) emerges, a pre-trained AI would be unable to diagnose this.

6.1.2 Imaging in the Cancer Pathway

To consider where in the clinical course imaging is performed and thus the opportunities in which to intervene, we can follow a typical patient pathway. A single cancer cell is insufficient to manifest symptoms, and so all patients can be expected to have an asymptomatic period until a cancer has grown large enough to disrupt normal body functions. After diagnosis, patients who proceed to treatment do so with the goal of either cure or palliation. Imaging plays an important part of monitoring the status of the cancer throughout the treatment. Even when treatment is immediately indicated, as in the case of a slow growing benign tumour, imaging is often employed as part of surveillance. It is important to note that a significant subset of cancer patients will have a very limited or non-existent amount of imaging data. This occurs in cancers where imaging serves no clinical use, such as in benign skin cancers cured with simple surgery.

Patients are diagnosed with cancer via screening services or because they have symptoms. Screening programmes aim to capture patients in a phase where their cancer is small and contained enough to be cured. The UK national breast screening programme is the only radiology-based programme, where women over the age of 50 and certain risk thresholds (such as a strong family history of the disease) are invited for regular mammograms. Mammograms are 2-dimensional radiographs that image each breast individually.

New patients with symptoms suspicious of cancer require investigations to confirm or exclude cancer. Three-dimensional imaging is not always necessary from the outset, especially if there are concerns regarding excess ionizing radiation. Investigations are directed to the anatomy of the associated symptom and the best modality for that anatomy. A headache can be investigated with an MRI of the head whereas a chest radiograph is the first step in investigating a persistent cough. If a cancer is diagnosed, completion of radiological staging is necessary for the cancer. This is also anatomically dependant on the primary cancer and its route of spread, but generally consists of regional or whole-body CT. Subsequent to initial treatment, patients will enter a follow up imaging schedule to (a) confirm treatment success and (b) monitor for any sign of recurrence. This schedule can be interrupted by new symptoms or clinical deterioration which may prompt an earlier re-assessment of the cancer status. Follow up imaging uses the same modality employed in initial staging, and thereby provides a longitudinal data-set within the same subject to chart the evolution of cancer as it undergoes treatment. As a consequence, many cancer patients will undergo significant amounts of imaging during their diagnosis and treatment. The stages of a cancer journey and some of the imaging used within are listed in Table 6.2.

Table 6.2 Clinical stages of cancer journey

Clinical course	Asymptomatic	Symptomatic	Post-treatment	Surveillance	Deterioration
Radiology indication	Screening, incidental finding	Diagnostics and staging	Response assessment	Monitoring	Disease re-assessment
Examples (Clinical indication)	Mammogram (National screening programme) CT lung (High risk smokers)	Chest radiograph (Persistent cough) Ultrasound (Breast lump investigation)	CT body (Re-evaluation of cancer load) MRI head (Brain cancer)	CT body (Re-evaluation of cancer load) MRI head (Brain cancer)	CT body (Re-evaluation of cancer load) MRI head (Brain cancer)

6.2 Cancer Biomarker Research

Disease results from physiological interplay between genetics and the environment detrimental to the host. Both normal and pathological phenotypes are the result of complex interactions between molecular pathways that are not yet fully understood. Biomarkers are attempts to find measurable indicators of a physiological state and changes to that state. These encompass most medical investigations across all modalities. They can be as simple as height and weight to complex genomic profiling of an excised cancer identifying mutations vulnerable to anti-cancer therapy. Biomarkers therefore have a role in the management of all clinical disease entities, aiding treatment decisions and constant research to update and innovate. The goal of biomarker research in cancer is to identify and quantify biological metrics which correlate with clinical outcomes and ultimately improve anti-cancer management.

Certain biomarkers are primarily of interest within their specialities, and cancer care plays host to a significant number of these. Examples are tumour markers which are naturally occurring molecules noted to be elevated in states of active cancer and have been present in clinical practice for at least fifty years. Imaging biomarkers in cancer are based on lesion recognition and detection but can also extend to knock-on effects cancer and its care has on non-cancer tissue. This includes radiograph-based screening mammograms for the early detection of breast cancer to ultrasound-based echocardiograms to assess chemotherapy toxicity on the heart.

The two main biomarker classifications are predictive and prognostic. Predictive biomarkers inform on the likely effect of a therapy. These are frequently molecular targets against which specific drugs can be deployed. Prognostic biomarkers inform on the overall outcome, such as the previously mentioned RECIST criteria used to assess response to treatment. Certain biomarkers can be classified as both, as in the staging systems which determine the extent to which the cancer has spread using cross-sectional imaging. In this instance, higher cancer stage is inversely correlated with both the likelihood of curative success of treatments as well as survival.

Relatively little in the way of biomarker research is translated into clinical practice [7]. They either do not measure relevant biological features or are limited to academic settings due to the lack of translational strategies. Cancer Research UK (CRUK) and the European Organisation for Research and Treatment of Cancer (EORTC) lists two translational gaps that must be traversed for imaging biomarkers in particular to reach clinical utility [8]. The first requires the biomarker to be a biologically grounded, able to withstand clinically and technically reliable and cost-effective hypothesis testing. The second step ushering it into the routine management of patients with cancer with the necessary regulatory framework and regulations. Clinically translatable AI must cross these two gaps to deliver new biomarkers into routine practice.

6.3 Machine Learning Applications in Cancer Cross-Sectional Imaging

Although several ML algorithms such as random forest and support vector machine have been applied in radiology, convolutional neural networks have risen to dominate the field (CNN) [9, 10]. CNN are a variant of the deep neural network (DNN) inspired by the visual cortex of the brain particularly suited to spatial relationship and not reliant on hand-crafted features. Because DNNs would collapse the pixels within an image into a one-dimensional vector, important spatial information on how the pixels is orientated relative to each other is lost. A CNN in contrast would preserve the structure of an image because it can receive inputs as a two-dimensional array. Convolutional layers, the essential component of CNNs, will scan across an input image by subdividing it into a grid and summarising information in each grid space onto a node in a new layer. These nodes are assigned weights, which are adjusted according to the importance as the architecture learns the patterns common to the image dataset its interpreting. As the entire image is processed intact, it allows features to be captured from anywhere within the image [11]. A simple analogy here would be if a CNN were learning to identify pictures of "dogs", convolutional layers may capture and project "snout" and "collar" as nodes onto a new layer, of which "snouts" would be assigned a higher weight as they are more likely to represent "dog".

The architecture of a CNN that does the learning consists of convolutional layers followed by pooling layers, connected by a non-linear operation used as an activation function. The pooling layer performs dimensionality reduction by filtering only the maximum value (max pooling or MaxPool) or average value (average pooling) from each convolutional layer through to the next layer. In keeping with our "dog" CNN analogy, the activation function acts as a form of gatekeeper for the "snout" node generated in the convolutional layer. If there are insufficient "snout" pixels in the input image, then the corresponding "snout" node will not be activated and fire into the pooling layer. In this analogy the pooling layer captures the outputs of the "snout" and "collar" nodes and can summarise them into a "dog head" node. Thus, the feature learning section of a CNN will learn patterns within an image, which when connected onto a classification layer, allows predictions to be generated by mapping those features learned features to predetermined labels. A CNN trained on a dataset where pictures of dogs are paired with the breed can therefore learn to differentiate between them by the particular characteristics of each breed (Fig. 6.2).

An example of this architecture using the popular Python language machine learning library Tensorflow through the Keras application interface is illustrated in Box 1. The first convolutional layer accepts a 2D input image and extracts 32 features. The filter parameter give dimensionality to the output space of the next layer, while stride parameter specifies how fast the filter moves across the input image and thereby how big each grid being captured is. The activation function between the convolutional and pooling layers is specified as ReLu, and with the final activation to the output layer the logistic function 'softmax'. The first convolutional layer is

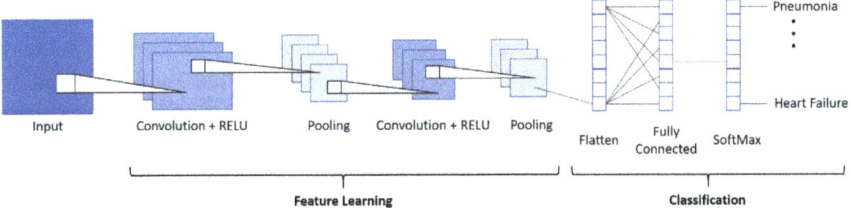

Fig. 6.2 Convolutional neural network architecture

downsampled by a pooling layer using the MaxPool method, followed by another convolutional and pooling layer pair now extracting 64 features. The output layer flattens the spatial information in a single dimensional vector which can be combined with class membership to derive predictions across *n* classes (5 in this case). The classification output segment can be replaced with a large range of desired tasks, such as semantic segmentation, whilst retaining the feature learning front half.

Box 1. Python Tensorflow CNN Architecture Example

```
import tensorflow as tf
def generate_model():

    model=tf.keras.Sequential([

        #first convolutional layer
        tf.keras.layers.Conv2D(32, filter_size=3, activation='relu'),
        tf.keras.layers.MaxPool2D(pool_size=2, strides=2),
        #second convolutional layer
        tf.keras.layers.Conv2D(64, filter_size=3, activation='relu'),
        tf.keras.layers.MaxPool2D(pool_size=2, strides=2),
        #fully connected classifier to 5 outputs
        tf.keras.layers.Flatten(),
        tf.keras.Dense(1024, activation='relu'),
        tf.keras.layers.Dense(5, activation='softmax').

]).
Return model.
```

CNNs optimises features using the same methodology as DNNs, using a cost function, gradient descent and backpropagation. A CNN architecture begins with random weightings distributed throughout the nodes in its architecture. As a CNN is fed new labelled data during training, the architecture is able to use a specified cost function (e.g. mean squared error) to measure the predicted output against the true value from the label and thus compute the magnitude of the error. Gradient descent, a function which uses derivatives to ascertain both the magnitude and size of the error, to correct this error. These corrections are then fed back through the nodes of the CNN in a process called backpropagation in order to adjust the sizes and magnitudes of the weights within each node in order to better align model with the correct prediction. CNNs typically undergo training, validation and testing on separate datasets like DNNs to avoid the biases inherent to a single dataset known as overfitting [12].

CNNs were originally noted for their ability to classifying hand-written digits [13]. They subsequently found further notoriety by halving the second-best error rate in the 2010 ImageNet challenge in the classification of 1000 image types [14]. More recently in medicine, CNNs continue their success in image-based tasks achieving dermatology specialist level classification on pictures of skin lesions, correctly classifying cancerous histopathology off slides and detecting diabetic retinopathy with a specificity of 95% [12, 15, 16]. Within radiology, CNNs can classify pathology on plain radiographs to near 100% [17]. To consider new applications in machine learning, we first explore the most common existing applications of ML in cancer care.

6.3.1 Lesion Detection/Classification

Because solid malignancies manifest radiologically through the presence of abnormal lesions, their accurate detection and interpretation forms the basis for any cancer related work. Within the treatment pathway, this starts in screening programmes where the patient is asymptomatic with no inciting concerns prompting a referral. These can be regarded as binary classification problems, where the goal of an algorithm is to classify cancer versus non-cancer. Up to 30% of cancers on mammograms can be missed by a reporting radiologist whereas CNNs have demonstrated 95.5+% accuracy on classifying mammography mass lesions across a range of mammogram databases [18, 19]. Similar trials using low-dose CT screening for lung cancer in smokers has using 3D-CNN achieving AUC of 0.94 by using the entire CT as an input [20]. The 3D approach requires a modified CNN architecture, which usually receives 2D images, as done by Setio et al. via a multi-stream CNN based on differently orientated 2D to simulate multiplanar reconstruction from each lung nodule candidate, subsequently converging in the fully connected layers to obtain classification [21].

In patients presenting with symptoms suspicious for cancer, the primary goal of radiological investigation is to confirm or exclude the presence of cancer, with the secondary goal to explore other causes of the symptoms. Radiologically, such as task is rarely clear-cut, and lesions may instead be graded on a risk scale. Prostate Imaging Reporting and Data System (PI-RADS) is a standard reporting system for which MRI prostates are assessed for the likelihood of cancer, but is subject to inter-reader variability [22]. When separated into a binary classifier, CNN was able to achieve AUC of 0.87 when using confirmed prostate cases for training [23]. An equivalent system, Breast Imaging Reporting and Data System (BI-RADS) exist for suspicious breast cancer lesions on imaging, and are graded between 0 and 5 depending on clinical suspicion [24]. It is also possible to combine lesion detection and classification. Huang et al. developed an automated end-to-end two-stage CNN, first for lesion detection to be followed by lesion classification on ultrasound images, achieving accuracies of 0.734–0.998 [25].

6.3.2 Segmentation

In cases of known cancer, being able to quantify the volume of disease can yield information on how fast the disease is progressing or how effective the treatment is. Current radiological response assessment is done using the RECIST criteria, which compares perpendicular measurements across the largest visualised lesions [5]. It is not practical to measure every single lesion every single time, as workload would scale with the number of lesions present, yet this may become necessary where a mixed response to treatment is encountered. Fully automated CNNs have been developed to automate semantic segmentation across a range of imaging modalities. This includes primary tumours on brain MRIs and locoregional lymph node spread on the background of normal anatomy on chest CTs [26, 27].

Delineation of normal organs is a routine time-consuming task in radiotherapy planning, allowing for the treatment software to calculate radiation dose and thus risk of radiation toxicity. Atlas-based software to automate organ segmentation has existed for decades, as normal anatomy is homogeneous to a degree [28, 29]. However, tumours are morphologically heterogenous, and the clinical judgement used to decide on whether tumour is appropriately targeted has seen some success in ML equivalents [30]. Instead, where entire tissue regions require radiation, segmentation via CNN can be brought in as a machine "second check" as part of a quality assurance purpose [31]. Being able to track cancer volume over time allows for monitoring after treatment, either for recurrence in cases of cure or treatment response in incurable cases.

When comparing predicted segmentation tasks against segmentation done by experts, the two most common scores used are Jaccard and Dice, represented visually in Box 2 [32]. These measure the trade-off between overlap and miss in related by slightly different ways. No one index is uniformly superior, but familiarity is important due to their use as a loss function for segmentation.

Box 2. Comparison of Jaccard and Dice Indices

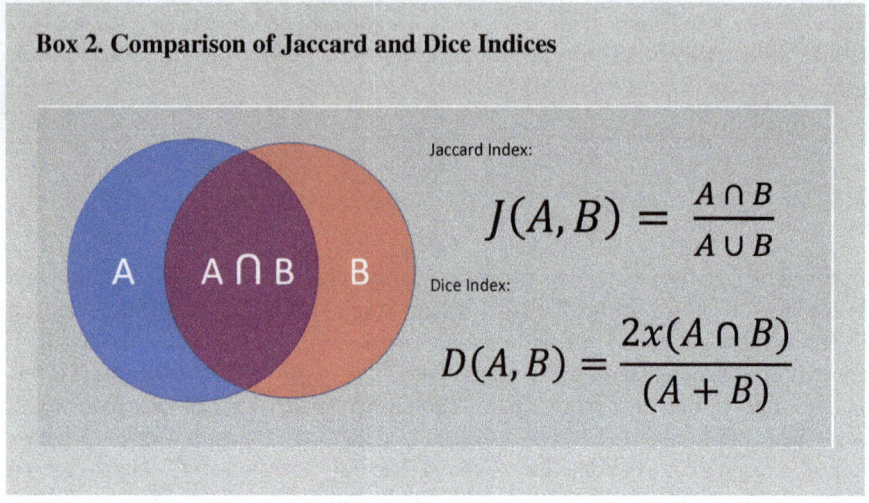

6.3.3 Cancer-Related Radiomics

Cancers can affect the body in ways beyond their mere physical presence. This can result in hormonal imbalances, inflammation and metabolic changes brought on by additional molecular signals from the tumour. These features can be extracted from medical imaging including through the use of ML algorithms and are termed collectively as radiomics. These can be divided into semantic features, which are describable by a radiologist in terms of dimensions and morphology, and agnostic features which are mathematically extracted quantitative descriptors [33].

Semantic features existed prior to computational exploitation, with prior examples such as tumour-related swelling predicting their severity grade [34]. Another example is a by-product of Positron Emission (PET) Scans, which measure radioisotope tagged glucose uptake on a scan. Metabolically active organs such as the brain or processes such as infection or cancer will demonstrate quantifiably higher activity over other tissues. Measuring metabolic characteristics on PET imaging been linked to outcomes such as chemotherapy responsiveness, as metabolically active tissues with a high turn-over rate are particularly vulnerable [35]. Agnostic features on the other hand result from deep learning methods yielding mathematical products such as fractal dimensions, and can be used across serial CT imaging to predict treatment response from lung cancer using a combined CNN with a recurrent neural network [36]. Agnostic features within the peritumoral region can also be used to strengthen the prediction of the tumour itself [37].

The dangers of radiomics, and especially with agnostic features include the "curse of dimensionality" where analysis in high-dimensional settings can be responsible for overfitting [38]. Features stability and dimensionality reduction are important priorities when relying on deep methods and may simplify models towards clinical applicability and explicability. A general rule-of-thumb is to have at least ten times more samples than free parameters [39].

6.4 Preparing Radiology Data for Machine Learning

AI algorithms require large repository of pre-processed data in order to achieve success. Supervised AI methods further require expert-derived labelling to achieve ground truth, all of which are costly both in terms of money and time. Large, well prepared and well annotated databases are valued due to the "garbage in, garbage out" principle, where biases and poorly prepared training data will result in a poor predictive tool. Digital Imaging and Communications in Medicine (DICOM) is an international non-proprietary data interchange protocol, digital image format and file structure that sees the widest use in the UK healthcare system and allows compatibility between different manufacturers. The Picture Archiving and Communication System (PACS) consists of medical imaging capture and viewing equipment, data archives and the distribution network. These two systems form the basis on which medical imaging data is captured, viewed and shared in the majority of UK based systems.

The workflow for obtaining and preparing medical imaging data for machine learning is summarised as follows [40]. Researches hoping to access medical data for machine learning purposes will need to take several steps to obtain and prepare the data before subjecting it to any computational analysis. As the data involves human participants, a combination of an ethics board review and informed consent is required for permission to access the images. Subject to this, the unprocessed data is typically geographically locked, with each health centre only able to access images obtained locally. Multi-institutional studies are likely to have to replicate ethics and access processes for each individual site, and possibly each principal investigator. Most systems have built-in software able to run queries on archived data to filter in and or out desired data. This step is crucial in completing the dataset as it is can easily exclude entire subsections of imaging data.

After access and acquisition, images need to have identifiable DICOM metadata and annotation removed and be transferred to a dedicated research storage. The resultant database should be examined for bias (e.g. sampling via single-institution or demography) and homogenized. Medical images are typically sampled at excess to the 300 by 300-pixel dimensions used for popular CNN architectures [14, 41]. Down sampling may be necessary as training on high-resolution datasets requires a high processing power, however this may result in loss of high-dimensional features. Thresholding of image pixel values, as in the case of the basic Hounsfield Unit in CT, can help restrict reconstruction to only certain tissues of interest. Accurate ground truth definition requires the input from domain experts. Manual labelling is costly but often a necessity, though alternatives include methods to extract labels from medical reports of the images [42].

This lengthy process explains why adequately annotated datasets are so costly to generate and thus valuable for machine learning. Partial solutions include transfer learning, where a model has been pre-trained from a natural image dataset [43]. An alternative is augmentation, where image manipulation such as rotation, axial flipping and deformation are applied to existing databases in order to artificially increase sample size. General adversarial networks have even been successful in generating synthetic datasets based on existing images to increase the training pool [44].

6.5 Example of Biomarker Discovery: Sarcopenia in Cancer

We give an example of how an imaging biomarker in cancer care has been developed. A by-product of visualising cancer in the body is the capture of normal body anatomy, which currently does not undergo additional routine assessment. Cachexia is the catabolic or wasting effect cancer has on the body via hormonal, inflammatory and metabolic changes. Cachexia has a worse prognostic impact on cancer outcomes in terms of survival, treatment toxicity and post-operative complications [45, 46]. The resultant muscle and fat loss form the biological basis for imaging biomarker development. Pathological muscle loss is known as sarcopenia, an entity originating in geriatric medicine as a marker for frailty where it has been linked to worse mortality [47].

Sarcopenia has historically been investigated radiologically using regional dual energy X-ray absorptiometry (DEXA), an ionizing investigation with minimal radiation dose yielding 2-dimensional representation of fat and non-fat tissue. Reference ranges for sarcopenia in non-cancer population use appendicular values as subjecting arms and legs to radiation is more acceptable than the head, torso or abdomen which house vital organs. More advanced cross-sectional imaging such as CT and MRI reconstruct anatomic structure in a superior fashion but leads to excess radiation exposure and is expensive to implement in population-based sarcopenia studies on otherwise healthy individuals. Fortunately, these advanced cross-sectional studies are part of routine cancer imaging, allowing the window of opportunity for incidental sarcopenia evaluation.

6.5.1 Defining Cancer Sarcopenia

Prado et al. conducted one of the earliest studies exploring the effect of sarcopenia in cancer on which many subsequent studies are based, and thus bears examining in more detail [48]. The methodology is based on work by the same group correlating the skeletal muscle index (skeletal muscle cross-section divided by height squared) to whole body Fat Free Mass (FFM) on DEXA in lung and GI cancer patients [49]. The correlation between the L3 skeletal muscle index (L3SMI) and whole body DEXA was measured at $r = 0.94$ with the following relationship: Whole body FFM (kg) $= 0.30 \times$ [skeletal muscle at L3 using CT (cm^2)] $+ 6.06$ [49]. Prado et al. adopted this measure in their study on the effect of sarcopenic *obesity* in cancer, evaluating 250 patients with BMI ≥ 30 and a diagnosis of lung or gastrointestinal (GI) cancer. Using overall survival as their endpoint, they derived sex-specific cut-offs (male: 52.4 cm^2/m^2; female: 38.5 cm^2/m^2) via optimum stratification under which lean body mass had a Hazard Ratio (HR) of 4.2 for mortality. In their study, 15% of the patient population was considered sarcopenic by the derived sex-specific cut-offs. The Prado et al. cut-offs have since been used in different cancer subgroups including renal, head and neck, hepatocellular, breast and ovarian [50–54]. The survival derived cut-offs for sarcopenia has also been used to measure other outcomes such as disease free progression, treatment toxicity, post-operative complication and post-operative length of stay [53–56]. These studies have not always found that sarcopenia as defined by Prado et al. impacts outcomes, particularly among the curative sub-population (as opposed to the metastatic). Prado et al.'s work was further expanded in the same population of GI and Lung cancer patients without the obesity criteria, deriving BMI- and sex- stratified cut-offs for sarcopenia using the same methodology now yielding significant for overall survival (male BMI ≥ 25: 53 cm^2/m^2, BMI < 25: 43 cm^2/m^2; female: 41 cm^2/m^2) [57] with sarcopenic patients now constituting 40.9% of the study population.

Skeletal muscle mass is a product of height, genetics, activity, hormone levels and diet, peaking in the third decade [58]. The derivation of L3SMI using height squared as denominator minimises correlation between the index and height across age, sex, ethnicity and study populations and brings the value in line with similar indices such as BMI [59]. Remaining within the same disease group and the establishment of sex- stratified cut-offs controls for study population and sex. Age can yield a difference of 4.8–10.2 cm^2/m^2 when comparing across decades in the same cancer study population [60]. The effect of ethnicity is widely variable depending on whether the study reference range originate in the same ethno-geographic region. L3SMI ranges between 28.6 and 38.9 cm^2/m^2 in women and 32.5–55.8 cm^2/m^2 in men depending on whether studies are performed in eastern Asia or on western populations [61, 62]. Because the original cancer sarcopenia work was done in western populations, studies have either applied these to both western or eastern populations or made a conscious effort to isolate ethnic effects by applying eastern criteria to eastern populations. Western criteria are generally higher, and when applied to an eastern population would erroneously lead to a higher prevalence and thereby minimise its impact on study outcomes. Wu et al. demonstrated statistical significance of L3SMI sarcopenia in a Chinese pancreatic cancer population using east Asian criteria but no significance when applying Prado et al.'s criteria in the same population, with a prevalence of 11% and 66.4% respectively depending on criterion used [63].

There is methodological variance in the definition of L3SMI sarcopenia in the wider cancer sarcopenia literature, defining cut-offs by median, tertiles, 5th centile from a separate healthy control population, as well as rates of loss [64–67]. Alternatives to abdominal sarcopenia assessment can be found in studies which limit themselves to assessment of the largest muscle alone, the psoas [68–70]. Because not all tumour types require imaging of the abdomen, attempts to interpret radiological sarcopenia elsewhere anatomically has been made in the thorax, neck and in the muscles of the head [71–73]. Finally, the integration of other semantic sarcopenia radiomics such as muscle attenuation (to assess muscle quality) and fat volume/attenuation to yield a more complete body morphometric picture has yielded mixed results as predictive biomarkers [54, 65, 74, 75].

Outcome based optimal binary cut-off has statistically utility as it offers a simple interpretation of the effect measure with relative risk and odds ratios and makes data summarization more efficient. Clinically binary thresholds are also advantageous in simplifying risk classification into high-versus low risk and produces a practical clinical tool for establishing biological thresholds, thus assisting treatment decisions by establishing prognosis. Despite sarcopenia not being consistently defined, an international consensus panel on cancer cachexia proposes L3SMI values of 55.4 and 38.9 cm^2/m^2 for men and women [76]. This is in reference to sarcopenia thresholds in non-cancer literature using the formulae relating L3SMI to body and limb DEXA values that informed the Prado et al. work. This is on the higher side of values typical for the western population and must be taken into consideration if applied to e.g. east Asian populations.

6.5.2 Scalable Solutions to Radiological Sarcopenia Assessment

Manually measuring cross-sectional skeletal muscle area is not feasible in clinical practice. Current software packages such as OsirisX (Pixmeo, Switzerland) and SliceOmatic (TomoVision, Montreal, Canada) can semi-automate segmentation of medical imaging with comparable accuracy [77]. The workflow involved requires manual selection of slices within imaging files and feeding these to through the segmentation process of the software after specifying tissue parameters. These systems are thus not fully automated but have had their segmentations validated in cancer populations [78]. OsirisX software was used to assist Lee et al. in the generation of ground truth segmentations upon which to train a CNN in a cohort of lung cancer patients. They compared convolutional layer granularity (by stride variation) and grayscale definition (by varying windowing across Hounsfield Units) and were able to train their model on 250 images to extract semantic markers such as muscle shape and texture better than semi-automated methods [79]. Although they achieved a Dice coefficient of 0.92, a drop-off in performance in cases with higher BMI was noted, possibly owing to segmentation misinterpretation between muscle and soft tissue oedema. Dabiri et al. achieved slightly higher Dice co-efficient of 0.98 using 6621 pre-extracted CT slices from three cancer datasets using an architecture combining CNN, which performs better on coarse features, with a U-net (a type of CNN) that better extracts the finer boundaries [80]. Dong et al. added agnostic feature generation to slice-based semantic radiomics by applying PyRadiomics, an open-source platform capable of extracting a large panel of engineered features from medical imaging [81]. Using L3SMI to define sarcopenia, they examined a single slice at T12 in the CT of 99 lung cancer patients. 851 shape, first-order intensity statistics, texture and wavelet features were extracted and reduced to five by in large part due to dimensionality reduction owing to sharing a high correlation magnitude. They were ultimately able to achieve specificity, sensitivity and area under curve scores of 0.944, 0.833 and 0.889 respectively.

Previous studies have relied on pre-localised slices as inputs for their models. To automate the process of extracting radiomics from a single slice of cross-sectional imaging, landmark localisation is needed as an additional step. Burns et al. designed a two-stage process whereby a U-net received pixel matrix converted DICOM images of CT chest, abdomen and pelvis scans, first segmenting individual vertebrae along the longitudinal axis of the spine, followed by skeletal muscle segmentation at desired spinal levels [82]. The model was trained de novo against 102 manually segmented scans as ground truth with five-fold cross-validation achieving a Dice coefficient at 0.938. Kanavati et al. constructed a similar architecture with a connected two-step U-Net for L3 slice detection and segmentation in a larger aggregated cancer dataset of 1070 CTs with additional augmentation [83]. They optimised computational efficacy by only reconstructing a limited 2D Maximum Intensity Projection sagittal slice for L3 detection, subsequently achieving Dice coefficient of 0.96 in threefold cross validation.

Moving beyond single slice analysis, 3D skeletal muscle volume definition is more computationally ambitious and limited by the lack of whole-body imaging in clinical practice. Standard cancer imaging to evaluate systemic disease is still limited to the thorax, abdomen and pelvis as metastatic disease tends to manifest centrally rather than in the limbs. Whole body imaging is therefore most encountered in PET scans which automatically images a patient entirely. This method also hypothesises that appendicular skeletal muscle plays as important a role as central skeletal muscle, which lacks the evidence base of e.g. the L3SMI biomarker. Blanc-Durand et al. used a CNN trained on the low-CT dose component of 189 PET scans in lung cancer patients to auto-segment body morphology in terms of skeletal muscle and adipose tissue achieving Dice coefficients of 0.91–0.95 [84]. With a reasonable graphical processing unit (GTX1080Ti), they managed to infer a volume of $256 \times 256 \times 300$ voxels in only 3 s. Unlike previous studies, this group went on to validate their model in clinical outcomes, finding prognostic significance in adipose tissue ratios (but not in skeletal muscle).

6.5.3 Remaining Translational Gaps

Multiple studies have demonstrated the ability to automate the localisation and segmentation of sarcopenia biomarkers. Although this addresses scalability, these studies remain weak regarding lack of clinical outcomes. Until this is done, errors and their source may remain in the computational models. For instance, localisation tasks can miss due to the presence of transitional vertebrae, anatomically variants present in between 4 and 30% of individuals [85]. Kavanati et al. was the only group who chose to acknowledge their presence but was unable to account for their variant, ultimately excluding them in their training data [83].

Although sarcopenia research has yet to fully cross the second biomarker translational gap for clinical implementation, there now exists a solid body of work around which regulation can be generated if a consensus approach for sarcopenia assessment is reached. The existence of international consensus criteria exist suffers from demographic weaknesses that risk over-representing sarcopenia in ethnic populations who natively harbour less skeletal muscle. Overall, there has been ongoing advances in developing cancer sarcopenia as a radiological biomarker, from the recognition and application of population-specific parameters to the improving efficiency and accuracy of computational models automating radiological analysis.

6.6 Conclusion

The vast amount of imaging data generated by cancer services is fertile ground for biomarker development. Bearing in mind the purpose and role imaging fits within cancer care pathways allows the unused imaging by-products to be repurposed in the most optimal fashion. Radiology data lends itself to computational analysis which can automate high dimensional feature extraction and analysis. Despite existing in abundance, imaging data is locked behind decentralisation and regulatory barriers. Much of cancer imaging work is retrospective due to decreased risk and the practicality of accessing an existing database. This can be the starting ground for any hypothesis generating biomarker research, but ultimately needs to be validated in prospective work.

Research questions needs to be grounded in biology, with domain experts guiding feature selection, provide ground truth labels and keep the work clinically relevant. Clinically relevant work can then seek computational solutions, from basic tasks such as segmentation to deeper learning in the form of feature selection as demonstrated in the examples in this chapter. Partnerships between data scientists who understand and can leverage the best computational architectures is essential for project success. We therefore advocate for clinician-data science partnerships for the best chance of success.

References

1. Lumbreras, B., Donat, L., Hernandez-Aguade, I.: Incidental findings in imaging diagnostic tests: a systematic review. Br. J. Radiol. **83**(988), 276–289 (2010). Available from: https://doi.org/10.1259/bjr/98067945. Available from: https://www.ncbi.nlm.nih.gov/pubmed/20335439
2. Pickhardt, P.J., Kim, D.H., Meiners, R.J., Wyatt, K.S., Hanson, M.E., Barlow, D.S., et al.: Colorectal and extracolonic cancers detected at screening CT colonography in 10 286 asymptomatic adults. Radiology **255**(1), 83–88 (2010)
3. Operational Information for Commissioning. Diagnostic Imaging Dataset Annual Statistical Release 2016/17. National Health Service (2017)
4. Reardon, S.: Rise of the robot radiologists. Nature **576**, 55 (2019)
5. Eisenhauer, E.A, Therasse, P., Bogaerts, J., Schwartz, L.H., Sargent, D., Ford, R., et al.: New response evaluation criteria in solid tumours: revised RECIST guideline (version 1.1). Eur. J. Cancer (1990) **45**(2), 228–247 (2009). Available from: https://doi.org/10.1016/j.ejca.2008.10.026. Available from https://search.datacite.org/works/
6. Mettler, F.A., Walter, H., Yoshizumi, T.T., Mahesh, M.: Effective doses in radiology and diagnostic nuclear medicine: a catalog. Radiology **248**(1), 254–263 (2008)
7. Poste, G.: Bring on the biomarkers. Nature **469**, 156–157 (2011)
8. O'Connor, J.P.B., Aboagye, E.O., Adams, J.E., Aerts, Hugo, J.W.L., Barrington, S.F., Beer, A.J., et al.: Imaging biomarker roadmap for cancer studies. Nat. Rev. Clin. Oncol. **14**(3), 169–186 (2016). Available from: https://doi.org/10.1038/nrclinonc.2016.162. Available from: https://search.datacite.org/works/
9. Sarica, A., Cerasa, A., Quattrone, A.: Random forest algorithm for the classification of neuroimaging data in Alzheimer's disease: a systematic review. Front. Media SA (2017)
10. Lao, Z., Shen, D., Liu, D., Jawad, A.F., Melhem, E.R., Launer, L.J., et al.: Computer-assisted segmentation of white matter lesions in 3D MR images using support vector machine. Acad. Radiol. **15**(3), 300–313 (2008). Available from: https://doi.org/10.1016/j.acra.2007.10.012. Available from: https://www.clinicalkey.es/playcontent/1-s2.0-S1076633207005831
11. Yamashita, R., Nishio, M., Do, R.K.G., Togashi, K.: Convolutional neural networks: an overview and application in radiology. Insights into Imaging **9**(4), 611–629 (2018). Available from: https://doi.org/10.1007/s13244-018-0639-9. Available from: https://search.datacite.org/works/
12. Rakhlin, A., Shvets, A., Iglovikov, V., Kalinin, A.A.: Deep convolutional neural networks for breast cancer histology image analysis. Cold Spring Harbor Laboratory (2018). Available from: https://explore.openaire.eu/search/publication?articleId=sharebioRxiv::97119dc2e35c1a0874f0ca5a51203e58
13. Lecun, Y., Bottou, L., Bengio, Y., Haffner, P.: Gradient-based learning applied to document recognition. Proc. IEEE **86**(11), 2278–2324 (1998). Available from: https://doi.org/10.1109/5.726791. Available from: https://ieeexplore.ieee.org/document/726791
14. Krizhevsky, A., Sutskever, I., Hinton, G.: ImageNet classification with deep convolutional neural networks. In: NIPS 12 Proceedings of the 25th International Conference on Neural Information Processing Systems, December (2012)
15. Esteva, A., Kuprel, B., Novoa, R.A., Ko, J., Swetter, S.M., Blau, H.M., et al.: Dermatologist-level classification of skin cancer with deep neural networks. Nature (London) **542**(7639), 115–118 (2017). Available from: https://doi.org/10.1038/nature21056. Available from: https://search.datacite.org/works/
16. De Fauw, J., Ledsam, J.R., Romera-Paredes, B., Nikolov, S., Tomasev, N., Blackwell, S., et al.: Clinically applicable deep learning for diagnosis and referral in retinal disease. Nat. Med. **24**(9), 1342–1350 (2018). Available from: https://doi.org/10.1038/s41591-018-0107-6. Available from: https://search.datacite.org/works/
17. Rajkomar, A., Lingam, S., Taylor, A.G., Blum, M., Mongan, J.: High-throughput classification of radiographs using deep convolutional neural networks. J. Digit. Imaging **30**(1), 95–101 (2016). Available from: https://doi.org/10.1007/s10278-016-9914-9. Available from: https://search.datacite.org/works/

18. Chougrad, H., Zouaki, H., Alheyane, O.: Deep convolutional neural networks for breast cancer screening. Comput. Methods Programs Biomed. **157**, 19–30 (2018). Available from: https://doi.org/10.1016/j.cmpb.2018.01.011. Available from: https://search.datacite.org/works/
19. Ekpo, E.U., Alakhras, M., Brennan, P.: Errors in mammography cannot be solved through technology alone. Asian Pac. J. Cancer Prev. **19**, 291–301 (2018). Available from: https://doi.org/10.22034/APJCP.2018.19.2.291
20. Ardila, D., Kiraly, A.P., Bharadwaj, S., Choi, B., Reicher, J.J., Peng, L., et al.: End-to-end lung cancer screening with three-dimensional deep learning on low-dose chest computed tomography. Nat. Med. **25**(6), 954–961 (2019). Available from: https://doi.org/10.1038/s41591-019-0447-x. Available from: https://www.ncbi.nlm.nih.gov/pubmed/31110349
21. Setio, A.A.A., Ciompi, F., Litjens, G., Gerke, P., Jacobs, C., van Riel, S.J., et al.: Pulmonary nodule detection in CT images: false positive reduction using multi-view convolutional networks. IEEE Trans. Med. Imaging **35**(5), 1160–1169 (2016). Available from: https://doi.org/10.1109/TMI.2016.2536809. Available from: https://ieeexplore.ieee.org/document/7422783
22. Rosenkrantz, A.B., Ginocchio, L.A., Cornfeld, D., Froemming, A.T., Gupta, R.T., Turkbey, B., et al.: Interobserver reproducibility of the PI-RADS version 2 Lexicon: a multicenter study of six experienced prostate radiologists. Radiology **280**(3), 793–804 (2016). Available from: https://doi.org/10.1148/radiol.2016152542. Available from: https://www.ncbi.nlm.nih.gov/pubmed/27035179
23. Yoo, S., Gujrathi, I., Haider, M.A., Khalvati, F.: Prostate cancer detection using deep convolutional neural networks. Springer Science and Business Media LLC (2019)
24. Mendelson, E.B., Berg, W.A., Merritt, C.R.B.: Toward a standardized breast ultrasound lexicon, BI-RADS: ultrasound. Semin. Roentgenol. **36**(3), 217–225 (2001). Available from: https://doi.org/10.1053/sroe.2001.25125
25. Huang, Y., Han, L., Dou, H., Luo, H., Yuan, Z., Liu, Q., et al.: Two-stage CNNs for computerized BI-RADS categorization in breast ultrasound images. Springer Science and Business Media LLC (2019)
26. Bouget, D., Jørgensen, A.A., Kiss, G., Leira, H.O., Langø, T.: Semantic segmentation and detection of mediastinal lymph nodes and anatomical structures in CT data for lung cancer staging. Springer Science and Business Media LLC (2019)
27. Dong, H., Yang, G., Liu, F., Mo, Y., Guo, Y.: Automatic brain tumor detection and segmentation using U-net based fully convolutional networks (2011)
28. Bondiau, P., Malandain, G., Chanalet, S., Marcy, P., Habrand, J., Fauchon, F., et al.: Atlas-based automatic segmentation of MR images: validation study on the brainstem in radiotherapy context. Int. J. Radiat. Oncol. Biol. Phys. **61**(1), 289–298 (2005). Available from: https://doi.org/10.1016/j.ijrobp.2004.08.055
29. Kim, N., Chang, J.S., Kim, Y.B., Kim, J.S.: Atlas-based auto-segmentation for postoperative radiotherapy planning in endometrial and cervical cancers. Springer Science and Business Media LLC (2020)
30. Men, K., Dai, J., Li, Y.: Automatic segmentation of the clinical target volume and organs at risk in the planning CT for rectal cancer using deep dilated convolutional neural networks
31. Chen, X., Men, K., Chen, B., Tang, Y., Zhang, T., Wang, S., et al.: CNN-based quality assurance for automatic segmentation of breast cancer in radiotherapy. Front. Oncol. **10**, 524 (2020). Available from: https://doi.org/10.3389/fonc.2020.00524. Available from: https://www.ncbi.nlm.nih.gov/pubmed/32426272
32. Bertels, J., Eelbode, T., Berman, M., Vandermeulen, D., Maes, F., Bisschops, R., et al.: Optimizing the dice score and Jaccard index for medical image segmentation: theory & practice. arXiv (2019). Available from: http://bvbr.bib-bvb.de:8991/F?func=service&doc_library=BVB01&local_base=BVB01&doc_number=030192982&sequence=000001&line_number=0001&func_code=DB_RECORDS&service_type=MEDIA
33. Gillies, R.J., Kinahan, P.E., Hricak, H.: Radiomics: images are more than pictures, they are data. Radiology **278**(2), 563–577 (2016). Available from: https://doi.org/10.1148/radiol.2015151169. Available from: https://www.ncbi.nlm.nih.gov/pubmed/26579733

34. Asari, S., Makabe, T., Katayama, S., Itoh, T., Tsuchida, S., Ohmoto, T.: Assessment of the pathological grade of astrocytic gliomas using an MRI score. Neuroradiology **36**(4), 308–310 (1994). Available from: https://doi.org/10.1007/BF00593267. Available from: https://www.ncbi.nlm.nih.gov/pubmed/8065577
35. Mamede, M., Abreu-E-Lima, P., Oliva, M.R., Nosé, V., Mamon, H., Gerbaudo, V.H.: FDG-PET/CT tumor segmentation-derived indices of metabolic activity to assess response to neoadjuvant therapy and progression-free survival in esophageal cancer: correlation with histopathology results. Am. J. Clin. Oncol. **30**(4), 377–388 (2007). Available from: https://doi.org/10.1097/COC.0b013e31803993f8. Available from: https://www.ncbi.nlm.nih.gov/pubmed/17762438
36. Xu, Y., Hosny, A., Zeleznik, R., Parmar, C., Coroller, T., Franco, I., et al.: Deep learning predicts lung cancer treatment response from serial medical imaging. Clin. Cancer Res. **25**(11), 3266–3275 (2019). Available from: https://doi.org/10.1158/1078-0432.CCR-18-2495. Available from: https://www.narcis.nl/publication/RecordID/oai:cris.maastrichtuniversity.nl:publications%2F83373506-ea66-4d5d-a602-42cb665907f9
37. Sun, Q., Lin, X., Zhao, Y., Li, L., Yan, K., Liang, D., et al.: t Forget the Peritumoral region. Frontiers Media, SA (2020)
38. Altman, N., Krzywinski, M.: The curse(s) of dimensionality. Nat. Methods **15**(6), 399–400 (2018). Available from: https://doi.org/10.1038/s41592-018-0019-x. Available from: https://www.ncbi.nlm.nih.gov/pubmed/29855577
39. Peeken, J.C., Bernhofer, M., Wiestler, B., Goldberg, T., Cremers, D., Rost, B., et al.: Radiomics in radiooncology—challenging the medical physicist. Physica medica **48**, 27–36 (2018). Available from: https://doi.org/10.1016/j.ejmp.2018.03.012
40. Willemink, M.J., Koszek, W.A., Hardell, C., Wu, J., Fleischmann, D., Harvey, H., et al.: Preparing medical imaging data for machine learning. Radiology **295**(1), 4–15 (2020). Available from: https://doi.org/10.1148/radiol.2020192224. Available from: https://www.ncbi.nlm.nih.gov/pubmed/32068507
41. Szegedy, C., Liu, W., Jia, Y., Sermanet, P., Reed, S., Anguelov, D., et al.: Going deeper with convolutions. In: 2015 IEEE Conference on Computer Vision and Pattern Recognition (CVPR), pp. 1–9. IEEE. Available from: https://ieeexplore.ieee.org/document/7298594. Available from: https://doi.org/10.1109/CVPR.2015.7298594
42. Wang, X., Peng, Y., Lu, L., Lu, Z., Bagheri, M., Summers, R.M.: ChestX-Ray8: Hospital-scale chest X-Ray database and benchmarks on weakly-supervised classification and localization of common thorax diseases. In: 2017 IEEE Conference on Computer Vision and Pattern Recognition (CVPR), July 2017, pp. 3462–3471. IEEE. Available from: https://ieeexplore.ieee.org/document/8099852. Available from: https://doi.org/10.1109/CVPR.2017.369
43. Shin, H., Roth, H.R., Gao, M., Lu, L., Xu, Z., Nogues, I., et al.: Deep convolutional neural networks for computer-aided detection: CNN architectures, dataset characteristics and transfer learning. IEEE Trans. Med. Imaging **35**(5), 1285–1298 (2016). Available from: https://doi.org/10.1109/TMI.2016.2528162. Available from: https://ieeexplore.ieee.org/document/7404017
44. Frid-Adar, M., Diamant, I., Klang, E., Amitai, M., Goldberger, J., Greenspan, H.: GAN-based synthetic medical image augmentation for increased CNN performance in liver lesion classification. Neurocomputing (Amsterdam) **321**, 321–331 (2018). Available from: https://doi.org/10.1016/j.neucom.2018.09.013
45. Zhang, X., Dou, Q., Zeng, Y., Yang, Y., Cheng, A.S.K., Zhang, W.: Sarcopenia as a predictor of mortality in women with breast cancer: a meta-analysis and systematic review. BMC Cancer **20**(1), 172 (2020). Available from: https://doi.org/10.1186/s12885-020-6645-6. Available from: https://www.ncbi.nlm.nih.gov/pubmed/32131764
46. Nishimura, J.M., Ansari, A.Z., D'Souza, D.M., Moffatt-Bruce, S.D., Merritt, R.E., Kneuertz, P.J.: Computed tomography-assessed skeletal muscle mass as a predictor of outcomes in lung cancer surgery. Ann. Thoracic Surg. **108**(5), 1555–1564 (2019). Available from: https://doi.org/10.1016/j.athoracsur.2019.04.090
47. Arango-Lopera, V.E., Arroyo, P., Gutierrez-Robledo, L.M., Perez-Zepeda, M.U., Cesari, M.: Mortality as an adverse outcome of sarcopenia. J. Nutr. Health Aging **17**(3), 260–262 (2013)

48. Prado, C.M.M., Lieff, J.R., Mccargar, L.J., Reiman, T., Sawyer, M.B., Martin, L., et al.: Prevalence and clinical implications of sarcopenic obesity in patients with solid tumours of the respiratory and gastrointestinal tracts: a population-based study. Lancet Oncol. **9**, 629–635 (2008). Available from: https://doi.org/10.1016/S1470
49. Mourtzakis, M., Prado, C.M.M., Lieffers, J.R., Reiman, T., McCargar, L.J., Baracos, V.E.: A practical and precise approach to quantification of body composition in cancer patients using computed tomography images acquired during routine care. Appl. Physiol. Nutr. Metab. **33**(5), 997–1006 (2008). Available from: https://doi.org/10.1139/H08-075. Available from: http://www.ingentaconnect.com/content/nrc/apnm/2008/00000033/00000005/art00018
50. Fattouh, M., Chang, G.Y., Ow, T.J., Shifteh, K., Rosenblatt, G., Patel, V.M., et al.: Association between pretreatment obesity, sarcopenia, and survival in patients with head and neck cancer. Wiley (2018)
51. Ataseven, B., Luengo, T.G., Du Bois, A., Waltering, K., Traut, A., Heitz, F., et al.: Skeletal muscle attenuation (Sarcopenia) predicts reduced overall survival in patients with advanced Epithelial Ovarian Cancer undergoing primary debulking surgery (2018)
52. Antoun, S., Baracos, V.E., Birdsell, L., Escudier, B., Sawyer, M.B.: Low body mass index and sarcopenia associated with dose-limiting toxicity of sorafenib in patients with renal cell carcinoma. Ann. Oncol. **21**(8), 1594–1598 (2010). Available from: https://doi.org/10.1093/annonc/mdp605
53. Seror, M., Sartoris, R., Hobeika, C., Bouattour, M., Paradis, V., Rautou, P., et al.: Computed tomography-derived liver surface nodularity and sarcopenia as prognostic factors in patients with resectable metabolic syndrome-related hepatocellular carcinoma. Ann. Surg. Oncol. (2020)
54. Omarini, C., Palumbo, P., Pecchi, A., Draisci, S., Balduzzi, S., Nasso, C., et al.: Predictive role of body composition parameters in operable breast cancer patients treated with neoadjuvant chemotherapy. Cancer Manage. Res. **11**, 9563–9569 (2019). Available from: https://doi.org/10.2147/cmar.s216034
55. Tsukioka, T., Izumi, N., Mizuguchi, S., Kyukwang, C., Komatsu, H., Toda, M., et al.: Positive correlation between sarcopenia and elevation of neutrophil/lymphocyte ration in pathological stage IIIA (N2-positive) non-small cell lung cancer patients. General Thoracic Cardiovascular Surg. **66**(12), 716–722 (2018). Available from: https://doi.org/10.1007/s11748-018-0985-z. Available from: https://www.ncbi.nlm.nih.gov/pubmed/30105630
56. Basile, D., Parnofiello, A., Vitale, M.G., Cortiula, F., Gerratana, L., Fanotto, V., et al.: The IMPACT study: early loss of skeletal muscle mass in advanced pancreatic cancer patients. Wiley (2019)
57. Martin, L., Birdsell, L., MacDonald, N., Reiman, T., Clandinin, T.M., McCargar, L.J., et al.: cancer cachexia in the age of obesity: skeletal muscle depletion is a powerful prognostic factor, independent of body mass index. J. Clin. Oncol. **31**(12), 1539–1547 (2013). Available from: https://doi.org/10.1200/JCO.2012.45.2722. Available from: http://jco.ascopubs.org/content/31/12/1539.abstract
58. Heymsfield, S.B., Gonzalez, M.C., Lu, J., Jia, G., Zheng, J.: Skeletal muscle mass and quality: evolution of modern measurement concepts in the context of sarcopenia. Proc. Nutr. Soc. **74**(4), 355–366 (2015). Available from: https://doi.org/10.1017/S0029665115000129
59. Baumgartner, R.N., Koehler, K.M., Gallagher, D., Romero, L., Heymstleld, S.B., Ross, R.R., et al.: Am. J. Epidemiol. Copyright O 1998 by The Johns Hopkins University School of Hygiene and Pubfic Health All rights reserved (1998)
60. Xiao, J., Caan, B.J., Cespedes Feliciano, E.M., Meyerhardt, J.A., Kroenke, C.H., Baracos, V.E., et al.: The association of medical and demographic characteristics with sarcopenia and low muscle radiodensity in patients with nonmetastatic colorectal cancer. Am. J. Clin Nutr. **109**(3), 615–625 (2019). Available from: https://doi.org/10.1093/ajcn/nqy328. Available from: https://www.ncbi.nlm.nih.gov/pubmed/30850836
61. Zheng, Z., Lu, J., Zheng, C., Li, P., Xie, J., Wang, J., et al.: A novel prognostic scoring system based on preoperative sarcopenia predicts the long-term outcome for patients after R0 resection for gastric cancer: experiences of a high-volume center. Ann. Surg. Oncol. **24**(7), 1795–1803

(2017). Available from: https://doi.org/10.1245/s10434-017-5813-7. Available from: https://www.ncbi.nlm.nih.gov/pubmed/28213789
62. Lanic, H., Kraut-Tauzia, J., Modzelewski, R., Clatot, F., Mareschal, S., Picquenot, J.M., et al.: Sarcopenia is an independent prognostic factor in elderly patients with diffuse large B-cell lymphoma treated with immunochemotherapy. Leukemia lymphoma **55**(4), 817–823 (2014). Available from: https://doi.org/10.3109/10428194.2013.816421. Available from: http://www.tandfonline.com/doi/abs/
63. Wu, C., Chang, M., Lyadov, V.K., Liang, P., Chen, C., Shih, T.T., et al.: Comparing Western and Eastern criteria for sarcopenia and their association with survival in patients with pancreatic cancer. Clin. Nutr. (Edinburgh, Scotland) **38**(2), 862–869 (2019). Available from: https://doi.org/10.1016/j.clnu.2018.02.016
64. Alwani, M.M., Jones, A.J., Novinger, L.J., Pittelkow, E., Bonetto, A., Sim, M.W., et al.: Impact of sarcopenia on outcomes of autologous head and neck free tissue reconstruction. J. Reconstr. Microsurg. **36**, 369–378 (2020)
65. Shirdel, M., Andersson, F., Myte, R., Axelsson, J., Rutegard, M., Blomqvist, L., et al.: Body composition measured by computed tomography is associated with colorectal cancer survival, also in early-stage disease. Acta Oncologia. **7**(59), 799–808 (2020)
66. Higashi, T., Higashi, T., Hayashi, H., Hayashi, H., Taki, K., Taki, K., et al.: Sarcopenia, but not visceral fat amount, is a risk factor of postoperative complications after major hepatectomy. Int. J. Clin. Oncol. **21**(2), 310–319 (2016). Available from: https://doi.org/10.1007/s10147-015-0898-0. Available from: https://www.ncbi.nlm.nih.gov/pubmed/26338271
67. Petrova, M.P., Donev, I.S., Radanova, M.A., Eneva, M.I., Dimitrova, E.G., Valchev GN, et al. Sarcopenia and high NLR are associated with the development of hyperprogressive disease after second-line pembrolizumab in patients with non-small-cell lung cancer. Clin. Exp. Immunol. **202**(3), 353–362 (2020). Available from: https://doi.org/10.1111/cei.13505. Available from: https://onlinelibrary.wiley.com/doi/abs/
68. Chakedis, J., Spolverato, G., Beal, E., Woelfel, I., Bagante, F., Merath, K., et al.: Pre-operative sarcopenia identifies patients at risk for poor survival after resection of biliary tract cancers. J. Gastrointest. Surg. **22**(10), 1697–1708 (2018). Available from: https://doi.org/10.1007/s11605-018-3802-1. Available from: https://www.ncbi.nlm.nih.gov/pubmed/29855867
69. Conrad, L.B., Awdeh, H., Acosta-Torres, S., Conrad, S.A., Bailey, A.A., Miller, D.S., et al.: Pre-operative core muscle index in combination with hypoalbuminemia is associated with poor prognosis in advanced ovarian cancer. J. Surg. Oncol. **117**(5), 1020–1028 (2018). Available from: https://doi.org/10.1002/jso.24990. Available from: https://onlinelibrary.wiley.com/doi/abs/
70. Zakaria, H.M., Massie, L., Basheer, A., Boyce-Fappiano, D., Elibe, E., Schultz, L., et al.: Application of morphometrics as a predictor for survival in female patients with breast cancer spinal metastasis: a retrospective cohort study. Spine J. **18**(10), 1798–1803 (2018). Available from: https://doi.org/10.1016/j.spinee.2018.03.007
71. Furtner, J., Berghoff, A.S., Albtoush, O.M., Woitek, R., Asenbaum, U., Prayer, D., et al.: Survival prediction using temporal muscle thickness measurements on cranial magnetic resonance images in patients with newly diagnosed brain metastases
72. Swartz, J.E., Pothen, A.J., Wegner, I., Smid, E.J., Swart, K.M.A., de Bree, R., et al.: Feasibility of using head and neck CT imaging to assess skeletal muscle mass in head and neck cancer patients. Oral Oncol. **62**, 28–33 (2016). Available from: https://doi.org/10.1016/j.oraloncology.2016.09.006. Available from: https://www.clinicalkey.es/playcontent/1-s2.0-S1368837516301634
73. Sealy, M.J., Dechaphunkul, T., van der Schans, C.P., Krijnen, W.P., Roodenburg, J.L.N., Walker, J., et al.: Low muscle mass is associated with early termination of chemotherapy related to toxicity in patients with head and neck cancer. Clin. Nutr. (Edinburgh, Scotland) 39(2), 501–509 (2020). Available from: https://doi.org/10.1016/j.clnu.2019.02.029
74. Ní Bhuachalla, É.B., Daly, L.E., Power, D.G., Cushen, S.J., Maceneaney, P., Ryan, A.M.: Computed tomography diagnosed cachexia and sarcopenia in 725 oncology patients: is nutritional screening capturing hidden malnutrition? Wiley (2017)

75. Srpcic, M., Jordan, T., Popuri, K., Sok, M.: Sarcopenia and myosteatosis at presentation adversely affect survival after esophagectomy for esophageal cancer. Walter de Gruyter GmbH (2020)
76. Fearon, K., Strasser, F., Anker, S.D., Bosaeus, I., Bruera, E., Fainsinger, R.L., et al.: Definition and classification of cancer cachexia: an international consensus. Lancet Oncol. **12**, 489–495 (2011). Available from: https://doi.org/10.1016/S1470
77. Rollins, K.E., Awwad, A., Macdonald, I.A., Lobo, D.N.: A comparison of two different software packages for analysis of body composition using computed tomography images. Nutrition (Burbank, Los Angeles County, Calif.) **57**, 92–96 (2019). Available from: https://doi.org/10.1016/j.nut.2018.06.003
78. Feliciano, E.M.C., Popuri, K., Cobzas, D., Baracos, V.E., Beg, M.F., Khan, A.D., et al.: Evaluation of automated computed tomography segmentation to assess body composition and mortality associations in cancer patients. J. Cachexia, Sarcopenia Muscle **11**(5) (2020). Available from: https://doi.org/10.1002/jcsm.12573
79. Lee, H., Troschel, F., Tajmir, S., Fuchs, G., Mario, J., Fintelmann, F., et al.: Pixel-level deep segmentation: artificial intelligence quantifies muscle on computed tomography for body morphometric analysis. J. Digit Imaging **30**(4), 487–498 (2017). Available from: https://doi.org/10.1007/s10278-017-9988-z. Available from: https://www.ncbi.nlm.nih.gov/pubmed/28653123
80. Dabiri, S., Popuri, K., Cespedes Feliciano, E.M., Caan, B.J., Baracos, V.E., Beg, M.F.: Muscle segmentation in axial computed tomography (CT) images at the lumbar (L3) and thoracic (T4) levels for body composition analysis. Comput. Med. Imaging Graph. **75**, 47–55 (2019). Available from: https://doi.org/10.1016/j.compmedimag.2019.04.007
81. Dong, X., Dan, X., Yawen, A., Haibo, X., Huan, L., Mengqi, T., et al.: Identifying sarcopenia in advanced non-small cell lung cancer patients using skeletal muscle CT radiomics and machine learning. Thoracic Cancer **11**(9), 2650–2659 (2020). Available from: https://doi.org/10.1111/1759-7714.13598. Available from: https://onlinelibrary.wiley.com/doi/abs/
82. Burns, J.E., Yao, J., Chalhoub, D., Chen, J.J., Summers, R.M.: A machine learning algorithm to estimate sarcopenia on abdominal CT. Acad. Radiol. **27**(3), 311–320 (2020). Available from: https://doi.org/10.1016/j.acra.2019.03.011
83. Kanavati, F., Islam, S., Arain, Z., Aboagye, E.O., Rockall, A.: Fully-automated deep learning slice-based muscle estimation from CT images for sarcopenia assessment (2020). Available from: https://arxiv.org/abs/2006.06432
84. Blanc-Durand, P., Campedel, L., Sébastien Mule, A., Jegou, S., Luciani, A., Pigneur, F., et al.: Prognostic value of anthropometric measures extracted from whole-body CT using deep learning in patients with non-small-cell lung cancer. Imaging Inf. Artif. Intell. **30**, 3528–3537 (2020)
85. Carrino, J.A., Campbell, J., Paul, D., Lin, D.C., Morrison, W.B., Schweitzer, M.E., Flanders, A.E., et al.: Effect of spinal segment variants on numbering vertebral levels at lumbar MR imaging. Radiology **259**(1), 196–202 (2011). Available from: https://doi.org/10.1148/radiol.11081511. Available from https://www.ncbi.nlm.nih.gov/pubmed/21436097

Chapter 7
Automatic Detection of LST-Type Polyp by CNN Using Depth Map

Yuji Iwahori, Shota Miyazaki, Hiroyasu Usami, M. K. Bhuyan, Boonserm Kijsirikul, Aili Wang, Naotaka Ogasawara, and Kunio Kasugai

Abstract Lateral Spreading Tumor (LST) type flat polyps are sometimes overlooked and difficult to be detected among many lesions. This paper proposes a CNN model of multiple input and multiple output structure to detect LST-type polyp with high accuracy, which is based on U-Net architecture for the segmentation. Not only the original endoscope image but also depth map is also used to the original CNN structure of 2 inputs and 4 outputs. Here, proposed method obtains 3D shape from the original endoscope image and creates the depth map under the condition of point light source illumination and perspective projection. Higher accuracy of 85% was obtained for the detection of LST-type polyp by the proposed method. It is shown that the multiple input-output structure of U-Net model gives the higher performance of segmentation problem using both of original endoscope image and depth map.

Y. Iwahori (✉) · S. Miyazaki · H. Usami
Department of Computer Science, Chubu University, Kasugai 487-8501, Japan
e-mail: iwahori@isc.chubu.ac.jp

H. Usami
e-mail: usami@isc.chubu.ac.jp

M. K. Bhuyan
Department of Electronics and Electrical Engineering, Indian Institute of Technology Guwahati, Assam 781039, India
e-mail: mkb@iitg.ac.in

B. Kijsirikul
Department of Computer Engineering, Chulalongkorn University, 254 Phayathai Road, Pathumwan, Bangkok 10330, Thailand
e-mail: Boonserm.K@chula.ac.th

A. Wang
Harbin University of Science and Technology, 52 Xuefu Rd, Nangang, Harbin, China
e-mail: aili925@hrbust.edu.cn

N. Ogasawara · K. Kasugai
Department of Gastroenterology, Aichi Medical University, Nagakute, Aichi 480-1195, Japan
e-mail: nogasa@aichi-med-u.ac.jp

K. Kasugai
e-mail: kuku3487@aichi-med-u.ac.jp

© The Author(s), under exclusive license to Springer Nature Switzerland AG 2022
C.-P. Lim et al. (eds.), *Handbook of Artificial Intelligence in Healthcare*,
Intelligent Systems Reference Library 211,
https://doi.org/10.1007/978-3-030-79161-2_7

Keywords LST-type polyp · U-Net · Segmentation · 3D shape · Endoscope image

7.1 Introduction

An endoscope is used to detect polyps in the medical field. These diagnosis are performed for internal organs such as the stomach and intestines to find the abnormal parts such as bleeding, inflammation, and ulcer and so on. Polyps generally form all elevated lesions and there is a risk to become cancerous later. Therefore, it is important to detect polyp in the early stage and perform excision and follow-up. Polyp which is found by the diagnosis using an endoscopy may have a variety of sizes and shapes, so medical doctors may overlook polyps due to factors such as lack of experiences or diagnosis for the long time.

Lateral Spreading Tumor (LST) type flat polyps are sometimes overlooked and difficult to be detected especially among many lesions. LST-type polyp is a lesion on the intestinal wall unlike a normal rounded polyp and it is defined as a tumor larger than 10 mm that is spread laterally along the intestinal wall. This is a typical form of non-polypoid colon tumor. Therefore, it is required to detect LST-type polyp automatically from the image sequences taken by endoscope to prevent the overlook as a support for medical doctor's diagnosis.

Hwang et al. [1] and Ooto et al. [2] propose methods to detect polyps automatically from endoscope images. Hwang et al. [1] assumes a rounded shape of polyp and elliptical fitting is applied based on the polyp shape characteristics.

However, these methods are not effective for the shape characteristics of LST-type polyps since polyp is specified using region segmentation using edges detected from endoscope images. There is some possibility that whole part of LST-type polyp is not included in one image and there is a problem the method cannot be applied.

Ooto et al. [2] applies morphology processing and construct a likelihood map from the edge information and color information obtained from endoscope image. Features are extracted from Convolutional Neural Network (CNN) and SVM is used to detect polyp regions. Although this method makes it possible to identify the polyps by distinguishing between the polyps and intestinal walls to obtain edge information, there is a problem in constructing a likelihood map when LST-type polyp exists along the intestinal walls.

Miyazaki et al. [3] proposed a method to detect LST-type polyps. In Miyazaki et al. [3], U-Net in Ronneberger et al. [4] is used as a neural network which integrates and learns both of local features and global location information. Here, LST-type polyps are detected for each patch. However, the method in Miyazaki et al. [3] has the difficulty to distinguish between the intestinal wall and polyps from the shape characteristics of LST-type polyps, and the output of U-Net has many over detection results. It is necessary to solve the problem to distinguish between the intestinal walls and polyps.

In the field of general object recognition in dealing with CNN, the results become more accurate in the method which uses not only RGB images but also Depth images (Depth Map) at the same time as proposed in Zhang et al. [5] and Lai et al. [6].

To estimate the depth information, there are Godard et al. [7] and Gordon et al. [8] as the method that enables unsupervised learning of depth information. These approaches are useful for the general condition such as car view scene or landscape scene using learning of KITTI training set. Although the endoscope image dataset has recently often used to detect polyp, the approach to estimate the depth map is in very limited situation and it is required based on the endoscope environment.

So this paper proposes a new method to recover the 3D shape of a polyp from the endoscope image to obtain the depth map to improve the detection performance of LST-type polyp. Proposed method estimates the depth information from the viewpoint using Eikonal equation that expresses the image intensity equation and estimates the depth information at an interesting trial point using equation obtained from both of optical constraint a geometrical constraint. Modified Eikonal equation is derived under the conditions of point light source illumination and perspective projection. Using the modified Eikonal equation, a framework of Fast Marching Method (FMM) proposed by Kimmel et al. [10] is applied to recover the whole shape of image including polyps. Depth map is derived from the height of the recovered shape of polyp.

This paper uses a polyp RGB image and depth map which represents the relative 3D shape information using U-Net and RGB image and depth image are integrated and used to the multiple input and output of CNN structure to detect LST-type polyps with the higher performance.

7.2 Background

Proposed method uses an endoscope image which was taken under a white light source. Specular reflection components are removed and almost Lambertian reflectance image is generated. to recover 3D shape under the assumption of Lambertian reflectance image. Height Z is obtained using the method and a depth map is created. Obtained depth map is used with the original endoscope image as the input of the constructed CNN to detect polyps for each patch as output and the final detection result is provided. Flow of the proposed method is shown as follows.

Step 1   Removal of specular reflectance components and generation of Lambertian image
Step 2   Recovering 3D shape of endoscopic images and creating depth map
Step 3   Construction of a CNN using a depth map obtained in Step 2
Step 4   Detection result for each patch from the output of Step 3 and final integration of results

Fig. 7.1 Example of interpolation result

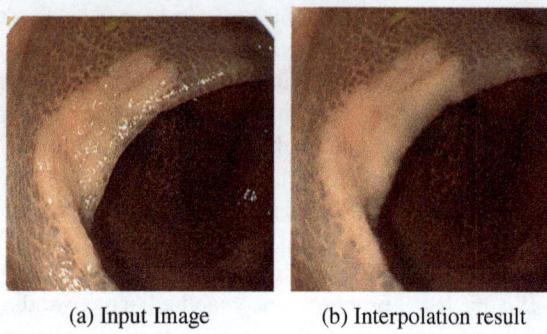

(a) Input Image (b) Interpolation result

7.2.1 Removal of Specular Reflectance Components and Generation of Lambertian Images

Proposed method recovers 3D shape of polyp and creates the depth map for the original image. First the original RGB image is converted to the gray scale Lambertian image to recover the 3D shape under the assumption of Lambertian image.

Here, a method of Ikeda et al. [9] is used to remove the specular reflectance component and generate Lambertian image. In Ikeda et al. [9], Fast Fourier Transform and region detection using color component are used to detect the specular component region.

In the region detection using FFT, which component is the least in the image among the RGB components is determined, then FFT is applied to the component so that only the high frequency components are remained, Next, a threshold is used to blue or green which has a low component in endoscope image and pixels with strong specular reflectance component are detected. Mask image is generated by applying logical OR operation with expansion processing and specular component region is interpolated based on the generated mask image. Interpolation method is applied to leave edge information as much as possible for 8 neighbor points around the interesting point. Filter which is distributed with the coefficients is applied based on the weight of the distance. Interpolation is done by taking sum of 8 neighboring points and result of interpolation is shown in Fig. 7.1 as an example.

The color system of the interpolated image is converted from RGB to HSV. Then, classification is performed for each reflectance using H histogram of color information and processing of uniform reflectance is performed using the ratio of V. The procedure of uniform reflectance is as follows.

Step 1 Perform classification using H histogram.
Step 2 Two points are taken on the boundary of the largest class and the class of interest, and ratio of V is calculated.
Step 3 Point with the shortest distance from the interesting point is extracted and interest point is classified into the largest class.

Fig. 7.2 Example of generated Lambertian image

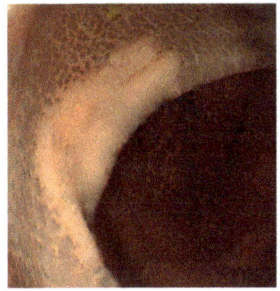 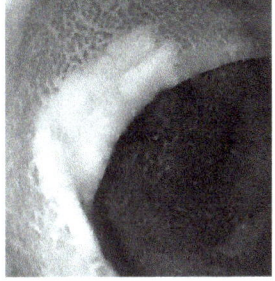

(a) Input image

(b) After applying uniform reflectance processing

Step 4   Do the same processing for the all class to make the uniform reflectance from the largest class where the value of H is close.

Generated Lambertian image is shown in Fig. 7.2.

7.2.2 Recovering 3D Shape and Creating Depth Map

Observed image intensity E under the assumption of Lambertian reflectance is represented by the depth Z, surface gradient parameters $(p, q) = (\partial Z/\partial X, \partial Z/\partial Y)$ and reflectance factor C. From this relation, optical constraint equation represented as Eq. (7.1) can be derived to represent the depth Z with other parameters. While the relationship between Z and (p, q) at the neighboring points is similar and representing the depth Z with the integral relations using (p, q) gives the geometrical constraint equation in Eq. (7.2). x, y are the observed image coordinates and f is the focal length of the lens.

$$Z_1 = \sqrt{CV(-px - qy + f)/E(p^2 + q^2 + 1)^{\frac{1}{2}}} \tag{7.1}$$

where E is image intensity and $V = f^2/(x^2 + y^2 + f^2)^{\frac{3}{2}}$.

$$Z_2 = Z_k(f - px_k - qy_k)/(f - px_t - qy_t) \tag{7.2}$$

Both of Z should be the same at each point and equalizing two right terms and rearranging gives the form of Eikonal equation. Here, the framework of FMM (Fast Marching Method) is used to solve the Eikonal equation.

Here, t ($trial$) represents an unknown interest point on the image, and k($known$) represents an known neighboring points of Z. C is a reflectance factor.

Z_1 and Z_2 should be equal and these can find the height Z at an interest point from these two equations. Therefore $Z_1 = Z_2$ and Eq. (7.3) is held. Since Eq. (7.2) uses known p and q and let $(p, q) = (p_k, q_k)$ in Eq. (7.3).

$$\sqrt{\frac{CV(-px - qy + f)}{E(p^2 + q^2 + 1)^{\frac{1}{2}}}} = \frac{Z_k(f - p_k x_k - q_k y_k)}{f - p_k x_t - q_k y_t} \tag{7.3}$$

Expanding Eq. (7.3) gives the form of Eq. (7.4).

$$\sqrt{p^2 + q^2} = \sqrt{(C/E)^2 A - 1} \tag{7.4}$$

where $A = \frac{V^2(f - p_k x_t - q_k y_t)^6}{Z_k^4 (f - p_k x_k - q_k y_k)^4}$.

The depth Z can be calculated by Eq. (7.5).

$$Z_{ij} = \begin{cases} \frac{(Z_a + Z_b + \sqrt{2 f_{ij} - (Z_a - Z_b)^2}}{2} & (|Z_a - Z_b| < f_{ij}) \\ min(Z_a, Z_b) + f_{ij} & (|Z_a - Z_b| \geq f_{ij}) \end{cases} \tag{7.5}$$

where $Z_a = min(Z_{i-1,j}, Z_{i+1,j})$, $Z_b = min(Z_{i,j-1}, Z_{i,j+1})$ and f_{ij} is the right term of Eq. (7.4). Procedure of polyp shape recovery is as follows based on the Eikonal equation.

Step 1 Set the pixel with the maximum intensity value as known and the initial point, Set the gradient parameters by $(p, q) = (-\frac{x}{f}, -\frac{y}{f})$ and set the depth Z using Eq. (7.1). Let the point of be $Z = \infty$ for other points except the initial point.

Step 2 Set $trial$ for 4 neighboring points around the initial point and Z at these four neighboring points of interest are calculated using Eq. (7.5) using the (p, q) at the initial point.

Step 3 Z at four neighboring points calculated in Step 2 is used to update (p, q) for one of four points using the difference of Z at two points. This updated (p, q) are used to calculate Z of the neighboring $trial$ point, where X and Y of $trial$ point are the world coordinates using $(X, Y) = (\frac{Z}{f} x, \frac{Z}{f} y)$.

$$p_+ = \frac{Z_{i+1,j} - Z_{i,j}}{X_{i+1,j} - X_{i,j}}, \quad p_- = \frac{Z_{i,j} - Z_{i-1,j}}{X_{i,j} - X_{i-1,j}} \tag{7.6}$$

$$q_+ = \frac{Z_{i,j+1} - Z_{i,j}}{Y_{i,j+1} - Y_{i,j}}, \quad q_- = \frac{Z_{i,j} - Z_{i,j-1}}{Y_{i,j} - Y_{i,j-1}} \tag{7.7}$$

Step 4 Z of $trial$ point is updated using (p, q) obtained by Eq. (7.5) in Step 3.

Step 5   Let the pixel which gives the minimum value of Z be *known*.
Step 6   Repeat Step 2 to Step 5 until Z of all pixels are calculated.

3D shape recovery for endoscope image is done by obtaining Z distribution. Z distribution obtained by the above steps procedure is used to create the depth map. Value of depth map is normalized between 0 and 1 and it is assumed the depth map is relative information. of Z. The depth map is used to the multiple input CNN constructed based U-Nets. The validity of recovering Z was confirmed using simulation model of a hemisphere. Simulated hemisphere was created under the condition of point light source illumination and perspective projection. Light source is located at the coordinate (0,0,0) which is the same point as the viewpoint (center of the lens). It was assumed that the radius of hemisphere R=5[mm] and focal length f is 10 [mm] and the reflectance factor is 22950. The center of hemisphere is located at (0,0,15) and simulation image was generated using Eq. (7.8). Depth Z from viewpoint is calculated using Eq. (7.9). Result of depth map for the hemisphere is shown in Fig. 7.3.

$$E = C \frac{f^2(-px - qy + f)}{(x^2 + y^2 + f^2)^{\frac{3}{2}} Z^2 (p^2 + q^2 + 1)^{\frac{1}{2}}} \qquad (7.8)$$

$$Z = \frac{f^2 Z_0 - \sqrt{f^4 Z_0^2 - f^2(x^2 + y^2 + f^2)(Z_0 - R^2)}}{(x^2 + y^2 + f^2)} \qquad (7.9)$$

From the result, the average error of height Z was 0.2672 [mm] in Fig. 7.3. It is shown that 3D recovery for the simulation was done with high precision. In the actual environment, Fig. 7.2 shows an input image where the focal length $f = 10$ [mm] and the reflectance factor $C = 84291$. Figure 7.4b shows the depth map. Depth map in this paper is the relative depth information and it is assumed the value of C is treated as known in the experiment.

7.3 Construction of U-Net Using Depth Map

7.3.1 *Preprocessing and Construction of Dataset*

In this paper, the following processing is done for the training data set given to CNN.
- Grayscale image conversion
- Contrast Limited Adaptive Histogram Equalization (CLAHE)

Endoscope image after the above processings and the corresponding depth map created from Z are used. The processed images are shown in Fig. 7.5a, and b. Then

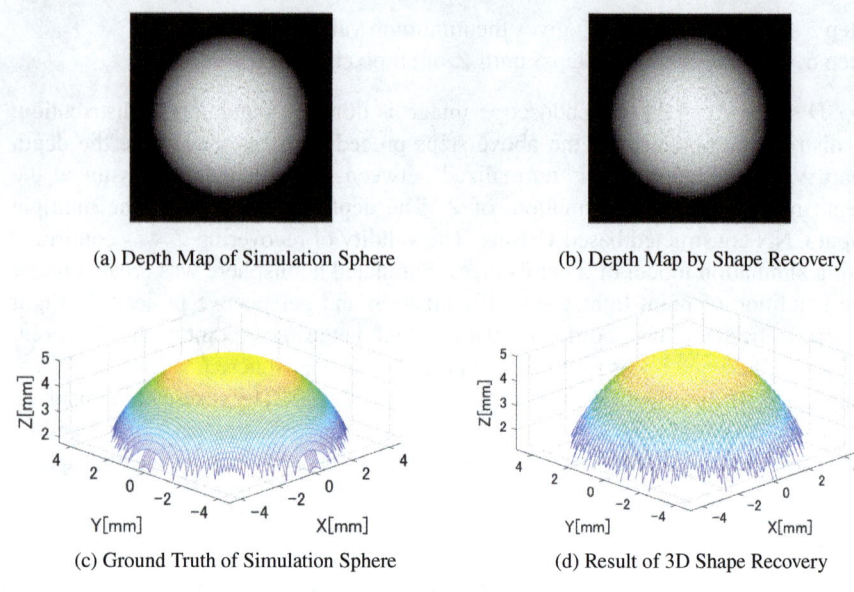

Fig. 7.3 3D shape and depth map

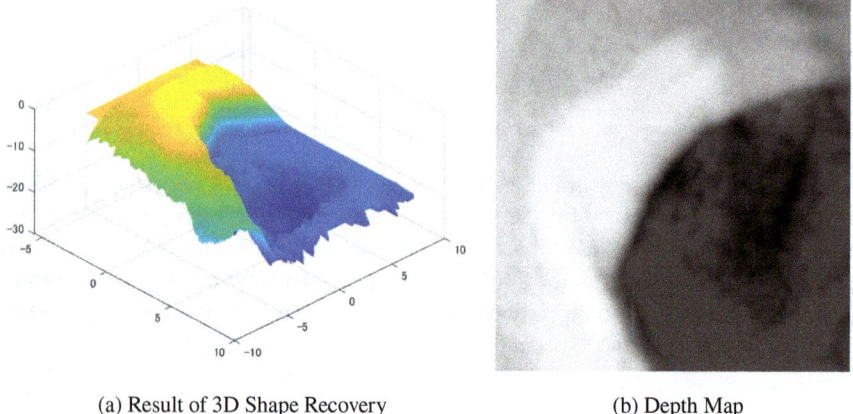

Fig. 7.4 Result of 3D shape recovery and created depth map

the random patch of 48×48 pixels are created as shown in Figs. 7.6a, b. Here, original endoscope image includes unnecessary region in the four corners of each image as shown in Fig. 7.5c, and only the target region is used to the created patch where unnecessary region is removed.

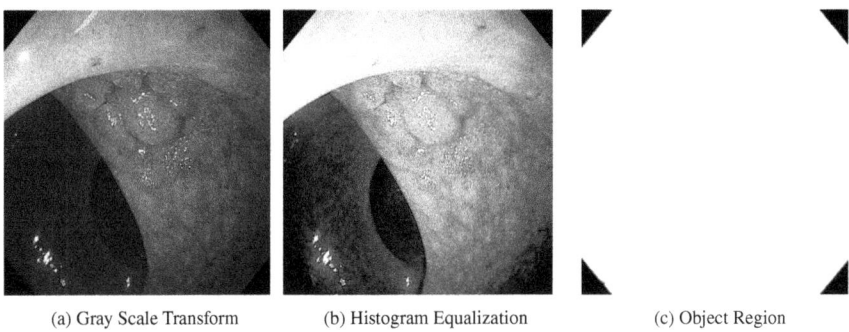

(a) Gray Scale Transform (b) Histogram Equalization (c) Object Region

Fig. 7.5 Preprocessing

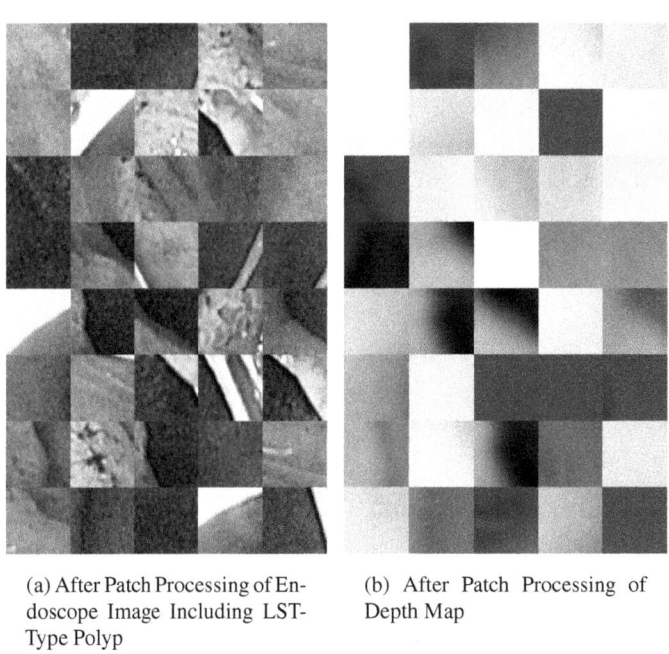

(a) After Patch Processing of Endoscope Image Including LST-Type Polyp

(b) After Patch Processing of Depth Map

Fig. 7.6 Example of patch processing

7.3.2 Construction of CNN Model Using U-Net Structure

This method constructs the CNN using the U-Net structure of Ronneberger et al. [4]. Based on the consideration of resolution of input image used in the experiment, U-Net structure is constructed by reducing the number of layers as shown in Fig. 7.7. Both of endoscope image and the corresponding depth map are used, so the input layer has two inputs. CNN used in this method is shown in Fig,7.8. Further, 2 inputs and multiple outputs CNN is constructed to increase the treated information. CNN

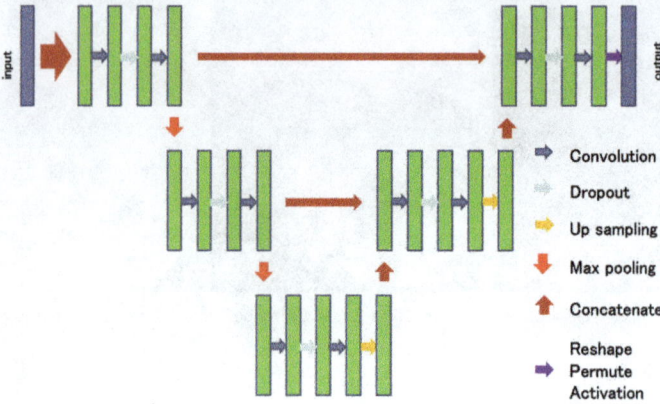

Fig. 7.7 U-Net structure with reduced layers

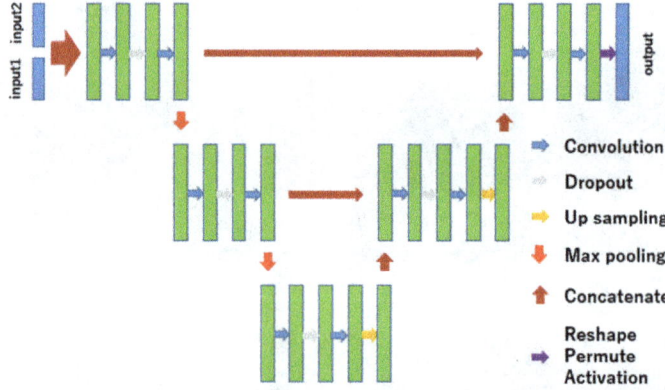

Fig. 7.8 2 inputs and 1 output CNN structure based on U-Net

is constructed using U-Net structure and number of layers of U-Net is reduced based on the image resolution of input image. Input layers consist of two layers, one of which is the patch image and the other of which is the patch image of depth map. In addition, depth map is used to input and the output obtained from the downsampling in the U-Net structure is used to the upsampling in the structure. Similarly endoscope image and depth map are replaced in the corresponding layers and a total of four kinds of output are prepared and used for the learning. Figure 7.9 shows the overview of constructed CNN.

7.3.2.1 2 Inputs and 1 Output CNN

2 Inputs and 1 Output CNN is constructed with the following structure.

7 Automatic Detection of LST-Type Polyp by CNN Using Depth Map

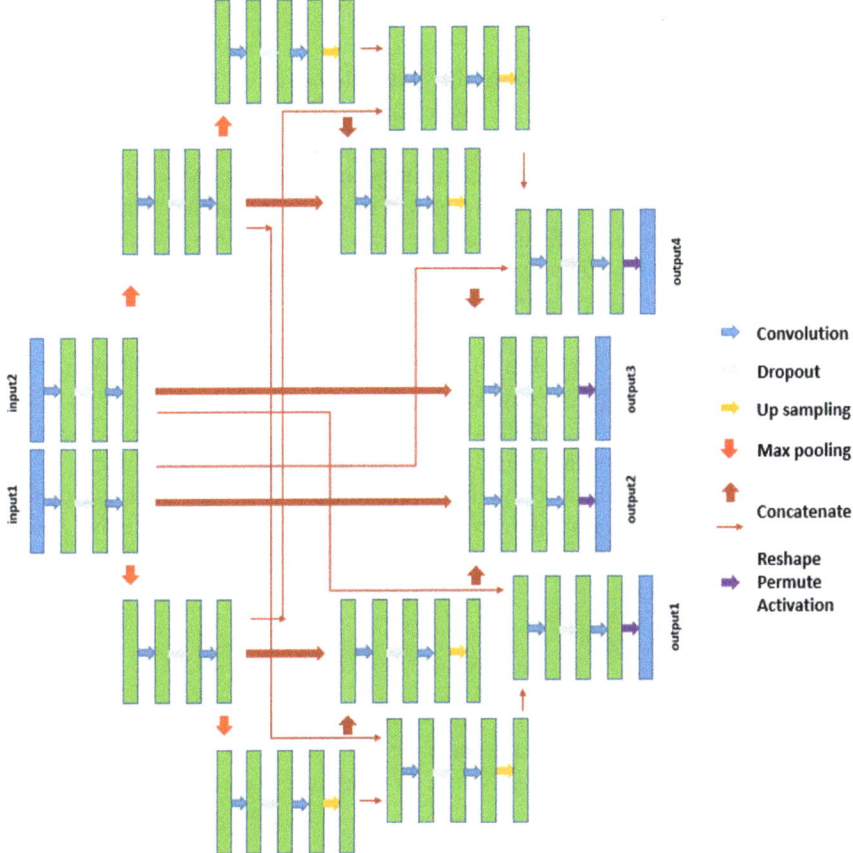

Fig. 7.9 2 inputs and 4 outputs CNN structure based on U-Net

Two inputs are connected in the channel direction in input layer and the structure consists of three layers. Here each layer consists of convolutional layer for Encoder, Dropout and convolutional layer which means one block with pooling layers.

Decoder part is upsampled from the bottom layer and it combines with the corresponding above layer. In the final block, the array is changed after sandwiching the convolution layer and the dimension of the input is replaced, and output is obtained via ReLU function.

Kernel size of all the convolutional layers in each block are 3×3 and that of convolution layer for the output layer is 1×1. Pooling layer performs max pooling with 2×2 windows and striding. Upsampling is also done with 2×2 windows.

7.3.2.2 2 Inputs and 4 Outputs CNN

Two inputs and 4 outputs CNN is constructed with the following structure.

Two inputs are connected in the channel direction in input layer and the structure consists of three layers. Here each layer consists of convolutional layer for Encoder, Dropout and convolutional layer which means one block with pooling layers.

Decoder part is upsampled from the bottom layer and it combines with the corresponding above layer. In the final block, the array is changed after sandwiching the convolution layer and the dimension of the input is replaced, and output is obtained via ReLU function. This processing is done in two cases of input 1 and input 2 and two outputs are obtained.

Encoder part of input 1 and Decoder part of input 2 is connected and in the final block, the array is changed after sandwiching the convolution layer and the dimension of the input is replaced, and output is obtained via ReLU function. Replacing input 1 and input 2 and 2 outputs are added and a total of 4 outputs are provided.

Kernel size of all the convolutional layers in each block are 3×3 and that of convolution layer for the output layer is 1×1. Pooling layer performs max pooling with 2×2 windows and striding. Upsampling is also done with 2×2 windows.

7.4 Experiment

Experiment was done to evaluate the performance of these proposed CNN structures for the detection of LST-type polyp image from actual endoscope image.

7.4.1 Evaluation Method

In the accuracy evaluation, patch based evaluation is applied for the detection by stetting the desired patch size. This evaluation is used for the final detection result.

Patch of 20×20 pixels is applied for the output of constructed CNN, thresholding for the output value is used for the patch based output of CNN structures and the judgment is done from the result whether polyp is included or not in the patch image.

Detection performance of 2 inputs and 4 outputs CNN derives 4 kinds of outputs for the patch based polyp detection. Here voting processing is introduced to provide the final judgment by integrating the outputs for the LST-type polyp detection.

Flow of the accuracy evaluation is shown in Fig. 7.10.

Sensitivity, Specificity and Accuracy was used for the evaluation indexes.

True Positive (TP) is the number of polyps judged to be polyps, True Negative (TN) is number of non-polyps judged to be non-polyps, False Positive (FP) is the number of polyps judged to non-polyp, and False Negative (FN) is number of non-polyp judged to polyp.

7 Automatic Detection of LST-Type Polyp by CNN Using Depth Map

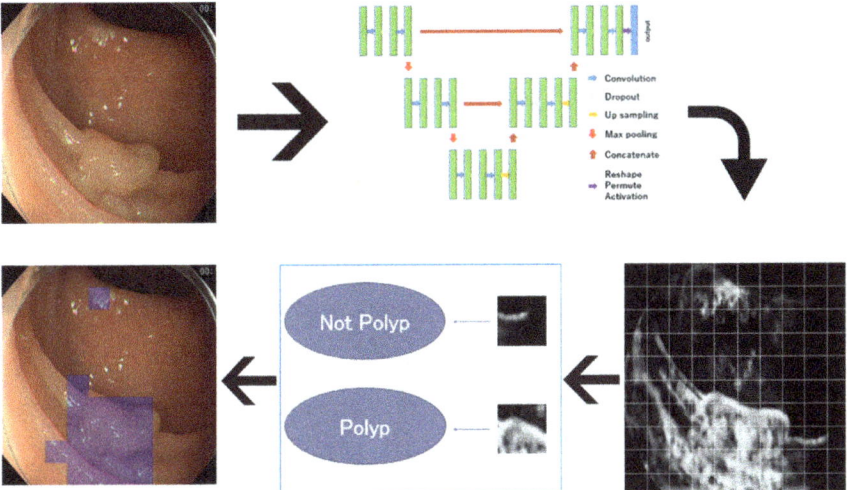

Fig. 7.10 Flow of accuracy evaluation

Sensitivity is the correct ratio of polyp judged to polyp. Specificity is the correct ratio of non-polyp judged to non-polyp. Accuracy is the correct ratio of the whole cases of judgment.

$$Sensitivity = \frac{TP}{TP + FP} \tag{7.10}$$

$$Specificity = \frac{TN}{TN + FN} \tag{7.11}$$

$$Accuracy = \frac{TP + TN}{TP + FP + TN + FN} \tag{7.12}$$

7.4.2 Detection Experiment

The dataset used in the experiment was taken under a white light source of endoscope. Endoscope images including LST-type polyps were used and the corresponding depth map images were created using our original algorithm.

20 images were randomly selected and used for the evaluation of test images while the remaining 50 images were used for the learning of CNN.

Learning dataset was created by making 190,000 patch images of 48×48 pixels in addition to the pre-processing for the original endoscope images.

Simultaneously mask images as shown in Fig. 7.5b were prepared as patch image of 48×48 pixels. This mask image is used as a correct label image. Learning procedure used Categorical Cross Entropy for the loss function and Stochastic FGradient

Fig. 7.11 Results of output

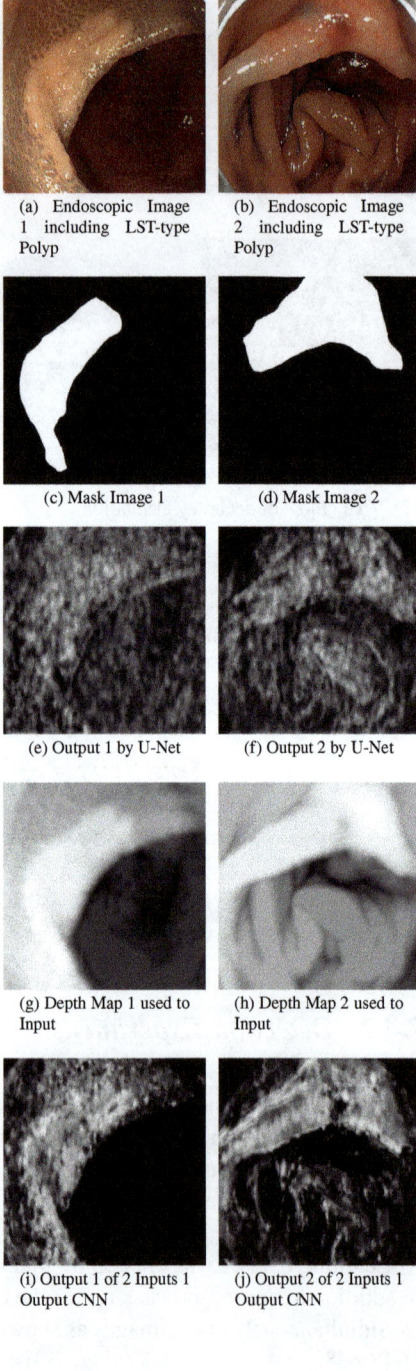

7 Automatic Detection of LST-Type Polyp by CNN Using Depth Map

Fig. 7.12 Detection results

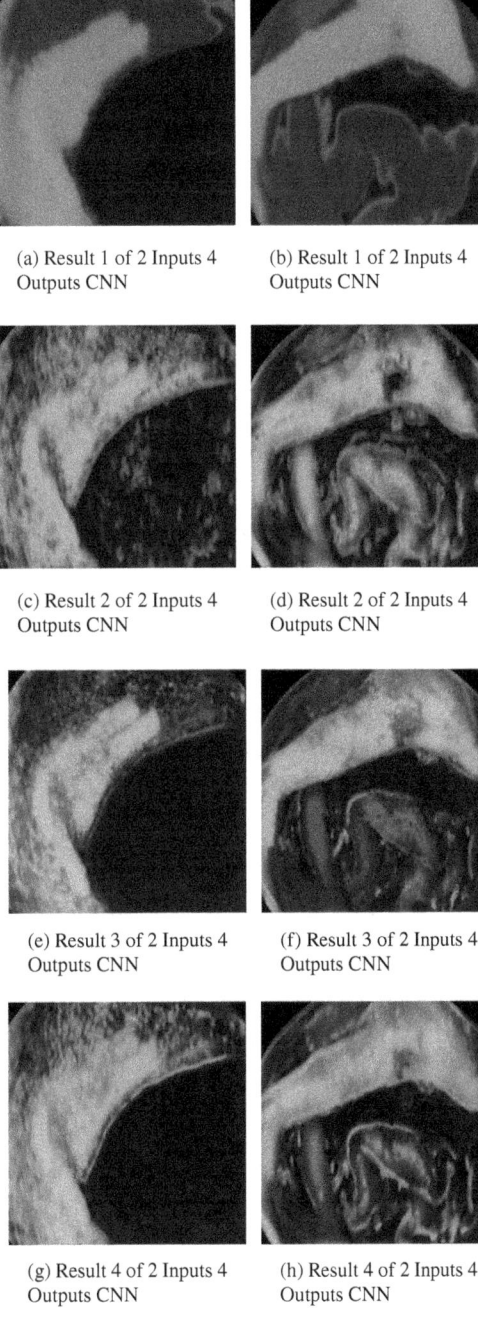

(a) Result 1 of 2 Inputs 4 Outputs CNN

(b) Result 1 of 2 Inputs 4 Outputs CNN

(c) Result 2 of 2 Inputs 4 Outputs CNN

(d) Result 2 of 2 Inputs 4 Outputs CNN

(e) Result 3 of 2 Inputs 4 Outputs CNN

(f) Result 3 of 2 Inputs 4 Outputs CNN

(g) Result 4 of 2 Inputs 4 Outputs CNN

(h) Result 4 of 2 Inputs 4 Outputs CNN

Decent (SGD) for the optimization. Initial value of learning rate was 0.1, batch size was 32, and number of maximum learning epochs was 150, 150, 400 for each of U-Net, 2 Inputs and 1 Output CNN, 2 Input and 4 Output CNN. Learning time using GTX 1080 Ti (as GPU) was 27,691[sec], 108,752[sec], 229,204[sec], respectively and detection time of the output in the test was 219[sec], 227[sec], 1,037[sec], respectively.

Detection results as outputs by these constructed CNN are shown in Fig. 7.11, Fig. 7.12, respectively.

As a quantitative evaluation, the results show that there are many results which do not include polyp when only endoscope image is used as input as shown in Figs. 7.11 and 7.12. However, it is shown that adding the depth map information is useful from the observations that there is the higher accuracy of polyp detection on around the inner part of large intestine or there is a large difference from the polyp and intestinal wall. Figure 7.12 shows the outputs of depth map and endoscope image are different and it shows different patches are strongly detected respectively. Integration of these results can provide more robust outputs and LST-type polyp can be detected more exactly. Detection results of (1) 1 output U-Net, (2) 2 inputs and 1 output CNN, (3) 2 inputs and 4 output CNN are shown in Table 7.1.

Table 7.1 suggests that both of Sensitivity and Accuracy are higher values in the case when depth map is added than the case when it is not used and detection ratio increased. Integration by 2 inputs and 4 outputs CNN suppresses the over detection rather than the case of connection of channel direction in input layer. As a result, it is shown that whole correct ratio also increased. This represents adding and using depth map plays an important role to detect LST-type polyp in comparison with the use of only the endoscope image. It was confirmed that the proposed method is useful from these results.

Final detection results by Sect. 7.4.2 are shown in Figs. 7.13 and 7.14, respectively. Ground Truth is shown in Fig. 7.13c, d and these are created by section 7.4.2 from the mask image shown in Fig. 7.11c, d.

Figure 7.13 shows over detection except polyp is seen when depth map is not used to input. When depth map is used to input, over detection region is suppressed and detection ratio of polyp increases.

Figure 7.14 also shows the more suppressions of over detection than the case of 1 output and improvement of detection is confirmed at around the region where some non-detection region existed and overall the detection ratio was also improved.

If patch size becomes smaller then it becomes possible to detect more detailed results, while the processing time needs more and these are advantage and disadvantage respectively. It is also considered that increasing the number of endoscope images can make it possible to improve the accuracy for the detection of LST-type polyp.

Fig. 7.13 Final output 1

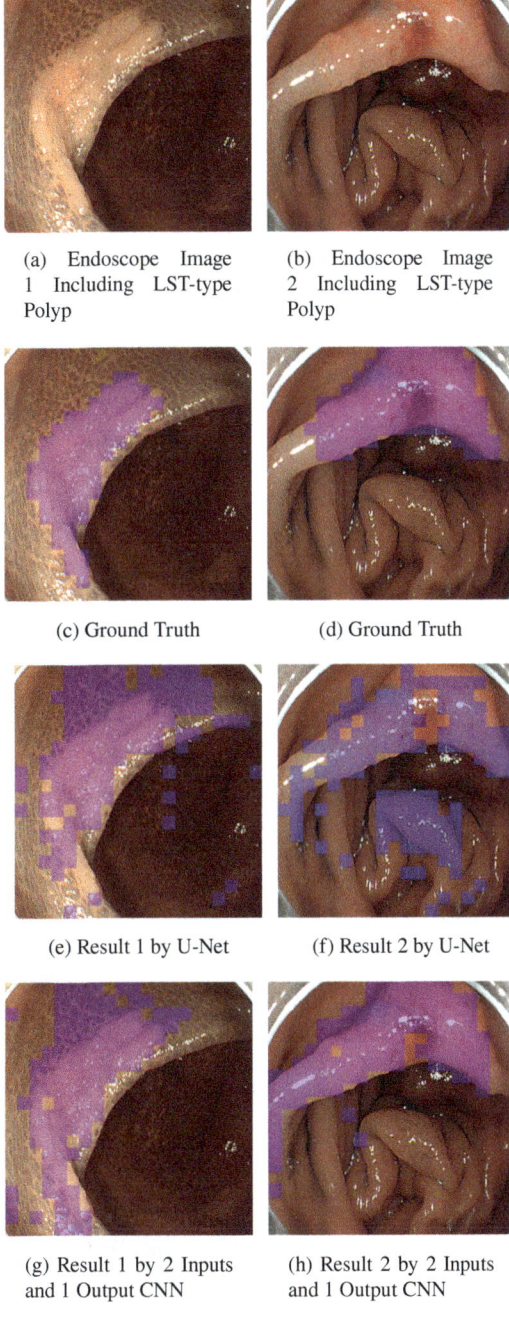

(a) Endoscope Image 1 Including LST-type Polyp

(b) Endoscope Image 2 Including LST-type Polyp

(c) Ground Truth

(d) Ground Truth

(e) Result 1 by U-Net

(f) Result 2 by U-Net

(g) Result 1 by 2 Inputs and 1 Output CNN

(h) Result 2 by 2 Inputs and 1 Output CNN

Fig. 7.14 Final output 2

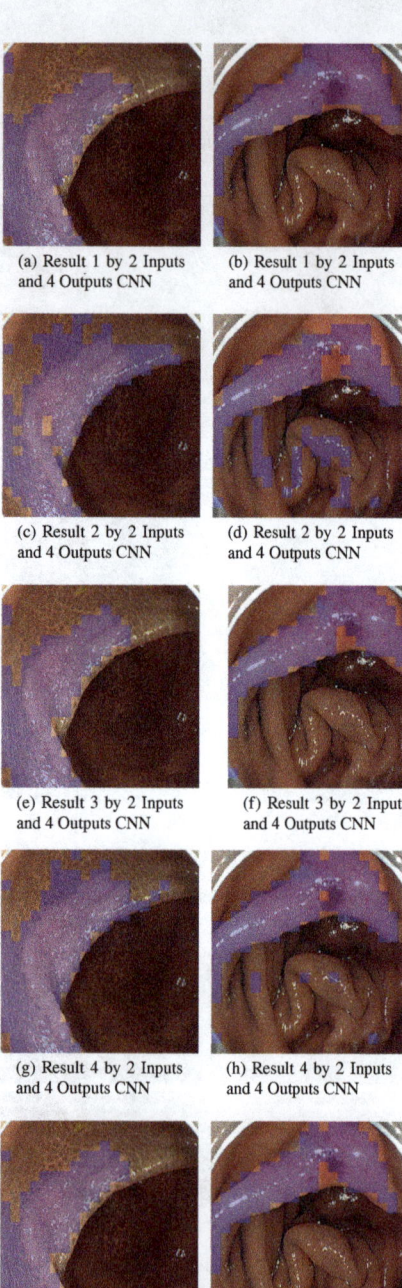

Table 7.1 Accuracy evaluation (%)

	TP	FP	TN	FN	Sensitivity	Specificity	Accuracy
(1)	1309	747	5125	819	63.67	86.22	80.43
(2)	1419	637	5265	679	69.02	88.57	83.55
(3)	1495	561	5324	620	72.71	89.56	85.24

7.5 Conclusion

This paper proposed a new method to detect the LST-type polyp with high accuracy. 2 inputs and 4 outputs CNN structure was created with depth map in addition to the original endoscope image. Comparative experiment was performed to evaluate the effectiveness of the proposed method from the cases of only one endoscope image with U-Net and other 2 inputs and multiple outputs CNNs by adding the depth map information. It is confirmed that integration of outputs gives more robust result and detection ratio was improved with adding the depth information.

Using 2 inputs and getting 4 outputs with input image and depth map provides the higher accuracy rather than the case when input image and depth map are just connected and 1 output is obtained. Voting processing was introduced to raise the detection ratio by integrating the outputs as one result.

Further subjects includes the improvement under the condition of the low cost and higher accuracy and improvement for the undetected and/or misclassification of LST-type polyp in addition to the parameter adjustment for each output layer of the constructed CNN structure.

Acknowledgements Iwahori's research is supported by Japan Society for the Promotion of Science (JSPS) Grant-in-Aid Scientific Research(C) (#20K11873) and Chubu University Grant. Usami's research is supported by JSPS Grant-in-Aid for Research Activity Start-up (#19K24370).

References

1. Hwang, S., Oh, J., Tavanapong, W., Wong, J., De Groen, P.C.: Polyp detection in colonoscopy video using elliptical shape feature. In: IEEE International Conference on Image Processing, 2007. ICIP 2007, vol. 2, pp. II–465. IEEE (2007)
2. Ooto, T., Usami, H., Iwahori, Y., Wang, A., Ogasawara, N., Kasugai, K.: Cost Reduction of Creating Likelihood Map for Automatic Polyp Detection Using Image Pyramid, pp. 204–209. CSII (2017)
3. Miyazaki, S., Ooto, T., Usami, H., Iwahori, Y., Kijsirikul, B., Kasugai, K.: Automatic Detection of LST-type Polyp using U-Net, P134, Poster, Intelligent Image Processing, WiNF 2018 Workshop (2018)

4. Ronneberger, O., Fischer, P., Brox, T.: U-net: convolutional networks for biomedical image segmentation. In: International Conference on Medical Image Computing and computer-Assisted Intervention, MICCAI, vol. 9351, pp. 234–241. Springer, LNCS (2015)
5. Zhang, J., Li, W., Ogunbona, P.O., Wang, P., Tang, C.: RGB-D-based action recognition datasets: A survey. Pattern Recognition **60**, 86–105 (2016)
6. Lai, K., Bo, L., Ren, X., Fox, D.: A large-scale hierarchical multi-view RGB-D object dataset. ICRA 1817–1824 (2011)
7. Godard, C., Aodha, O. M., Brostow. G.J.: Unsupervised monocular depth estimation with left-right consistency, pp. 270–279. CVPR (2017)
8. Gordon, A., Li, H., Jonschkowski, R., Angelova, A.: Depth from Videos in the Wild: Unsupervised Monocular Depth Learning from Unknown Cameras, pp. 1–17 (2019). arXiv https://arxiv.org/pdf/1904.04998.pdf
9. Ikeda, N., Usami, H., Iwahori, Y., Kijsirikul, B., Kasugai, K.: Generating Lambertian image by removing specular reflection component and difference of reflectance factor using HSV. In: Proceedings of ITC-CSCC 2016, T2-5, Computer Vision (2), pp. 547–550 (2016)
10. Kimmel, R., Sethian, J. A.: Optimal algorithm for shape from Shading and path planning. JMIV **14**, 237–244 (2001)

Chapter 8
Artificial Intelligence and Deep Learning, Important Tools in Assisting Gastroenterologists

M. Luca, A. Ciobanu, T. Barbu, and V. Drug

Abstract The incidence of colorectal cancers nowadays, with a high rate of mortality, justifies the effort of scientists from different disciplines in solving this problem. Early detection of pre-cancerous signs considerably increases the survival rate. Inter and intra-observer variability might be stated in lesions' diagnosis due to the patient's personal particularities, depending on colon cleansing degree or influenced by the expert's training, state of mind or attentiveness. Computer aided detection and diagnosis with special designed software, for different practical aspects, assisting endoscopy physicians, comes to reinforce the certitude of adopted decisions. Artificial intelligence, deep learning, graphic interfaces and the development of parallel computing devices, accelerated a lot the practical achievements in colon cancer prevention, during the latest years.

Keywords Artificial intelligence · Deep learning · Convolutional neural networks · Computer-aided diagnosis · Image processing · Video colonoscopy · Gastrointestinal endoscopy

8.1 Introduction

Intelligent techniques are important tools in the educational process, for training and assisting students and young physicians to recognizing malignant or non-malignant structures, since cancer is the second leading cause of death, after cardiovascular diseases, in the world [1].

M. Luca (✉) · A. Ciobanu · T. Barbu
Institute of Computer Science, Iași Branch, Romanian Academy, Bd. Carol I, Nr. 8, 700505 Iași, Romania
e-mail: mihaela.luca@iit.academiaromana-is.ro

V. Drug
University of Medicine and Pharmacy, "Gr. T. Popa", Iași, Romania

Institute of Gastroenterology and Hepathology, "Sf. Spiridon", Emergency Hospital, Iași, Romania

Referring to the cancer incidence and mortality based on the reports of the International Agency for Research on Cancer, GLOBOCAN 2020 states that, after the lung cancer (with an estimated 18% lethal cases), the colorectal cancer (CRC) is the second leading death cause (9.4%) worldwide [2].

This fully justifies the global concern and effort that scientists spend trying to use combined and assisted methods in CRC prevention and eradication [3].

After the preliminary non-invasive fecal tests, FIT—immunochemical test [4], DNA or FOBT—occult blood test, (which perform less [5]), follow the invasive ones: colonoscopy or the flexible sigmoidoscopy, the narrow band (NB) endoscopy, capsule endoscopy (CE) or computed tomography colonography (CTC). All these are indicated by the physician in correlation with more personal data (age, gender, genetics and patient's illness history).

Colonoscopy is still considered the golden standard for periodic surveys in CRC evaluations [6], under the American, European or Asia Pacific consensus statements. Most of the national or regional gastrointestinal endoscopy societies are affiliated to World Endoscopy Organization (WEO), in an effort of adopting the appropriated standards to be followed by anyone around the globe [3].

Note that, World Endoscopy Organization is reuniting professional societies from three geographical zones: "Asia–Pacific Society of Digestive Endoscopy" (A-PSDE), "European Society of Gastrointestinal Endoscopy" (ESGE) and "Inter-American Society of Digestive Endoscopy" (SIED) for both American continents. It also has two independent members SGA (Saudi Gastroenterology Association), IAGH (Iranian Association of Gastroenterology and Hepatology), and more collaborating societies: ASGE (American Society of Gastrointestinal Endoscopy), BSG (British Society of Gastroenterology), Gastroenterological Association of Thailand, Indonesian Society for Digestive Endoscopy, Japan Gastroenterological Endoscopy Society, Korean Society of Gastrointestinal Endoscopy, Gastroenterological Society of Singapore, Philippine Society of Digestive Endoscopy, "Asociación Colombiana de Endoscopía Digestiva", "Sociedade Brasileira de Endoscopia Digestiva" [3].

The Minimal Standard Terminology (MST) for gastrointestinal endoscopy was updated in 2016 [7].

8.2 Computer-Assisted Colonoscopy for CRC Early Detection

Colorectal cancer frequently develops in the large intestine of the lower gastrointestinal (GI) tract. It might develop from a benign little growth of glandular tissue, placed on the surface of the interior membrane of the colon, named adenomas [8]. Some of them may become malignant structures, transforming in colon cancer. Passing into the lymph vessels or blood these cells could transform in metastases. It is essential to stop them, early.

Automated detection of polyps is challenging, as this implies analyzing different shapes, sizes, colors and textures, sometimes partly covered by artefacts or anatomical particularities [9]. "The endoscopic appearance can be similar to protruded lesions, flat elevated lesions, and flat lesions ... images have noisy background with bleeding and endoluminal folds, which suppresses the accuracy of the detection process" [10].

The aim of a colonoscopy is to detect the prerequisites for possible colon cancers, identifying polyps, sessile serrated lesions, adenomas or the bleeding lesions. It is possible to recognize their nature using white light, chromo endoscopy, virtual chromo endoscopy (NBI-narrow band imaging [11]) and magnifying procedures [12–14].

Removing the polyps if possible (using the "resect and discard" strategy), referring to surgery if needed, and regularly surveying the incipient abnormalities, before evolving into cancer, are the targets of this exam.

Note that in NBI, light of specific wavelengths is used to enhance the cellular details and particular aspects of the mucosal surface: blue (440–460 nm) to detect capillary vessels near the surface of the membrane, while green (540–460 nm) is absorbed by the blood vessels located deeper within the mucosal layer [13].

The optical biopsy during the colonoscopy is ideal for efficient survey in colonoscopy [15]. Training young physicians to recognize precancerous sessile serrated lesions or adenomas upon their aspect is a worthwhile attempt.

In a very recent editorial [16] focusing on the problems and impressing results of applying artificial intelligence (AI) in video colonoscopy analysis, while speaking about the randomized studies made to objectively measure these benefits, they stated in a side-remark: "an embarrassing variability in adenoma detection rates (ADRs) across any series of endoscopists raises questions about the status of screening colonoscopy as a clinical standard... Low-detectors can miss up to 75% of neoplastic lesions as compared with high-detectors... indicating a general reluctance of some endoscopists to recognize their own underperformance" [16]. AI embedded in colonoscopy devices offers solutions around the world, and the randomized studies about its impact on the medical daily practice are opening "the new Silk Road" [16].

In the classical approach, computer aided detection (CAD) on video colonoscopies, was "based on very complex pattern recognition: color, discrete cosine transform (DCT), pixel's contrast relative to gray levels of vicinity pixels, J48 classifier, local binary patterns (LBPs) with strong illumination invariant texture primitives... histograms of binary patterns computed across regions were used to select features" [17], reminding only a few image processing methods from the numerous attempts.

More recent, artificial intelligence, which includes machine learning (ML), which, at its turn, includes deep learning (DL), took the place of these very difficult methods proposed only a few years ago, at the beginning of the last decade, replacing them with millions of repetitive convolutions, inside very deep structures.

DL is the new method which came to replace or to complete old classic methods that were used before. Seminal ideas in DL early arose in 1998 in Yann LeCun's paper [18], and they were developed only later [19, 20], due to possible parallel computing. Ideas quickly spread, not only due to the powerful deep learning networks, but also to the vision challenges on a fundamental image database ImageNet [21]. This came from Stanford vision lab, Stanford and Princeton Universities that planed to map all the world of objects. ImageNet [21], (containing 14,197,122 images, 21,841 indexed "synsets") is structured according to the "WordNet hierarchy (currently only the nouns), in which each node of the hierarchy is depicted by hundreds and thousands of images" [21, 22].

Winners of the ImageNet Large Scale Visual Recognition Challenge (ILSVRC) [23] contributed a lot to the DL networks diversification. Convolution neural networks (CNN) [19], AlexNet in 2012 [24], Inception (GoogLeNet) in 2014 [25], VGGNet [26], Xception [27], or Residual Networks ResNet [28] (recently applied in [29]), are only o few deep learning architectures which were recurrently used, afterward.

Thousands of papers were published and communicated in the image processing and object identification field in the last decade.

In gastrointestinal endoscopies the research subjects are diverging a lot: from offline video colonoscopy (using classic image processing and assessing), to real time adenoma and polyp detection using DL, from optic microscopy (to detect the possible malignant cellular content of the identified structures), to colon cleansing evaluation or to global evaluation of AI and ML impact on colonoscopies and gastroendoscopies in randomized control studies.

Deep learning used in analyzing video colonoscopies and Graphic Processing Units (GPU) together with dedicated software libraries, made a huge difference in designing real time video colonoscopy assisting devices.

8.2.1 Polyps' Semantic Segmentation

Several recent studies focus on segmentation of images in order to better serve the learning task for young physicians, trying to find the exact edges of the adenoma and serrated polyps with DL using fully convolutional neural networks (FCNN) [30–32] or based on self learning, on self-paced transfer networks [33].

A special remark has to be done referring to UNet [34] and UNet + + deep learning methods successfully applied in colon semantic segmentation [35], offering some of the best results.

A big step in rapid developing new techniques was made during the Medical Image Computing and Computer Assisted Intervention Conference, (MICCAI) [36], with the Endoscopic Vision Challenge and GIANA Sub-challenge on Gastrointestinal Image Analysis, which set the stage for an important competition on automatic assessing of the video colonoscopies [36].

8.2.2 Reviews and Meta-Analysis, Randomized Studies and AI Embedded Colonoscopy Devices

Among the reviews and meta-analysis in computer assisted video colonoscopies using the new domains of AI, ML and DL, which appeared in the last several years, we will select to cite only the papers published during the last year, 2020 [37–40], which covers very well this domain with its novelties.

Citing only a few papers published in the last two years [41–46] we may say that a lot of teams focused on using DL as primary tool in their systems, with impressing results. Therefore, random studies on numerous groups of patients with thousands of polyps detected [47–52] are necessary to evaluate the efficacy of AI methods on clinical cases and were published during the last three years. This game the start of a competition towards developing technical solutions embedded in the actual colonoscopy systems as Genius AI, Medtronic [53], Argus [54], Olympus' ENDO-AID, in combination with Evis X1 [55] or ENDOANGEL [50].

Our attempts in automatic video colonoscopy analysis comprise research in evaluating the colon cleansing degree, studying membrane surface aspects using LAB color space, with both classic methods, and deep learning, on Nvidia Jetson devices for polyp detection on our own image databases [56–62]. We are intending to further develop them in an interdisciplinary research project. We will discuss step by step some issues intricate in automatic computer assisted colonoscopy evaluation.

8.2.3 Well Structured Labeled Databases

Each learning method starts with a good database with well structured, labeled data. In a recent study regarding the development of automatic colonoscopies processing, it was underlined that there were very few well labeled databases available for research [63].

Some of the existing gastrointestinal (GI) image databases are CVC (more datasets) [64], ASU Mayo polyp database [65], Kvasir, Kvasir SEG—for polyps, and a few other datasets, an overview of them being given in a recent paper on the HyperKvasir [66]. HyperKvasir dataset contains 110,079 images and 374 videos from various GI examinations, resulting in 1 million images and frames in total, so significantly increasing the amount of labeled medical data for supervised learning and unlabeled data [66]. Current work in ML successfully tackles the challenge of lack of data in semi-supervised learning: "Instead of learning from a large set of annotated data, algorithms can now learn from sparsely labeled and unlabeled data" [66].

"Despite the new performance highs, the recent advanced segmentation models still require large, representative and high quality annotated datasets" [67], implying the need to focus on the techniques for handling imperfect medical image segmentation datasets (scarce, noisy, sparse, weak annotations, unreliable labels).

8.3 Dealing with Video Colonoscopy Frames

Video colonoscopy, sigmoidoscopy or colon capsule endoscopy, are techniques which deliver images registered inside the colon with one or more cameras, according to the structure of the devices we use. If a video colonoscopy is lasting 12 to 20 min or more, the video obtained might be split in tens of thousands of frames.

The quality of these images is affected by light reflection, speckles, water jets (for cleaning the surface of the colon), debris, fecal traces, mucus, undigested food residues or even traces of blood. When some of these are present, the images are only partly informative or completely non informative and, if possible, it is better to be discarded [60, 68–70]. Some examples of non-informative or even perturbing images might be observed in Fig. 8.1, presenting images selected from our own database (we have 17 anonymised video colonoscopies split in hundreds of thousands of images).

Accurate adenoma or polyps images need very effective colon cleansing, therefore degrees are estimated on bowel preparation scales as Boston Bowel Preparation Scale (BBPS) [71] or the Ottawa Scale [72], Aronchick Scale [73–75], standards in America, Chicago Bowel Preparation Scale (CBPS) [76], attributing either marks computed for every colonoscopy, or linguistic values (excellent, good, or fair), upon the conventions adopted by each country.

BBPS is a "10-point scale assessing", from 0 to 9, with marks attributed by convention, to each of the three main segments of the colon upon its state: 0 for unprepared colon, covered, impossible to be cleaned; 1 for partial covered areas of the colon segments, with solid residues or opaque liquid; 2 for minor residues staining, with still visible mucosa of the colon segment; 3 for well seeing the entire colon segment mucosa, no residual staining, no fragments, no opaque liquid [71].

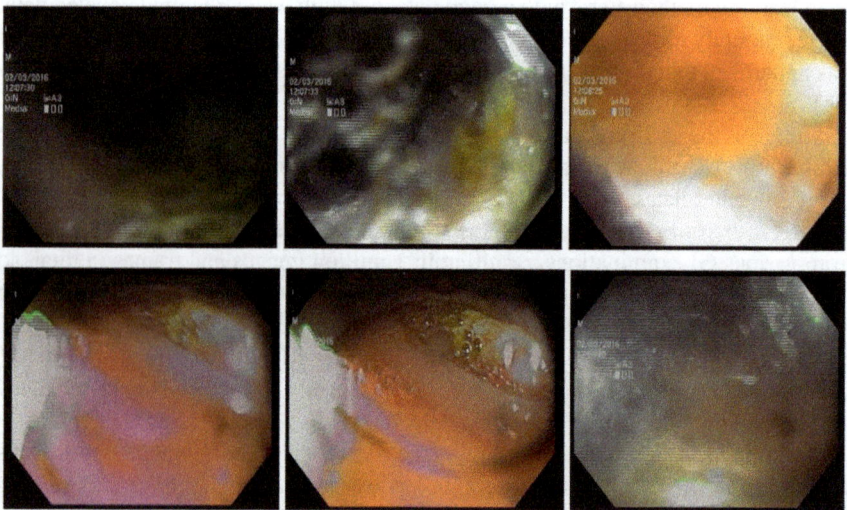

Fig. 8.1 Non-informative frames offering no clue for diagnosis

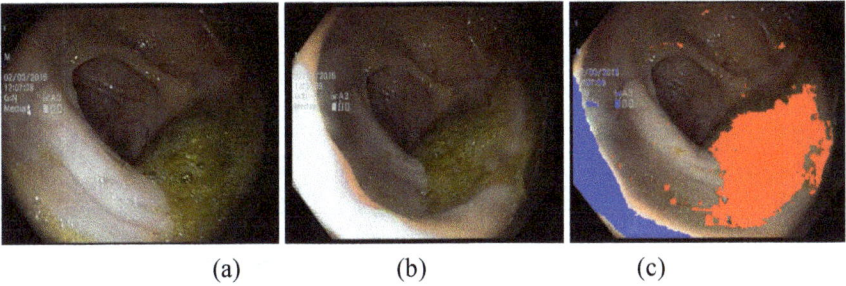

Fig. 8.2 Video colonoscopy frames partly covered with stool

This is important in order to decide upon the level of bowel preparation quality which requires an early repeated colonoscopy [77].

The scores might be also automatically computed using RGB colour space [78, 79], or La*b* colour space which has computational advantages for the automatic evaluation [61, 62]. Figure 8.2 depicts frames with covered areas, where we automatically identified the fecal content selecting the appropriated range of colours in La*b* colour space. In this colour space L represents the lightness, a* is the axis for green–red colours, and b* is the axis for blue–yellow colours. Moving up and down on the L axis we practically have nuances of the same (a*, b*) couple, defining a certain colour [59, 62]. Detecting the colour domain for each category of debris on the inner surface of the colon, we are able to detect, mark and count them on the entire surface exposed. In Fig. 8.2c we marked in red the traces of stool and with blue the light reflection on the membrane which makes it becoming white (artefact).

Image preprocessing and automatically discarding non-informative frames is an advisable operation [80], as sometimes, well trained deep learning networks are returning false positive (disturbing) results, due to the round shapes of the artefacts, similar to adenoma and polyps, in these images (see Figs. 8.3).

We stated that, for example, blurred regions of the highly illuminated frames, bubbles or even blood vessels network patterns (as we will further see), might be confused with polyps as in the situations presented in Figs. 8.3 and 8.4.

Discarding non-informative frames was done by classic computing methods [60, 69] which are unfortunately time consumers (entropy threshold computing on regions of the image is also one of these methods [81]).

Better results might be obtained training a DL network to recognize these images as artefacts, besides the training for polyps, adenoma and serrated polyps recognition, training it on non-informative frames, too [66].

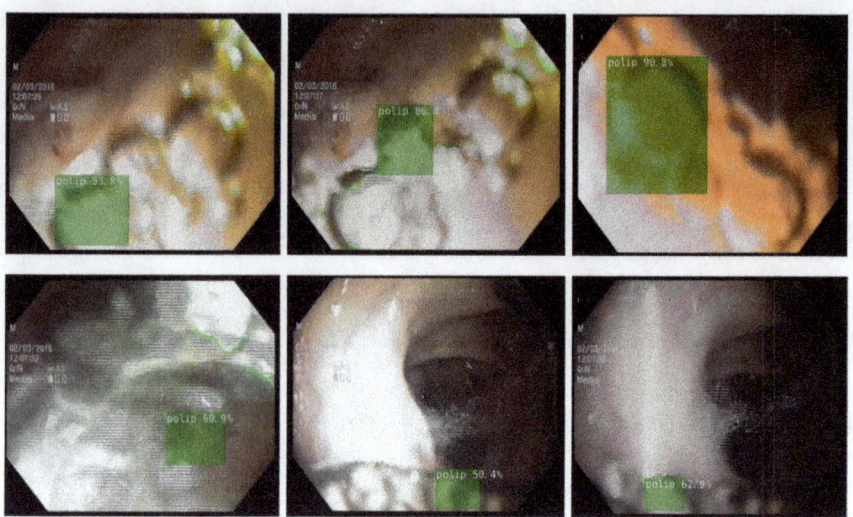

Fig. 8.3 Artefacts influencing polyp detection: bubbles are confused with the round shape of possible protrusions, with probabilities from 50.4% to 90.8%

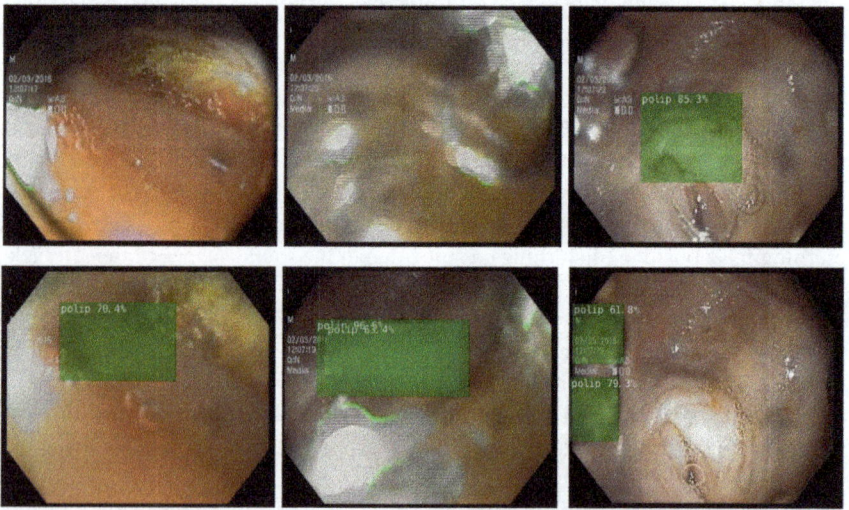

Fig. 8.4 False positive detection: blurred areas, light reflects, are confused with polyps

8.4 Deep Learning on Video Colonoscopies

As we have already mentioned, video colonoscopy images present artefacts, air bubbles, reflections, speckles, water jets, debris, fecal residues, and polyps, adenoma, malign structures, diverticula, membrane lesions, different textures on membrane

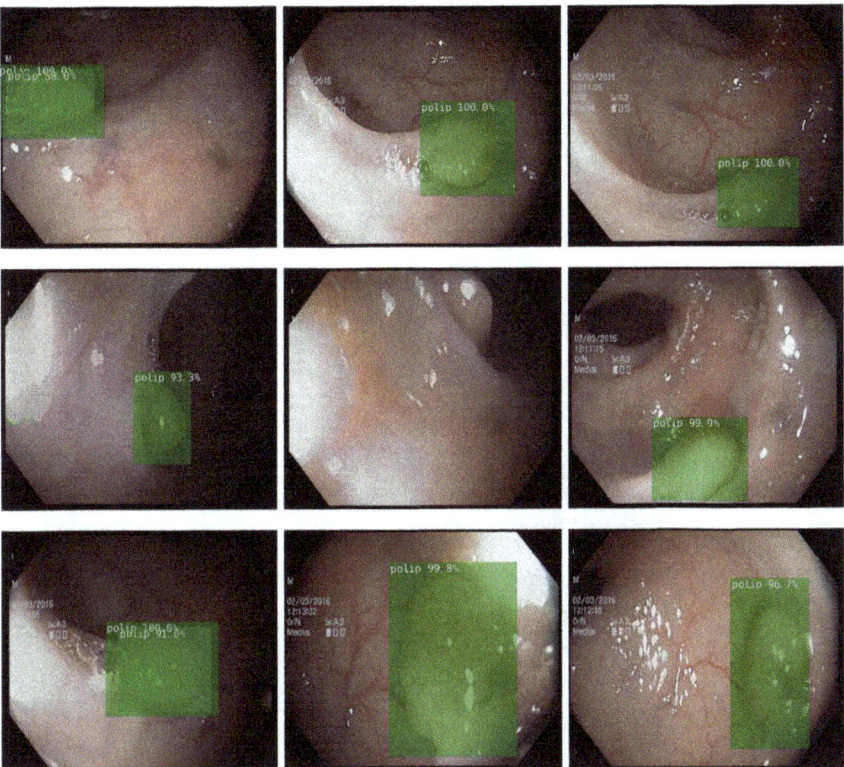

Fig. 8.5 Deep Learning using MobileNet on Jetson Xavier NX recognises the polyps. Very few false negative instances occurs

surface, folds, etc. Automatically dealing with all these aspects is a tough challenge shared among research teams worldwide. International competitions accelerated the discoveries in endoscopic vision, automatic polyp and abnormalities detection and gastrointestinal image analysis as MICCAI [36] or ILSVRC [23].

Open source publications, gastroenterology atlases and a few image databases, come to offer the much needed information, while endoscopists have still identified further needs for coping in acquiring and structuring labeled image databases [63].

Human experts might easily cope with the complex situations in search of the abnormal aspects on video colonoscopies, yet the computer must learn to recognize and discard the non informative content of the video colonoscopy or to use those frames, to learn from negative examples, too [67].

Improvements either enhance the technique diversifying optical devices, employing more angles and high quality cameras [11], using new cleansing methods and demanding better trained endoscopists [82], or obtain better diagnosis via artificial intelligence and deep learning on parallel computing devices. This facilitates real-time detection and dimensioning of polyps, adenoma, cancer or lesions.

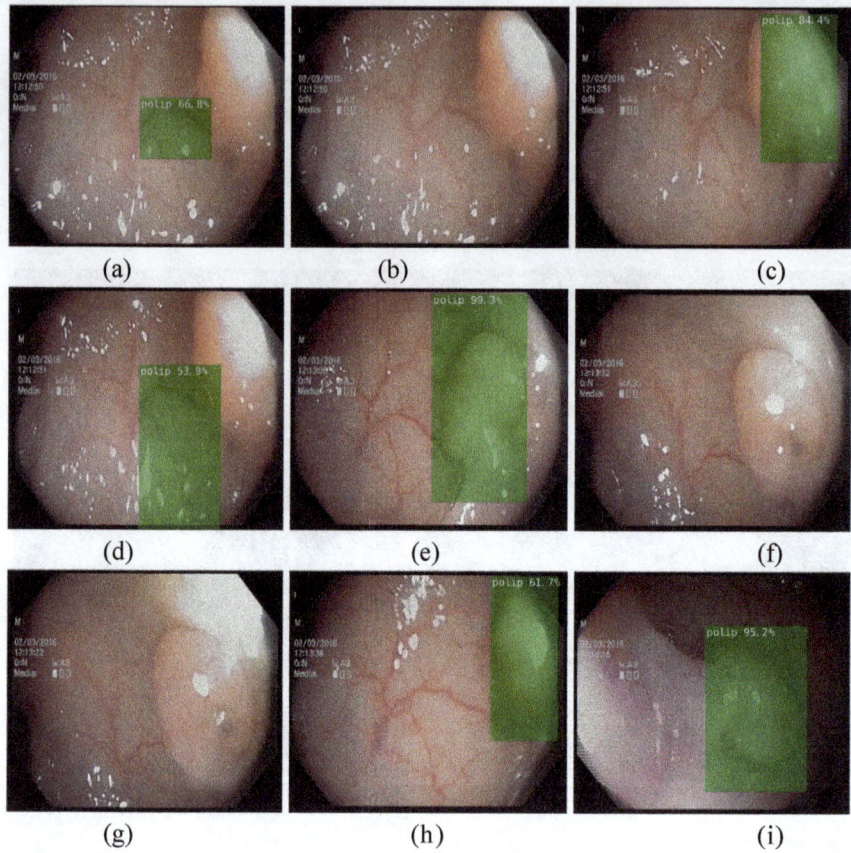

Fig. 8.6 Deep Learning using MobileNet correctly recognizes polyps as shown in **c, e, h, i**. False positive cases where the blood vessels network is confused with the a polyp shape **a, d**, and some non-identified instances **b, f, g** were observed

One of the deep learning networks often used in video colonoscopy polyp detection is the Convolutional Neural Network (CNN), working „in almost real-time with raw, unprocessed frames from the video sequence captured from the endoscope... to differentiate conventional adenomas from hyperplastic polyps" [42]. It was tested on colonoscopy frames "with already identified diminutive polyps with proven histology" [42]. Other DL architectures implied in automatic detection of polyps was ResNet [29]. "Exploring deep learning and transfer learning for colonic polyp classification" [83], is a paper which refers to 19 different DL architectures (CNN, GoogLeNet, VGG-VD16, VGG-VD19, AlexNet, etc.) comparing each other [83]. Yet, using a big number of simple convolutions it is not enough, as depthwise separable convolutions are making the difference [84, 85].

8.4.1 Deep Learning on Video Colonoscopies Using Nvidia Jetson Xavier

In order to find a practical method for video colonoscopy analysis, we used MobileNet, a deep learning network structure proposed in 2017 by a team from Google.Inc., [86]. As a novely, MobileNet uses depthwise separable convolutions with remarkable advantages, explained in [26, 27, 84, 85].

Compared to Inception V3, the number of operations and parameters for MobileNet, is almost 10 times smaller for a loss of around one percent in accuracy. This is due precisely to the fact that MobileNet uses "depthwise separable convolutions to build light weight deep neural networks" [86]. It has "two simple global hyper-parameters trading between latency and accuracy, allowing the model builder to choose the right sized model" [86]. As explained in [86, 87], to approach the MobileNet, the input tensor is split into channels and the kernel is split into channels, too. For each channel, the input is convolved with the corresponding filter (giving a 2D tensor) and finally the output tensors are stuck back together.

In depthwise separable convolution each channel is kept separate.

Each "Mobilenet block" contains: a 3×3 Depthwise Convolution, a BatchNorm (normalization) and ReLU (rectifying linear unit activation), then 1×1 Convolution, BatchNorm and ReLU again [86]. The network starts with a (Conv, BatchNorm, ReLU) block, continues with a series of "Mobilenet blocks" and closes with the Avg Pool and Fully Connected layers. All layers are followed by a BatchNorm and ReLU nonlinearity, as the diagram in MibileNets original paper shows [86, 87]. Counting depthwise and pointwise convolutions as separate layers, MobileNet has 28 layers.

We have run MobileNet on the Nvidia Jetson Xavier NX [88], with good results.

For the database we have 17 video anonymised colonoscopies. Every colonoscopy split into frames gives around 50.000 images. We have made a small, but relevant, selection of video sequences for our tests.

The MobileNet was already trained on usual objects and this knowledge was transferred by retraining it with polyp instances manually annotated on our colonoscopy frames [88–90]. The dataset was distributed as usual: 80% for training, 15% for validation and 5% for testing.

The results were surprisingly good, obtained after just 10 min of retraining the original MobileNet (Figs. 8.5 and 8.6).

Running MobileNet on Jetson Xavier NX makes this approach accessible for a large range of applications [88–90].

AI and DL helps especially for e-learning and for assisting physicians on their daily routine for computer-aided diagnosis, for polyp detection, localization amd classification [91–94].

Learning from the complexity of ImageNet, a common effort of the medical teams worldwide might help in creating a reliable labeled polyp and adenoma image database. It might be even more complex, with all the digestive pathology and relevant images for the gastrointestinal endoscopies.

Relying on this complex, well structured database, DL architectures, which are continuously developing, might give affordable and confident solutions, for training and for objective diagnosis.

8.5 Conclusions

Computer-aided detection, artificial intelligence, machine learning and deep learning in processing video colonoscopy have made a breakthrough compared to the classic methods. Automatic detection of polyps and adenomas on colonoscopy video frames has become a useful tool for training and assisting the physicians, towards objective evaluation. Deep learning is a new technique that makes possible the real time processing of colonoscopies with very good and consistent results.

Available hardware and software tools allow researchers to rapidly obtain excellent results. The only drawback is the necessity to construct large and consistent databases of annotated colonoscopy frames, containing different types of polyps and adenomas. This might take a lot of time and has to imply joint research teams of hardware engineers, image processing specialists and, of course, experienced endoscopists.

References

1. Ritchie, H.: "Causes of Death". Published online at OurWorldInData.org. Retrieved from: 'https://ourworldindata.org/causes-of-death', online resource accessed in Feb. 2021 (2018)
2. Sung, H., Ferlay, J., Siegel, R.L. et al.: Global Cancer Statistics 2020: GLOBOCAN Estimates of Incidence and Mortality Worldwide for 36 Cancers in 185 Countries, https://acsjournals.onlinelibrary.wiley.com/doi/full/https://doi.org/10.3322/caac.21660, online Feb. 2021. (2021)
3. World Endoscopy Organization previously known as OMED, https://www.worldendo.org/
4. Cross, A.J., Wooldrage, K., Robbins, E.C., et al.: Faecal immunochemical tests (FIT) versus colonoscopy for surveillance after screening and polypectomy: a diagnostic accuracy and cost-effectiveness study in Gut 2019; **68**, 1642–1652 (2019)
5. East, J.E., Vleugels, J.L., Roelandt, P., et al.: Advanced endoscopic imaging: European Society of Gastrointestinal Endoscopy (ESGE) technology review. Endoscopy **48**, 1029–1045 (2016). https://doi.org/10.1055/s-0042-118087
6. Petruzziello, L., Hassan, C., Alvaro, D., et al.: Appropriateness of the indication for colonoscopy: is the endoscopist' the 'gold standard'? J. Clin. Gastroenterol. **2012**(46), 590–594 (2012)
7. Aabakken, L., Rembacken, B., LeMoine, O., Kuznetsov, K., Rey, J.-F., Rösch, T., Eisen, G., Cotton, P., Fujino, M.: Minimal standard terminology for gastrointestinal endoscopy, MST3.0 https://www.worldendo.org/resources/minimal-standard-terminology-mst/, http://www.worldendo.org/wp-content/uploads/2016/08/160803_MST30.pdf (2016)
8. Messmann, H.: Atlas of Colonoscopy: Techniques, Diagnosis, Interventional Procedures, in Georg Thieme, Verlag, Stuttgart, Germany, http://www.thieme.com (2004)
9. Tajbakhsh, N., Gurudu, S.R., Liang, J.: Automated polyp detection in colonoscopy videos using shape and context information. IEEE Trans Med Imaging **35**, 630–644 (2016)

10. Sornapudi, S., Meng, F., Yi, S.: Region-based automated localization of colonoscopy and wireless capsule endoscopy polyps. Appl. Sci. **9**(12), 2404 (2019). https://www.mdpi.com/2076-3417/9/12/2404?type=check_update&version=1 https://doi.org/10.3390/app9122404
11. Ngu, W.S., Rees, C.: Can technology increase adenoma detection rate? in Therapeutic Advances in Gastroenterology, vol. 11, pp. 1–18, (2018) Creative Commun Attr. http://journals.sagepub.com/doi/full/https://doi.org/10.1177/1756283X17746311, (access June 2018) https://www.ncbi.nlm.nih.gov/pmc/articles/PMC5784538/#bibr60-1756283X17746311
12. Iwatate, M., Ikumoto, T., Hattori, S., Sano, W., Sano, Y., Fujimori, T., (2012), NBI and NBI Combined with Magnifying Colonoscopy, Review Article in Diagnostic and Therapeutic Endoscopy. Art. ID 173269, 11 pages, Hindawi Publ. Corp., https://doi.org/10.1155/2012/173269, https://downloads.hindawi.com/archive/2012/173269.pdf
13. OLYMPUS, Narrow Band Imaging (NBI): A New Wave of Diagnostic Possibilities. https://www.olympus-europa.com/
14. Su, M.Y., Hsu, C.M., Ho, Y.P., Chen, P.C., Lin, C.J., Chiu, C.T.: Comparative study of conventional colonoscopy, chromoendoscopy, and narrow-band imaging systems in differential diagnosis of neoplastic and nonneoplastic colonic polyps. Am J Gastroenterol. **101**(12): 2711–6 (2006). https://doi.org/10.1111/j.1572-0241.2006.00932.x. PMID: 17227517. https://pubmed.ncbi.nlm.nih.gov/17227517/
15. Zhang, Y., Chen, H.Y., Zhou, X.L., Pan, W.S., Zhou, X.X., Pan, H.H.: Diagnostic efficacy of the Japan Narrow-band-imaging Expert Team and Pit pattern classifications for colorectal lesions: A meta-analysis. World J Gastroenterol. **26**(40), 6279–6294 (2020). https://doi.org/10.3748/wjg.v26.i40.6279. PMID:33177800
16. Repici, A., Hassan, C.: Artificial intelligence for colonoscopy: the new Silk Road, Referring to Barua I et al. pp. 277–284 (2021), Editorial, Endoscopy 2021; 53: 285–287, DOI https://doi.org/10.1055/a-1367-1979 ISSN 0013–726X , Thieme © 2021
17. Geetha, K., Rajan, C.: Automatic colorectal polyp detection in colonoscopy video frames. Asian Pacific J. Cancer Prevent. **17**(11), 4869–4873 (2016). https://doi.org/10.22034/APJCP.2016.17.11.4869
18. LeCun, Y., Bottou, L., Bengio, Y., Haffner, P.: Gradient-based learning applied to document recognition. Proc. of the IEEE **86**(11), 2278–2324 (Nov. 1998). https://doi.org/10.1109/5.726791
19. LeCun, Y., Kavukcuoglu, K., Farabet, C.: Convolutional networks and applications in vision, in Circuits and Systems (ISCAS), Proc. of 2010 IEEE International Symposium on, pp. 253–256. IEEE, (2010)
20. LeCun, Y., Bengio, Y., Hinton, G.: Deep learning. Nature **521**(7553), 436–444 (2015). https://doi.org/10.1038/nature14539
21. ImageNet, http://www.image-net.org/ (actualized in March 2021).
22. Princeton University "About WordNet." WordNet. Princeton University. 2010.
23. Russakowsky, O., Deng, J., Su, H., et al.: ImageNet large scale visual recognition challenge. Int. J. Comput. Vision **115**, 211–252 (2015), https://www.researchgate.net/publication/265295439_ImageNet_Large_Scale_Visual_Recognition_Challenge, https://doi.org/10.1007/s11263-015-0816-y
24. Krizhevsky, A., Sutskever, I., Hinton, G.E.: ImageNet classification with deep convolutional neural networks. Adv. Neural Inf. Process Syst **2012**, 1097–1105 (2012)
25. Szegedy, C., Liu, W., Jia, Y., Sermanet, P., Reed, S., Anguelov, D., Erhan, D., Vanhoucke, V., Rabinovich, A.: Going Deeper with Convolutions (2014). https://arxiv.org/abs/1409.4842 (downloaded in Dec. 2020)
26. Simonyan, K., Zisserman, A.: Very Deep Convolutional Networks for Large-Scale Image Recognition, (VGG) (2014). https://arxiv.org/pdf/1409.1556.pdf (accessed in Dec. 2020).
27. Chollet, F.: Xception: Deep Learning with Depthwise Separable Convolution, (2017). https://arxiv.org/pdf/1610.02357.pdf (downloaded in Dec. 2020)
28. He, K., Zhang, X., Ren., Sun, J.: Deep Residual Learning for Image Recognition, ResNet, https://arxiv.org/abs/1512.03385 (downloaded in Dec. 2020)

29. Yang, Y.J., Cho, B.J., Lee, M.J., Kim, J.H., Lim, H., Bang, C.S., Jeong, H.M., Hong, J.T., Baik, G.H.: Automated classification of colorectal neoplasms in white-light colonoscopy images via deep learning. J. Clin. Med. **9**(5), 1593 (2020 May 24). https://doi.org/10.3390/jcm9051593. PMID:32456309;PMCID:PMC7291169
30. Brandao, P., Mazomenos, E., Ciuti, G., Cali'o, R., Bianchi, F., Menciassi, A., Dario, P., Koulaouzidis, A., Arezzo, A., Stoyanov, D.: Fully convolutional neural networks for polyp segmentation in colonoscopy. Appl. Sci. **9**(12), 2404 (2019) https://doi.org/10.3390/app912 2404.
31. Guo, Y., Bernal, J., Matuszewski, B.: Polyp segmentation with fully convolutional deep neural networks—extended evaluation study. J. Imaging. **6**(7), 69 (2020). https://doi.org/10.3390/jim aging6070069
32. Long, J., Shelhamer, E., Darrell, T.: Fully convolutional networks for semantic segmentation. In Proceedings of the IEEE Conference on Computer Vision and Pattern Recognition, pp. 3431–3440 (2015)
33. Yao, Y., Gou, S., Tian, R., Zhang, X., He S.: Automated classification and segmentation in colorectal images based on self-paced transfer network. BioMed Res. Int. 6683931 (2021). https://doi.org/10.1155/2021/6683931
34. Ronneberger, O., Fischer, P., Brox, T.: U-net: convolutional networks for biomedical image segmentation. In International Conference on Medical Image Computing and Computer-Assisted Intervention, pp. 234–241. Springer (2015)
35. Zhou, Z., Rahman Siddiquee, M.M., Tajbakhsh, N., Liang, J.: UNet++: a nested u-net architecture for medical image segmentation. In: Stoyanov D. et al. (eds.) Deep Learning in Medical Image Analysis and Multimodal Learning for Clinical Decision Support. DLMIA 2018, ML-CDS 2018. Lecture Notes in Computer Science, vol. 11045. Springer, Cham (2018). https://doi.org/10.1007/978-3-030-00889-5_1
36. MICCAI, Medical Image Computing and Computer Assisted Intervention Conference, www.miccai.org, Endoscopic Vision Challenge https://endovis.grand-challenge.org/endoscopic_v ision_challenge/ accessed in December 2020
37. Lui, T.K.L., Guo, C.-G., Leung, W.K.: Accuracy of artificial intelligence on histology prediction and detection of colorectal polyps: a systematic review and meta-analysis. Gastrointestinal Endoscopy **92**, 11–22.e6 (2020)
38. Hassan, C., Spadaccini, M., Iannone, A., Maselli, R., Jovani, M., Chandrasekar, V.T., Antonelli, G., Yu, H., Areia, M., Dinis-Ribeiro, M, Bhandari, P., Sharma, P., Rex, D.K., Rösch, T., Wallace, M., Repici, A.: Performance of artificial intelligence for colonoscopy regarding adenoma and polyp detection: a meta-analysis. Gastrointestinal Endoscopy 2021; **93**, 77–85 (2020). https://doi.org/10.1016/j.gie.2020.06.059. https://www.sciencedirect.com/science/article/abs/pii/S00 16510720345235
39. Barua, I., Vinsard, D., Jodal, H. et al.: Artificial intelligence for polyp detection during colonoscopy: a systematic review and meta-analysis. Endoscopy **53**, 277–284 (2020)
40. Sánchez-Peralta, L.F., Bote-Curiel, L., Picón, A., Sánchez-Margallo, F.M., Pagador, J.B.: Deep learning to find colorectal polyps in colonoscopy: a systematic literature review. Artific. Intell. Med. **108**, 101923 (2020), https://doi.org/10.1016/j.artmed.2020.101923
41. Trasolini, R., Byrne, M., (2020), Artificial intelligence and deep learning for small bowel capsule endoscopy, Review, in Digestive Endoscopy, Vol. 33, Issue 2, p.290–297, Wiley Online Library, https://onlinelibrary.wiley.com/doi/full/https://doi.org/10.1111/den.13896
42. Byrne, M.F., Chapados, N., Soudan, F., Oertel, C., Linares, P.M., Kelly, R., Iqbal, N., Chandelier, F., Rex, D.K.: Real-time differentiation of adenomatous and hyperplastic diminutive colorectal polyps during analysis of unaltered videos of standard colonoscopy using a deep learning model. Gut. **68**(1), 94–100 (2019). https://doi.org/10.1136/gutjnl-2017-314547. PMID:29066576;PMCID:PMC6839831
43. Poon, C.C.Y., Jiang, Y., Zhang, R., Lo, W.W.Y., et al.: AI-doscopist: a real-time deep-learning-based algorithm for localizing polyps in colonoscopy videos with edge computing devices. NPJ Digit Med. 2020 May 18; **3**, 73 (2020). https://doi.org/10.1038/s41746-020-0281-z, https://pub med.ncbi.nlm.nih.gov/32435701/

44. Misawa, M., Kudo, S.E., Mori, Y., Hotta, ., Ohtsuka, K., Matsuda, T., Saito, S., Kudo, T., Baba, T., Ishida, F., Itoh, H., Oda, M., Mori, K.: Development of a computer-aided detection system for colonoscopy and a publicly accessible large colonoscopy video database (with video). Gastrointestinal Endoscopy **31**, S0016–5107(20)34655–1 (2020). https://doi.org/10.1016/j.gie.2020.07.060. https://pubmed.ncbi.nlm.nih.gov/32745531/
45. Pannala, R., Krishnan, K., Melson, J., Parsi, M.A., Schulman, A.R., Sullivan, S., Trikudanathan, G., Trindade, A.J., Watson, R.R., Maple, J.T., Lichtenstein D.R.: Artificial intelligence in gastrointestinal endoscopy. VideoGIE. **5**(12), 598–613 (9 Nov 2020). https://doi.org/10.1016/j.vgie.2020.08.013. https://www.ncbi.nlm.nih.gov/pmc/articles/PMC7732722/
46. Becq, A., Chandnani, M., Bharadwaj, S., Baran, B., Ernest-Suarez, K,, Gabr, M., Glissen-Brown, J., Sawhney, M., Pleskow, D.K., Berzin, T.M.: Effectiveness of a deep-learning polyp detection system in prospectively collected colonoscopy videos with variable bowel preparation quality. J. Clin. Gastroenterol. **54**(6), 554–557 (2020 Jul). https://doi.org/10.1097/MCG.0000000000001272. https://pubmed.ncbi.nlm.nih.gov/31789758/
47. Repici, A., Badalamenti, M., Maselli, R., et al.: Efficacy of real-time computer-aided detection of colorectal neoplasia in a randomized trial. Gastroenterol. **2020**(159), 512–520 (2020)
48. Wang, P., Berzin, T.M., Glissen Brown, J.R., et al.: (2019) Real-time automatic detection system increases colonoscopic polyp and adenoma detection rates: a prospective randomized controlled study. Gut **68**, 1813–1819 (2019)
49. Wang, P., Liu, X., Berzin, T.M., et al.: Effect of a deep-learning computer-aided detection system on adenoma detection during colonoscopy (CADe-DB trial): a double-blind randomised study. Lancet Gastroenterol Hepatol **5**, 343–351 (2020), https://pubmed.ncbi.nlm.nih.gov/31981517/
50. Gong, D., Wu, L., Zhang, J., et al.: Detection of colorectal adenomas with a real-time computer-aided system (ENDOANGEL): a randomized controlled study. Lancet Gastroenterol Hepatol **5**, 352–361 (2020)
51. Hassan, C., Wallace, M.B., Sharma, P., Maselli, R., Craviotto, V., Spadaccini, M., Repici, A.: New artificial intelligence system: first validation study versus experienced endoscopists for colorectal polyp detection. Gut **69**, 799–800 (2020)
52. Liu, W.N., Zhang, Y.Y., Bian, X.Q., et al.: Study on detection rate of polyps and adenomas in artificial-intelligence-aided colonoscopy. Saudi J. Gastroenterol. **26**, 13–19 (2020)
53. GI Genius™ Intelligent Endoscopy Module | Medtronic https://www.medtronic.com/covidien/en-us/products/gastrointestinal-artificial-intelligence/gi-genius-intelligent-endoscopy.html, (accessed in December 2020)
54. ARGUS Technology to Support Polyp Detection & Sizing www.argusml.com, (accessed in December 2020)
55. ENDO-AID, EvisX1, Olympus, Fierce Biotech, Medtech, https://www.fiercebiotech.com/medtech/olympus-to-roll-out-colonoscopy-ai-for-spotting-lesions-polyps-real-time, (accessed in December2020)
56. Ciobanu, A., Luca, M., Drug, V.: Objective method for colon cleansing evaluation using color CIELAB features, in International Conference on e-Health and Bioengineering (EHB), Iași, 29–30 Oct. 2020, pp. 1–4, publ. IEEE (2020), https://doi.org/10.1109/EHB50910.2020.9280110, https://ieeexplore.ieee.org/document/9280110/ Corpus ID: 228098537
57. Luca, M., Barbu, T., Ciobanu, A.: An overview on computer processing for endoscopy and colonoscopy videos, In: Balas, V., Jain, L., Balas, M., Shahbazova, S. (eds.) Soft Computing Applications, First online 18 Aug. 2020, Advances in Intelligent Systems and Computing, vol. 1222. Springer, Cham (2020). https://doi.org/10.1007/978-3-030-52190-5_1
58. Ciobanu, A., Luca, M., Drug, V., Tulceanu, V.: Steps towards computer-assisted classification of colonoscopy video frames, 6th IEEE International Conference on E-health and Bioengineering – EHB Sinaia, Romania, (2017)
59. Luca, M., Ciobanu, A., Drug, V.: Colonoscopy videos: towards automatic assessing of the bowels cleansing degree. In: Várkonyi-Kóczy, A.R. (ed.) Engineering for Sustainable Future, Book Series: Lecture Notes in Networks and Systems, Springer Intern. Publ., Springer Professional "Technik", (2020). https://doi.org/10.1007/978-3-030-36841-8_28.

60. Luca, M., Ciobanu, A.: Polyp detection in video colonoscopy using deep learning, to appear in Journal of Intelligent and Fuzzy Systems, in 2021 (2021)
61. Luca, M., Ciobanu, A., Drug, V.: LAB Automatic evaluation of colon cleansing, ESGE Days 2019, ePP50, abstract volume, p. 145 (2019)
62. Ciobanu, A., Costin, M., Barbu, T.: Image categorization based on computationally economic LAB colour features. In Balas, V., Fodor, J., Várkonyi-Kóczy, A., Dombi, J., Jain, L. (eds.) Soft Computing Applications. Advances in Intelligent Systems and Computing, Springer, Berlin, Heidelberg, vol. 195, pp 585–593 (2013)
63. Ahmad, O.F., Mori, Y., Misawa, M., et al.: Endoscopy establishing key research questions for the implementation of artificial intelligence in colonoscopy—a modified Delphi method, Endoscopy (9 Nov 2020). https://doi.org/10.1055/a-1306-7590
64. CVC Colon DB http://www.cvc.uab.es/CVC-Colon/index.php/databases/ , http://mv.cvc.uab.es/projects/colon-qa/cvccolondb, CVC ClinicDB, https://polyp.grand-challenge.org/site/Polyp/CVCClinicDB/ (accessed in Dec 2020)
65. ASU Mayo DB https://polyp.grand-challenge.org/site/polyp/asumayo/ accessed June 2020
66. 66. HyperKvasir Borgli, H., Thambawita, V., Smedsrud, P.H., Hicks, S., et al.: HyperKvasir, a comprehensive multi-class image and video dataset for gastrointestinal endoscopy. Scientific Data 7, Art. Nr. 283 (2020). https://doi.org/10.1038/s41597-020-00622-yhttps://www.nature.com/articles/s41597-020-00622-y.pdf
67. Tajbakhsh N., Jeyaseelan L.,, Li Q., Chiang J. N., Wu Z., Ding X., (2020) Embracing Imperfect Datasets: A Review of Deep Learning Solutions for Medical Image Segmentation, in Medical Image Analysis Vol. 63: 101693, 2020, https://doi.org/10.1016/j.media.2020.101693
68. Ballesteros, C., Trujillo, M., Mazo, C.: Automatic classification of non-informative frames in colonoscopy videos, 6th IEEE Latin-American Conference on Networked and Electronic Media (LACNEM 2015), Medellin, pp. 1–5 (2015). https://doi.org/10.1049/ic.2015.0307
69. Tajbakhsh, N., Chi, C., Sharma, H., Wu, Q., Gurudu, S.R., Liang, J.: Automatic assessment of image informativeness in colonoscopy, in Abdominal Imaging. Computational and Clinical Applications, pp. 151–158, Springer (2014)
70. Oh, J., Hwang, S., Lee, J., Tavanapong, W., Wong, J., de Groen, P.C.: Informative frame classification for endoscopy video. Med. Img. Anal **11**(2), 110–127 (2007)
71. Calderwood, A.H., Jacobson, B.C.: Comprehensive validation of the boston bowel preparation scale. Gastrointest. Endosc. **2010**(72), 686–692 (2010)
72. Rostom, A., Jolicoeur, E.: Validation of a new scale for the assessment of bowel preparation quality in Gastrointestinal. Endoscopy **2004**(59), 482–486 (2004)
73. Aronchick, C.A., Lipshutz, W.H., Wright, S.H., et al.: A novel tableted purgative for colonoscopic preparation: efficacy and safety comparisons with Colyte and Fleet Phospho-Soda. Gastrointest. Endosc. **52**, 346–352 (2000)
74. Gerard, D.P., Foster, D.B., Raiser, M.W., Holden, J.L., Karrison, T.G.: Validation of a new bowel preparation scale for measuring colon cleansing for colonoscopy: the Chicago bowel preparation scale. Clin. Transl. Gastroenterol. **4**(12), e43n (2013)
75. Hassan, C., East, J., Radaelli, F. et al.: Bowel preparation for colonoscopy: European Society of Gastrointestinal Endoscopy (ESGE) Guideline—Update (2019). https://www.esge.com/bowel-preparation-for-colonoscopy-esge-guideline-update-2019/
76. Kaminski, M.F., Thomas-Gibson, S., Bugajski, M. et al.: Performance measures for lower gastrointestinal endoscopy: an European Society of Gastrointestinal Endoscopy ESGE Quality Improvement Initiative. Endoscopy **49**, 378–397 (2017). https://www.esge.com/performance-measures-for-lower-gastrointestinal-endoscopy/
77. Clark, B.T., Rustagi, T., Laine, L.: What level of bowel prep quality requires early repeat colonoscopy: systematic review and meta-analysis of the impact of preparation quality on adenoma detection rate. Am. J. Gastroenterol. **109**, 1714–23 (2014). PMID: 25135006. https://doi.org/10.1038/ajg.2014.232
78. Muthukudage, J.K., Oh, J.H., Tavanapong, W., Wong, J., de Groen, P.C.: Color Based Stool Region Detection in Colonoscopy Videos for Quality Measurements. In: Ho, Y.-S. (ed.) PSIVT 2011, Part I, LNCS 7087, pp. 61–72. Springer, Berlin Heidelberg (2011)

79. Hwang, S., Oh, J., Tavanapong, W., Wong, J., de Groen, P.C.: Stool detection in colonoscopy videos, in Proc. of Intern. Conference of the IEEE Eng. in Medicine and Biology Society (EMBS 2008), Vancouver, British Columbia, Canada, pp. 3004–3007 (2008)
80. Sánchez-González, A., García-Zapirain, Soto, B.: Colonoscopy Image Pre-Processing for the Development of Computer-Aided Diagnostic Tools (2017). https://doi.org/10.5772/67842, https://www.intechopen.com/books/surgical-robotics/colonoscopy-image-pre-processing-for-the-development-of-computer-aided-diagnostic-tools
81. Nagy, S., Sziová, B., Pipek, J.: On structural entropy and spatial filling factor analysis of colonoscopy pictures. Entropy **21**(3), 256 (2019). https://doi.org/10.3390/e21030256
82. Huang, Q., Fukami, N., Kashida, H., Takeuchi, T., Kogure, E., Kurahashi, T., Stahl, E., Kudo, Y., Kimata, H., Kudo, S.E.: Inter-observer and intra-observer consistency in the endoscopic assessment of colonic pit patterns. Gastrointest Endosc. **60**(4), 520–526 (2004). https://doi.org/10.1016/s0016-5107(04)01880-2. PMID: 15472672
83. E. Ribeiro, Uhl, A., Wimmer, G., Häfner, M.: Exploring deep learning and transfer learning for colonic polyp classification, Hindawi Publishing Corporation, Computational and Mathematical Methods, in Medicine, vol. 2016, open source, http://dx.doi.org/https://doi.org/10.1155/2016/6584725
84. Wang, C.F.: A Basic Introduction to Depthwise Separable Convolutions (2017). https://towardsdatascience.com/a-basic-introduction-to-separable-convolutions-b99ec3102728 (accessed in Nov 2020)
85. Bendersky, E.: Depthwise Separable Convolutions for Machine Learning (2018). https://eli.thegreenplace.net/2018/depthwise-separable-convolutions-for-machine-learning/(accessed in Nov 2020)
86. Howard, A.G., Zhu, M., Chen, B., Kalenichenko, D. et al.: MobileNets: Efficient Convolutional Neural Networks for Mobile Vision Applications (2017). https://arxiv.org/pdf/1704.04861.pdf (accessed in Nov 2020)
87. CNN Architectures—MobileNet implementation | Machine Learning Tokyo, MLT https://www.youtube.com/watch?v=4XyCFwOOHbM&t=273s (accessed in March)
88. Jetson Xavier, N.X., https://www.nvidia.com/en-us/autonomous-machines/embedded-systems/jetson-nano/ (accessed in November)
89. https://github.com/dusty-nv/jetson-inference (accessed in Nov 2020)
90. https://github.com/tzutalin/labelImg (accessed in Nov 2020)
91. Nogueira-Rodríguez, A., Domínguez-Carbajales, R., López-Fernández, H., Iglesias, A., Cubiella, J., Fdez-Riverola, F., Reboiro-Jato, M., Glez-Peña, D.: Deep neural networks approaches for detecting and classifying colorectal polyps. Neurocomputing **423**, 721–734 (2021), ISSN 0925–2312, https://doi.org/10.1016/j.neucom.2020.02.123
92. de Groen, P.C.: Using AI to improve adequacy of inspection in gastrointestinal endoscopy. Tech. Innovations Gastrointest. Endosc. **22**(2), 71–79 (2020)
93. Rex, D.K.: Can we do resect and discard with artificial intelligence-assisted colon polyp "optical biopsy?" Tech. Innovations Gastrointest. Endosc. **22**(2), 52–55 (2020). https://doi.org/10.1016/j.tgie.2019.150638
94. Byrne, M. (ed.).: Artificial intelligence in gastroenterology. Tech. Innovations Gastrointest. Endosc. **22**(2), 41–90 (2020). https://www.sciencedirect.com/journal/techniques-and-innovations-in-gastrointestinal-endoscopy/vol/22/issue/2

Chapter 9
Last Advances on Automatic Carotid Artery Analysis in Ultrasound Images: Towards Deep Learning

Maria del Mar Vila, Beatriz Remeseiro, Maria Grau, Roberto Elosua, and Laura Igual

Abstract Atherosclerosis is the main pathogenic process causing most Cardiovascular Diseases (CVDs). The Carotid Artery (CA) Ultrasound image is currently being used to detect the presence of subclinical atherosclerosis since it provides a measurement of the Intima Media Thickness (IMT) of the artery and can be used to identify the presence of atherosclerotic plaques. Moreover, it is well known that disruption of an atherosclerotic plaque plays a crucial role in the pathogenesis of

---

M. M. Vila (✉) · M. Grau · R. Elosua
Department Epidemiologia i Salut Pública, IMIM, Institut Hospital del Mar d'Investigacions Mèdiques, Dr. Aiguader 88, 08003 Barcelona, Spain
e-mail: mvila@imim.es; mvilamun10@alumnes.ub.edu

M. Grau
e-mail: mgrau@imim.es; mariagrau@ub.edu

R. Elosua
e-mail: relosua@imim.es

M. M. Vila · L. Igual
Department de Matemàtiques i Informàtica, Universitat de Barcelona, Gran via de les Corts Catalanes 585, 08007 Barcelona, Spain
e-mail: ligual@ub.edu

M. M. Vila · M. Grau
CIBER Epidemiología y Salud Pública, Instituto de Salud Carlos III, Monforte de Lemos 3-5, Pabellón 11, 28029 Madrid, Spain

B. Remeseiro
Department of Computer Science, Universidad de Oviedo, Campus de Gijón s/n, 33203 Gijón, Spain
e-mail: bremeseiro@uniovi.es

M. Grau
Department de Medicina, Universitat de Barcelona, Carrer Casanova 143, 08036 Barcelona, Spain

R. Elosua
CIBER Enfermedades Cardiovasculares, Instituto de Salud Carlos III, Monforte de Lemos 3-5, Pabellón 11, 28029 Madrid, Spain
Facultat de Medicina, Universitat de Vic-Universitat Central de Catalunya, Ctra. de Roda, 70, 08500 Vic, Barcelona, Spain

© The Author(s), under exclusive license to Springer Nature Switzerland AG 2022
C.-P. Lim et al. (eds.), *Handbook of Artificial Intelligence in Healthcare*, Intelligent Systems Reference Library 211,
https://doi.org/10.1007/978-3-030-79161-2_9

CVD events. Thus, the characterization of plaque morphology based on B-mode Ultrasound images is useful to assess the vulnerability of atherosclerotic lesions and for the CV risk assessment. Many image analysis techniques have been developed for the automatic segmentation of intima-media in CA, as well as for plaque characterization. Recently, Deep Learning has appeared to be a popular representation-based machine learning technique based on artificial neural networks, which are breaking records in many computer vision applications. In this chapter, we review the state-of-the-art of CA segmentation, plaque classification, and risk assessment in B-mode Ultrasound images with a focus on the last proposals based on Deep Learning. We summarize the most recent works in comprehensive tables to easily compare them and emphasize their strengths and weaknesses. Finally, we try to help to lay the foundation for the next steps taking advantage of the power of Deep Learning, also considering the challenges that this entails (Part of the content of this chapter was previously published in *Artificial Intelligence In Medicine* (https://doi.org/10.1016/j.artmed.2019.101784)).

Keywords Carotid artery segmentation · Ultrasound images · Intima media thickness · Carotid plaque detection · CV risk assessment · Machine learning · Deep learning

9.1 Introduction

Atherosclerosis is the main pathogenic process causing most Cardiovascular Diseases (CVDs). More precisely, atherosclerosis is a chronic inflammatory process characterized morphologically by an asymmetric focal thickening of the innermost layer of the artery (see Fig. 9.1). It starts early in life, progresses with age and usually appears with subclinical arterial wall alterations that precede cardiovascular clinical events.

Carotid Artery (CA) B-mode Ultrasound (US) image is currently being used to detect the burden of subclinical atherosclerosis since it provides a measurement of the Intima Media Thickness (IMT) of the artery. IMT is defined as the distance between Lumen-Intima (LI) and Media-Adventitia (MA) interfaces, and it is commonly estimated in the far wall of the CA [2]. A B-mode US is a cross-sectional image constructed from echoes that are generated by reflection of US waves at tissue boundaries. As a result, the B-mode US can show in a grayscale image the tissues and organ boundaries. In particular, the IMT measurement in the clinical examination requires the longitudinal view (in a plane parallel to the direction of the artery, see Fig. 9.2a), and the data source used for CA evaluation is a longitudinal B-mode US image, either in single images or videos. Videos are image sequences showing the two periods of the cardiac cycle (CC), diastole and systole, which present different characteristics related to the arteries' atherosclerosis health. Measurement of the CA IMT with B-mode US is a non-invasive, sensitive, and relatively inexpensive technique for the atherosclerotic risk evaluation. Moreover, the IMT measurement

9 Last Advances on Automatic Carotid Artery Analysis …

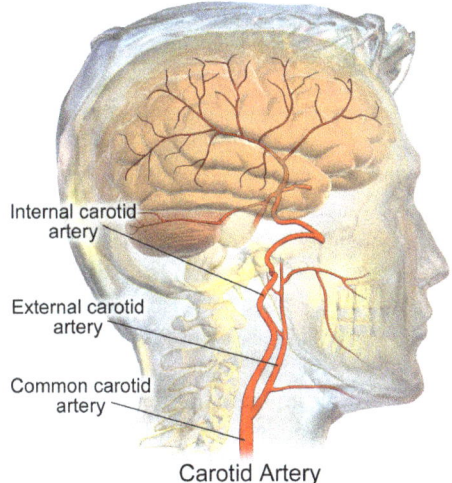

Fig. 9.1 Illustration of the carotid artery, the internal carotid artery and its different segments (common carotid artery, internal carotid artery, and external carotid artery). The bulb is the junction between these segments [1]

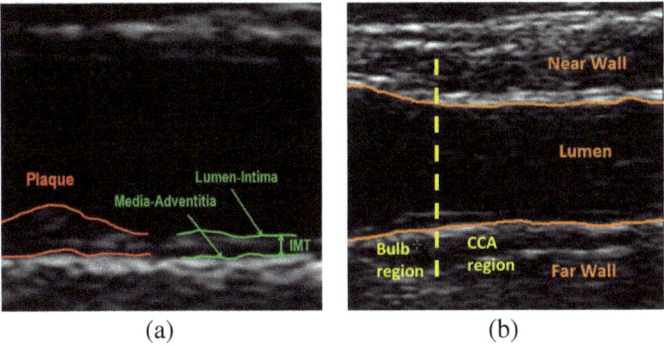

Fig. 9.2 Two examples of B-mode US CA images: (**a**) the red lines show the presence of atherosclerosis plaque and the green lines show the Intima Media Thickness (IMT) measurement; and (**b**) the five anatomical regions represented in a Common CA (CCA) B-mode US image

is considered as an indicator of the presence of plaque, as is stated in the Mannheim consensus [2]. This consensus defines a sufficient criterion for plaque detection: plaques are structures into the arterial lumen showing IMT > 1.5 mm.

Carotid arterial wall assessment may include different CA segments, the Common CA (CCA), the Internal CA (ICA), or Bulb segments of the CA (see Fig. 9.1). Atherosclerotic thickening and plaque are commonly found at the bifurcation of the CA and the beginning of the ICA, but only occasionally occur in the CCA. However, it is well known that noise represents the most prominent problem in US imaging and, in particular, noise is more evident in internal areas such as bulb or ICA. Therefore, most B-mode US studies are performed assessing the CCA due to its accessibility, which makes the quality of the CCA images better compared to those of other artery segments.

Furthermore, it is well known that the disruption of an atherosclerotic plaque plays a crucial role in the pathogenesis of CVD events. Plaque disruption is characterized by the content of lipid, muscle cells, and the thickness of the fibrous cap, among other factors [3]. Non-invasive CA B-mode US is a well-established method that helps to visualize and quantify atherosclerotic lesions. Therefore, B-mode US characterization of plaque morphology is useful in assessing the vulnerability of the atherosclerotic lesions. Moreover, plaque and also CA walls characterization can be used as a powerful tool for CV risk assessment and CV event prediction [4].

In this chapter, we review some automatic and semi-automatic techniques that have been recently introduced in the literature for CA segmentation, allowing for IMT measurement and plaque detection, as well as for CA plaque classification and risk assessment in 2D B-mode longitudinal images.

Among the automatic image analysis techniques used for CA analysis, recent efforts focus on Deep Learning (DL), a powerful set of techniques for training Neural Networks (NNs) composed of a high number of layers and parameters [5, 6]. DL has achieved so remarkable improvements last years that DL models have become the solution to many real-life computer vision problems (e.g., object recognition, high-end surveillance, facial recognition, license plate readers). Current developments in DL applied to medical image analysis achieved inconceivable results, matching human performance in applications such as image classification of skin lesions as benign lesions or malignant skin cancers [7], and detection and classification of arrhythmia at the cardiologist-level in ambulatory electrocardiograms [8].

The rest of this chapter is organized as follows. In Sect. 9.2, we first review the state-of-the-art of CA segmentation techniques in B-mode US and IMT estimation; and secondly, we revise a DL proposal for IMT estimation and plaque detection. In Sect. 9.3, we review the objectives related to characterization of B-mode US CA plaque images and the techniques proposed in the literature. Section 9.4 includes a discussion about the main open challenges in DL applied to this medical problem. Finally, Sect. 9.5 closes the chapter with our conclusions and future perspective.

9.2 Carotid Artery Segmentation and Intima Media Thickness Estimation in Ultrasound Images

As mentioned in the introduction, B-mode longitudinal US images are commonly used for IMT estimation. The IMT is conventionally measured manually by a trained operator from the B-mode US scan images. The methodology is highly user-dependent, time-consuming, tedious, and infeasible when using large image databases.

Several computerized techniques have been developed for automatically estimate the IMT measurement. The automatic IMT estimation procedure first requires a CA image interpretation, which consists in localizing the different anatomical components of the CA such as lumen, far wall, near wall, Bulb, and CCA (see Fig. 9.2b). In particular, Mannheim consensus [2] states that the IMT for CCA images is estimated 1cm distal from the Bulb, which reflects this necessity. As defined in Sect. 9.1, IMT estimation and plaque detection only needs the intima-media region segmentation (see Fig. 9.2a). We call Region of Interest (ROI) the bounding box in the image containing these interfaces. The LI and MA interfaces delimit the segmentation of the Carotid Intima-Media region (CIM region).

The difficulties in CA segmentation in B-mode US scan images come from the following issues:

1. These images have a low signal-to-noise ratio. It is well known that noise and the presence of speckles represent the most prominent problem in US imaging.
2. The acquisition of the US is user-dependent, and the quality of the image strongly depends on the scanner used and its settings.
3. The high variability in vessel morphology in general together with the variability due to atherosclerosis disease make the task difficult.

Basic techniques for CIM region delineation and plaque segmentation presented in the literature include, among others, Hough transform [9], edge detection [10, 11], active contours [12, 13], snakes [14, 15], and other solutions such as integrated approaches that combine several basic Machine Learning (ML) methods [16–18]. Review articles [19, 20] present more references of studies that use image processing, statistical methods, and basic ML techniques. A more recent review [21] shows the influence of automatic artificial intelligence techniques in clinical practice guidelines for CVD/stroke risk to improve patient outcomes. In particular, it shows how automated IMT measurement techniques have evolved in the last 15 years. It includes a quantitative search of the latest ML and DL techniques for this purpose, but the works are not reviewed. Conversely, in this chapter, we review and compare the proposals and their details. Moreover, we include a more in-depth summary of the latest proposals in the field and emphasize the advantages and challenges of DL techniques.

According to Loizou [20], the methods can be broadly classified into two categories. The first category includes techniques that require user interaction, i.e., semi-automatic; whereas the second one includes fully automatic methods. Semi-automatic approaches [11, 15] require user interaction for manual initialization to select the ROI and/or to correct wrong results during examination. In general, the manual ROI selection together with this type of interactions result in better performance. The best semi-automatic methods found in the literature for clinical practice are the ones that offer visual feedback during image acquisition instead of analyzing stored images [11].

In contrast, fully automatic methods [10, 12, 16–18, 22, 23] run without any initial setting or user interaction. The main advantage of these techniques is that they are able to process large amounts of data. Furthermore, they allow the reproducibility of results, and save time and resources. Preliminary efforts using ML [16–18] and DL [13, 22–25] in fully automatic IMT evaluation are presented in the literature. Lara et al. [26–28] proposed several IMT estimation methods using windowing processes on a ROI and a feed-forward network for pixel classification. Standard multi-layer perceptron (MLP) was introduced in [28], but the best results are obtained in [22] where an auto-encoder was also proposed for CA image interpretation. However, despite all these sophisticated techniques, these approaches do not outperform the snake-based method presented in [12]. For their part, Zhang et al. [18] proposed a two-step segmentation method of the CIM region based on patch-based classification and stacked sequential learning. Later, patch-based Convolutional Neural Networks (CNNs) were used in different steps for IMT estimation [23]. More specifically, this work uses US videos instead of a unique frame and adds an extra first step for selecting three end-diastolic ultrasound frames. Despite the DL advantages, ML techniques applied to IMT region segmentation are still present in the literature. For instance, Qian and Yang [17] presented an approach to automatically segment plaque that uses several ML methods and combines them in an iterative algorithm. Rajasekaran et al. [13] used a CNN for the detection of a ROI, although an active contour based snake algorithm was further used to extract the boundaries of LI and MA layers. Biswas et al. [24, 25] proposed two interesting approaches based on a combination of two DL models. Firstly, they used a method that consists of a convolutional encoder/decoder to first extract features and then created the segmented images from them [25]. In particular, the training system uses two kinds of gold standards, one for LI and other for MA, which lead to the design of two DL systems. However, the final stage of this approach still needs a ML-based "refinement" in order to increase the accuracy of the system. More recently, they proposed an interesting two-stage method based on two independent DL models [24]. In this case, one model uses a CNN with patch images as input to form the ROI, and the other model uses a Fully Convolutional Network (FCN) to segment the CIM region within that ROI. In particular, this DL approach uses patches instead of the whole image at once, allowing a better control of the small regions of the image. Despite the novelty of these proposals, they require a complex system because they are composed of two sophisticated DL models.

To the best of our knowledge, all the aforementioned DL segmentation techniques are two-step approaches that define separate methods to first locate the ROI (performed manually in the case of semi-automatic methods); and second, delineate the CIM region within the ROI. On the contrary, Vila et al. [29] presented a single-step DL approach for automatic CA image interpretation. This approach is based on semantic segmentation using Densely Connected Convolutional Networks (DenseNets) [30], which were designed to facilitate the training of very deep networks due to a reduction in the number of parameters and the reuse of feature maps. This proposal represents the first attempt in the literature to accurately segment and interpret the different anatomical components of the CA (lumen, far wall, near wall, Bulb, CIM region and CIM-Bulb region, see Fig. 9.4), which has demonstrated to be helpful in the proper estimation of the IMT. Using the segmented regions, a straightforward approach for IMT estimation and plaque detection is defined.

Table 9.1 Most recent/relevant techniques for CA segmentation and IMT estimation together with their main characteristics: author(s) and reference, year of publication, the segmentation method used, if the method is Semi-Automatic (SA) or Fully-Automatic (FA) ("(1)": one-step, and "(2)": two-step), the processing time per frame, the type of data as a Unique Frame (UF) or Video (V), the artery territory, the presence of plaque in the images of the data set, the number of images in the data set (N), if the images were acquired from different devices (Different Devices), and the mean IMT error in mm. Notice that NS means "Not Specified" in the referenced paper

Author	Year	Segmentation method	Method SA/FA	Proc. time per frame	Image modality	Artery territory	Presence of plaque	N	Different devices	Mean IMT Error (mm)
Faita et al. [11]	2008	Edge Detection	SA(2)	NS	V	CCA	No	150	No	0.001
Molinari et al. [16]	2012	Snakes (CALEX) Basic ML techniques	FA(2)	2s	UF	CCA	NS	885	No	0.022
Molinari et al. [10]	2012	Edge Detection	FA(2)	<15s	UF	CCA	NS	365	Yes	0.078
Loizou et al. [14]	2013	Snakes	SA(2)	28s	UF	CCA	Yes	20	No	0.065
Menchón-Lara et al. [22]	2015	NN Auto-Encoders	FA(2)	1.4s	UF	CCA	NS	55	No	0.018
Bastida-Jumilla et al.[12]	2015	Frequency-Domain Snakes	FA(2)	12.2s	UF	CCA	NS	46	No	0.014
Zhang et al. [18]	2015	Patch-based Basic ML techniques	FA(2)	NS	UF	CCA	Yes	100	Yes	1.37% (point-to-point relative error)
Shin et al. [23]	2016	CNN Patch-based	FA(2)	NS	V	CCA	NS	92	No	0.023 per interface (LI and MA)
Zhao et al. [15]	2017	Snakes	SA(2)	0.24s	V	NS	Yes	NS	Yes	0.053

(continued)

Table 9.1 (continued)

Author	Year	Segmentation Method	Method SA/FA	Proc. Time per Frame	Image Modality	Artery Territory	Presence of Plaque	N	Different Devices	Mean IMT Error (mm)
Qian et al. [17]	2018	Patch-based Basic ML techniques	FA(2)	6min	UF	CCA	Yes	29	No	0.34 (average point-to-point distance)
Biswas et al. [25]	2018	CNN	FA(2)	NS	UF	CCA	Yes	407	No	0.124
Rajasekaran et al. [13]	2019	CNN for ROI Active contour	FA(2)	NS	UF	NS	NS	500	No	0.066
Vila et al. [29]	2019	FCN Semantic Segmentation	FA(1)	0.79s	UF	CCA & Bulb	Yes	4,751 (CCA) 3,733 (Bulb)	Generalization Test	0.022 (CCA) 0.06 (Bulb)
Biswas et al. [24]	2020	CNN	FA(2)	NS	UF	CCA	Yes	250	No	0.0935

In Table 9.1, we summarize some relevant proposals for CIM segmentation and IMT estimation presented in the literature and compare several characteristics of every method. Let us comment on the different characteristics reported in Table 9.1.

- Column "Segmentation Method". Almost half of the recent methods are based on DL techniques. In particular, different architectures of NNs are adopted in 6 out of the 14 works reported.
- Column "Method SA/FA". It is worth mentioning that the Semi-Automatic (SA) methods do not achieve better results than the Fully-Automatic (FA) methods in all cases.
- Column "Proc. Time per Frame". The information of the processing time per frame is not provided in all the papers. It is important to note that even if the DL methods can take quite a long time to be trained (depending on the power of the hardware, GPU, and other properties), the important factor to consider is the time spent on testing, which is generally fast.
- Column "Image Modality". Regarding the image modality, there are several works which consider Video (V) instead of a Unique Frame (UF). The IMT estimation in the diastolic and systolic cycle separately is useful to analyze the health of the artery (see Sect. 9.1). Taking videos into account allows to analyze a specific period of the cardiac cycle as in [23]; or both periods [11, 15], making the assessment of the method more robust.
- Column "Artery Territory". Most of the presented works and reference values from the guidelines focus only on CCA images. The image quality of other territories, such as Bulb or ICA, is worse than CCA (poorer contrast and more affected by noise, see Sect. 9.1). Moreover, successful imaging depends on the anatomy of subjects. These facts make the segmentation of the CIM region in these other territories difficult. According to Table 9.1, only [29] deals with Bulb images. However, automatic segmentation of different territories would be very useful and should be addressed if there is a will to have an impact on clinical practice.
- Column "Presence of Plaque". The shape variability of the CIM region makes difficult the design of a robust segmentation method. In the non-plaque images (i.e., images in which the plaque does not appear), the CIM region is observed as a straight thin shape, whereas the presence of plaque leads to a focal thickening of the CIM region, resulting in an irregular shape (see Fig. 9.2a). As a consequence, most of the previous works found in the literature only face the problem of measuring the IMT within plaque-free regions and discard images with the presence of plaque. Some methods reported in Table 9.1 [14, 15, 18, 25, 25, 29] broaden the target and build a general method capable of accurately estimating IMT values even in the presence of plaque. This property makes the methods useful for data sets of population studies (such as the one considered in [29], Sect. 9.2.1.1). Moreover, the presence of plaque in the data set allows to evaluate the plaque detection ability of the proposals.
- Column "N". In terms of the number of images processed, the size of the considered data sets in the IMT estimation studies is quite small. Although these sample sizes guarantee an adequate level of study power, a large-scale study —such as the

one used in [29]— is required to carefully assess the effect of variability on segmentation performance, and also to evaluate the systems before their application in the real praxis.
- Column "Different Devices". The different devices and settings used for image acquisition provide data sets with different image characteristics. Dealing with these differences implies a difficult challenge for the robust segmentation of CA components and IMT estimation. For this reason, most of the methods in the literature use data sets provided by a single device. Conversely, the data sets used in [10, 15, 29] contain images from different clinical centers. In particular, Vila et al. [29] validated the robustness and generalization power of their method by applying it to a second data set, which contains images provided by a different equipment (see Sect. 9.2.1.1).
- Column "Mean IMT Error (mm)". A proper validation procedure should evaluate several proposals comparing the obtained IMT estimation with other state-of-the-art approaches to demonstrate the superior performance of the proposed method, as done in [29]. The direct comparison of the error values presented in Table 9.1 is not fair since these values are completely influenced by the considered data sets. Even so, we can highlight the results reported in [29], since only two FA methods [12, 22] reach minor errors, although these values could be influenced by the small size of their data sets.

9.2.1 Deep Learning Proposal for IMT Estimation and Plaque Detection

In this section, we review the approach presented in [29] that includes CIM region segmentation, IMT estimation, and plaque detection.

CA semantic segmentation is about solving the problem of separating the different anatomical components in the CA image; that is, obtaining a mask with six or four different labels, depending on whether CCA or Bulb images are being analyzed, respectively (see Fig. 9.4). For this purpose, the proposal uses a Semantic Segmentation (SS) algorithm that works in an end-to-end framework, instead of using image features such as shapes or pixel-based features. In particular, it uses Fully Convolutional Networks (FCN) [31], a particular type of Convolutional Neural Networks (CNN) that do not use fully-connected layers. Figure 9.3 depicts the workflow of this approach [29]: an image of any size is taken as input data and transformed to obtain a segmented image, with the same spatial resolution, through an inference, learning process. Figure 9.4 shows an example of two CA images (inputs to the SS model) and their corresponding segmented images (expected outputs of the SS model).

The selected architecture to solve the CA segmentation problem was the so-called Tiramisu [32], an extension of DenseNets to FCNs. Densely Connected Convolutional Networks (DenseNets) [30] are an extension of the well-known Residual Networks (ResNets) [33]. DenseNets have been designed to ease the training of very

9 Last Advances on Automatic Carotid Artery Analysis ...

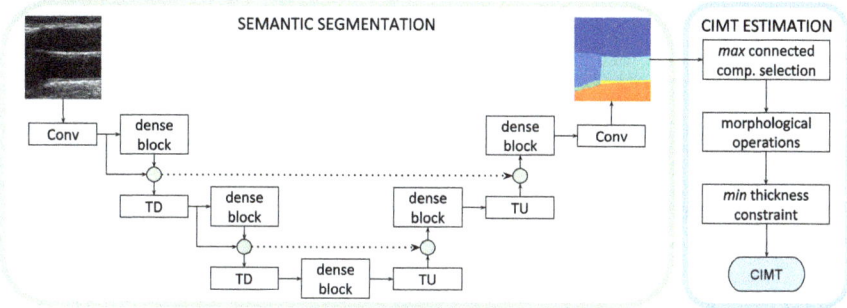

Fig. 9.3 Workflow of the method for semantic carotid artery segmentation and IMT estimation [29]. The SS model is composed of a down-sampling path with Transition Down (TD) blocks, and an up-sampling path with Transition Up (TU) blocks, both including dense blocks that create the feature maps. A Convolution (Conv) is applied at the input of the network as well as at the end, to generate the final segmentation. The small circles represent concatenations, and the dotted arrows are the skip connections

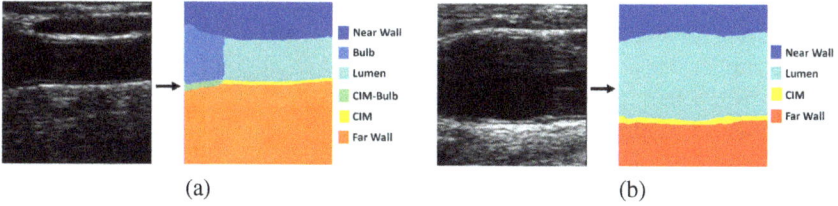

Fig. 9.4 Example of the input (left) and expected output (right) of the SS model for images of both territories: (**a**) CCA and (**b**) Bulb. The legend at right details the segmentation labels

deep networks, and present some characteristics that make them very appropriate for SS: parameter efficiency, implicit deep supervision, and feature reuse. The Tiramisu architecture (see Fig. 9.3, left) is composed of a down-sampling path with transition down (TD) blocks to extract coarse semantic features, and an up-sampling path with transition up (TU) blocks to recover the input image resolution at the output level. Both paths are connected by means of skip connections that allow the recovery of fine-grained information. They are defined by a sequence of dense blocks that contain a set of concatenated layers, as proposed in DenseNets. Dense blocks are composed of concatenated layers that include Batch Normalization, Rectified Linear Unit, 3×3 convolution, and Dropout. TD blocks are composed of Batch Normalization, Rectified Linear Unit, 1×1 convolution, Dropout, and 2×2 max-pooling. Finally, TU blocks are composed of 3×3 transposed convolution.

The output of the semantic segmentation is used to estimate the IMT: the CIM region is first selected from the obtained mask, and then the IMT measurement is computed as the mean from all the absolute distance between the two borders (LI and MA interfaces). Afterwards, each image is classified as containing plaque or non-plaque, using the IMT measurement and following the Mannheim consensus (see Sect. 9.1).

9.2.1.1 Data Sets

For the experiments, two data sets were considered: REGICOR and NEFRONA. The first data set was used to validate the IMT estimation and it consists of a sample 8,484 images corresponding to 2379 subjects from Girona's Heart Registry [34]. The second data set is formed by 27 images from Atherotrombotic Diseases Unit Detection Hospital Arnau de Vilanova and it is used for the generalization test. Both data sets were obtained with different types of equipment, frequencies, and resolutions. The Ground Truth (GT) for the IMT estimation was given by the Amsterdam Medical Center[1] (AMC), and they were obtained from a semi-automatic software e-track [35]. Besides the GT for IMT estimation and plaque detection, a segmentation GT was defined for a subset of the REGICOR images. In order to obtain it, an expert (Expert1) manually delineated and labeled the different regions of the original images, using six labels for CCA and four for Bulb (see Fig. 9.4). Since this manual task is complicated and time-consuming, only a representative subset of REGICOR images was labeled, including 159 CCA images (51 with plaque and 108 without plaque), and 172 Bulb images (68 with plaque and 104 without). The training set contains 141 images for the CCA and 155 images for the Bulb, while the rest is used for testing. A summary of the different experiments and data sets is presented in Table 9.2, and described in the next Section.

9.2.1.2 Experiments

Experiment 1: *Segmentation*
In order to validate the proposed segmentation method, six different approaches were applied to a subset of the REGICOR data set: four DenseNets models based on Tiramisu, the U-Net method [36], and a two-step approach based on the shallow method Random Forest (RF). Regarding the Tiramisu model, two different configurations were considered that varied the depth of the network: Tiramisu56 (a total of 56 layers, 4 per dense block) and Tiramisu103 (a total of 103 layers, from 4 to 12 per block). In order to show if the SS of several anatomical components helps in the CIM region segmentation, the results provided by the two Tiramisu models (Tiramisu56 and Tiramisu103) were also compared using only two labels (CIM region and *background*). This second approach is called Binary Segmentation (BS), whilst the one with all the labels is called Semantic Segmentation (SS). Notice that both approaches, BS and SS, were compared by considering two labels in the evaluation measure. In order to demonstrate the adequacy of using DenseNets, the U-Net was also considered in the experimentation. In this sense, it is worth pointing out that the main

---

[1] https://www.abc.uva.nl/research/institutes/institute-articles/academic-medical-center-amc.html.

Table 9.2 Summary of the different experiments carried out for validation purposes

Experiment 1: Segmentation
Purpose: comparison of different segmentation approaches
Data set: subset of REGICOR. GT: manually segmented images
images: 159 (CCA), 172 (Bulb). Train/test split: $\approx$ 90–10%
Performance measures: accuracy, specificity, sensitivity, precision, Dice coefficient
Experiment 2: IMT estimation
Purpose: comparison of different methods for IMT estimation
Data set: REGICOR. GT: IMT values
images: 8,484 (all of them used for validation)
Error measurement: correlation coefficient and Bland-Altman analysis
Experiment 3: Plaque detection
Purpose: comparison of different methods for plaque detection
Data set: REGICOR. GT: plaque detection (yes/no)
images: 8,484 (all of them used for validation)
Performance measures: accuracy, specificity, sensitivity

difference between U-Net and Tiramisu is that the first one uses standard convolutions instead of the dense blocks used in the DenseNet architecture. Finally, in order to compare the NNs with classical methods, a two-step approach based on RF was also considered. In particular, RF2 refers to the two-step approach in which a ROI is first automatically extracted (pre-processing) and then a patch-based RF (multi-class) is used for pixel-wise classification. In this case, a post-processing specifically designed for this method [18] can be applied, which is referred as RF2-PP.

All the NN models were trained using a GeForce Titan X (Pascal) 12GB GPU from NVIDIA. The models' weights were initialized using the HeUniform initialization [37], and the RMSprop algorithm [38] was used as optimizer. The training process was carried out in two steps, as in [32]: (1) pre-training with random cropping for data augmentation (crop dimension: 224×224 px), learning rate $1e-3$, and batch size 3; and (2) fine-tuning with full size images (image dimension: 470×445 px), learning rate $1e-4$, and batch size 1. The outputs were monitored using the pixel-wise accuracy and the Dice coefficient, with a patience of 100 during pre-training and 50 during fine-tuning.

A complete set of measures was used to evaluate the performance of the different models: the pixel-wise metrics accuracy (Acc.), specificity (Spec.), sensitivity (Sens.), precision (Prec.) and Dice coefficient (DC), considering the CIM region (positive) and the background (negative).

Results Fig. 9.5 depicts the comparison between the different segmentation approaches in CCA (top) and Bulb (bottom) test images. It can be seen that the different Tiramisu architectures clearly improve the RF2 results (mainly note the improvement in DC). Moreover, making the Tiramisu model deeper by increasing the number of parameters (from 56 to 103) does not improve the results, probably

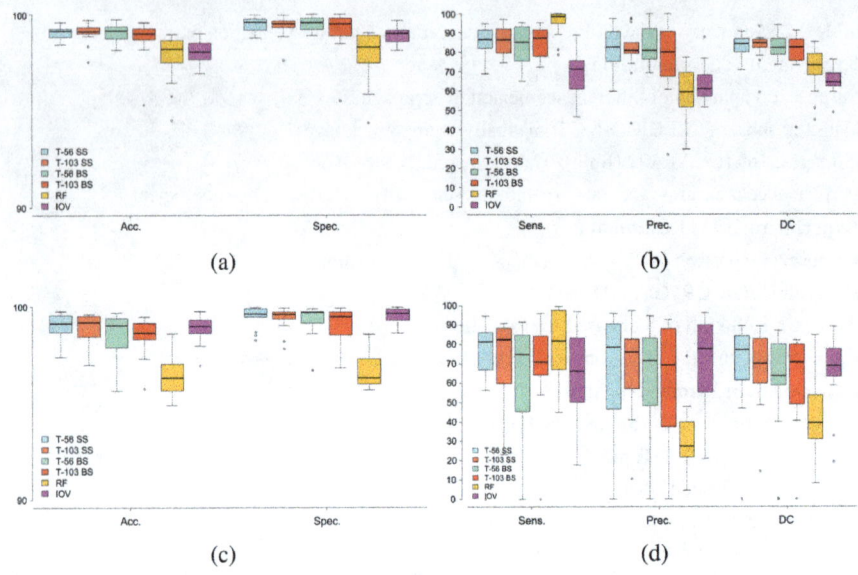

Fig. 9.5 Box-plot of metric results for the different segmentation methods and IOV: (left) accuracy and specificity, and (right) sensitivity, precision and Dice coefficient. The plots show the measurements for CCA images, (**a**) and (**b**); and Bulb images, (**c**) and (**d**). Note that the overlap measurements are split up for visualization purposes, using different scales in the abscissa axis

due to the size of the training set. Although the BS is equivalent to SS in CCA images, the semantic information is necessary (see the IMT estimation step in these images, Sect. 9.2). Note that the improvement using SS is more evident in Bulb images. Regarding U-Net, its results are slightly worse than Tiramisu103 BS and are not included in the graphic. Finally, the IOV results (considering Expert1 as GT, versus Expert2) are low compared with the automatic methods results, specially in terms of sensitivity and DC, in both CCA and Bulb images. These results and the high standard deviations show the difficulty of reproducing the CA results in clinical trials. It is worth noting that all the measures were computed using the Expert1's labels as GT, but the values are equivalent for the labels of Expert2.

Experiment 2: *IMT estimation*
With the aim of evaluating the method proposed by Vila et al. [29] in terms of IMT estimation over the REGICOR data set, they considered the correlation coefficient (cc) between the GT and the predicted IMT values as well as the Bland-Altman analysis. For a deep comparison, the methods used in *Experiment 1* (Tiramisu56, Tiramisu103 and RF2-PP) were considered together with other approaches found in the literature.

Results Fig. 9.6a shows the correlation between the IMT values (GT and predicted) in CCA images for the best method (i.e., "Tiramisu56 SS+IMT estimation"), which reaches a high cc of 0.81 (cc = 0.77 when applying only Tiramisu56 SS). The result is very similar to Tiramisu103 (cc = 0.80), in contrast to RF2-PP (cc = 0.72).

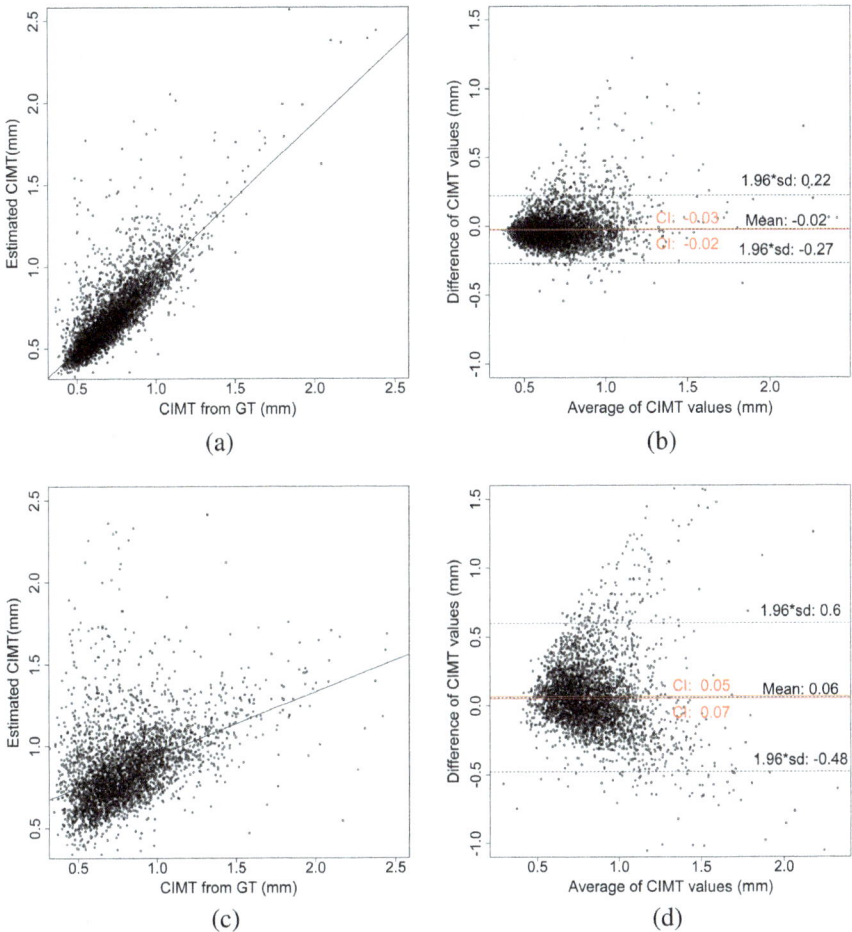

Fig. 9.6 Correlation between IMT values (left), and Bland-Altman analysis (right). Both plots show the relation between GT and the estimated values in CCA images, (**a**) and (**b**); and in Bulb images, (**c**) and (**d**). Red solid lines show the confidence intervals (CI) for the "mean of the differences" line

Regarding Bulb images (see Fig. 9.6c), "Tiramisu56 SS+IMT estimation" achieves a lower cc of 0.43 (cc = 0.34 when applying only Tiramisu56 SS), probably due to the worse quality of the images in Bulb, which makes the task more difficult in this territory. However, the proposal presented in [29] still outperforms RF2-PP, which only reaches a cc of 0.41.

In Fig. 9.6b, the Bland-Altman plot depicts the difference, in CCA images, between the IMT of the corresponding two values (estimated and GT) against the average of both values. This plot shows a high degree of agreement between the two measures, especially in the cases where the IMT is small (<0.5mm), which correspond to healthy population (i.e., without plaque) [34]. Furthermore, this plot shows that the predicted IMT is, on average, slightly underestimated (mean −0.02). The confidence intervals for the "mean of the differences line" (red line in Fig. 9.6) shows that this bias is statistically significant. Therefore, in order to achieve the interchangeability of the techniques this bias cannot be avoided.

The results are similar for Bland-Altman analysis in Bulb images (see Fig. 9.6d) and, in this case, the average slightly overestimates the IMT measure (the mean of the differences is 0.06 and this bias is also statistically significant). Column named "Mean IMT Error (mm)" in Table 9.1 compares the mean IMT error obtained with several methods found in the literature. It should be highlighted that the IMT error achieved with the approach by Vila et al. [29] is low compared with other fully automatic methods reviewed in the table. In particular, only some two-step methods [12, 22] reach a IMT error lower, but in a much smaller data set and only in one territory (CCA). In fact, the size of the data set used in [29] is much larger than the ones considered in the rest of papers (8484 versus 20 to 885 images). Note that, as can be seen in this column of Table 9.1, the IMT error is not always presented as the mean of the IMT error; in some cases, it is presented as point-to-point relative error, average point-to-point distance, or evaluating the mean error for each interface separately.

Fig. 9.7 shows qualitative examples of the CIM segmentation results and plaque detection for four CCA and four Bulb images. The first and third columns show examples of CIM region segmentation, outlined in green, in non-plaque images; whereas the second and the fourth columns show examples of images with plaque, outlined in red.

Finally, it is important to note that the processing time to estimate the IMT and detect a plaque is only 0.79 s, as can be also seen in Table 9.1 (column "Proc. Time per Frame").

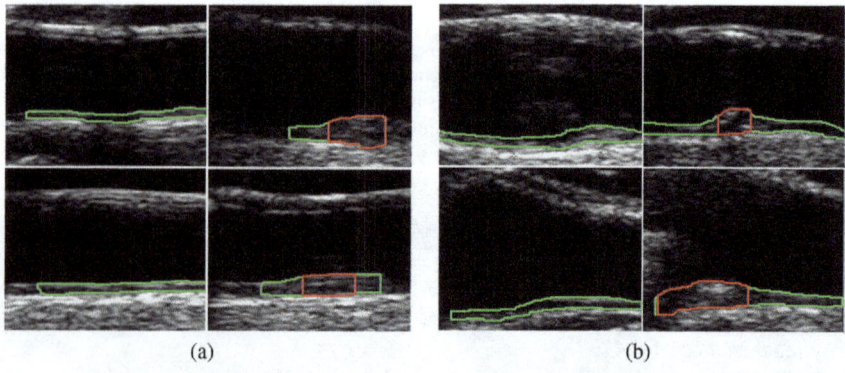

Fig. 9.7 Qualitative results of the CIM segmentation for eight different images: (**a**) CCA images, and (**b**) Bulb images. Green lines are the CIM region boundaries and red lines the detected plaque boundaries. Images are cropped for visualization purposes

Table 9.3 Results of plaque detection in REGICOR images for different methods, the number of plaques in each territory and the following validation measures: accuracy (Acc.), sensitivity (Sens.), and specificity (Spec.)

Territory Images	Method	# Plaques/Total images	Acc.	Sens.	Spec.
CCA	RF2	50/4,722	50.05%	100.00%	49.00%
	RF2-PP	50/4,722	94.08%	86.00%	94.16%
	NN method [29]	50/4,751	96.45%	80.00%	96.63%
Bulb	RF2	240/3,539	35.09%	98.33%	30.49%
	RF2-PP	240/3,539	78.50%	69.58%	79.15%
	NN method [29]	264/3,733	78.09%	78.32%	75.00%

Experiment 3: *Plaque detection* Here we present the evaluation of the method proposed by Vila et al. [29] in terms of plaque detection over the REGICOR data set, including a comparison with the two-step approaches (RF2 and RF2-PP). For this purpose, the following metrics were used, considering the presence of plaque as positive and the absence of plaque as negative: accuracy (Acc.), specificity (Spec.), and sensitivity (Sens.).

Results: Table 9.3 includes the plaque detection results in CCA and Bulb images, showing a promising performance, mostly in CCA. The smaller number of plaques in the data set gives lower sensitivity values than specificity values. Regarding Bulb images, there is still large room for improvement, probably due to the poorer quality of these images, as commented before. Note that the RF2 method needs a sophisticated post-processing to achieve similar results to the ones provided by the NN method [29]. Figure 9.7 shows qualitative examples of the plaque detection results.

9.3 Carotid Artery Plaque Classification and Risk Assessment in 2D CA Ultrasound Images

As it has been introduced in Sect. 9.1, atherosclerosis is characterized by focal thickenings of the innermost layer of the artery, which is reflected in the artery walls. Since the tissue of CA walls provides information about the patients' arteries and cardiovascular health, the study of CA US plaque images has been considered of clinical relevance. The long induction period of atherosclerosis makes it suitable for the study of subclinical disease for preventive purposes. Thus, there are several medical interests related to the characterization of the atherosclerotic plaque in CA. For example, tools that can monitor atherosclerosis can also improve diagnosis and subsequent treatment [39]. Moreover, early identification of vulnerable, rupture-prone atherosclerotic plaques is a vigorous research field because not all carotid plaques are necessarily harmful and carotid surgery carries a considerable risk for the patient. The main purpose of the methods developed in this field is to create an image-based system that characterizes the atherosclerotic plaque and the carotid artery walls. Given CA US images, the challenges of these methods can be mainly grouped in four different objectives (see Sect. 9.3.2 for more details):

- *Objective 1*: classification of individuals with or without presence of symptoms.
- *Objective 2*: cardiovascular risk stratification.
- *Objective 3*: prediction of risk of future cardiovascular events.
- *Objective 4*: classification of tissue components.

Several techniques can be found in the literature to deal with these objectives. Sharma et al. [40] provided the first state-of-the-art review to comprehend the field of ultrasonic vascular morphology tissue classification. In particular, they revised different ML techniques in tissue morphology and classification using US imaging. More recently, Saba et al. [21] provided some guidelines of artificial intelligence-based methods for IMT and carotid plaque measurements, and discussed how they could be used as calculators for risk stratification assessment and prediction of events.

Table 9.4 summarizes some relevant works from the literature related to plaque and CA wall characterization in US longitudinal images (see Appendix for the abbreviations). The remainder of this section is devoted to discussing the information contained in Table 9.4: the properties of the data used in the different studies, the objectives of the different works, the considered image features, the used methods and the results.

9.3.1 Data Properties: Transversal/Follow-Up, Different Devices, Image Modality, Artery Territory, Number of Samples and Ground Truth

CA US images' characterization means to extract image patterns that describe or classify the atherosclerotic plaque and the carotid artery walls in order to solve any of the four mentioned objectives. Most of the studies focus on plaque characterization of a single frame of B-mode US 2D longitudinal images from the CA [4, 41–52] (see "Unique Frame" (UF) in column "Image Modality" from Table 9.4). This is because US imaging is a non-expensive and non-invasive technique for CA visualization that has been extensively used to examine atherosclerosis of a patient (see Sect. 9.2). Different image modalities are also used in the literature, as in [53], where the scans of the CCA, the Bulb, and the ICA are performed bilaterally in three different longitudinal projections, as well as transversal projections to analyze the entire plaque (see "4Fs (3 lon. & 1 transv." in column "Image Modality" from Table 9.4). Other studies include the information of the CA appearance during the cardiac cycle. In these cases, the specific instants (systole and diastole) are analyzed separately [54] (see "2F (sys. & diast.)" in column "Image Modality" from Table 9.4), or together, adding the information of the mechanical interactions from image sequences [55] (see "Video" in column "Image Modality" from Table 9.4).

Regarding the artery territory, in contrast to the research works reviewed in Sect. 9.2, the images used in some of these studies belong to ICA and Bulb (see column "Artery Territory" Table 9.4). This is because plaques occur only occasionally in the other regions of the artery. Besides, not all studies focus on the CIM region. Near wall characterization also adds information of the entire artery [4, 52] (see "CCA (far & near wall)" in column "Artery territory" from Table 9.4).

The GT in the revised literature is closely related to the objective of the particular work (see column "Ground Truth" from Table 9.4). The GT in *Objective 1* is based on clinical symptoms, which means whether the individual whose image is analyzed suffered any symptom related to CVDs or not [41, 42, 44, 50, 51, 54, 55]. The GT for the *Objective 2* is a previous risk stratification using the lumen diameter, which is a factor related to atherosclerosis [4, 52]. For the *Objective 3*, the methods are validated using the events occurred in a period of time [45, 46, 53], except in [49]. In this last paper, the validation is a comparison of the risk stratification (done using several cardiovascular risk factors) obtained from several risk prediction functions. Finally, the GT used for *Objective 4* is obtained from an endarterectomy (i.e., a surgical process that removes a sample of plaque) [47] or from a tissue component classification done by an expert [48].

The size of the data sets (see column "N" from Table 9.4) are similar to the studies presented in Sect. 9.2. The largest data set is the one presented in [46] with 1,121 subjects included in their Follow-Up (FU) study. Note that in the studies for the *Objective 4* the samples are small compared to the sample size of the other studies. This could be due because the endarterectomy used in the GT from [47] is aggressive for the patient, and the manual classification for the GT in [48] is tedious and very time-consuming.

Regarding the acquisition devices (see column "Different Devices" from Table 9.4), most of the works use data sets provided by a single device. In contrast, the images used in [44] and in [55] were obtained from two different types of equipment. Despite the challenge they present, their proposals result in most robust methods for risk prediction (*Objective 3*) [44] and for the classification of the presence or absence of past CV symptoms (*Objective 1*) [55].

9.3.2 Work Objectives

The details of the four objectives faced in the literature are explained below. There is a particular interest in the study of atherosclerotic plaques for clinical decision making. More specifically, it is crucial to identify plaques that are vulnerable to rupture because they lead to clinical events [56]. Efficient classification techniques are needed to determine the CV risk using CA US images.

Table 9.4 Most recent/relevant techniques for CA plaque characterization together with their main characteristics: author and reference, year of publication, if the method includes follow-up measurements, if the data set contains images acquired from different devices, the type of data as a Unique Frame or Video, the artery territory, the objectives of the proposal method, the image features used, the method, the number of subjects of the data set (N), the results, and the ground truth used. Notice that NS means "Not Specified" in the referenced paper

Author	Year	Transversal/ Follow-up	Different devices	Image modality	Artery territory	Work objective	Image features	Methods	N	Results	Ground truth
Gronholdt et al. [45]	2001	FU (4.4 years)	No	UF	NS	Risk prediction of events (3)	GSM	Statistics Cox, Kaplan Meier	246 plaques 111 asym & 135 sym	Relative risk 3.1 between 2 plaque types	44 events in 4.4 years
Brajesh et al. [47]	2002	T	No	UF	ICA	Mult. class.: 5 tissues (4)	PDA, GSM	Statistics Spearman	20 plaques (19 patients) 7sym & 13 asym	Spearman cc: 0.7	Endarterectomy
Stoitsis et al. [51]	2006	T	No	UF	NS	Bin. class.: symp/asymp (1)	FT	Statistics Bootstrap	19 plaques 10 sym & 9 asym	Significant Bootstrap p-value in 3 features	Based on the clinical symptoms
Nikolaos et al. [54]	2011	T	No	2F (sys. & diast.)	NS	Bin. class.: symp/asymp (1)	GSM, WT FS: div. value	SVM, PNN	20 plaques 11 symp & 9 asym	Acc: 90% (diast.) 75% (syst.)	Based on the clinical symptoms
Kyriacou et al. [46]	2012	FU (4 years)	No	UF	ICA	Risk prediction of events (3)	TPA, GSM, pdf and cdf	SVM, PNN	1121 patients	Acc 77%	Events with 157 death

(continued)

Table 9.4 (continued)

Author	Year	Transversal/follow-up	Different devices	Image modality	Artery territory	Work objective	Image features	Methods	N	Results	Ground truth
Acharya et al. [43]	2012	T	No	UF	ICA	Bin. class.: symp/asymp (1)	WT FS: t-test	SVM	346 plaques 150 asym & 196 sym	Acc 83.7%	Based on the clinical symptoms
Irie et al. [53]	2013	FU (4.6 years)	No	4Fs(3 lon. & 1 transv.)	CCA, Bulb, ICA	Risk prediction of events (3)	TPA, plaque shape. GSM	Statistics AUC. Cox	287 patients	AUC 0.82%	34 Events during 55 months
Acharya et al. [44]	2013	T	Yes	UF	CCA	Bin. class.: symp/asymp (1)	GLCM FS: t-test	SVM,kNN,PNN DT,GMM,NBC	146/346 plaques 44/196 sym & 102/150 asym	Acc 93.1% and 85.3%	Based on the clinical symptoms
Acharya et al. [41]	2013	T	No	UF	Bulb	Bin. class.: symp/asymp (1)	GLCM, RLM,WT, HOS FS: t-test	SVM	146 plaques (99 patients)	Acc 91.7%	Based on the clinical symptoms
Acharya et al. [50]	2013	T	No	UF	CCA	Bin. class.: symp/asymp (1)	LBP, GLCM, RLM,WT, HOS FS: t-test, kullback, div. value	SVM	160 plaques 110 asym & 50 sym	Acc 90.7%	Based on the clinical symptoms

(continued)

Table 9.4 (continued)

Author	Year	Transversal/ follow-up	Different devices	Image modality	Artery territory	Work objective	Image features	Methods	N	Results	Ground truth
Gastounioti et al. [55]	2014	T	Yes	Video	NS	Bin. class.: symp/asymp (1)	kinematic features FS: Fisher, Wilcoxon, PCA	SVM, kNN, PNN DT, DA	56 plaques 28sym & 28 asym	Acc 88%	Based on the clinical symptoms
Acharya et al. [42]	2015	T	No	UF	CCA	Bin. class.: symp/asymp (1)	IMT, IMTv. GL using HOS. FS: ANOVA	SVM,kNN,PNN	118 plaques (59 patients)	Acc 99.1%	Based on the clinical symptoms
Lekadir et al. [48]	2017	T	No	UF	NS	Mult. class.: 3 tissues (4)	Patch based (end-to-end)	CNN	56 plaques	Acc 78.5% patch based Mean cc area 0.91%	Clinician expert
Araki et al. [52]	2017	T	No	UF	CCA(far & near wall)	Risk stratification (2)	GLCM, RLM	SVM	407 plaques	Acc 99%	Lumen diameter for risk stratification
Saba et al. [4]	2017	T	No	UF	CCA(far & near wall)	Risk stratification (2)	GLCM, RLM	PCA, SVM	407 plaques	Acc 98.83%	Lumen diameter for risk stratification
Khanna et al. [49]	2019	FU (10 years)	No	UF	CCA	Risk prediction of events (3)	CUSIP in two periods of time	Statistics AUC	202 images for period	AUC 0.92.7%	Risk stratification with risk functions

- **Objective 1**: There are image-based techniques for binary classification of plaques: symptomatic and asymptomatic [41–44, 50, 51, 54, 55] (see "Bin. class.: symp/asymp" in column "Work Objective" from Table 9.4). Symptomatic plaques are from patients who have suffered any cerebrovascular event. In contrast, asymptomatic plaques are from patients who have not experienced any of these diseases.
- **Objective 2**: In the recent literature, some attempts have appeared to assess the CV risk of subjects using CA image features. This is carried out by solving a classification problem between two ranges: low and high risk [4, 52] (see "Risk stratification" in column "Work Objective" from Table 9.4).
- **Objective 3**: Despite the advances in imaging modalities and identifying plaque vulnerability characteristics, such as its composition, few of these plaques rupture and even fewer lead to clinical events [56]. Therefore, it is important to perform studies to evaluate the individual risk that entails atherosclerosis evolution. This fact has motivated several studies to analyze the CA in a longitudinal study in order to predict the occurrence of CV events during a period [45, 46, 49, 53] (see "Risk prediction of events" in column "Work Objective" from Table 9.4). Longitudinal studies involve repeated observations of the same subjects during a period of time (see "Follow-Up" (FU) in column "Transversal/Follow-Up" from Table 9.4).
- **Objective 4**: It is established that the composition of atherosclerotic plaque is related to CVD [3]. Some proposals in the literature deal with the classification of the plaque components (generally lipid, fibromuscular, and calcium). This classification is usually performed by an expert [57, 58] or using image-based techniques built on the gray intensity levels from the plaque region [47, 48] (see "Mult. class." in the column "Work Objective" from Table 9.4). These image based-techniques address the classification problem with a multi-class classification method [47, 48]. The number of studies related to this objective are relatively small probably because the GT is difficult to obtain, either because it requires surgery [47] or it is manually obtained [48].

9.3.3 Image Features

The features used in the literature to characterize atherosclerotic tissue are, in general, based on gray intensity values (see column "Image Features" from Table 9.4). The most standard feature is the Grayscale Median (GSM) method [4, 47, 52–54]. The technique proposed in [47] for the *Objective 2* is a combination of GSM and Pixel Distribution Analysis (PDA). However, it demonstrates an agreement between these image features and histologic measurements. The studies proposed in [4, 52] presented good accuracies for risk stratification using GSM features. The estimation of the spatial distribution of gray levels is a suitable technique for texture analysis. Gray Level Co-occurrence Matrix (GLCM) [59] and Run Length Matrix (RLM) [60] methods based on gray level values are used to examine the texture in CA US images [44]. For a more objective analysis, the group of Acharya et al. [41, 44, 50] developed novel integrated indices using a combination of significant features to deal with

Objective 1. As a result, they concluded that grayscale features based on a combination of trace transform [61] and texture properties are suitable for the classification of symptomatic and asymptomatic plaques. Another different approach using the information of the pixel intensity values and their distribution is the tissue classification method (*Objective 4*) proposed in [48]. In contrast to the other proposals, the image feature used in this case is the entire patch around the pixel that is used as the input to the model.

Frequency-based approaches, such as the ones based on Wavelet Transforms (WT), can decompose the frequency content of the image and, consequently, reveal texture characteristics from different materials of the plaque [41, 43, 50, 51, 54]. Several studies present a scale-frequency approach showing that WT features are a good alternative for the characterization of plaque tissue between the symptomatic and asymptomatic groups (*Objective 1*). In this sense, Tsiaparas et al. [54] demonstrated that WT features are more accurate than "traditional" features as GSM, since they capture both the frequency and spatial content of the image. For their part, Stoitsis et al. [51] conducted a study comparing several frequency-based texture analysis based on WT and Fourier Transform (FT) for the plaque classification. The methods presented in [41–43, 50] use a combination of some techniques mentioned above such as GLCM, RLM and WT resulting in good accuracies for the binary classification of the *Objective 1*. In particular, Acharya et al. [50] also used a gray-based feature texture known as Local Binary Pattern (LBP), whilst [41, 42, 50] added the features extracted by the Higher-Order Spectra (HOS) technique [62], which provides high noise immunity.

Some studies use quantitative measures from atherosclerotic plaque to compare them with the occurrence of CVD or other pathologies during the FU period [46, 53]. Since IMT and IMT variability may be associated with atherosclerosis symptomatology (see Sect. 9.2), the most common image-based phenotypes use for CA US images characterization include: IMT average, IMT maximum, IMT minimum, IMT Variability (IMTv), and Total Plaque Area (TPA) [21]. To the best of our knowledge, the most recent work proposed in this field is [49], which presents an image-based method to provide a 10-year risk calculator based on the fusion of Cardiovascular Risk Factors (CVRFs) and changes in the mentioned carotid image-based phenotypes.

For the *Objective 1*, common statistical methods are used in the literature in order to select the relevant features for the binary discrimination. These methods are Student's t-test [41, 43, 44], ANOVA test [42], and Divergence value to rank the features [50, 54]. An interesting work that combines three different selection strategies is presented in [55]. These strategies are Fisher discriminant ratio, Wilcoxon rank-sum test, and Principal Component Analysis (PCA), and were used to select the features that are able to better discriminate the two groups. In particular, the features used in this study are kinematic features of the arterial wall estimated with the motion analysis from B-mode US image sequences, occurring during the cardiac cycle.

9.3.4 Methods and Results

Different methods have been proposed in the literature to deal with the different types of image features for the respective objectives (see column "Methods" from Table 9.4). Several statistical methods are used in order to characterize the atherosclerotic plaque and/or CA wall features. For example, the comparisons between PDA predictions for different tissue components with the histologic analysis of plaques (*Objective 4*) are done using Spearman coefficient of correlation in [47]. In order to determine the discriminatory value of texture features from the two groups for *Objective 1*, the bootstrap method was used in [51]. This method compares the mean values of the features extracted from each group. As a result, three texture features were found to significantly discriminate between symptomatic and asymptomatic plaques. All three features correspond to texture patterns in the horizontal direction, indicating that horizontal texture patterns characterize the atherosclerotic plaque. Kaplan-Meier analysis and Cox regression are statistical methods employed in survival studies to predict events in longitudinal studies as the ones used for the *Objective 3*. In particular, these two methods were used in [45], whilst Cox regression was used in [53]. Also, the Area Under the Curve (AUC) was used to validate the same objective in [49, 53]. In this case, AUC measures the ability of the binary classifier in risk stratification for the validation in [49] (see "Ground Truth" column from Table 9.4) and in risk prediction of events in [53]. In particular, using the AUC, Khanna et al. [49] concluded that the addition of the image-based phenypes to the classical CVRFs outperforms the ten currently available conventional cardiovascular risk calculators.

On the other hand, the basic ML methods presented for the *Objective 1* are supervised classifiers based on the assumption that each of these features belong to two distinct classes: symptomatic and asymptomatic. In these cases the classification methods are: k-Nearest Neighbor (kNN) [42, 44, 55], Decision Trees (DT) [44, 55], Discriminant Analysis (DA) [55], Gaussian Mixture Model (GMM) [44], and Naïve Bayes classifier (NBC) [44]. The most common ML method used in the revised literature is Support Vector Machine (SVM), used for classification in *Objective 1* [41–44, 50, 54, 55] and for risk stratification in *Objective 2* [4, 52]. DL strategies as Probabilistic Neural Networks are also used for *Objective 1* [42, 44, 54, 55] and for risk prediction in *Objective 3* [46]. These DL strategies use hand-crafted feature vectors as input to the network and a traditional pipeline design, instead of using the raw image as input and allowing an end-to-end learning. For their part, Lekadir et al. [48] is the only DL approach proposed in the literature that performs end-to-end learning using a CNN with image patches as the input to the model. This approach does multi-class classification of each pixel of the plaque into a tissue component. The entire patch adds all the information around the pixel that is analyzed by the model. Then, the CNN chooses automatically the relevant information optimal to the discrimination of the different plaque constituents resulting in good accuracy results and correlation.

Note that there is no fair way to do a general comparison of the results (see "Results" column from Table 9.4) because the validation methods, the GT, and the data sets are different in each proposal.

9.4 Discussion: Challenges in Deep Learning

There is no doubt that DL techniques are revolutionized the field of medical imaging, as it was prognosticated in recent publications [63, 64]. Although there are still several open issues to be addressed, DL has already demonstrated significant potential to overcome human performance in selected tasks, such as medical image segmentation [65]. Moreover, DL provides key information in the clinical decision-making process [7, 8].

Currently, the main challenges of DL in medical imaging are mainly related to data quality and quantity for building reliable and generalizable DL models, as well as the design of new models for maximum transparency and dependability.

The success or failure of a DL system mainly depends on the number and quality of available medical image data. The images are used by DL networks during training to extract informative features for identifying the presence of a target structure or disease. However, many fields of medicine still lack of proper big data sets necessary for training and validating DL models. The ability to use data of high quality, adequate quantity and proper annotations is the way to achieve *good* DL systems in the future. The creation of rich data sets for multi-center and multi-scanner/device DL evaluation is crucial for DL research in medical imaging. Initiatives in the data collection and publication of these data sets are even more valuable for benchmarking. Data augmentation and data synthesis is also an important challenge in DL and has attracted significant attention over the past years [66].

Another major cause of concern and obstacle towards the trustful application of DL is the lack of understanding of the way DL models predict a final outcome. The black box nature of these methods makes them difficult to understand for clinicians who may become skeptical and reluctant to adopt them, despite the good performance usually achieved. Therefore, explainability and interpretability strategies [67] along with uncertainty quantification [68] are gaining popularity in the attempt to shed light on black box methods and improve transparency, trust, and believability. A DL model for medical diagnosis should not only care about the accuracy, but also about how explainable the model is and how certain the prediction is. If the uncertainty is too high, practitioners should be notified in order to take this information into account in the final decision-making process.

9.5 Conclusions and Future Perspective

This chapter presents a review of the literature on CA segmentation, IMT estimation, CA plaque classification, and risk assessment in CA Ultrasound images. The review provides two main novelties with respect to previous reviews. First, we summarized the main literature in tables with the main characteristics of the works to provide a comprehensive and synthetic comparison, and emphasize the deficiencies and shortcomings of the different proposals. Second, we focused on the advancements in novel DL techniques. For CA image segmentation, we found several proposals based on DL; however, we highlighted the limited number or non-existence of contributions based on DL (traditional and end-to-end learning pipeline designs) in some of the four reviewed objectives on CA plaque classification and risk assessment. We also discussed the challenges that must be faced up in order to make the field of medical imaging in general, and therefore the analysis of CA images in particular, moves towards DL. Moreover, we revised a recent DL proposal for IMT estimation and plaque detection in order to give an illustration of the power of these novel techniques.

There is still much to explore in DL techniques to characterize the CA's plaque and walls. In fact, there is no DL works for US CA image characterization in longitudinal studies. We have seen that, in general, the image information of plaque or artery walls, such as gray value, texture, and even morphology, improves the atherosclerosis evaluation. Thus, it would be interesting to explore DL methods such as CNN, which are end-to-end and can automatically extract relevant information from the entire image for specific purposes as assessing CV risk and the prediction of events. Moreover, NNs allow integrating other risk factors, such as clinical data, which are very relevant for predicting cardiovascular events in longitudinal studies and big data sets. This could also be another potential line of research.

In general, we note that currently, the existing data sets used in publications are limited in number and multi-center or multi-scanner/device perspective. This makes difficult to validate the proposals extensively beyond showing error metrics, to show their generalization power and to build approaches robust to different scenarios. Moreover, it is necessary to extend the segmentation of plaque to other territories of the CA if there is a real will to fully automate the whole posterior process of plaque characterization/classification and risk assessment.

Acknowledgements This work was partially supported by the Spanish Ministry of Economy and Competitiveness through the Instituto de Salud Carlos III-FEDER (CIBERCV CB16/11/00246), the Spanish Ministry of Science, Innovation and Universities (grant RTI2018-095232-B-C21) and the Catalan Government (grant SGR1742).

9.6 Appendix

List of acronyms/abbreviations used in the chapter:

AUC Area under the curve
asymp Asymptomatic
CA Carotid artery
CC Cardiac cycle
cc correlation coefficient
CCA Common carotid artery
CIM Carotid intima-media
CVD Cardiovascular disease
CVRF Cardiovascular risk factor
cdf cumulative density function
CUSIP Carotid ultrasound image-based phenotypes
DA Discriminant analysis
div. Divergence
DL Deep learning
DT Decision trees
F Frame
FT Fourier transform
FS Feature selection
FU Follow-up
GL Gray level
GLCM Gray level co-occurrence matrix
GMM Gaussian mixture model
GSM Grayscale median
GT Ground truth
HOS Higher order spectra
ICA Internal carotid artery
IMT Intima media thickness
IMTv IMT variability
kNN k-Nearest neighbor
Kullback Kullback-Leiber
LBP Local binary pattern
LI Lumen-intima
long. Longitudinal (image projections)
MA Media-adventitia
ML Machine learning
N Number
NN Neural network
NBC Naive Bayes classifier
NS Not specified
PCA Pixel component analysis
PDA Pixel distribution analysis
pdf probability density function
PNN Probabilistic neural networks
RFR Framingham risk score
RLM Run length matrix

ROI Region of interest
SVM Support vector machine
symp symptomatic
T Transversal (studies)
transv. Transversal (image projections)
TPA Total plaque area
UF Unique frame
US Ultrasound
V Video
WT Wavelet transform

References

1. Blausen.com staff (2014) Medical gallery of Blausen Medical 2014. WikiJournal Med. **1**(2). https://doi.org/10.15347/wjm/2014.010. ISSN 2002-4436. [CC BY 3.0 (https://creativecommons.org/licenses/by/3.0)], from Wikimedia Commons. Carotid arteries (2014)
2. Touboul, P.-J., Hennerici, M.G., Meairs, S., Adams, H., Amarenco, P., et al.: Mannheim carotid intima-media thickness and plaque consensus (2004–2006-2011). Cardiovascular Dis. **34**(4), 290–296 (2012)
3. Falk, E.: Pathogenesis of atherosclerosis. J. Am. Coll. Cardiol. **47**, C7–C12 (2006, Supplement, 8)
4. Saba, l., Jain, P.K., Suri, H.S., Ikeda, N., Araki, T., Singh, B.K., Nicolaides, A., Shafique, S., Gupta, A., Laird, J.R., et al.: Plaque tissue morphology-based stroke risk stratification using carotid ultrasound: a polling-based pca learning paradigm. J. Med. Syst. **41**(6), 98 (2017)
5. LeCun, Y., Bengio, Y., Hinton, G.: Deep learning. Nature **521**(7553), 436–444 (2015)
6. Ravì, D., Wong, C., Deligianni, F., Berthelot, M., Andreu-Perez, J., Lo, B., Yang, G.-Z.: Deep learning for health informatics. IEEE J. Biomed. Health Inf. **21**(1), 4–21 (2016)
7. Esteva, A., Kuprel, B., Novoa, R.A., Ko, J., Swetter, S.M., Blau, H.M., Thrun, S.: Dermatologist-level classification of skin cancer with deep neural networks. Nature **542**(7639), 115–118 (2017)
8. Hannun, A.Y., Rajpurkar, P., Haghpanahi, M., Tison, G.H., Bourn, C., Turakhia, M.P., Andrew, Y.N.: Cardiologist-level arrhythmia detection and classification in ambulatory electrocardiograms using a deep neural network. Nat. Med. **25**(1), 65–69 (2019)
9. Xu, X., Zhou, Y., Cheng, Xi., Song, E., Li, G.: Ultrasound intima-media segmentation using hough transform and dual snake model. Comput. Med. Imaging Graphics **36**(3), 248–258 (2012)
10. Molinari, F., Pattichis, C.S., Zeng, G., Saba, L., Acharya, U.R., Sanfilippo, R., Nicolaides, A., Suri, J.S.: Completely automated multiresolution edge snapper—a new technique for an accurate carotid ultrasound IMT measurement: clinical validation and benchmarking on a multi-institutional database. IEEE Trans. Image Process. **21**(3), 1211–1222 (2011)
11. Faita, F., Gemignani, V., Bianchini, E., Giannarelli, C., Ghiadoni, L., Demi, M.: Real-time measurement system for evaluation of the Carotid Intima-media thickness with a robust edge operator. J. Ultrasound Med. **27**(9), 1353–1361 (2008)
12. Bastida-Jumilla, M.C., Menchón-Lara, R.M., Morales-Sánchez, J., Verdú-Monedero, R., Larrey-Ruiz, J., Sancho-Gómez, J.L.: Frequency-domain active contours solution to evalu-

ate intima-media thickness of the common carotid artery. Biomed. Signal Process. Control, **16**(Complete), 68–79 (2015)
13. Rajasekaran, C., Jayanthi, K.B., Sudha, S., Kuchelar, S.: Automated diagnosis of cardiovascular disease through measurement of Intima media thickness using deep neural networks. In: Annual International Conference of the IEEE Engineering in Medicine and Biology Society, 6636–6639 (2019)
14. Loizou, C.P., Kasparis, T., Spyrou, C., and Marios Pantziaris. Integrated system for the complete segmentation of the common Carotid Artery cifurcation in ultrasound images. In: Papadopoulos, H., Andreou, A.S., Iliadis, L., Maglogiannis, I. (eds) Artificial Intelligence Applications and Innovations, pp. 292–301 (2013)
15. Zhao, S., Gao, Z., Zhang, H., Xie, Y., Luo, J., Ghista, D., Wei, Z., Bi, Xiaojun, Xiong, Huahua, Chenchu, Xu, et al.: Robust segmentation of intima-media borders with different morphologies and dynamics during the cardiac cycle. IEEE J. Biomed. Health Inf. **22**(5), 1571–1582 (2017)
16. Molinari, F., Meiburger, K.M., Saba, L., Acharya, U.R., Famiglietti, L., Georgiou, N., Nicolaides, A., Mamidi, R.S., Kuper, H., Suri, J.S.: Automated carotid IMT measurement and its validation in low contrast ultrasound database of 885 patient Indian population epidemiological study: results of AtheroEdge® software pp. 209–219 (2014)
17. Qian, C., Yang, X.: An integrated method for atherosclerotic carotid plaque segmentation in ultrasound image. Comput. Methods Programs Biomed. **153**, 19–32 (2018)
18. Zhang, C., Vila, M.M., Radeva, P, Elosua, R., Grau, M., Betriu, A., Fernandez-Giraldez, E., Igual, L.: Carotid artery segmentation in ultrasound images. In: MICCAI Workshop on Computing and Visualization for Intravascular Imaging and Computer Assisted Stenting (2015)
19. Molinari, F., Zeng, G., Suri, J.S.: A state of the art review on intima-media thickness (IMT) measurement and wall segmentation techniques for carotid ultrasound. Comput. Methods Programs Biomed. **100**(3), 201–221 (2010)
20. Loizou, Christos P.: A review of ultrasound common carotid artery image and video segmentation techniques. Med. Biol. Eng. Comput. **52**(12), 1073–1093 (2014)
21. Saba, L., Jamthikar, A., Khanna, N.N., Gupta, D., Viskovic, K., Suri, H.S,. Gupta, A., Mavrogeni, S., Turk, M., Laird, J.R., Pareek, G., Miner, M., Sfikakis, P.P., Protogerou, A., Kitas, G.D., Viswanathan, V., Nicolaides, A., Bhatt, D.L., Suri, J.S.: Global perspective on carotid intima-media thickness and plaque: should the current measurement guidelines be revisited? Int. Angiol. **38**(6):451–465 (2019)
22. Menchón-Lara, R.M., Sancho-Gómez, J-L.: Fully automatic segmentation of ultrasound common carotid artery images based on machine learning. Neurocomputing **151**, 161 – 167 (2015)
23. Shin, J.Y., Tajbakhsh, N., Hurst, R.T., Kendall, C.B., Liang, J.: Automating carotid intima-media thickness video interpretation with convolutional neural networks. In: IEEE Conference on Computer Vision and Pattern Recognition, pp. 2526–2535 (2016)
24. Biswas, M., Saba, L., Chakrabartty, S., Khanna, N.N., Song, H., Suri, H.S., Sfikakis, P.P., Mavrogeni, S., Viskovic, K., Laird, J.R., Cuadrado-Godia, E., Nicolaides, A., Sharma, A., Viswanathan, V., Protogerou, A., Kitas, G., Pareek, G., Miner, Martin, Suri, Jasjit S.: Two-stage artificial intelligence model for jointly measurement of atherosclerotic wall thickness and plaque burden in carotid ultrasound: A screening tool for cardiovascular/stroke risk assessment. Comput. Biol. Med. **123** (2020)
25. Biswas, M., Kuppili, V., Araki, T., Edla, D.R., Godia, E.C., Saba, L., Suri, H.S., Omerzu, T., Laird, J.R., Khanna, N.N., et al.: Deep learning strategy for accurate carotid intima-media thickness measurement: an ultrasound study on Japanese diabetic cohort. Comput. Biol. Med. **98**, 100–117 (2018)
26. Menchón-Lara, R., Bastida-Jumilla, M., Larrey-Ruiz, J., Verdu-Monedero, R., Morales-Sànchez, J., Sancho-Gómez, J.: Measurement of Carotid Intima-Media Thickness in ultrasound images by means of an automatic segmentation process based on machine learning. In: Eurocon, pp. 2086–2093 (2013)
27. Menchón-Lara, R., Sancho-Gómez, J.: Ultrasound image processing based on machine learning for the fully automatic evaluation of the Carotid Intima-Media Thickness. In: 12th International Workshop on Content-Based Multimedia Indexing, pp. 1–4 (2014)

28. Rosa-María Menchón-Lara, María-Consuelo Bastida-Jumilla, Juan Morales-Sánchez, and José-Luis Sancho-Gómez. Automatic detection of the intima-media thickness in ultrasound images of the common carotid artery using neural networks. Med. Biol. Eng. Comput. **52**:, 169–181 (2014)
29. del Mar Vila, M., Remeseiro, B., Grau, M., Elosua, R., Betriu, A., Fernandez-Giraldez, E., Igual, L.: Semantic segmentation with DenseNets for carotid artery ultrasound plaque segmentation and CIMT estimation. Artif. Intell. Med. **103**, 101784 (2020)
30. Huang, G., Liu, Z., Weinberger, K.Q., van der Maaten, L.: Densely connected convolutional networks. In: IEEE Conference on Computer Vision and Pattern Recognition, pp. 4700–4708 (2017)
31. Shelhamer, E., Long, ., Darrell, T.: Fully convolutional networks for semantic segmentation. IEEE Trans. Pattern Anal. Mach. Intell. **39**(4), 640–651 (2017)
32. Jégou, S., Drozdzal, M., Vazquez, D., Romero, A., Bengio, Y.: The one hundred layers Tiramisu: fully convolutional DenseNets for semantic segmentation. In: IEEE Conference on Computer Vision and Pattern Recognition Workshops, pp. 1175–1183 (2017)
33. He, K., Zhang, X., Ren, S, Sun, J.: Deep residual learning for image recognition. In: IEEE Conference on Computer Vision and Pattern Recognition, pp. 770–778 (2016)
34. Grau, Maria, Subirana, Isaac, Agis, David, Ramos, Rafel, et al.: Grosor íntima-media carotídeo en población española: valores de referencia y asociación con los factores de riesgo cardiovascular. Revista Española de Cardiología **65**(12), 1086–1093 (2012)
35. de Groot, E., Hovingh, G.K., Wiegman, A., Duriez, P., Smit, A.J., Fruchart, J.-C., Kastelein, J.J.P.: Measurement of arterial wall thickness as a surrogate marker for atherosclerosis. Circulation 109(23 suppl 1), III–33 (2004)
36. Ronneberger, O., Fischer, P., Brox, T.: U-net: Convolutional networks for biomedical image segmentation. In: International Conference on Medical Image Computing and Computer-Assisted Intervention, pp. 234–241 (2015)
37. He, K., Zhang, X., Ren, S., Sun, J.: Delving deep into rectifiers: surpassing human-level performance on imagenet classification. In: IEEE International Conference on Computer Vision, pp. 1026–1034 (2015)
38. Tieleman, T., Hinton, G.: RMSProp adaptive learning. Neural Networks for Machine Learning, COURSERA (2012)
39. Lahoz, C., Mostaza, J.M.: Atherosclerosis as a systemic disease. Revista Española de Cardiología (English edition) **60**, 184 – 195 (2007)
40. Sharma, A.D., Gupta, A., Kumar, P.K., Rajan, J., Saba, L., Nobutaka, I., Laird, J.R., Nicolades, A., Suri, J.S.: A review on carotid ultrasound atherosclerotic tissue characterization and stroke risk stratification in machine learning framework. Curr. atherosclerosis Rep. **17**(9), 1–13 (2015)
41. Acharya, U.R., Faust, O., Sree, S.V., Alvin, A.P.C., Krishnamurthi, G., Seabra, JC.R., Sanches, J., Suri, J.S., Understanding symptomatology of atherosclerotic plaque by image-based tissue characterization. Comput. Methods Programs Biomed. **110**(1), 66 – 75 (2013)
42. Acharya, U.R., Sree, S.V., Molinari, F., Saba, L., Nicolaides, A., Suri, J.S.: An automated technique for carotid far wall classification using grayscale features and wall thickness variability. J. Clin. Ultrasound **43**(5), 302–311 (2015)
43. Acharya, U.R., Faust, O., Sree, S.V., Molinari, F., Saba, L., Nicolaides, A., Suri, J.S.: An Accurate and Generalized Approach to Plaque Characterization in 346 Carotid Ultrasound Scans. IEEE Transactions on Instrumentation and Measurement **61**(4), 1045–1053 (2012)
44. U.Rajendra Acharya, MuthuRamaKrishnan Mookiah, S. Vinitha Sree, David Afonso, Joao Sanches, Shoaib Shafique, Andrew Nicolaides, L.M. Pedro, J. Fernandes e Fernandes, and JasjitS. Suri. Atherosclerotic plaque tissue characterization in 2D ultrasound longitudinal carotid scans for automated classification: a paradigm for stroke risk assessment. *Medical Biological Engineering Computing*, 51(5):513–523, 2013
45. Gronholdt, Marie-Louise M., Nordestgaard, Børge G., Schroeder, Torben V., Vorstrup, Sissel, Sillesen, Henrik: Ultrasonic Echolucent Carotid Plaques Predict Future Strokes. Circulation **104**(1), 68–73 (2001)

46. Kyriacou, E.C., Petroudi, S., Pattichis, C.S., Pattichis, M.S., Griffin, M., Kakkos, S., Nicolaides, A.: Prediction of high-risk asymptomatic carotid plaques based on ultrasonic image features. IEEE Trans. Inf. Technol. Biomed. **16**(5), 966–73 (2012)
47. Lal, B.K., Hobson II, R.W., Pappas, P.J., Kubicka, R., Hameed, M., Chakhtura, E.Y., Jamil, Z., Padberg F.T., Jr., Haser, P.B., Durán, W.N.: Pixel distribution analysis of b-mode ultrasound scan images predicts histologic features of atherosclerotic carotid plaques. J. Vascular Surg. **35**(6), 1210 – 1217 (2002)
48. K. Lekadir, A. Galimzianova, À. Betriu, M. del Mar Vila, L. Igual, D. L. Rubin, E. Fernández, P. Radeva, and S. Napel. A Convolutional Neural Network for Automatic Characterization of Plaque Composition in Carotid Ultrasound. IEEE J. Biomed. Health Inf/ **21**(1), 48–55 (2017)
49. Khanna, N.N., Jamthikar, A.D., Gupta, D., Nicolaides, A., Araki, T., Saba, L., Cuadrado-Godia, E., Sharma, A., Omerzu, T., Suri, H.S., et al. Performance evaluation of 10-year ultrasound image-based stroke/cardiovascular (CV) risk calculator by comparing against ten conventional CV risk calculators: a diabetic study. Comput. Biol. Med. **105** 125–143 (2019)
50. Acharya, U.R., Krishnan, M.M.R., Sree, S.V., Sanches, J., Shafique, S., Nicolaides, A., Pedro, L.M., Suri, J.S.: Plaque tissue characterization and classification in ultrasound carotid scans: a paradigm for vascular feature amalgamation. IEEE Trans. Instrum. Measur. **62**(2), 392–400 (2013)
51. Stoitsis, J., Tsiaparas, N., Golemati, S., Nikita, K.S.: Characterization of carotid atherosclerotic plaques using frequency-based texture analysis and bootstrap. In: 8th Annual International Conference of the IEEE Engineering in Medicine and Biology Society, pp. 2392–2395 (2006)
52. Araki, T., Jain, P.K., Suri, H.S., Londhe, N.D., Ikeda, N., El-Baz, A., Shrivastava, V.K., Saba, L., Nicolaides, A., Shafique, S., et al.: Stroke risk stratification and its validation using ultrasonic echolucent carotid wall plaque morphology: a machine learning paradigm. Comput. in Biol. Med. **80**, 77–96 (2017)
53. Irie, Y., Katakami, N., Kaneto, H., Takahara, M., Nishio, M., Kasami, R., Sakamoto, K., Umayahara, Y., Sumitsuji, S., Ueda, Y., Kosugi, K., Shimomura, I.: The utility of ultrasonic tissue characterization of carotid plaque in the prediction of cardiovascular events in diabetic patients. Atherosclerosis **230**(2), 399–405 (2013)
54. Tsiaparas, N.N., Golemati, S., Andreadis, I.I., Stoitsis, J.S., Valavanis, I.K., Nikita, K.S.: Comparison of multiresolution features for texture classification of carotid atherosclerosis from b-mode ultrasound. IEEE Trans. Inf. Technol. Biomed. **15**, 130–137 (2011)
55. Gastounioti, A., Makrodimitris, S., Golemati, S., Kadoglou, N.P.E., Liapis, C.D., Nikita, K.S.: A novel computerized tool to stratify risk in carotid atherosclerosis using kinematic features of the arterial wall. IEEE J. Biomed. Health Inf. **19**(3), 1137–1145 (2014)
56. Toutouzas, G., Benetos, G., Karanasos, A., Chatzizisis, Y.S.,. Giannopoulos, A.A., Tousoulis, D.: Vulnerable plaque imaging: updates on new pathobiological mechanisms. Eur. Heart J. **36**(45), 3147–3154 (2015)
57. Kern, R., Szabo, K., Hennerici, M., Meairs, S.: Characterization of carotid artery plaques using real-time compound B-mode ultrasound. Stroke **35**(4), 870–875 (2004)
58. Schulte-Altedorneburg, G., Droste, D.W., Haas, N., Kemény, V., Nabavi, D.G., Füzesi, L., Ringelstein, E.B.: Preoperative B-mode ultrasound plaque appearance compared with carotid endarterectomy specimen histology. Acta Neurol. Scand. **101**(3), 188–194 (2000)
59. Carstensen, J.M.: Description and simulation of visual texture. Ph.D. thesis, Technical University of DenmarkDanmarks Tekniske Universitet, Department of Informatics and Mathematical Modeling, Institut for Informatik og Matematisk Modellering (1992)
60. Galloway, Mary M.: Texture analysis using gray level run lengths. Comput. Graph. Image Process. **4**(2), 172–179 (1975)
61. Kadyrov, A., Petrou, M.: The trace transform and its applications. IEEE Trans. Pattern Anal. Mach. Intell. **23**(8), 811–828 (2001)
62. Nikias, C.L., Mendel, J.M.: Signal processing with higher-order spectra. IEEE Signal Process. Mag. **10**(3), 10–37 (1993)
63. Yasaka, K., Abe, Y.: Deep learning and artificial intelligence in radiology: current applications and future directions. PLOS Med. **15**(11), 1–4 (2018, November)

64. Pesapane, Filippo, Codari, Marina, Sardanelli, Francesco: Artificial intelligence in medical imaging: threat or opportunity? Radiologists again at the forefront of innovation in medicine. Eur. Radiol. Exp. **2**(1), 35 (2018)
65. Lei, T., Wang, R., Wan, Y., Du, X., Meng, H., Nandi, A.K.: Medical image segmentation using deep learning: a survey. arXiv preprint arXiv:2009.13120 (2020)
66. Shorten, C., Khoshgoftaar, T.M..: A survey on image data augmentation for deep learning. J. Big Data **6**(1),60 (2019)
67. Arrieta, A.B., Díaz-Rodríguez, N., Del Ser, J., Bennetot, A., Tabik, S., Barbado, A., García, S., Gil-López, S., Molina, D., Benjamins, R., et al.: Explainable Artificial Intelligence (XAI): oncepts, taxonomies, opportunities and challenges toward responsible AI. Inf. Fusion **58**, 82–115 (2020)
68. Abdar, M., Pourpanah, F., Hussain, S., Rezazadegan, D., Liu, L., Ghavamzadeh, L., Fieguth, P., Khosravi, A., Acharya, U.R., Makarenkov, V., et al.: A review of uncertainty quantification in deep learning: techniques, applications and challenges. arXiv preprint arXiv:2011.06225 (2020)

Chapter 10
Radiomics and Its Application in Predicting Microvascular Invasion of Hepatocellular Carcinoma

Weibin Wang, Qingqing Chen, Risheng Deng, Fang Wang, Yutaro Iwamoto, Lanfen Lin, Hongjie Hu, Ruofeng Tong, and Yen-Wei Chen

Abstract Hepatocellular carcinoma (HCC) is a global health concern, with increasing morbidity and mortality rates in the world. Microvascular invasion (MVI) is a major cause of early postoperative recurrence of HCC. Predicting MVI before surgery can help doctors develop treatment plans. However, the diagnosis of MVI depends on postoperative pathological verification, which is difficult to predict before surgery. In recent years, more researchers have used radiomics to solve clinical problems. In this study, we used radiomics to predict MVI. We propose a fusion model that combines clinical and radiomics magnetic resonance imaging data to predict MVI of HCC. At present, our fusion prediction model achieves 72.60% accuracy and 0.7607 area under the curve (AUC). In this chapter, we first introduce fundamentals of radiomics and then we present our MVI prediction method using radiomics.

Keywords Microvascular invasion · Radiomics · Fusion prediction model

---

W. Wang · Y. Iwamoto · Y.-W. Chen (✉)
Graduate School of Information Science and Engineering, Ritsumeikan University, Kusatsu 525-8577, Shiga, Japan
e-mail: chen@is.ritsumei.ac.jp

Q. Chen · F. Wang · H. Hu
Department of Radiology, Sir Run Run Shaw Hospital, Zhejiang University, Hangzhou 310000, Zhejiang, China

R. Deng · L. Lin · R. Tong · Y.-W. Chen
College of Computer Science and Technology, Zhejiang University, Hangzhou 310000, Zhejiang, China

R. Tong · Y.-W. Chen
Research Center for Healthcare Data Science, Zhejiang Lab, Hangzhou, Zhejiang, China

© The Author(s), under exclusive license to Springer Nature Switzerland AG 2022
C.-P. Lim et al. (eds.), *Handbook of Artificial Intelligence in Healthcare*, Intelligent Systems Reference Library 211, https://doi.org/10.1007/978-3-030-79161-2_10

10.1 Introduction

10.1.1 What is Radiomics

Medical imaging refers to the technology and process of obtaining internal tissue images of the human body in a non-invasive manner. Common medical imaging techniques include X-ray, computerized tomography (CT), positron emission tomography (PET), magnetic resonance imaging (MRI), medical ultrasonography, mammography and angiography. Traditional evaluation of medical images mainly relies on semantic features such as typical density/intensity patterns [1]. However, further assessments are largely limited by both the unavailability of examination machines and poor resolution of observers' eyes [2]. Different doctors may have different assessments of the same image.

Radiomics is an emerging technique for medical imaging analysis, which was first described in 2012 by Lambin et al. [3] to convert CT/MRI/PET imaging data into a high-dimensional and hundreds of quantitative radiomics signatures comprising 2D/3D shape-based features, first-order statistics and other mid-level texture patterns [4]. This quantitative analysis method eliminates the assessment differences between doctors. Moreover, it can be calculated in batches according to feature extraction algorithms, saving doctors' evaluation time.

A simple radiomics pipeline with medical images is shown in Fig. 10.1.

The processing flow of radiomics is summarized into the following parts: image data acquisition; tumour area calibration; tumour area segmentation; feature extraction and quantification; feature selection; classification and prediction. In Fig. 10.1, we simplified the first three parts into one. After acquiring the region of interest, we extract features from images. Radiomics uses features such as shapes, textures

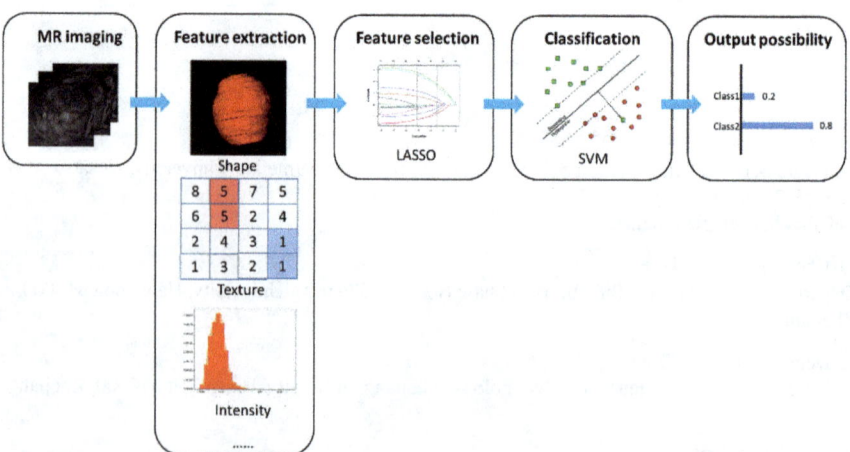

Fig. 10.1 Simple radiomics pipeline

and intensity to represent images. Generally, hundreds of extracted features have several redundant features. Therefore, filtering out these features using different feature selection methods is necessary. In computer vision, after the feature selection process, a classifier (e.g. support vector machine [5] and random forest [6]) is usually used to make predictions.

Overall, radiomics extracts information from images (CT, MRI, PET, etc.) in a high-throughput manner and uses deeper mining, prediction and analysis of a large amount of image data to help doctors make the most accurate diagnosis. Radiomics can be intuitively understood as transforming visual image information into deep-level features for quantitative research.

10.1.2 What Has Been Achieved in Medical Image Analysis Using Radiomics

With the advancement of technology and improvement of research, radiomics has made several new advances in CT, MRI, PET and gene fusion. The number of first-order and second-order statistics, textures and wavelet features has reached thousands. The number of theoretical methods for extracting features is also increasing. The number of publications on radiomics has been increasing since 2012 [7], as shown in Fig. 10.2. More studies have demonstrated the effectiveness and clinical applicability of radiomics. In 2016, Radiology published an authoritative review of radiomics. This review re-emphasises the core idea of radiomics 'converting digital images into mineable data' and points out that this conversion from image to data will become normal for future clinical image analysis. Some studies have shown that radiomics features can be used as prognostic imaging markers for tumour therapy assessment [8–10].

A method for predicting distant metastasis based on CT image radiomics shows that among 635 image features, 35 image features can be used as predictors of distant metastasis. The consistency index is above 0.6, and the false discovery rate is below 0.05 [13]. The above-mentioned research embodies the characteristics of radiomics as a prognostic indicator of clinical prediction. Extracting a large number

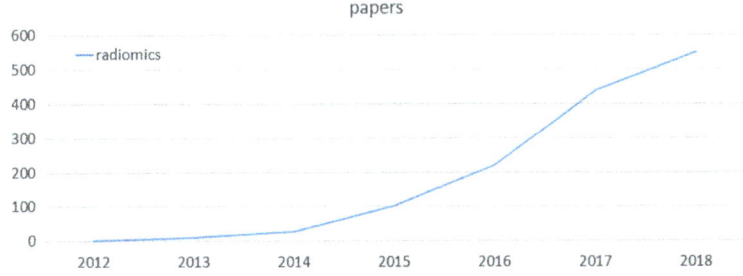

Fig. 10.2 Publication statistics of radiomics

of features from MRI for research has become one of the research hotspots at this stage. For example, in the study of brain glioma, radiomics was used in the diagnosis of malignant glioma, the formulation of pre-surgical programmes and the monitoring after treatment [14].

With the gradual increase in the incidence of breast cancer, there is also a need for an effective method to achieve accurate diagnosis and analysis of breast cancer. To solve this problem, radiomics has also been widely used in MRI diagnosis of breast cancer [15].

Zhou et al. extracted 300 features (hand-crafted low-level features) from CT images, selected 21 features and predicted the recurrence of hepatocellular carcinoma (HCC) using the least absolute shrinkage and selection operator (LASSO) logic regression method [16]. Ning et al. also proposed a method for predicting the early recurrence of HCC using CT-based radiomics signature [17]. Both of their studies demonstrated that radiomics signature is effective and is a potential biomarker for preoperative prediction of early recurrence of HCC. At the same time, radiomics features are used to construct a prediction model. Texture, as a biomarker of internal tumour heterogeneity, can help physicians conduct a more in-depth analysis of pathology. They also found that combining extracted CT image features and clinical data can effectively improve the accuracy of a prediction model.

Traditional imaging diagnoses mainly rely on the judgement of physicians, whereas radiomics analyse data based on data and extracts high-dimensional image features as new biomarkers to help clinical decision making. Using radiomics features to predict mutant epidermal growth factor receptor, it has been reported in the literature that the combination of five radiomics feature sets and clinical features such as pathological grading and smoking can be used to predict mutations using only clinical features. The area under the curve increased from 0.667 to 0.709 [18].

Generally, the extraction of large-scale radiomics features depends on computer vision and image processing technology, and low-level image feature descriptions are used to define the shape, clarity, compactness and visual appearance of tumours. Therefore, a large number of radiomics features can realise medical data integration. On the other hand, radiomics transforms cross-sectional image arrays into quantifiable features, laying the foundation for constructing an imaging genomics framework. This framework integrates knowledge from different fields and draws inferences about the causal relationship between them. The application of radiomics is not limited to the above-mentioned areas.

10.1.3 Application of Radiomics in Hepatocellular Carcinoma

HCC is a global health problem, with increasing morbidity and mortality rates in the world [19]. American Association for the Study of Liver Diseases, European Association for the Study of the Liver and The Asian Pacific Association for the

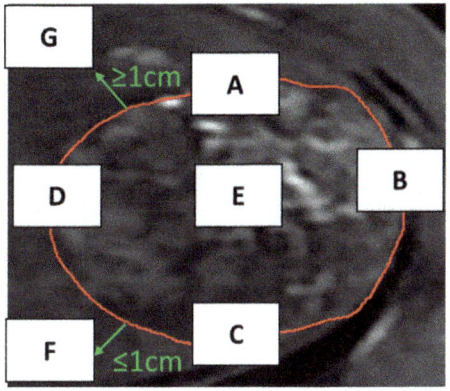

Fig. 10.3 There are seven points A–F that need to be tested through postoperative microscopic examination. ABCD: Tumour and liver tissue boundary. E: Inside the tumour. F: Near tumour area ($\leq$1CM). G: Distant tumour area ($\geq$1CM). If no MVI is found at all points, the patient is considered to have no MVI, otherwise, the patient has MVI

Study of the Liver have all updated their official guidelines on the management of HCC based on 'Expert Consensus' [20, 21]. With the development of radiomics in recent years, a growing number of radiomics methods have been embedded in clinical practice for HCC diagnosis, staging, treatment response assessment and prognosis prediction.

Microvascular invasion (MVI) of HCC is the main factor affecting the recurrence and survival of patients after surgery [22]. MVI results can only be obtained through pathology after resection, which is difficult to predict before surgery. Postoperative microscopic examination can detect MVI. The specific test standards are shown in Fig. 10.3. Preoperative determination of the presence or absence of MVI can guide the scope of surgical resection and post-operative follow-up.

Studies based on clinical indicators (baseline data), CT/MRI imaging findings (semantic features) or radiomics features have been proposed to predict MVI of HCC. Z. Lei et al. used preoperative clinical indicators to analyse whether HCC patients had MVI [23]. Chen et al. used semantic features from MRI images to determine whether HCC patients have MVI before surgery [24]; Zhang extracted radiomics features from MRI images to predict whether there is MVI in HCC patients [25]. Lei only used clinical data and ignored medical imaging information. The Li-Rads method used by J. Chen relies too much on doctors' experience and requires manual analysis of patient images, which takes a lot of time for doctors. R. Zhang used radiomics to quantitatively extract features, but they did not use all information of multiphase MRI.

The purpose of our study is to propose an effective model for predicting MVI of HCC patients. The contributions of our study are as follows:

(1) We use radiomics to extract features of multiphase MRI and compared the performance of different phases.
(2) We compare the prediction performance of a radiomics model and clinical model.
(3) We combine clinical data and radiomics features to establish a fusion model.

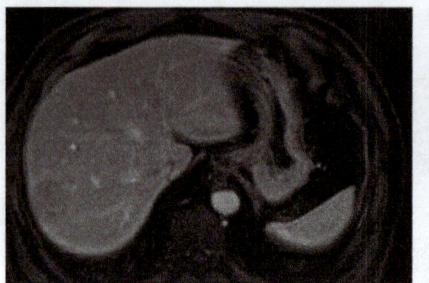 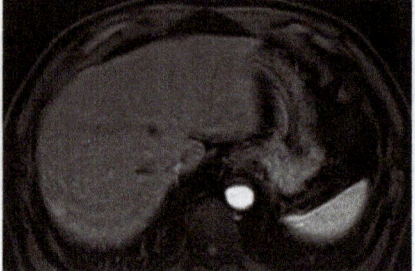

Fig. 10.4 Normal liver image (left) and liver image with artefact (right)

10.2 Radiomics Signature and Prediction Model

In this section, we introduce the process of radiomics in detail and the challenges in the process. We introduce the radiomics process according to the following five parts: acquisition of image data; calibration and segmentation of tumour regions; feature extraction and quantification; feature selection; classification and prediction.

10.2.1 Medical Image Acquisition

There are strict standards for radiomics selection of patient images for experiments. Patients' shaking or breathing during the scan can cause blurred images and artefacts, as shown in Fig. 10.4. Blurred images and artefact images cannot be used in radiomics. This is different from deep learning methods, which allow noisy images.

Modern hospital imaging equipment differs greatly in image acquisition and reconstruction protocols (different modal data and different image layer thickness). Doctors do not have a unified standard to regulate this process. Incoming data of radiomics need to have the same or similar acquisition parameters to ensure that the data will not be affected by a model and parameters. Although there are many cancer patients in the world, the data of patients with cancer are relatively small in each hospital. Radiomics research needs to find data that strictly meet the enrolment conditions to ensure data consistency. The data available are still not sufficient. Therefore, radiomics research should find a compromise between the amount of available data and the entry criteria to ensure the basic amount of data.

10.2.2 Calibration and Segmentation of Tumour Regions

Image segmentation is the first step of radiomics, which separates the tumour area from other tissues to facilitate the next step of tumour feature extraction. Owing to the heterogeneity and irregularity of tumours, precise segmentation of specific tumours is a huge challenge. In the field of medical image segmentation, sometimes multiple doctors are required to label and correct the same image. This takes a significant amount of time for doctors. For example, it takes an average of 1 h for a doctor to mark an infected area of an HCC patient. If there are 100 patients, this is already a terrible workload. Figure 10.5 is the manually annotated MRI of an HCC patient.

Although a variety of segmentation algorithms have been applied to tumour area calibration in recent years, manually traced segmentations are often used as the gold standard (ground truth). However, artificial segmentation will inevitably result in differences in segmented images in labelling due to variations among individuals. High-precision automatic specific tumour segmentation algorithm will be a challenge that radiomics needs to tackle in the future.

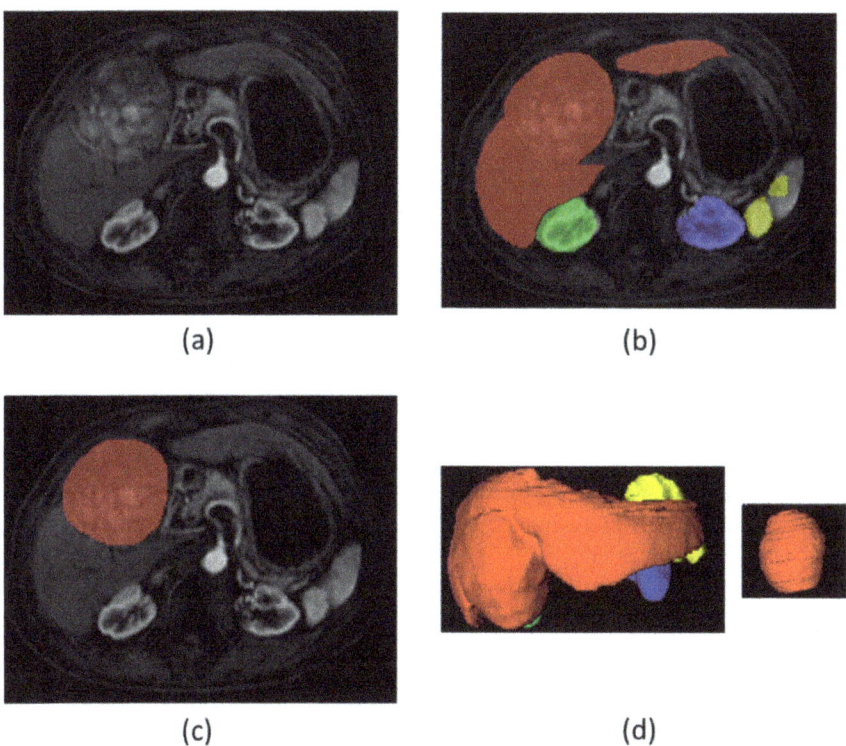

Fig. 10.5 Manually annotated liver MRI. **a** Original MRI. The red label in **b** is the liver area, and the labels of other colours are other tissues and organs. The liver area contains normal liver parenchyma and tumour. The red label in **c** is the tumour area. **d** 3D view

10.2.3 Feature Extraction and Quantification

Radiomics features are artificially defined. Most features defined below comply with feature definitions as described by the Imaging Biomarker Standardization Initiative. Zwanenburg et al. summarised these features [26]. These features include shape feature, first-order statistics, gray level co-occurrence matrix (GLCM), gray level dependence matrix (GLDM), gray level run length matrix (GLRLM), gray level size zone matrix (GLSZM) and neighbouring gray tone difference matrix.

For example, calculating the surface area feature, which is one of the shape features.

$$A_i = \frac{1}{2}|a_ib_i \times a_ic_i| \tag{10.1}$$

$$A = \sum_{i=1}^{N_f} A_i \tag{10.2}$$

where a_ib_i and a_ic_i are edges of the ith triangle in the mesh, formed by vertices a_i, b_i and c_i. To calculate the surface area, first, the surface area A_i of each triangle in the mesh is calculated (10.1). The total surface area is then obtained by taking the sum of all calculated sub-areas (10.2).

There are hundreds of radiomics features, and it takes too much time to write computer programmes for each of them. Van Griethuysen and others encapsulated these features into a library [27]; we only need to use this library to automatically calculate these features. Their codes are open source, and it is convenient to use this library with Python.

However, as we mentioned in Sect. 10.2.2, annotated images will be different because they are annotated by different radiologists. Therefore, we will require a radiologist to annotate more than 20% of the total sample. Another radiologist needs to annotate all samples. To ensure the reliability of the features extracted from the annotated images, we usually conduct an intraclass correlation coefficient (ICC) test first. ICC is used to evaluate the reliability between multiple measurements on the same subject. For example, we extracted two sets of radiomics features and calculated their ICC values based on images annotated by two radiologists, as shown in Table 10.1.

ICC is calculated as follows:

$$ICC = \frac{(MS_{group} - MS_{error})/m}{\frac{MS_{group} - MS_{error}}{m} + MS_{error}} \tag{10.3}$$

$$MS_{group} = \frac{SS_{group}}{n-1} \tag{10.4}$$

Table 10.1 Two sets of radiomics features extracted from the same image annotated by two radiologists

Group	Radiologist A	Radiologist B	n_j	$\overline{X_j}$
Feature 1	0.84	0.85	2	0.845
Feature 2	0.59	0.61	2	0.60
Feature 3	20.65	21.17	2	20.91
Feature 4	34.60	34.44	2	34.52
Feature 5	39.82	39.82	2	39.82
n_i	5	5	10 (N)	
$\overline{X_i}$	19.30	19.38	19.34($\bar{X}$)	

*The bold numbers in the table are original data, and the rest are obtained by calculating these data

$$MS_{error} = \frac{SS_{error}}{N - n - 1} \quad (10.5)$$

$$SS_{group} = \sum_j n_j (\overline{X_j} - \bar{X})^2 \quad (10.6)$$

$$SS_{error} = \sum_i \sum_j (X_{ij} - \overline{X_i} - \overline{X_j} + \bar{X})^2 \quad (10.7)$$

where i and j represent the row and column coordinates of data in Table 10.1, respectively. m represents the number of radiologists. N represents the size of the original data. $\overline{X_i}$, $\overline{X_j}$ and $\bar{X}$ are the average values of the row, column and overall data, respectively. The ICC value is between 0 and 1. If the ICC value is less than 0.8, the consistency of extracted features is poor. In contrast, the consistency of a feature is good if the ICC value greater than 0.8. We typically retain features with an ICC value greater than 0.8 and discard the rest.

10.2.4 Feature Selection

As there are numerous extracted radiomics features, we need to select the relevant features from the high-dimensional data. Feature selection is one of the key steps in radiomics, which will directly influence subsequent training of models. Hence, it is critical to choose an effective feature selection method. This section mainly introduces two commonly used methods.

Least Absolute Shrinkage and Selection Operator (LASSO). LASSO is a linear regression method [28]. It is used in the fields of statistics and machine learning. This regression method can also select relevant features that are important for classification. LASSO minimises the slope of a linear function with the lowest loss because it is based on linear regression (residual; a sum-mation of the distance between a linear graph and the inspected data). The LASSO regression model works based on the following Lagrangian form:

$$\min_{\beta \in \mathbb{R}^p} \left\{ \frac{1}{N} \left(\left(\sum_{i=1}^{N} y_i - \sum_{j=1}^{M} \beta_j X_{ij} \right) \right)^2 - \lambda \sum_{j=1}^{M} |\beta_j| \right\} \quad (10.8)$$

Here, N represents the number of patients, and M represents the number of features. X_{ij} represents the j-th feature at the i-th patient; y_iy represents the outcome (with class labels, 1 for ER and 0 for NER) of the i-th patient; β_j represents the slope of the graph (coefficient) at the j-th feature; λ represents the effectiveness required to balance the first and second terms.

Solving Eq. (10.8), we have to determine λ and calculate and check the highest suitable result. Then, we find β_j (Coefficient) by minimising the equation. Only important clinical features that correlated with y or class label will produce non-zero coefficients, enabling us to rule out all features with zero coefficients.

Random forest. A random forest (RF) is a machine learning method that can accomplish both classification and feature selection tasks [6]. The basic idea of an RF is to use a voting mechanism of multiple decision trees to improve a model. We assume that an RF uses k decision trees, then a certain number of sample subsets must be randomly generated to train each tree. If all samples are used to train k decision trees, the characteristics of local samples will be ignored, which is not good for the generalization ability of the model. As a result, the RF model performs very well in a classification problem; the modelling process of an RF is shown in Fig. 10.6.

In addition, while constructing an RF, the importance of each feature can also be calculated on basis of a certain index (such as the reduction of average impurity). We can select the more important features by sorting the features based on their score. Figure 10.7 shows a visualisation picture of 17 features sorted using an RF method. We implement this method on Python using Scikit-learn (a machine learning library tool) [29].

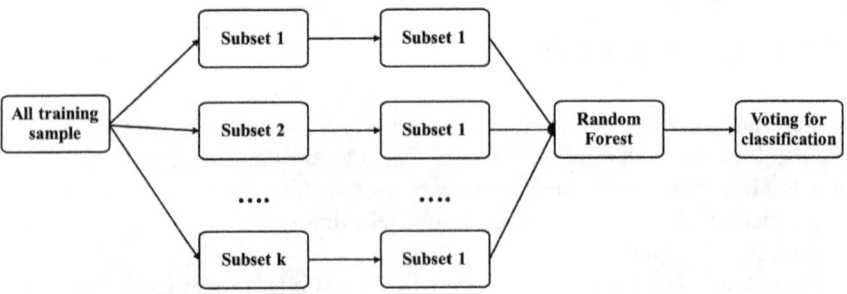

Fig. 10.6 Process of a random forest

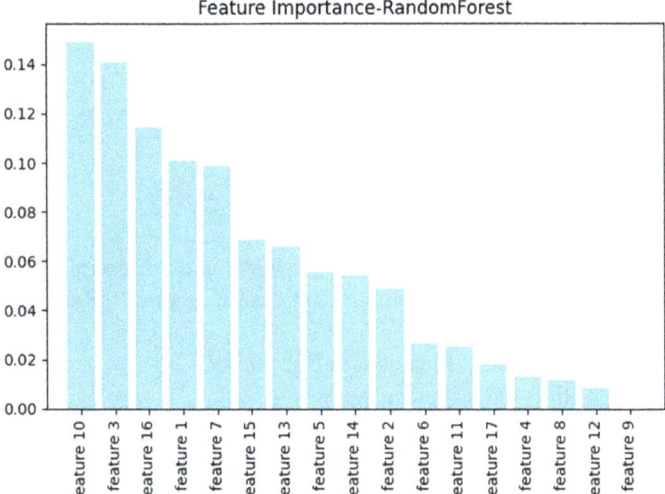

Fig. 10.7 Features sorted by importance score using random forest

Radiomics should select high-quality features based on data characteristics (such as data redundancy and the number of samples). Generally, a small sample dataset should conform to the following selection rules according to the feature number n:

(1) If $n < 10$, then select 75% of features.
(2) If $10 < n < 75$, then select 40% of features.
(3) If $75 < n < 100$, then select 10% of features.
(4) If $100 < n < 1000$, then select 3% of features.
(5) If $n > 1000$, then select less than 25 features.

10.2.5 Classification and Prediction

Researchers have used several machine learning techniques in the medical field. Support vector machines (SVMs) and RFs are important machine learning classification methods. Researchers typically use these two classifiers to build a prediction model using radiomics features.

Support Vector Machine (SVM). SVM is a generalised linear classifier for binary classification of data in supervised learning [5]. For a linearly separable dataset, a linear classifier can be obtained: $h(x) = \text{sign}(w^T x)$. Maximise the distance to classify the minimum distance of the hyperplane under the premise of classifying all training data as much as possible. Suppose the hyperplane equation is $w^T x' + b = 0$ and assuming any two points on the plane is x' and x", then both points satisfy $w^T x' = -b$; $wTx" = -b$; w is the normal vector of the hyperplane, then $w^T(x" - x') = 0$. Distance definition from point to hyperplane:

$$f(x) = \left|\frac{w^T}{w(x-x')}\right| = \frac{1}{w}\left|w^T x + b\right| \qquad (10.9)$$

The SVM can be expressed as $max f(x)$, subject to every $y_n(w^T x_n + b) > 0$,

$$\max f(x) = \min_{n=1,\ldots N} \frac{1}{w} y_n(w^T x + b) \qquad (10.10)$$

Random forest (RF). An RF is a classifier that contains multiple decision trees and uses multiple trees to train and predict samples [6]. Figure 10.8 shows a decision tree.

This tree divides the space, as shown in Fig. 10.9.

The process of RF is the following steps:

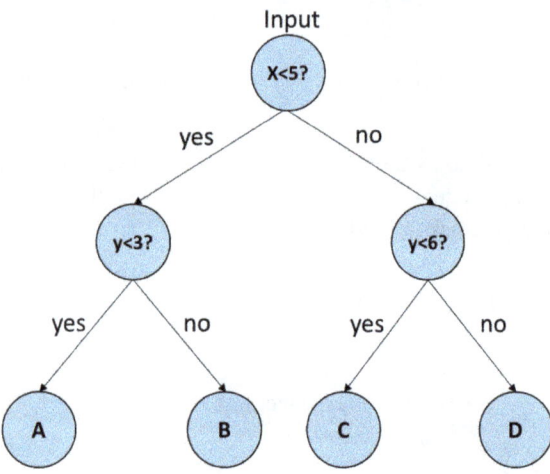

Fig. 10.8 Decision tree

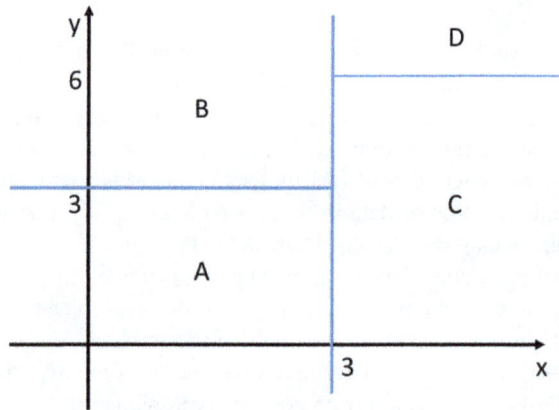

Fig. 10.9 A divided space using a decision tree in Cartesian coordinates

1. Import data and convert features to float form,
2. Divide the dataset into n parts for easy cross-validation,
3. Construct a subset of data (random sampling) and select the optimal features under the specified number of features (assuming m, tuning),
4. Construct a decision tree (depth of the decision tree),
5. Create RFs (a combination of multiple decision trees),
6. Input the test set and output the predictions.

The subtree in an RF randomly selects a subset of features from all available features. Then, it selects the best feature from the randomly selected features. This can help distinguish decision trees in an RF and to improve classification performance.

10.2.6 Material and Clinical Model

The medical images and clinical data used in this study were collected from Sir Run Run Shaw Hospital, China. A total of 247 patients were used in our experiments. We used the Chi-square test to select clinical data. Clinical features with the p-value less than 0.05 were included in the experiments. The selected clinical features of patients are listed in Table 10.2.

Multiphase MRI includes non-contrast enhanced (NC), arterial (ART), portal venous (PV) and delay (DL) phases by injecting a contrast agent. Tumour and liver manifestations will be different in different phases, implying that multiphase MRI provides more information than the only MRI, as shown in Fig. 10.10.

After selecting seven impact factors from 29 clinical features using the Chi-square test method, we used SVM and RF classifiers to build clinical models, as shown in Fig. 10.11.

Table 10.2 Clinical features of patients on admission

Features	Chi-Square	P
Tumour location	6.899	0.009
Long Trail	8.141	0.004
Halo enhancement	25.831	< 0.001
Blood vessels	4.349	0.037
Mosaic	12.597	< 0.001
Nodular protrusion	15.511	< 0.001
Border invasion	6.396	0.011

*P = p-value

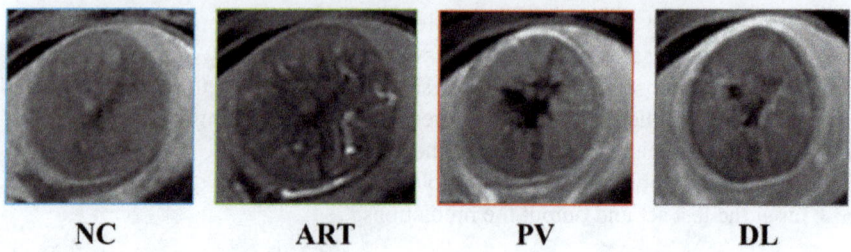

Fig. 10.10 Example images of HCC over four phases

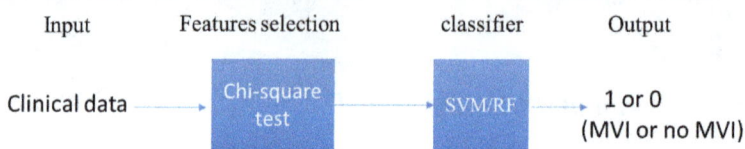

Fig. 10.11 Flow of clinical models

10.2.7 Radiomics Model and Fusion Model for Predicting MVI

From each phase of multiphase MRI, we extract 100 radiomics features, including shape feature (14 features), first-order statistics (18 features), GLCM (22 features), GLDM (14 features), GLRLM (16 features), and GLSZM (16 features). After extracting the features, we use LASSO to select the relevant features. The NC, ART, PV and DL phases have eight, nine, eight and eight features, respectively. Similarly, we also train SVM and RF classifiers on features from the different phases and compare the performance of the models (classifiers).

To make full use of the different feature types, we fuse the selected clinical features and multiphase radiomics MRI features. Thus, 40 features were used to develop the fusion model, as shown in Fig. 10.12.

10.3 Experiment

10.3.1 Experimental Result

In our experiments, 247 MRI images were collected from 2012 to 2019 at Sir Run Run Shaw Hospital, Zhejiang University, China. Each multiphase MRI image contains four phases (NC, ART, PV and DL). The resolution of the CT images is 512 × 512 pixels, and the thickness of each slice is 2.2 mm. The experimental data were marked and categorised by experienced radiologists. In our experiments, we randomly split

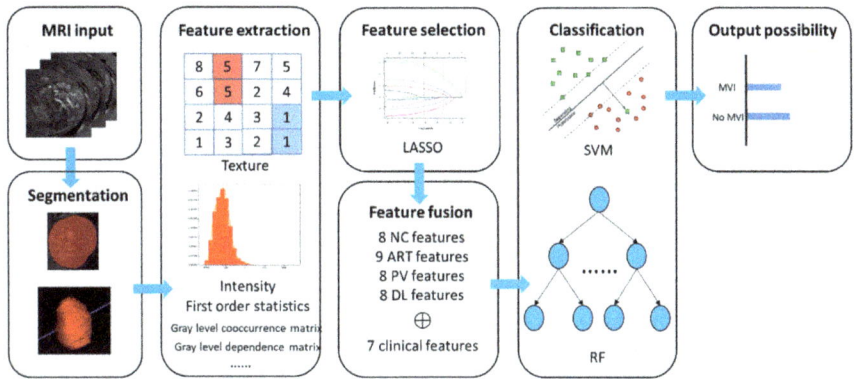

Fig. 10.12 Flow of fusion model

the 247 patient data points into training and test datasets, of which 174 data points were in the training dataset and 73 data points were in the test dataset. We used these two datasets to perform our comparative experiments to verify the effectiveness of our proposed method.

For image pre-processing, we resample the MRI images. Voxels in each MRI image volume were resampled to $1.0 \times 1.0 \times 1.0$ mm^3. Then, we use Z-score (0–1) to normalise the images. Finally, we remove image outliers.

Firstly, we conducted experiments using single-phase MRI and clinical data. The comparison results are shown in Table 10.3. In the comparative experiments, the accuracy of the clinical model is 68.49%; the accuracy of the radiomics models (four single-phase models) is 67.12% (NC), 65.75% (ART), 64.38% (PV) and 68.49% (DL). We can see that the accuracy of the clinical model and single-phase radiomics model is similar. However, the AUC of the DL radiomics model is 2% higher than the clinical model. The results show that the radiomics model achieves better results.

Because different results were achieved for liver tumours in different phases, we compared the four-phase radiomics models. Experimental results showed that the accuracy and AUC of the model trained in the DL phase (68.49% and 0.7282)

Table 10.3 Comparison results of different features

Features	Acc	AUC	Sen	Spec
NC	67.12%	0.6313	88.89%	32.14%
ART	65.75%	0.6646	86.67%	32.14%
PV	64.38%	0.6849	75.56%	46.43%
DL	68.49%	0.7282	88.89%	35.71%
Clinical	68.49%	0.7087	86.67%	39.29%
Fusion	72.60%	0.7607	86.67%	50.00%

*Acc: accuracy; AUC: area under the receiver operating characteristics curve; Sen: Sensitivity; Spec: specificity

were higher than those of models trained in the other three phases. To effectively use all information about a patient, we combine the four-phase and clinical data. The classification accuracy and AUC (72.60% and 0.7607) of the fusion model, which was trained using both the four-phase and clinical data, are higher than those of the single-phase radiomics and clinical models, indicating that the fusion of the four-phase radiomics and clinical data can effectively im-prove prediction performance.

10.3.2 The Direction of Future Progress

In 2012, the original radiomics method only used statistics and machine learning. Deep learning had made no progress in this area before then. In recent years, deep convolutional neural networks (DCNNs) have achieved state-of-the-art classification accuracy on ImageNet [30]. The high-level feature representation of DCNNs has proven to be superior to hand-crafted low-level and mid-level features [31–33]. Several studies have applied DCNNs to medical images of the liver. Bi et al. used ResNet to segment liver lesions and finished fourth in the ISBI 2017 Liver Tumour Segmentation Challenge [34]. Liang et al. proposed a DCNN with global and local pathways for focal liver lesions classification [35, 36]. These studies demonstrated the effectiveness of DCNNs in the field of medical image analysis.

Deep learning may outperform radiomics in terms of feature extraction. However, the features extracted using deep learning have one shortcoming: they are not interpretable. Although deep learning has demonstrated its superiority, it cannot be explained in clinical medicine. One of the important factors limiting the application of deep learning is the scarcity of medical data samples.

In summary, combining the interpretability advantages of radiomics with the powerful feature extraction ability of deep learning will be an attractive research topic in the future.

10.4 Conclusion

As AI's potential capability has been increasingly demonstrated, radiomics-based imaging quantitative approaches can capture important information for diagnostic, predictive and prognostic purposes in medicine. However, the transition of these computational methods to clinical and generalisation models necessitates further investigation. In the future, we intend to explore the combination of deep learning and radiomics.

Acknowledgements We would like to thank Sir Run Run Shaw Hospital for providing medical data and helpful advice on this research. This work is supported in part by the Grant-in-Aid for Scientific Research from the Japanese Ministry for Education, Science, Culture and Sports (MEXT) under the Grant Nos. 20KK0234, 21H03470, 20K21821 in part by Major Scientific Research Project of Zhejiang Lab under the Grant No. 2020ND8AD01..

References

1. Roberts, L.R., et al.: Imaging for the diagnosis of hepatocellular carcinoma: a systematic review and meta-analysis. Hepatology. **67**(1), 401–421 (2017)
2. Verma, V., et al.: The rise of radiomics and implications for oncologic management. JNCI: J. Natl. Cancer Inst. **109**(7), 441–3 (2017)
3. Lambin, P., et al.: Radiomics: extracting more information from medical images using advanced feature analysis. Eur J Cancer **48**(4), 441–6 (2012)
4. Gillies, R.J., Kinahan, P.E., Hricak, H.: Radiomics: images are more than pictures, they are data. Radiology. **278**(2), 563–577 (2016)
5. Chang, C., Lin, C.: LIBSVM: a library for support vector machines. ACM Trans. Intell. Syst. Technol. (TIST), **2**(3), 27(2011)
6. Breiman, L.: Random forests. Mach. Learn. **45**(1), 5–32 (2001)
7. Liu, Z., Wang, S., Di Dong, J.W., et al.: The applications of radiomics in precision diagnosis and treatment of oncology: opportunities and challenges. Theranostics **9**(5), 1303 (2019)
8. Braman, N.M., Etesami, M., Prasanna, P., et al.: Intratumoral and peritumoral radiomics for the pretreatment prediction of pathological complete response to neoadjuvant chemotherapy based on breast DCE-MRI. Breast Cancer Res. **19**(1), 57 (2017)
9. Kuo, M.D., Jamshidi, N.: Behind the numbers: decoding molecular phenotypes with radiogenomics—guiding principles and technical considerations. Radiology **270**(2), 320–325 (2014)
10. Huang, Y., Liang, C., He, L., et al.: Development and validation of a radiomics nomogram for preoperative prediction of lymph node metastasis in colorectal cancer. Sci. Found. China, pp. 2157–2164 (2016)
11. Kickingereder, P., Burth, S., Wick, A., et al.: Radiomic profiling of glioblastoma: identifying an imaging predictor of patient survival with improved performance over established clinical and radiologic risk models. Radiology **280**(3), 880–889 (2016)
12. Ma, X., Wei, J., Gu, D., et al.: Preoperative radiomics nomogram for microvascular invasion prediction in hepatocellular carcinoma using contrast-enhanced CT. Euro. Radiol., pp. 1–11 (2019)
13. Aerts, H.J., Velazquez, E.R., Leijenaar, R.T., Parmar, C., Grossmann, P., Carvalho, S., et al.: Decoding tumour phenotype by noninvasive imaging using a quantitative radiomics approach. Nat Commun **5**, 4006 (2014)
14. Lao, J., Chen, Y., Li, Z.C., et al.: A deep learning-based radiomics model for prediction of survival in glioblastoma multiforme. Sci. Rep. **7**(1), 1–8 (2017)
15. Valdora, F., Houssami, N., Rossi, F., et al.: Rapid review: radiomics and breast cancer. Breast Cancer Res. Treat. **169**(2), 217–229 (2018)
16. Zhou, Y., He, L., Huang, Y., et al.: CT-based radiomics signature: a potential biomarker for preoperative prediction of early recurrence in hepatocellular carcinoma. Abdominal Radiol. **42**(6), 1695–1704 (2017)
17. Ning, P., Gao, F., Hai, J., et al.: Application of CT radiomics in prediction of early recurrence in hepatocellular carcinoma. Abdominal Radiol. **45**(2) (2020)
18. Yang, X., Dong, X., Wang, J., et al.: Computed tomography-based radiomics signature: a potential indicator of epidermal growth factor receptor mutation in pulmonary adenocarcinoma appearing as a subsolid nodule. The Oncologist **24**(11), 1156–1164 (2019)
19. Njei, B., et al.: Emerging trends in hepatocellular carcinoma incidence and mortality. Hepatology. **61**(1), 191–199 (2015)

20. Forner, A., Reig, M., Bruix, J.: Hepatocellular carcinoma. Lancet **391**(10127), 1301–1314 (2018)
21. McGlynn, K.A., Petrick, J.L., London, W.T.: Global epidemiology of hepatocellular carcinoma. Clinics Liver Disease **19**(2), 223–238 (2015)
22. Hirokawa, Hayashi, M., Miyamoto, Y., et al.: Outcomes and predictors of microvascular invasion of solitary hepatocellular carcinoma. Hepatol. Res. **44**(8), 846–853 (2014)
23. Lei, Z., Li, J., Wu, D., et al.: Nomogram for preoperative estimation of microvascular invasion risk in hepatitis B Virus–related hepatocellular carcinoma within the milan criteria. JAMA Surg **151**, 356–358 (2016)
24. Chen, J., Zhou, J., Kuang, S., et al.: Liver imaging reporting and data system category 5 (LI-RADS LR-5): MRI predictors of microvascular invasion and recurrence after hepatectomy for hepatocellular carcinoma. Am. J. Roentgenol., pp. 1–10 (2019)
25. Zhang, R., Xu, L., Wen, X., et al.: A nomogram based on bi-regional radiomics features from multimodal magnetic resonance imaging for preoperative prediction of microvascular invasion in hepatocellular carcinoma. Quant Imaging Med Surg. **9**, 1503–1515 (2019)
26. Zwanenburg, A., Leger, S., Vallières, M., et al.: Image biomarker standardisation initiative-feature definitions. Radiotherapy Oncol. (2016)
27. Griethuysen, J., Fedorov, A., Parmar, C., et al.: Computational radiomics system to decode the radiographic phenotype. Cancer Res. **77**(21), 104–107 (2017)
28. Zou, H.: The adaptive lasso and its oracle properties. J. Am. Stat. Assoc. **101**(476), 1418–1429 (2006)
29. Pedregosa, F., Varoquaux, G., Gramfort, A., et al.: Scikit-learn: machine learning in Python. J. Mach. Learn. Res. **12**, 2825–2830 (2011)
30. Deng, J., et al.: Imagenet: a large-scale hierarchical image database. Computer Vision and Pattern Recognition, IEEE Conference (2009)
31. Krizhevsky, A., Sutskever, I., Hinton, G.E.: Imagenet classification with deep convolutional neural networks. Adv. Neural Inf. Process. Syst. pp. 1097–1105 (2012)
32. Szegedy, C., Liu, W., Jia, Y., et al.: Going deeper with convolutions. Proceedings of the IEEE Conference on Computer Vision and Pattern Recognition, pp. 1–9 (2015)
33. He, K., et al.: Deep residual learning for image recognition. Proceedings of the IEEE Conference on Computer Vision and Pattern Recognition (2016)
34. Bi, L., Kim, J., Kumar, A., et al.: Automatic Liver Lesion Detection using Cascaded Deep Residual Networks (2017)
35. Liang, D., et al.: Combining convolutional and recurrent neural networks for classification of focal liver lesions in multi-Phase CT images. International Conference on Medical Image Computing and Computer Assisted Intervention (2018)
36. Liang, D., et al.: Residual convolutional neural networks with global and local path-ways for classification of focal liver lesions. Pacific Rim International Conference on Artificial Intelligence, Springer, Cham (2018)

Chapter 11
Artificial Intelligence in Remote Photoplethysmography: Remote Heart Rate Estimation from Video Images

Zhaolin Qiu, Lanfen Lin, Hao Sun, Jiaqing Liu, and Yen-Wei Chen

Abstract This chapter aims to introduce remote heart rate estimation from video images, which is considered to be a cost-effective and comfortable method with great potential to become a supplementary medical modality or for daily health care. The principle of remote photoplethysmography signal extraction via video is first illustrated alongside early attempts to perform heart rate estimation. Next, mathematical models and computational algorithms based on these methods are discussed for solving movement artifacts and illumination changes. Deep learning methods are then reviewed, and a general overview of the datasets available for remote photoplethysmography learning is furnished.

Keywords Heart rate estimation · Remote photoplethysmography · Video image · Face · Deep learning

11.1 Introduction

Heart rate is a significant indicator of human health. It refers to the number of heartbeats per minute and can reflect the health of a person's heart activity. According to the occasion of heart rate measurement, the measurement can be generally divided into resting heart rate and maximum heart rate. Normally, heart rate should be within a certain range. High, low, or irregular resting heart rate may be a warning of some physical disease, which thus makes it valuable physical data to be monitored in

---

Z. Qiu · L. Lin · H. Sun · Y.-W. Chen (✉)
College of Computer Science and Technology, Zhejiang University, Hangzhou, China
e-mail: chen@is.ritsumei.ac.jp

L. Lin
e-mail: llf@zju.edu.cn

J. Liu · Y.-W. Chen
College of Information Science and Engineering, Ritsumeikan University, Kyoto, Japan

Y.-W. Chen
Zhejiang Lab, Research Center for Healthcare Data Science, Hangzhou, China

© The Author(s), under exclusive license to Springer Nature Switzerland AG 2022
C.-P. Lim et al. (eds.), *Handbook of Artificial Intelligence in Healthcare*,
Intelligent Systems Reference Library 211,
https://doi.org/10.1007/978-3-030-79161-2_11

clinical medicine. Maximum heart rate is generally utilized as a measure of physical performance, especially in athletes, as the heart beats faster during exercise, whereas more athletic individuals will generally have a lower increase in heart rate. Hence, heart rate is an essential indicator for both clinical care and personal health.

Traditional methods of heart rate measurement are usually contact-based. For instance, clinical observation of heart rate in real-time via electrocardiogram (ECG) requires the patient to wear an adhesive gel patch or chest strap to record electrical activities of the heart at all times. Although recording an ECG has been experimentally shown as a safe and painless procedure [1], patients can still experience skin irritation and discomfort.

Photoplethysmography (PPG) offers an alternative to heart rate measurement in a non-invasive manner. A pulse oximeter uses a light-emitting diode (LED) to illuminate the skin and then measures the amount of light transmitted or reflected in the LED. Changes in light volume caused by pressure pulses are then detected, based on which blood oxygen saturation is measurable, while heart rate is calculated from periodic fluctuations in the arteries. Since blood flow of the skin can be regulated by several physiological systems, PPG additionally serves to monitor respiratory rate, hypovolemia, and multiple other physiological signals. However, a pulse oximeter spring clip needs to be attached to fingertips or earlobes, causing pain during prolonged use.

Typically, PPG measurements using pulse oximetry require specific LED light sources, but experiments have shown that pulse measurements can be acquired by a camera that treats ordinary ambient light as the illumination source [2]. This leads to the possibility of non-contact PPG measurements, which is known as remote PPG (rPPG). The non-contact approach, once feasible, is low-cost and convenient, causing little or no discomfort to subjects, or even senselessly performed under fully automated conditions. Consequently, this attractive solution has induced many scholars to carry out researches and breakthroughs during the past decade. The basic idea of the non-contact remote PPG is to record the subjects' skin by a video camera, analyze the captured video and extrapolate the PPG signal via some algorithms, obtain physiological signals such as heart rate by then.

This chapter reviews the various methodologies for remote PPG measurement in the past decades. Mathematical modeling or computational algorithm-based methods will be presented first, which perform theoretical analysis or modeling of the acquired skin video to explore the association between changes in skin color and PPG signals. Then we will introduce some methods with deep learning based on which the raw video information is converted into a specific representation by a manual construction or a neural network, driving the neural network to recover the correlation between the representation and rPPG or heart rate through a rich volume of data. Datasets for the currently popular rPPG and remote heart rate trials are shown in the following part.

11.2 Naive Methods

Verkruysse et al. [2] demonstrated experimentally the feasibility of skin videos based on ambient light recordings. An inexpensive digital camera was used to capture facial areas of subjects in different resting postures (sitting, standing, lying) under sunlight or lamplight. After manually selecting the region of interest (ROI) of faces from the videos, for each frame the average of pixel colors within the ROI is calculated to obtain the raw signal named Pixel Values. Calculating the average is a common method to mitigate the influence of noises on facial colors to enhance the Signal Noise Ratio (SNR). Digital filtering is applied to the original signal, followed by Fast Fourier Transform as the time domain processing, which is widely used in single processing and also rPPG extraction [3, 4]. It is shown that the curves of heart rate and respiration rate can be seen dramatically in the processed color change information. This experiment revealed the potential of remote PPG and new algorithms have been proposed to improve the accuracy of remote estimation of heart rate and other physiological signals for more than a decade.

Some intriguing conclusions from the experiments are noteworthy in that the amplitude and shape exhibited in different color channels of RGB are not the same. The strongest plethysmographic signal is in the G channel, although the respiration rate signal is sometimes more dominant in the R or B channel. However, since the three channels have different signal shapes, the authors suggest that there may be some complementary relationships among the three color channels. In addition, movement artifacts are found to be an essential cause of noises in the experiments, due to the variation of light that causes large fluctuations in skin color when the subject's head is in motion, imposing obstacles and challenges to the prediction of remote physiological signals.

11.3 Blind Signal Separation

Despite the fact that rPPG-based methods have been proven possible, there are still challenges in their application as physiological signals such as heart rate embodied in the color changes on the skin appear excessively fragile and are highly susceptible to noise interference such as illumination and motion. Therefore, some scholars have tried to separate these disturbing factors, namely Blind Signal Separation (BSS).

11.3.1 Independent Component Analysis

Independent Component Analysis (ICA) is a widely accepted methodology that attempts to segregate heart rate signals, respiratory rate signals from noises. Poh et al. [5] proposed a fully automated method applicable to face color video recordings, which is based on automatic face tracking while separating the color channel blind sources into independent components. In their experiments, subjects are allowed to have small movements, so as to demonstrate that their algorithm is able to cope with movement artifacts; and to be present in one video at the same time, as to support that their algorithm can be used for multiple simultaneous measurements. Independent component analysis attempts to decompose the three color channels into three separate elementary signal sources:

$$x(t) = \mathbf{A}s(t) \qquad (11.1)$$

$$\hat{s}(t) = \mathbf{W}x(t) \qquad (11.2)$$

where $s(t)$ is the signal from the assumed three independent sources, which are converted by the matrix $\mathbf{A}$ to compose the resulting $x(t)$, i.e., the acquired RGB three-channel signals. The conversion matrix $\mathbf{W}$ is the inverse matrix of $\mathbf{A}$, which calculates the estimated value $\hat{s}(t)$ of the signals emitted by the three independent sources. An iterative method is used to maximize or minimize a particular cost function measuring non-Gaussianity such as kurtosis, negentropy, or mutual information so as to discern independent sources. In the experimental results, three signals derived from ICA necessarily contain a highly correlated signal with heart rate, indicating that the heart rate signal can be extracted by ICA.

In later works, Poh et al. [6] used ICA to estimate heart rate, respiratory rate, and heart rate variability. Using a five-band digital camera, McDuff et al. [7] obtained better results by experimentally comparing different combinations of color channels with ICA. Lam and Kuno [8] proposed a selection random patches-based approach to select multiple regions for ICA independently, which are fused together by a voting mechanism to improve the robustness of the model to motion and illumination changes to some extent. Single-channel independent component analysis, i.e., SCICA, is used by Yu et al. [9] to demonstrate that heart rate signals can also be decomposed from single-channel color signals (Fig. 11.1).

11.3.2 Principal Component Analysis

In addition to ICA, Principal Component Analysis, or Karhunen–Loeve Transformation, is also a powerful tool for signal analysis and processing. It identifies the principal patterns in the data and represents it in such a dimension making It highlights the similarities and dissimilarities of the data across hidden dimensions. Similar to ICA, PCA involves the same decomposition of the original multi-channel signal into a series of single-channel signals. In PCA, the first channel of the decomposition is required to point to the direction with the greatest variability in the original data, the second channel to the next largest direction, and so forth. Lewandowska et al. [10] experimentally demonstrated that PCA can also be applied as an algorithm for

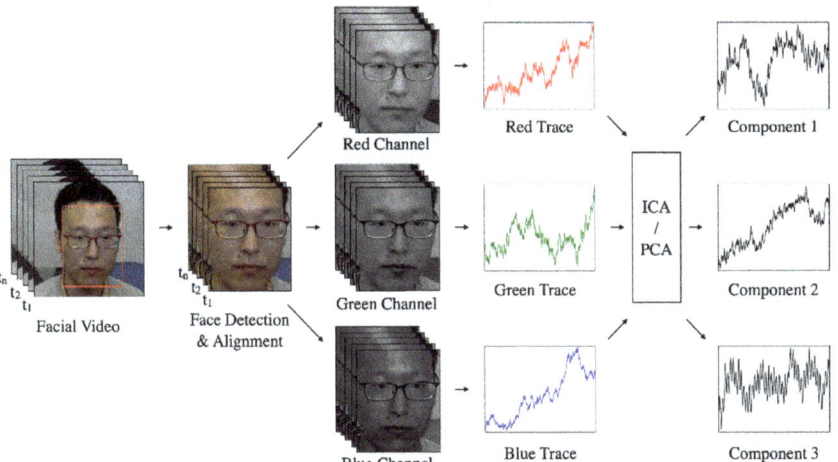

Fig. 11.1 Procedure of ICA and PCA

BSS in the context of remote heart rate prediction, with a comparison to the signal extracted by ICA.

11.3.3 Joint Blind Signal Separation

As face video datasets have grown richer, multiple-ROI methods have been proposed to make the most of these data, which makes Joint Blind Signal Separation (JBSS) possible. JBSS is an extension of the common ICA- or PCA-based BSS, which not only finds the components of independent sources at the multichannel level, but also extends the process to multi-ROI, i.e., finding independent sources in the multichannel multi-ROI dimension.

Guo et al. [11] firstly used JBSS in the task of predicting heart rate from face videos, and obtained the predicted Blood Volume Pulse (BVP) signal through the three steps of Facial Landmarks Estimation and Sub-region Construction, Independent Vector Analysis by JBSS, and Source Signal Selection via Normalized Cut, achieving better results than the ICA-only method in Heart Rate and Heart Rate Variability estimation.

Later, Qi et al. [12] proposed a new algorithm for remote heart rate testing by exploring correlations among facial subregion data sets using a JBSS-based approach, and tests performed on the publicly available dataset DEAP [13] similarly demonstrated the superiority of JBSS over the ICA-based BSS approach.

11.4 Modelling

Many of the earlier methods are based on the foundation that the subject needs to maintain a static resting posture under constant light. In practice, the ambient lighting is likely to change momentarily, and slight head movements and postural adjustments impact the performance of these methods. To make remote heart rate measurements practical and automated, environment interference needs to be eliminated, thus some researchers start experimenting with methods to avoid the effects of light, motion, and camera factors.

11.4.1 CHROM

To address the errors caused by motion, de Haan et al. [14] proposed a chrominance-based method (CHROM). By analyzing the skin color at rest and in a motion change state, the diffuse and specular reflectance components of light on the skin surface are considered, and the relative positions of the camera, skin, and light source in space can be estimated by modeling, thus eliminating motion artifacts. It is shown that CHROM achieves higher accuracy and robustness in various cases from stationary to moderate motion such as bicycle to vigorous motion such as stepping.

Later, de Haan et al. [15] proposed another chrominance-based method. They demonstrated that the different absorption spectra of arterial blood and bloodless skin cause the variations to occur along a very specific vector in a normalized RGB-space. Consequently, this feature can be used to design a specific "signature" to distinguish between color variations caused by pulses and those caused by motion artifacts, thus eliminating the effects caused by the latter. The experimental results of this method in diverse motion scenes are further enhanced than CHROM [14], with higher accuracy and improved SNR.

11.4.2 Illumination Rectification

Li et al. [16] tried to correct for different illumination. They hypothesized that the change of skin color in ROI consists only of the impulse signal of the skin and the change of ambient illumination, so the change caused by ambient illumination needs to be compensated. And the ambient light can be manifested from non-skin background region, as the background region is usually the same light source as the skin region. Therefore the color of the surrounding area is used as a reference to add a compensation to the skin color:

$$\mathbf{g}_{\text{IR}} = \mathbf{g}_{\text{face}} - h\mathbf{g}_{\text{bg}} \qquad (11.3)$$

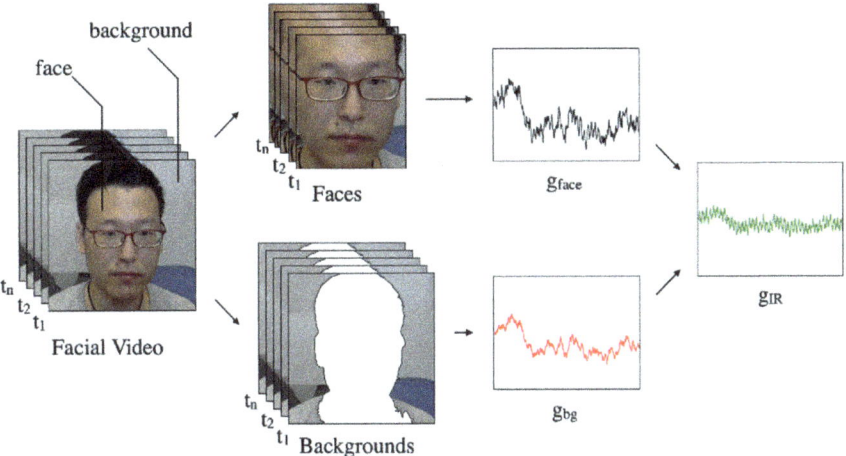

Fig. 11.2 Illumination rectification methods by Li et al. [16]

In order to find the h that minimizes the error, the authors used the Normalized Least Mean Square (NLMS) adaptive filter iteratively. The Distance Regularized Level Set Evolution (DRLSE) method is used to segment the ambient background region, thus enabling the correction of skin color according to ambient lighting (Fig. 11.2).

11.4.3 2SR, POS

Wang et al. [17] observed that the spatially redundant information obtained when sampling multiple regions of the skin using a single camera can be used to distinguish between pulse signals and motion-induced noise. They proposed a motion-compensated pixel-to-pixel pulse extraction, spatial pruning, and temporal filtering to extract the rPPG signal. Experiments conducted with 36 subjects demonstrate the feasibility of the pixel-track-complete approach, significantly improving the robustness to motion and the performance of the algorithm.

Soon after, Wang et al. [18] combined the spatially redundant pixels of the camera with the assumption of a well-defined skin mask and proposed the Spatial Subspace Rotation (2SR) algorithm to estimate the spatial subspace of skin color and measure its temporal rotation to extract the pulse signal. The algorithm is superior in that it does not require a priori knowledge of skin color and pulse signal, and it is experimentally shown that given a well-defined skin mask, 2SR performs better than ICA-based methods, as well as the CHROM [14] method, and the algorithm is easy to implement and extend.

In a later work, Wang et al. [19] investigated a new biological feature: the relative pulsatile amplitude, and employed it for the first time to design an efficient rPPG filtering method called Amplitude-Selective Filtering (ASF), which can be widely used in various rPPG methods and has been shown to have good results in sports scenarios such as fitness.

Recently, Wang et al. [20] proposed a Plane-Orthogonal-to-Skin (POS) operator, which defines a plane orthogonal to the skin-tone in the temporally normalized RGB space, thus enabling the extraction of rPPG signals. In this paper, the authors elaborate and compare the principles of the above algorithmic methods with existing rPPG methods. The experiments include videos with different skin tones, different light intensities, and different degrees of motion, and are compared with methods modeled by algorithms such as BSS [6], CHROM [14], and 2SR [18], where the superiority of the POS algorithm is demonstrated.

11.4.4 Motion Reduction

Some other methods are also being tried to compensate for the motion-induced errors. For example, Li et al. [16] took measures to deal with non-rigid motion within the ROI caused by expression changes, etc., since such motion would bring convex during the filtering process and influence the distribution of power spectral density. They divided the signal into segments and directly removed the segments with a standard deviation distribution of 95%. This approach, although simple and effective, is applicable only to some small expression changes of the subjects in a strictly controlled experimental setting, and is less powerful for complex motions in real scenes.

To overcome motion artifacts, Yu et al. [9] proposed a method of planar motion compensation and evidenced that the method could overcome motion artifacts and extract heart rate and respiration rate even under high-intensity exercise by measuring pulses of 12 subjects before, during and after cycling.

Feng et al. [21] considered the skin as a Lambertian radiator and analyzed the ROI of the face from the radiometry perspective. In their approach, an adaptive color difference operation between the red channel and the green channel is considered to reduce the interference of motion artifacts, and a bandpass filter is proposed to further remove residual motion artifacts based on the characteristics of the PPG signal. The experiment supports their idea and performs better in capturing the heart rate of subjects in motion.

11.5 Deep Learning

Modeling methods can grasp the relationship between skin color and environmental factors, and to a certain degree reduce the error and influence caused by lighting, movement and other factors, but these modeling methods usually have some limitations. However, some limitations are usually associated with these modeling methods.

They perform well in a particular environment, but may not function as well as traditional methods when the assumptions and premises of other models do not hold.

As more datasets containing videos of subjects' faces taken in different environments, real-time heart rate, respiration rate, and PPG and ECG signals became available, data-driven approaches became more valued. With the development of machine learning and deep learning, they are also soon noticed to be used to learn the pattern of skin color changes. And these methods generally have a stronger generalization capability, i.e., they are not bound by the preconditions and assumptions of modeling methods and can be used in a variety of complex and extreme environments.

Some of the early attempts to use this data-driven approach are the support vector regression used by Hsu et al. [22] and the Self-Adaptive Matrix Completion method by Tulyakov et al. [23]. The former uses intermediate features from the traditional Fourier transform, the Independent Component Analysis used by Poh et al. [5] and the chrominance-based approach proposed by de Haan et al. [14]. These features are fed into Support Vector Regression (SVR) for heart rate regression. The experimental results show the power and potential of the machine learning approach, which is significantly more effective than straightforward traditional methods. The latter method solves the problem of incomplete synchronization of chromatic features in different facial regions and the problem that facial motion and facial expressions can cause strong interference of chromatic features by adaptive matrix derivation method to a certain extent, and achieves satisfactory results on public datasets.

As computer performance increases, deep learning can be considered to extract deeper features or to perform regression. These methods use deep learning methods such as CNNs [24–30], RNNs [24, 30], and attention mechanisms [29, 30]. Some popular learning-based methods are presented below, divided into a feature extraction and expression section, which attempts to construct expressions from which neural networks can extract impulse signals, and an interference separation section, which attempts to separate impersonation signals from interference signals through neural networks. Comparative experiments [31, 32] are often conducted to contrast the advantages and disadvantages between deep learning methods and traditional methods.

11.5.1 Feature Extraction and Representation

To feed facial video information into a neural network, information needs to be extracted by means of feature extraction or to construct a specific representation of the video information. A conventional way is to use hand-craft features directly, which is based on some intermediate representations in the algorithms and modeling approaches mentioned in the previous section. For example, Hsu et al. [22] combined the intermediate features of FFT, ICA [5], and CHROM based algorithms [14] and modeling methods and input them into a support vector machine for regression. Hsu et al. [33] preprocessed the face detection region using the algorithm and obtained

2D Time–Frequency Representations, which are input to the deep learning model VGG-15 as images.

The Spatial–temporal Map proposed by Niu et al. [24] is a typical example of heart rate representation. In this paper, it is pointed out that the only useful information in the face video is the change of skin color caused by the change of blood volume and blood oxygenation, so the representation needs to be carefully constructed to achieve the adequate representation of this information. They divided the face region into 5 * 5 regions and averaged the skin color for each region across channels to reduce the impression of noise. In a later work, Niu et al. [25] extended this to a Multi-Scale Spatial–Temporal Map (Fig. 11.3).

After converting the skin color signal into an image, the heart rate can be extracted using the neural network used for image inputs. Another Spatiotemporal Representation was proposed by Song et al. [26]. They acquired the color changes of three ROIs on the skin and obtained the estimation curves of three BVP signals by the traditional rPPG method. The spatiotemporal feature images of the colored stripes are obtained by transforming the BVP signals obtained from the three ROIs as three channels with a Toeplitz matrix. The deep neural network used for the images easily extracts from them the variation pattern in the streak map and thus predicts the heart rate values (Fig. 11.4).

Another approach is to use a neural network to process the video information directly and extract the features from the video. Spetlik et al. [27] used an end-to-end heart rate convolutional neural network consisting of an extractor and an heart rate

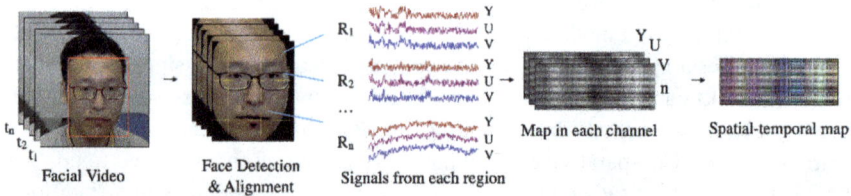

Fig. 11.3 Spatial–temporal Map by Niu et al. [24]

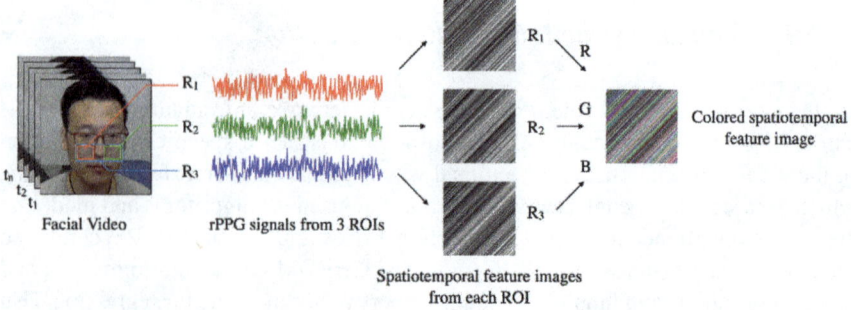

Fig. 11.4 Colored spatiotemporal feature image proposed by Song et al. [26]

estimator to do this. Where the extractor is responsible for extracting features from the sequence of face images against it, while the estimator regresses these features and finally outputs the heart rate.

11.5.2 Interference Separation and Signal Enhancement

Since skin color changes are susceptible to environmental interference, model-based algorithms try to separate out components that are not related to the impulse signal. However, these model-based methods make certain assumptions and may not satisfy the model prerequisites in realistic scenarios. At this point, deep learning demonstrates its capabilities. Algorithms have emerged that attempt to separate impulse signals from irrelevant signals or to augment impulse signals.

Niu et al. [25] applied a cross-verified feature disentangling strategy to a pair of videos with simultaneous inputs through an encoder-decoder structure. Specifically, the model seeks to separate the impulse signal and the impulse-independent signal in the video by the encoder, which can be recovered using a symmetric encoder. The impulse-independent parts of the two videos are exchanged during the recovery, achieving the purpose of cross-verified. The reconstructed implicit features are fed into the Physiological estimator later, and the rPPG signal and heart rate are estimated by CNN network (Fig. 11.5).

Yu et al. [28] have designed an end-to-end deep learning-based video enhancement method to extract rPPG signals in cases where the video quality is quite low or highly compressed. The method consists of a Spatio-Temporal Video Enhancement Network (STVEN) and an rPPG network (rPPGNet) for rPPG signal recovery. Experimental results show that the method achieves excellent performance for the case of highly compressed video.

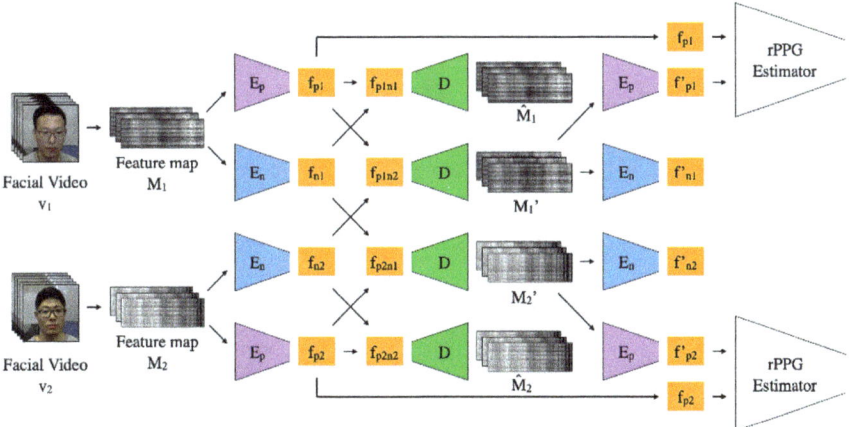

Fig. 11.5 Cross-verified feature disentangling strategy proposed by Niu et al. [25]

11.6 Popular Datasets for rPPG Learning

Prediction methods for rPPG signals, especially deep learning methods, rely on a large amount of training data from various environments and scenes. On the one hand, algorithm-based and modeling approaches need to consider various complex environmental factors to make their proposed algorithms have better performance. On the other hand, the training of neural networks must depend on a large volume of data, and more complex kinds of videos are beneficial to improve the robustness of the trained models. This section presents the more popular datasets that contain real-time observations of video of faces, heart rate, or physiological signals such as PPG, ECG, etc., for existing methods to study and evaluate. An overview of datasets is illustrated in Table 11.1.

- The DEAP dataset [13] is a collection of 32 subjects who participated in an experiment to analyze human emotions by recording their EEG and surrounding Peripheral physiological signals. Votes on the stimulated music videos are also collected and scored on Arousal, Valence, Dominance, Liking, and Familiarity. From the ECG signals and Peripheral physiological signals galvanic skin response (GSR), Blood volume pressure, Respiration pattern, Skin temperature, electromyogram (EMG) and electrooculogram (EOG).
- MAHNOB-HCI [34] is a multimodal emotional stimulus dataset that records face videos, audio signals, eye gaze data, and peripheral/central nervous system physiological signals while subjects watch different videos. The experiments were conducted under controlled conditions, where subjects were asked not to move as much as possible and the lighting was controlled. The database was mainly used for affective calculations, while heart rate could be extracted from the provided EEG signals, allowing the dataset to be used for remote heart rate (HR) estimation.
- The MMSE-HR dataset [35] is a multimodal corpus that involved 140 subjects. To evoke a range of real emotions, the experiment induced emotional changes in different ways, including conversations, watching movie clips, games, and

Table 11.1 Overview of popular datasets for rPPG learning

Dataset	# Subjects	# Videos	Motion	Illumination	Ground truth
DEAP	32	880	Expression	Controlled	EEG
MAHNOB-HCI	27	527	Slight movement	Controlled	EEG
MMSE-HR	40	102	Stable	Controlled	HR
PFF	10	104	Random	Varied	HR
VIPL-HR	107	3130	Stable/large	Varied	HR, SpO$_2$
OBF	106	424	Slight movement	Controlled	HR, HRV
ECG-Fitness	17	204	Exercising	Natural/artificial	ECG, HR
UBFC-RPPG	43	43	/	/	HR

physical stimulation. Data were acquired by a variety of sensors on the face, including heart rate, blood pressure, and other physiological signals.
- The PFF dataset [33] is designed specifically for remote heart rate prediction containing 104 videos of 10 subjects. In considering the natural situation, the videos are captured with random head movements, expression changes, and different lighting conditions, and different recording equipment.
- VIPL-HR [36] is a large-scale heart rate dataset for remote heart rate estimation. It controls a variety of different experimental conditions, including subject head movements, illumination changes, and different recording devices. In addition to color RGB video, near-infrared (NIR) video is also provided for the experimental set, and the dataset contains real-time heart rate, SpO_2, and BVP waveforms as ground truth.
- The OBF dataset [37] collects a large number of facial videos and physiological signals from healthy subjects as well as from patients with atrial fibrillation. Experiments on this dataset have shown that HRV extracted from video can be used for atrial fibrillation detection.
- ECG-Fitness [27] is a challenging dataset that records ECGs of subjects while performing different activities (speaking, rowing, cycling, elliptical trainer exercising). The video contains strenuous exercise, thus making it more challenging to predict physiological metrics such as rPPG signal or heart rate. Three light sources were considered, including natural light, 400 W halogen light, and 30 W led light. 204 videos from 17 subjects are included in the dataset.
- The UBFC-RPPG dataset [38] consists of 43 videos taken by 43 subjects that are required to engage in a time-sensitive mathematical game to elicit different heart rate variations. Heart rate was measured by a finger-clip pulse oximeter.

11.7 Future

The low cost, comfort and convenience, and growing accuracy of rPPG via video make it a strong potential and promising technology. Future developments in the technology and applications of rPPG will include the following topics.

Deep Learning Methods Combined with Traditional Algorithms

The existing research trend is increasingly shifting from traditional algorithm-based and modeling approaches to methods using deep learning. Methods using deep learning have surpassed some traditional methods in terms of results (error, correlation, and other metrics), and the errors are gradually becoming smaller, as can be seen in the comparison of hand-craft methods with learning-based methods conducted by J Hernandez-Ortega et al. However, there is still something to think about and learn from the model-based approaches. It may be a future direction to consider using the features obtained from modeling, combining them with techniques such as neural networks, and optimizing and adapting deep learning methods using the prior knowledge obtained from model-based methods.

Multimodal with Simultaneous Prediction of Multiple Physiological Signals

It has been experimentally shown that multiple signals such as heart rate, respiration rate, etc. can be extracted from the rPPG signal, while if an infrared camera/sensor is used, heart rate, respiration rate, body temperature, etc. can be measured simultaneously. Combined with the expression captured by the camera, expression recognition can be performed on the face, thus enabling multimodal emotion prediction. Multi-modality is also a mainstream direction of emotion prediction today, and adding multimodal information of heart rate and respiration in this field may also become a relatively unique idea.

Challenging More Difficult Datasets

Although there are many datasets collected by scholars, on the one hand many of them are collected for some specific environments, such as controlled laboratory environments, while on the other hand the quality and standards of the datasets vary individually. A complex environmental dataset collected in a natural environment is needed, and considering that heart rate collection devices as ground truth may not be portable, a commercial device such as a fitness bracelet can be used for real-time acquisition to obtain video in a real complex environment and its corresponding heart rate information. In conclusion, datasets determine to some extent the upper limit and bottleneck of application development in this field, therefore more difficult datasets are desired.

Applications in Personal Health Care

Heart rate information can be used in the daily health care of personal life. For example, an infrared camera can be used to capture the face while sleeping to detect heart rate, which can be used to assist in detecting sleep quality and thus suggesting sleep improvements. Although there are currently some solutions based on contact measurement, sleep detection will be facilitated to some extent by non-contact measurement methods. It is also advantageous to combine this method of sleep detection with a sound-based approach to achieve multimodal monitoring. The same reasoning can be implemented for exercise center rate monitoring, which will be more comfortable and convenient than the contact method.

Security Applications

With the monitoring of physiological signals such as heart rate, it is possible to identify whether the person passing through the face detection in front of the camera is a real person or a mask, thus improving the security of face detection technology. Moreover, the technology can be used for lie detection, only need to add the algorithm in the room's camera to observe its heart rate in real time, without the need to measure the signal of its heart rate through the polygraph, thus this method will be more convenient and practical.

Medical Assistance

When the rPPG signal has similar accuracy to traditional contact measurements, it can be used in the medical field. Patients who require 24-h monitoring can be remotely monitored for various physiological signals, thus eliminating the need to wear uncomfortable devices for long periods of time. Measuring physiological signals via video can also make telemedicine possible, although there is still a long way to go before it is fully realized. In addition, non-contact measurement and monitoring can be done senselessly for face-to-face consultation, counseling or observation of some psychological disorders, which may be offensive and unpleasant to patients if measured through contact.

Acknowledgements This work was supported in part by Major Scientific Research Project of Zhejiang Lab under the Grant No. 2020ND8AD01.

References

1. https://stanfordhealthcare.org/medical-tests/e/ekg/risks.html
2. Verkruysse, W., Svaasand, L.O., Stuart Nelson, J.: Remote plethysmographic imaging using ambient light. Opt. Express **16**(26) 21434–21445 (2008)
3. Kumar, M., Veeraraghavan, A., Sabharwal, A.: DistancePPG: robust non-contact vital signs monitoring using a camera. Biomed. Opt. Express **6**(5), 1565–1588 (2015)
4. Niu, X., et al.: Continuous heart rate measurement from face: a robust rppg approach with distribution learning. In: 2017 IEEE International Joint Conference on Biometrics (IJCB). IEEE, 2017
5. Poh, M.-Z., McDuff, D.J., Picard, R.W.: Non-contact, automated cardiac pulse measurements using video imaging and blind source separation. Opt. Express **18**(10), 10762–10774 (2010)
6. Poh, M.-Z., McDuff, D.J., Picard, R.W.: Advancements in noncontact, multiparameter physiological measurements using a webcam. IEEE Trans. Biomed. Eng. **58**(1), 7–11 (2010)
7. McDuff, D., Gontarek, S., Picard, R.W.: Improvements in remote cardiopulmonary measurement using a five band digital camera. IEEE Trans. Biomed. Eng. **61**(10), 2593–2601 (2014)
8. Lam, A., Kuno, Y.: Robust heart rate measurement from video using select random patches. In: Proceedings of the IEEE International Conference on Computer Vision, 2015.
9. Yu, S., et al.: Motion-compensated noncontact imaging photoplethysmography to monitor cardiorespiratory status during exercise. J. Biomed. Opt. **16**(7), 077010 (2011)
10. Lewandowska, M., et al.: Measuring pulse rate with a webcam—a non-contact method for evaluating cardiac activity. In: *2011 Federated Conference on Computer Science and Information Systems (FedCSIS)*. IEEE, 2011.
11. Guo, Z., Jane Wang, Z., Shen, Z.: Physiological parameter monitoring of drivers based on video data and independent vector analysis. In: 2014 IEEE International Conference on Acoustics, Speech and Signal Processing (ICASSP). IEEE, 2014.
12. Qi, H., et al.: Video-based human heart rate measurement using joint blind source separation. Biomed. Signal Process. Control **31**, 309–320 (2017)
13. Koelstra, S., et al.: Deap: a database for emotion analysis; using physiological signals. In: IEEE Trans. Affect. Comput. **3**(1), 18–31 (2011)
14. De Haan, G., Jeanne, V.: Robust pulse rate from chrominance-based rPPG. IEEE Trans. Biomed. Eng. **60**(10), 2878–2886 (2013)

15. De Haan, G., Van Leest, A.: Improved motion robustness of remote-PPG by using the blood volume pulse signature. Physiol. Measur. **35**(9), 1913 (2014)
16. Li, X., et al.: Remote heart rate measurement from face videos under realistic situations. In: Proceedings of the IEEE Conference on Computer Vision and Pattern Recognition, 2014
17. Wang, Wenjin, Sander Stuijk, and De Haan, G.: Exploiting spatial redundancy of image sensor for motion robust rPPG. IEEE Trans. Biomed. Eng. **62**(2), 415–425 (2014)
18. Wang, W., Stuijk, S., De Haan, G.: A novel algorithm for remote photoplethysmography: spatial subspace rotation. IEEE Trans. Biomed. Eng. **63**(9), 1974–1984 (2015)
19. Wang, W., et al.: Amplitude-selective filtering for remote-PPG. Biomed. Opt. Express **8**(3), 1965–1980 (2017)
20. Wang, W., et al.: Algorithmic principles of remote PPG. IEEE Trans. Biomed. Eng. **64**(7), 1479–1491 (2016)
21. Feng, L., et al.: Motion-resistant remote imaging photoplethysmography based on the optical properties of skin. IEEE Trans. Circuits Syst. Video Technol. **25**(5), 879–891 (2014)
22. Hsu, Y.C., Lin, Y.-L., Hsu, W.: Learning-based heart rate detection from remote photoplethysmography features. In: 2014 IEEE International Conference on Acoustics, Speech and Signal Processing (ICASSP). IEEE, 2014.
23. Tulyakov, S., et al.: Self-adaptive matrix completion for heart rate estimation from face videos under realistic conditions. In: Proceedings of the IEEE Conference on Computer Vision and Pattern Recognition, 2016.
24. Niu, X., et al.: Rhythmnet: End-to-end heart rate estimation from face via spatial-temporal representation. IEEE Trans. Image Process. **29**, 2409–2423 (2019)
25. Niu, X., et al.: Video-based remote physiological measurement via cross-verified feature disentangling. In: European Conference on Computer Vision. Springer, Cham, 2020.
26. Song, R., et al.: Heart rate estimation from facial videos using a spatiotemporal representation with convolutional neural networks. IEEE Trans. Instrum. Measur. **69**(10), 7411–7421 (2020)
27. Spetlik, R., et al.: Visual heart rate estimation with convolutional neural network. In: British Machine Vision Conference, 2018.
28. Yu, Z., et al.: Remote heart rate measurement from highly compressed facial videos: an end-to-end deep learning solution with video enhancement. In: Proceedings of the IEEE/CVF International Conference on Computer Vision, 2019.
29. Chen, W., McDuff, D.: Deepphys: video-based physiological measurement using convolutional attention networks. In: Proceedings of the European Conference on Computer Vision (ECCV). 2018
30. Niu, X., et al.: Robust remote heart rate estimation from face utilizing spatial-temporal attention. In: 2019 14th IEEE International Conference on Automatic Face & Gesture Recognition (FG 2019). IEEE, 2019
31. Hernandez-Ortega, et al.: A comparative evaluation of heart rate estimation methods using face videos. arXiv:2005.11101 (2020)
32. Song, R., et al.: New insights on super-high resolution for video-based heart rate estimation with a semi-blind source separation method. Comput. Biol. Med. **116**, 103535 (2020)
33. Hsu, G.-S., Ambikapathi, A.M.: Chen, M.-S.: Deep learning with time-frequency representation for pulse estimation from facial videos. In: 2017 IEEE International Joint Conference on Biometrics (IJCB). IEEE, 2017.
34. Soleymani, M., et al.: A multimodal database for affect recognition and implicit tagging. In: IEEE Trans. Affect. Comput. **3**(1), 42–55 (2011)
35. Zhang, Z., et al.: Multimodal spontaneous emotion corpus for human behavior analysis. In: Proceedings of the IEEE Conference on Computer Vision and Pattern Recognition, 2016.
36. Niu, X., et al.: VIPL-HR: A multi-modal database for pulse estimation from less-constrained face video. In: Asian Conference on Computer Vision. Springer, Cham, 2018.

37. Li, X., et al.: The OBF database: a large face video database for remote physiological signal measurement and atrial fibrillation detection. In: 2018 13th IEEE International Conference on Automatic Face & Gesture Recognition (FG 2018). IEEE, 2018.
38. Bobbia, S., et al.: Unsupervised skin tissue segmentation for remote photoplethysmography. Pattern Recogn. Lett. **124**, 82–90 (2019)

Part II
Advances in AI for Healthcare Information and Data Analytics

Chapter 12
Mining Data to Deal with Epidemics: Case Studies to Demonstrate Real World AI Applications

Christina Nousi, Paraskevi Belogianni, Paraskevas Koukaras, and Christos Tjortjis

Abstract The massive growth of Big Data kickstarted a new era for data analytics and knowledge discovery. Data mining algorithms are employed to analyze different types of data, which reside in complex information networks. Researchers focus on producing usable knowledge by taking advantage of opportunities in various domains (e.g., healthcare, social media, energy etc.). Epidemics and disease outbreaks raised concerns about effective infectious disease management in communities around the world. Therefore, they encourage the use of AI methods for management and prevention, in order to mitigate disease spread, and contain outbreaks. This work engages in *predictive* analytics, utilizing classification, as well as *descriptive* analytics utilizing association rule mining and clustering, which are widely used in healthcare and medicine, either for predicting outbreaks or for extracting usable information from healthcare and medical data. Certain steps need to be considered when attempting to perform data analysis, such as data extraction, cleaning, preprocessing, transformation, interpretation and evaluation. The experimental part of this chapter integrates widely used datasets retrieved from the UCI Machine Learning Repository related with the healthcare domain. This chapter offers a literature review on data mining in epidemics, while thoroughly discussing all the aforementioned concepts. It also presents a complete process/cycle of the required steps to analyze data retrieved from healthcare and medical sources. Hence, the research questions addressed can be summarized to the following: Q1. Which are the pervasive types of analytics involving the domains of medicine and healthcare? Q2. How is data mining performed

---

C. Nousi · P. Belogianni · P. Koukaras · C. Tjortjis (✉)
The Data Mining and Analytics Research Group, School of Science and Technology, International Hellenic University, 57001 Thessaloniki, Greece
e-mail: c.tjortjis@ihu.edu.gr

C. Nousi
e-mail: cnousi@ihu.edu.gr

P. Belogianni
e-mail: pbelogianni@ihu.edu.gr

P. Koukaras
e-mail: p.koukaras@ihu.edu.gr

© The Author(s), under exclusive license to Springer Nature Switzerland AG 2022
C.-P. Lim et al. (eds.), *Handbook of Artificial Intelligence in Healthcare*,
Intelligent Systems Reference Library 211,
https://doi.org/10.1007/978-3-030-79161-2_12

in the fields of healthcare and medicine? Q3. Which are the widespread techniques and methods utilized? These questions are discussed and elaborated, through a concise, informative and educational narration.

Keywords Data mining (DM) · Artificial intelligence (AI) · Machine learning (ML) · Supervised/unsupervised learning · Epidemics · Healthcare

Term Definition Table

Term	Definition
API (Application Programming Interface)	A set of functions and protocols that enables the data transmission and communication between software applications.
Data mining algorithms	Mathematical and computational expressions of patterns found in datasets.
Data point	An observation derived from a set of one or more measurements, presented either numerically or graphically.
Feature	An attribute or variable of a dataset that can be used for analysis.
Instance	A subset of the overall dataset or a single row of data.

12.1 Introduction

An epidemic is defined as a rapid, highly contagious disease that is likely to spread into the entire population in a short period of time. If the contagion measurement reaches the outbreak level, an epidemic is capable to even wipe out the population. It can be triggered by various factors, such as changes in the ecology of the host population, genetic changes and emerging pathogens. It can be restricted to one location but in the case of spreading to other countries or continents it can be characterized as a pandemic [1].

According to the Atlanta Center for Disease control "epidemic is the occurrence of more cases of disease, injury, or other health condition than expected in a given area or among a specific group of persons during a particular period. Usually, the cases are presumed to have a common cause or to be related to one another in some way." These contagious diseases can cause major economic, health and social impacts. It is believed to be the one of the major factors that had caused the 43% of life lost globally. Some of the best known examples in the world are dengue, yellow fever, cholera, diphtheria, influenza, bird flu, malaria, Ebola and many others [2].

The recent increases in global travel and the interconnected nature of modern life have led to an increased focus on the threat of epidemic diseases. Public health officials need accurate information on time, concerning disease outbreaks in order to take action and establish measures to contain them. Traditional disease surveillance techniques, such as reporting from clinicians can take more than a week to collect and distribute, so turning to more contemporary and timely sources of information is a current priority [3].

Various data sources must be considered and analyzed to support epidemic management. These sources can be categorized into traditional and contemporary means. The first category involves information that can be found in hospital records, laboratories and research centers, in public health authorities or the World Health Organization (WHO) and in meteorology departments [2]. Medical records are increasingly stored in medical databases and may serve as the basis for data mining. The second category refers to data collected from sensors and biosensors, social media and microblogs, phone calls and internet search queries [2]. For tracking certain behaviors, social media can also provide information that is often undocumented [4]. By implementing techniques like web and text mining on these data, that are mainly semi-structured or unstructured, it is possible to extract valuable information. For this aim, sentiment analysis, which can be described as a process of identification of feelings and emotions from texts, speeches and social media posts can be implemented with a view to revealing hidden facts and evidence. These data can provide past medical information and can also be used for understanding the current medical scenario. Early detection of a disease's activity can reduce its impact.

The advance of new technologies offers rapid identification of epidemics and new methods in predicting, preventing and controlling epidemic outbreaks [5]. There are many approaches that deal with epidemics, such as the use of data mining techniques, hybrid models, and time series analysis [2]. This chapter examines extensively data mining for dealing with epidemics.

Epidemic outbreaks had led the global community to raise concerns over infectious disease management, preventing and handling methods to diminish disease dissemination and to restrict infected areas. Various techniques are used in order to deal with epidemics and forecast their outcomes [6]. The fundamental aim of this chapter is to present an overview of current research involving data mining techniques. A brief summarization of data mining algorithms for classification, clustering, and association rules as well as their respective advantages is also introduced. Finally, several cases in which data mining techniques were implemented with a view to dealing with epidemics are presented.

12.1.1 Goal and Research Questions

The research goal of this chapter is to review the state of the art concerning mining data for epidemics, and experimentally verify the utility of Data Mining for dealing with epidemics. Thus, we focused on three research questions; (Q1): What is data mining? (Q2) Which are the techniques and methods of data mining? (Q3) In which cases of epidemics data mining techniques have been used? The first question aims to provide a brief overview of the term "data mining". The second research question focuses on its techniques and methods and, finally, the last question concentrates on specific case studies in which Knowledge Discovery techniques have been used to deal with several epidemic diseases. We tackle these questions respectively in Sects. 1.1.2, 1.1.3 and 1.3.

The literature survey was conducted by reviewing research publications in the fields of data mining, epidemics, and health care. We shortlisted 108 research articles. After removing duplicates and evaluating the abstract, and the year of publication, the number was decreased to 43. Eventually, after examining the content, we report on 23 articles, while referencing 41 sources in total.

12.1.2 Introduction to Data Mining

Data mining, the core analysis step of Knowledge Discovery in Databases (KDD) is the exploration and analysis of large data sets to discover meaningful patterns by combining methods from statistics and Artificial Intelligence (AI) with database management [7, 8]. The goal is to gain novel insights and innovative understanding of large datasets which can used to support decision making. Data mining can also enable the generation of scientific hypotheses from large experimental data sets and from the literature [9, 10].

It is worth highlighting the relationship between data mining KDD as the two terms have been used interchangeably [9]. A typical KDD process is shown in Fig. 12.1. Based on Fig. 12.1, the KDD process consists of an iterative sequence of steps, as follows [11]:

1. Selection: Selecting data relevant to the analysis task from the database on which exploration is about to pe performed
2. Preprocessing: Removing noisy and inconsistent data, dealing with missing values and so on. As part of exploratory analysis, we often use data visualization techniques such as graphs and plots. These provide a clearer overview of the data and reveal information that is important for understanding the dataset.
3. Transformation: Transforming data into appropriate forms for mining, use dimensionality reduction or other transformation methods
4. Data mining: Selecting a data mining algorithm, which is appropriate to identify and extract patterns in the data.

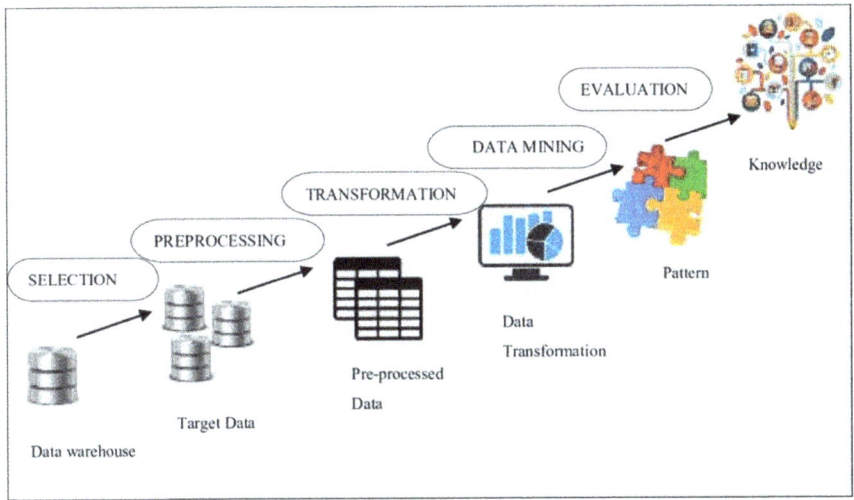

Fig. 12.1 KDD process [11]

5. Interpretation/Evaluation: Interpreting patterns into knowledge by removing redundant or irrelevant ones. Translating useful patterns into terms that are human-understandable. This step can also involve visualization techniques and offers an enhanced explanatory data analysis. These techniques are often embedded in dashboards that assist understanding the extracted information.

Data mining was firstly introduced in 1990s as a new approach to data analysis and knowledge discovery. It is a combination of old and modern methods, and its purpose is to find patterns which may be hidden in large datasets [12]. The first ACM Conference on Knowledge Discovery and Data Mining was held in 1995 in the USA and the term "data mining" was, initially, registered for the 2010 Medical Subjects Headings in late 2009 [9]. The process roots back to a mixture of machine learning, classical statistics and AI.

Machine Learning is the study of computer algorithms which focuses on making predictions [13]. There are some data mining techniques which are widely used for predicting epidemics. Support Vector Machine (SVM), Naïve Bayes, Decision Trees and Artificial Neural Networks (ANN) are some of the major classifiers used for predicting epidemic diseases such as Ebola and outbreaks of influenza [14].

Statistics is the base of most technologies on which data mining is built upon. Some of the main terms used in data mining are standard variance, regression analysis, cluster analysis, confidence intervals, standard deviation and distribution. All the above "tools" help the data analysis and the identification of patterns and relations [12].

AI uses heuristics to simulate a system. Its behavior attempts to approximate human ability to think and decide on their own [12]. It comprises methods that can modify algorithms and create new ones to provide the ability to computers or robots to perform tasks commonly associated with intelligent beings. AI refers to the simulation of human intelligence by machines that are programmed to think like humans and mimic their actions. The ideal characteristic of AI is its ability to rationalize and take actions that have the best chance of achieving a specific goal [15].

12.1.3 Data Mining Techniques

Data mining algorithms are very effective on complex datasets with a large number of attributes and samples. With respect to knowledge discovery, they explore and explain high-dimensional problems in which traditional statistical methods often fail [16]. Different techniques are needed to find several kinds of patterns. Based on the kind of patterns to be mined, tasks in data mining can be categorized into classification, clustering, association, regression and summarization [17]. All these methods are either predictive or descriptive data mining tasks, as shown in Fig. 12.2 [18].

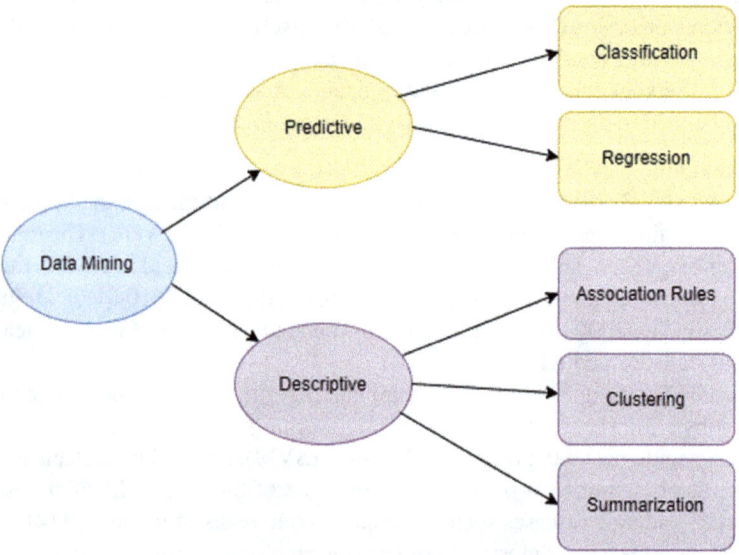

Fig. 12.2 Data mining techniques

12.1.3.1 Predictive Modeling

Predictive modeling is a process of using known variables or fields in the dataset to predict unknown or future values [19]. It is widely known as supervised learning. Such predictive mining tasks are classification and regression.

Classification is one of the main data mining tasks and it in its simplest form is the ordering of data into groups or classes. It predicts categorical class labels, discrete or nominal [20]. It classifies each data point into predefined classes (class label) based on the training set [21]. It is a form of supervised learning, in which the training set is accompanied by labels indicating the class of observations [22, 23]. The difference between clustering and classification is that classification uses predefined classes, while clustering establishes such classes or groups.

Regression is a supervised learning method for predicting numerical values, which can find a function that describes the data. The simplest form of regression is the linear one, which is used to find the line that best fits the data. Linear regression can be done using the least squares method. Non-linear regression is also possible, but it is mostly introduced when the given data are better described using non-linear functions. Examples of non-linear methods are exponential, cyclical, polynomial and Gaussian functions [7].

12.1.3.2 Descriptive Modeling

Descriptive modeling describes the real—world events and relationships between the data points, and focuses on finding patterns [19]. The most common term to describe this type of modeling is unsupervised learning. Some descriptive data mining task are clustering, association rule and summarization.

Clustering is the data mining task which divides the data into groups (clusters) in a way that the data points in the same groups have similar characteristics with each other but are dissimilar to data points in other groups [21]. It is unsupervised learning, as the class labels of training data do not exist and learning is performed by observations and not by examples, as with supervised learning [18]. It involves the identification of groups based on certain characteristics, though without reference to any predefined group information [24].

Association rule mining is another data mining task which aims to find interesting relations between variables in large databases [18]. In particular, this technique finds patterns, associations and correlations and, also, it generates rules among attributes [21, 25–29].

Summarization is the generalization or abstraction of data and it belongs to the unsupervised learning methods. A set of relevant data is abstracted and summarized, resulting to a small subset, which gives a general overview of the data. The most common ways of summarizing data into tables are frequency distribution, relative frequency distribution and relative frequency distribution tables [18]. Some of the prementioned techniques such as classification, clustering and association rules are mainly used to extract knowledge for analyzing and predicting various epidemic outbreaks [21]. These data mining task will be examined in more depth in the next section where real case studies of implementation of the methods are presented.

12.1.4 Chapter Overview

The next section, reviewing the literature, presents various algorithms used for classification, clustering, and association rule mining with a view to deal with epidemics and disease outbreaks. Future extensions could include other popular methods such as summarization and regression. During our preliminary experimentation process the selected dataset proved to be more suitable for the reported data mining techniques. The identified use cases are associated with diseases such as Ebola, Mumps, Measles, Cholera and Dengue fever. Section 1.3 briefly presents our methodology, experimental results are summarized in Sect. 1.4, and finally Sect. 1.5 concludes this chapter.

In general, data mining processes involve, *selection and identification* of correct information sources. Then, it entails *data extraction,* most commonly by utilizing a *database or APIs* for data retrieval. Once data are available, *cleaning, preprocessing and transformation* are performed, which involve dealing with noise, outliers, sampling, missing values, duplicate data and/or aggregation, feature selection, feature extraction, discretization and more. The next step deals with data *analysis, such as classification,* clustering, and association rule mining; depending on the task there are diverse techniques and methodologies. The final step is the *interpretation and evaluation,* which address the visualization of results, attempting to enhance human perception, easing the process of clarification and extraction of valuable/meaningful information, therefore knowledge. Also, experiments are discussed while reporting on methods proven to be informative for knowledge extraction, generating prospects for future work.

12.2 Literature Review

This section contains a description of several case studies. Disease outbreak detection differs from prediction in that the evidence of the incipient outbreak is already present, though, not yet obvious. Thanks to data mining, several epidemics have been dealt with, in order to decrease losses in human life. Researching and forecasting epidemic outbreaks before they happen helps to prevent the epidemic spread and build control mechanisms. In this chapter, some major epidemic outbreaks, which have been handled with the use of data mining, are reviewed.

12.2.1 Dengue Fever Analysis and Prediction with Classification and Association Rules

Dengue is an acute febrile disease of humans caused by a single-stranded RNA flavivirus transmitted by mosquitoes. These mosquitoes thrive in tropical urban areas by breeding in uncovered containers capable of holding rainwater, such as tires, buckets and flower pots [30]. This is the main reason why its appearance is more often and severe in tropical climate countries, such as Malaysia, Indonesia and Thailand [31].

The first case study focuses on discovering a predictive model for detecting a dengue outbreak, based on classification techniques. The dataset used, was collected from the Public Health Department, Selangor State. The selected attributes are year, week of the year, cumulative week from year 2003 till 2010, number of dengue fever incidents for current week, number of dengue hemorrhagic fever for current week, total number of cases in current week, maximum, minimum and average temperature value, humidity value, rainfall, month, age, sex, race, work, address, district office in charge, district and outbreak [31]. The case study uses two classes, the "existence of outbreak" class and "non-outbreak" class [31].

The target class is the outbreak attribute, which is produced by calculating the average of dengue cases over the previous and current week, and compare these values with the number of current dengue cases. If the value of cases for the current week is higher than the previous, then it is classified as an outbreak (1), otherwise it is classified as a non-outbreak (0). The data classified as outbreak (1) comprise 3087 cases and 2894 non-outbreak (0) [31].

Three classifiers were used to achieve better accuracy. The first was a Decision Tree Classifier, categorizing data in the form of a tree structure. The second was a Neural Network, the Multilayer Perceptron Network (MLP), mapping input data into the appropriate output and adjusting the weights. The last was based on Rough Set Theory, in order to deal with uncertain, noisy and incomplete data. Moreover, the tenfold cross validation (10—CV) method was applied, in which the dataset was split into test set and train set in percentages of 10% and 90% respectively, performing 10 iterations, to ensure that results are not random [31]. All models resulted in good performance using accuracy (ACC), ROC curves, MSE (Mean Square Error) and F-score as metrics for evaluation [31].

The second case tries to predict a dengue outbreak by describing a novel prediction method which utilizes Fuzzy Association Rule Mining (FARM) to extract relationships between clinical, meteorological, climatic, and socio-political data from Peru in the form of rules [30]. The data were obtained from the Peruvian Ministry of Health and only cases marked as "probable" and "confirmed" were included. The main attributes considered were the rainfall rate, temperature, altitude, and demographics. The next step was to extract rules from data using FARM, automatically build classifiers and select the best one based on performance.

The automated method built three different fuzzy association rule models predicting incidents as "no outbreak" and "outbreak" for the future [2]. It produced a dengue outbreak prediction four to seven weeks in advance, giving the opportunity to public health officials to mediate and perhaps mitigate its repercussions on time [30]. In general, the study results in the assumption that the approach could be extended for other geographical regions and other environmentally influenced infections, since the variables used are widely available for most, if not all countries.

12.2.2 Mumps Analysis with Clustering and Association Rules

In this case study, both clustering and association rules have been applied, to develop a better epidemiological model for mumps and help epidemiologists predict future outbreaks [32]. The case is illustrated through a study of the mumps virus in Scotland, in years 2004–2015. Mumps is a contagious disease which is caused by a virus, causing swelling of the parotid salivary glands in the face, and a risk of sterility in adult males. Despite the existence of vaccines, mumps is still dominant throughout the world [32].

The dataset used, consisted of mumps cases in Scotland from 2004 to 2015 and the selected attributes were age, sex, NHS Board, year, week, report date and MMR status (measles—mumps—rubella). The data were preprocessed, so that unknown and missing values were replaced by the median ones [32].

The first method used, was clustering with a view to choosing optimal parameters and features and improving the model structure. The aim of clustering was to group individuals with similar features, based on the infected cases [32]. The algorithm used, was K-means and the number of clusters defined, was two. By plotting the week attribute versus the MMR status attribute, it was observed that most of instances have been clustered from week 1 to week 26 and from week 41 to the last week of the year [32].

As the clusters were defined, association rules were applied to each cluster to understand and identify the common features in each cluster. The algorithm used, was Apriori. Applying Apriori, the study presented the existence of strong correlations among seasonality, MMR vaccination and age [32].

12.2.3 Cholera Analysis with Classification and Association Rules

This case study concentrates on detecting risk areas of cholera in Mopti region, Mali (West Africa), along the Niger River [20]. The database related to the risk areas, was combined with environment, climate and health data. Cholera is a contagious epidemic disease, often fatal, usually caused from infected water supplies. The case study's vision was to determine the impact of the Niger River on the cholera epidemic during rain periods [20].

Firstly, classification was introduced, applying the K-Nearest Neighbor (KNN) algorithm, to categorize the observations between the two target classes, the "existence of risk areas" and "no risk areas". After classification, Association rules were generated by Apriori which concluded that the level of Niger River has an impact on the variation of cholera epidemic rate in Mopti [20]. In particularly, it was presumed that the higher the river level was, the higher the water was contaminated. In addition, it was also conducted that when the confirmed cases were low, then, the risk area was also low [20].

12.2.4 Measles Analysis with Classification

Measles is a high contagious disease caused by Morbilivirus. The symptoms are fever, cough, runny nose, and inflamed eyes. It infects only humans who have not been vaccinated [19]. The World Health Organization (WHO) estimates that measles in one of the biggest epidemic killer, as 1.6 million people die from measles each year in developing countries. The goal of this case study was to predict the occurrence of measles outbreaks in Ethiopia, using data mining techniques [19]. The required data were collected from the WHO measles database, covering the period from 2006 to 2011. The initial dataset consists of 26,103 records and 44 attributes. After preprocessing, it was reduced to 15,631 records and 9 attributes [19]. The selected attributes are Datatype, Provinceofresidence, Sex, Vx_Status, Season, Urbanrural, Age_Cat, Measlesigm and Outbreak. The target class is the outbreak attribute, which indicates the existence of measles in Ethiopia [19].

The algorithms used were J48 decision tree (C4.5) and Naïve Bayes in order to acquire high levels of accuracy. The experiments for both algorithms were conducted using 70% split options and tenfold cross validation. Then we compared the results of these two methods. For J48 the 70% split test method led in slightly better accuracy reaching a score of 97.06%. The model presented a great performance and tended to be statistically significant. Thus, it is evident that in general, the selected attributes play, an important role in prediction [19]. Furthermore, for Naïve Bayes, a different number of attributes was tested, again using both 70% split option and tenfold cross validation. The best performance was achieved using 9 attributes and 70% split test options, reaching 93.1% accuracy [19].

To sum up, the overall score of J48 decision trees (C4.5) including accuracy, sensitivity and area under the ROC curve was higher than the score of Naïve Bayes, which constitutes a better model for the specific experiment. The study concludes, that, in case the accuracy is really high, it is feasible to predict the occurrence of measles outbreaks in different Ethiopian Regions and as a result prevent the spread of measles [19].

12.2.5 Ebola Analysis with Clustering

Ebola is an infectious and frequently fatal disease. The virus can be transmitted when someone contacts contagious people's fluids, such as blood, faeces and vomit. The fatality rate of Ebola ranged from 25 to 90% in previous outbreaks. In 2014, a huge Ebola outbreak spread out in West Africa. Generally, the most affected countries are Guinea, Sierra Leone and Liberia [33].

The researchers, in this case study, used K-means clustering, to understand the spreading process during the outbreak and detect the geographic pattern of an Ebola epidemic from 1 January 2014 to 30 March 2016 [33]. Particularly, the data points were categorized into 15 clusters, in which the size of the cluster corresponded to the number of districts, which suffered from Ebola. These clusters varied in size. Plotting the geographical space versus the timeline attribute indicated that Sierra Leon had the most observed Ebola cases, as well as the highest relative risk [33].

To conclude, this case study presented a framework that examines Ebola outbreak patterns from 2014 to 2016. This framework aimed to help minimizing the mortality of Ebola outbreaks and deal with other epidemics in the future [33].

12.3 Methodology

Having reviewed several prominent case studies in the literature, we decided to engage in predictive analytics, such as classification, as well as descriptive analytics, such as association rule mining and clustering, widely used in healthcare and medicine, either for predicting outbreaks or for extracting usable information from healthcare and medical data.

12.3.1 Methodology Outline

We conducted experiments on a dataset extracted by the UCI Machine Learning Repository regarding hepatitis. The aim is to inform the reader about a wide range of available options regarding data mining techniques, while enabling knowledge extraction from healthcare data.

The experiments showcase classification using a variety of algorithms, as well as clustering and association rule mining with different parameters. Classification was performed with Decision Trees, K-NN, Random Forest, Naïve Bayes, Deep Learning, Gradient Boosting and Voting classifier; we report the results for comparative reasons. Clustering experimentations included, K-Means, Expectation Maximization Clustering, DBSCAN and K-Medoids with a variety of distance calculation measures, such as Euclidean Distance, Canberra Distance, Inner Product Similarity and Manhattan Distance. Association rule mining was performed using FP-Growth; we report strong rules based on support and confidence values.

12.4 Experiments

12.4.1 Dataset

The dataset is about hepatitis and it was selected from the UCI Machine Learning Repository. It contains 155 instances and 20 attributes, mostly categorical some integer or real. Our aim was to determine whether the person lives or dies. So, the class attribute is binary, corresponding to live or die. 32 instances belong to the "die" class and 123 to the "live" class. For experimentation we used RapidMiner.

12.4.2 Classification

The first step was to import the dataset and preprocess it in a way that all polynomial attributes were transformed into integers, and missing values replaced by either the average feature value in the case of numerical ones, or the mode value in the case of categorical ones. Furthermore, in order to perform classification, we changed the target class from integer to string, so as the type would be nominal. After that, classification was implemented to test the accuracy of predicted values. Figure 12.3 presents the process of the Decision Tree Classifier.

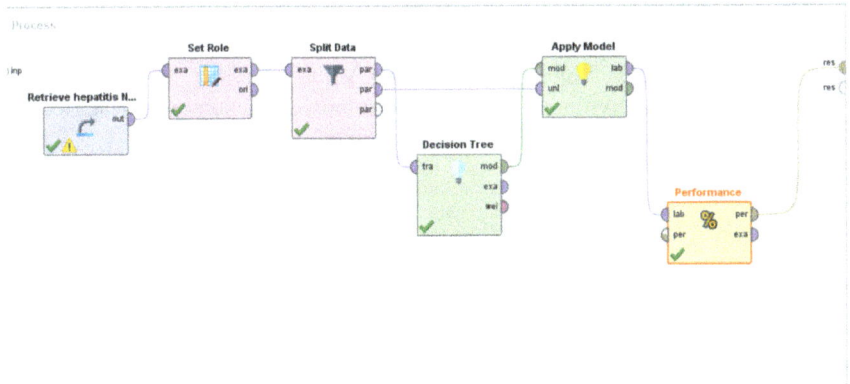

Fig. 12.3 Decision tree classification flow example

Table 12.1 Classifier accuracy

Classifier	Accuracy with fivefold cross-validation (%)	Standard deviation (%)	Squared error
Decision trees	79.65	±3.90	0.185 ± 0.040
K-NN	75.97	±7.43	0.196 ± 0.040
Random forest and random tree	**81.52**	±4.40	0.112 ± 0.021
Naïve Bayes	72.34	±15.88	0.255 ± 0.152
Deep learning	**83.38**	±3.86	0.140 ± 0.012
Gradient boosted trees	78.70	±4.08	0.144 ± 0.011
Voting classifier	**83.29**	±6.32	0.125 ± 0.045

The next step was to implement a 5-k fold cross validation and test different models. The performance of each classifier was measured in terms of accuracy. Accuracy is the ratio of true positives and true negatives divided by the total instances. This means that the accuracy shows the total number of instances that have been correctly classified by the trained classifier when tested with unseen data [34]. The formula of accuracy is:

$$Accuracy = (TP + TN) / (TP + FP + TN + FN) \tag{12.1}$$

where TP (true positive) shows a correct positive prediction of "die" class, TN (true negative) occurs when a person is correctly classified as "live" class, FP (false positive) shows the false prediction when a healthy patient is predicted to have died from hepatitis, and FN (false negative) is the worst-case decision where a patient who died from hepatitis is assigned to the "live" class [34].

The models we tested are: Decision Trees, K-NN, Random Forest, Naïve Bayes, Deep Learning, Gradient Boosted Trees and a Voting classifier, which combines the best performing algorithms. Their results in terms of accuracy for each of the algorithms are depicted in Table 12.1, with the top three values in bold.

12.4.2.1 Decision Trees

Decision Tree is a model that generates a tree-like structure that represents a set of decisions. It can be used to resolve both classification and regression problems. The method of "divide and conquer" is applied to construct a binary tree. The variable for the root node is selected based on its predictive significance represented by its p-value and the tree is divided into sub-trees. Next, following the same procedure the sub trees are further separated until the leaf node is reached. After the construction of the tree, rules can be extracted by crossing over each branch of the tree [34].

12.4.2.2 K-NN

K-Nearest-Neighbor (KNN) was originally introduced by Drs. E. Fix and J. L. Hodges Jr, in an unpublished technical report written for the U.S. Air Force School of Aviation Medicine [35]. KNN is the simplest supervised learning algorithm and it is a non-parametric method used both for classification and regression. It belongs to the category of "lazy" algorithms [36]. KNN mostly measures the difference or the similarity between two instances x and y by computing the distance using Euclidian, Manhattan or Minkowski measures for continuous variables and hamming for categorical variables. The most popular distance function, the Euclidean distance d (x, y) is:

$$d(x, y) = \sqrt{\sum_{i=1}^{n}(a_i(x) - a_i(y))^2} \tag{12.2}$$

KNN calculates the minimum distance from the query point instance to the train data, with a view to determining its K-nearest neighbors. There are many ways of selecting the k-value, but the simplest one is to run the algorithm many times with different k values and select the one with the greatest accuracy [37]. It only stores instances of the training data in the feature space, and the class of an instance is determined based on the majority votes from its neighbors. An instance is labeled with the class most common among its neighbors [38].

12.4.2.3 Random Forest

Random forests (RF) are an ensemble learning technique that can support classification and regression. They consist of multiple individual decision trees which are created randomly. Random forest searches for the best feature among a random subset of features in order to use it as a splitting criterion for each node. To classify an instance, each tree in the forest votes for a class, then the votes of different trees are integrated, and a class is predicted for each sample. The model chooses the class that has receive the most votes over all the trees in the forest [39]. One major advantage of this model over traditional decision trees is that it overcomes the problem of overfitting and delivers high performance and prediction accuracy. During training, the algorithm constructs many individual decision trees. Predictions from all trees are pooled to make the final prediction, which in the case of classification is the mode of the classes. As they use a collection of results to make a final decision, they are referred to as Ensemble techniques [38].

12.4.2.4 Naïve Bayes

Bayes theorem provides a way to calculate the probability of a hypothesis based on its prior probability, the probabilities of observing various data given the hypothesis, and the observed data itself. Naïve Bayes is a probabilistic algorithm based on Bayes theorem that can be used in a variety of classification tasks. It adopts the idea of complete variables independence, which means that the presence or absence of one feature is unrelated to the presence or absence of the others. It considers that all attributes independently contribute to the probability that the instance belongs to a certain class and bases its predictions for new instances based on the analysis of their ancestors. The model outputs a probability score, which shows that the observation belongs to a certain class [38].

12.4.2.5 Deep Learning

Deep Learning is based on Artificial Neural Networks and is inspired by the human brain. It is a function that processes data and creates patterns for use in decision making. Learning can be supervised, semi-supervised or unsupervised. Deep learning involves a set of models built using neural networks. A neural network takes in inputs, which are then processed in hidden layers using weights that are adjusted during training. Then the model produces a prediction.

12.4.2.6 Gradient Boosting

Boosted trees is a powerful ensemble-based supervised learning predictive technique, based on boosting. It converts a set of weak learners into a stronger learner. The idea is to build models from individual "weak learners" in an iterative way with a view to performing better than random guessing. As weak learner we consider any algorithm that can perform at least a little better than random solutions. In boosting, the individual models are built sequentially by putting more weight on instances with wrong predictions and high errors. Gradient Boosting focuses on the instances which are hard to correctly predict. Then use the strong learner's remaining errors (pseudo-residuals) to train the model so that it can learn from past mistakes. In Stochastic Gradient Boosting we train each ensemble on a subset of the training set, which can help improve model generalizability. The gradient is used to minimize a loss function. In each round of training, a weak learner is built, and its predictions are compared to the expected correct outcome. The distance between prediction and truth represents the error rate of the model. These errors can now be used to calculate the gradient [38].

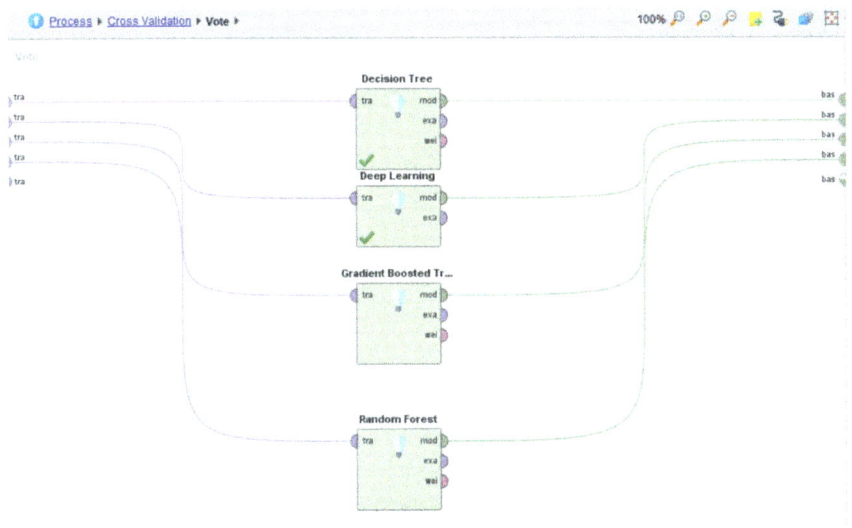

Fig. 12.4 Ensemble learning example

12.4.2.7 Voting Classifier

It is a combination of predictions of learning models. This algorithm typically uses a standard method, such as a tree classifier and categorizes each observation to the class receiving the largest number of votes or predictions. The process is depicted in Fig. 12.4.

12.4.3 Clustering

Clustering is the data mining task which divides the data into groups (clusters) in a way that the data points in the same groups have similar characteristics with each other but are dissimilar to the data points in other groups [21]. It is unsupervised learning, as the class labels of training data do not exist and learning is performed by observations rather than examples, as in supervised learning [18]. It involves the identification of groups based on certain characteristics, without reference to any predefined group information.

12.4.3.1 1st Experiment

Clustering was implemented to the dataset, as depicted in Table 12.2, in order to construct groups with similar characteristics. First, the hepatitis dataset was imported to RapidMiner and underwent cleaning. We selected auto cleansing for removing low

Table 12.2 Dataset overview

Class	Att2	Att3	Att4	Att5	Att6	Att7	Att8
2	30	2	1	2	2	2	2
2	50	1	1	2	1	2	2
2	78	1	2	2	1	2	2
2	31	1	?	1	2	2	2
2	34	1	2	2	2	2	2
2	34	1	2	2	2	2	2
1	51	1	1	2	1	2	1

quality columns and replacing missing values. Then, attributes with two values, 1 and 2, indicating yes and no respectively, were defined as categorical. All in all, only the second attribute was numerical, all others being categorical.

Then, we created the clustering flow, as shown in Fig. 12.5. To begin with, the class attribute was removed because we wanted to perform clustering, which is unsupervised learning. Then, the categorical values were converted to numerical ones because it is not feasible to calculate Euclidean distance having the categorical values as parameters. The data were normalized so as to achieve equalization of the range and data variability.

To find the optimal parameters for our model, we used the 'Optimize Parameters (Grid)" operator. We selected to optimize the number of clusters, k, and the measures to use. The measures selected were Euclidean Distance, Canberra Distance, Inner Product Similarity and Manhattan Distance. We see that the optimized value for k is 8 (Table 12.3), although we know that the number of classes is two: live and die.

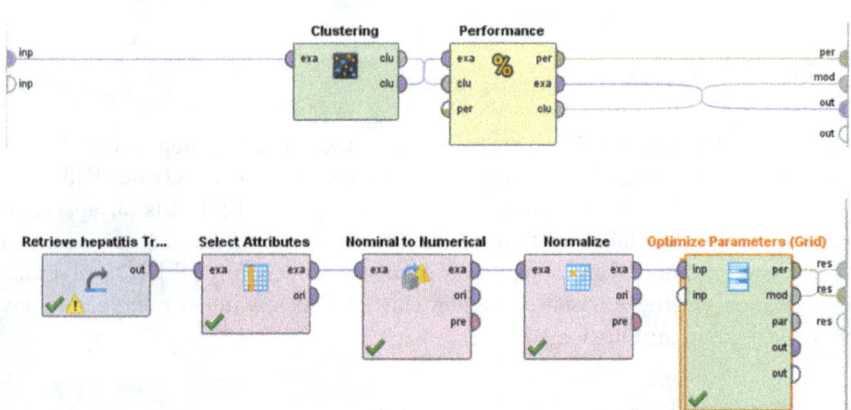

Fig. 12.5 Clustering flow

Table 12.3 Clusters for the 1st experiment

Cluster	Items
0	30
1	27
2	56
3	16
4	1
5	15
6	4
7	6
Sum of items	155

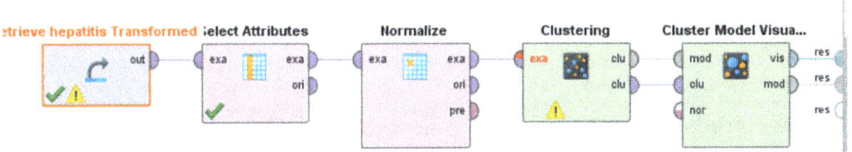

Fig. 12.6 Clustering flow using MixedEuclidean distance

Table 12.4 Cluster for the 2nd experiment

Cluster	Items
0	61
1	94
Sum of items	155

12.4.3.2 2nd Experiment

Knowing the right answer, that the number of classes is two, we set k = 2. Inside the clustering operator, on the measure type, we set the MixedMeasures parameter as there are categorical, real and integer values and the selected measure to calculate the distance between the data points is the MixedEuclideanDistance, shown in Fig. 12.6.

The result shows that the data are divided into two clusters, with cluster 0 consisting of 61 items and clusters 1 of 94 (Table 12.4). However, we know that the die and live class comprise 34 and 123 cases respectively.

12.4.3.3 3rd Experiment

To achieve a better result, we applied PCA for removing variables that may be less useful. PCA is a useful technique for the compression and classification of data, which aims to reduce the number of dimensions, without much loss of information

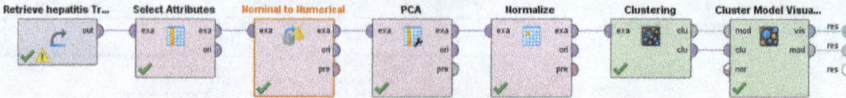

Fig. 12.7 Clustering flow using PCA

Table 12.5 Clusters for the 3rd experiment

Cluster	Items
0	37
1	118
Sum of items	155

[40]. Indeed, the distribution of data points into the clusters is really close to the original one, as shown in Fig. 12.7 and Table 12.5.

12.4.3.4 4th Experiment

Finally, we applied different types of clustering algorithms, using the flow in the 3rd experiment. Results are shown in Table 12.6.

To conclude, k-means algorithm is the most valid as it approximates the original class distribution of the data. Class die comprises 34 cases and the live class 123. Applying PCA, normalizing the data and performing k-means, cluster 0, which corresponds to the class die, consists of 37 items and cluster 1, which corresponds to the class live, consists of 118 items. For the sake of brevity, we omit other common clustering algorithms such as hierarchical clustering. Our scope is to present representative and diversified results based on our dataset. Also, clustering algorithms were executed using the default parameters, as presented in the official documentation of RapidMiner.

Table 12.6 Clustering model types

Clustering algorithm	Cluster model
K-means	Cluster 0: 37 items Cluster1: 118 items
Expectation maximization clustering	Cluster 0: 106 items Cluster1: 49 items
DBSCAN	Cluster 0: 3 items Cluster1: 152 items
K-medoids	Cluster 0: 56 items Cluster1: 99 items

12.4.4 Association Rule Mining

The next step was to apply association rule mining to the dataset after creating a subset of only the categorical values, with a view to finding patterns that connect certain characteristics with each other. Association rule is a data mining task which aims to find interesting relations between variables [21]. In particular, this technique finds patterns, associations and correlations and, also, it generates rules [21]. Figure 12.8 shows the procedure we used. We utilized FP-Growth for frequent item extraction and tested different levels of support and confidence.

An example of the rules extracted with support = 70% and confidence = 80% is depicted in Table 12.7. 10 rules were created, and it is important to explain that

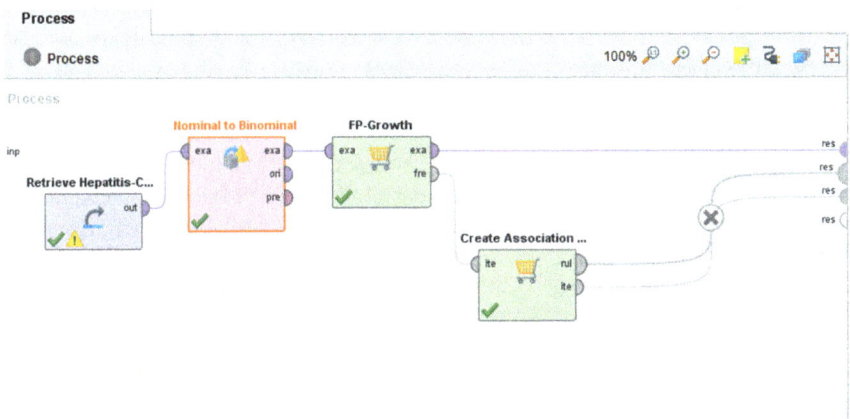

Fig. 12.8 Association rules flow

Table 12.7 Association rules with minimum support = 70% and confidence = 80%

Premises	Conclusion	Support	Confidence
SEX = 1	VARICES = 2	0.761	0.849
SEX = 1	ANTIVIRALS = 2	0.768	0.856
ASCITES = 2	SEX = 1	0.742	0.885
ANOREXIA = 2	SEX = 1	0.703	0.893
ANOREXIA = 2	VARICES = 2	0.703	0.893
VARICES = 2	SEX = 1	0.761	0.894
SPLEEN PALPABLE = 2	SEX = 1	0.703	0.908
ANTIVIRALS = 2	SEX = 1	0.768	0.908
VARICES = 2	ASCITES = 2	0.774	0.909
SPLEEN PALPABLE = 2	VARICES = 2	0.710	0.917
ASCITES = 2	VARICES = 2	0.774	0.923

Table 12.8 Association rules for different support and confidence levels

Support (%)	Confidence (%)	Number of association rules
50	70	505
50	80	294
50	90	86
60	70	105
60	80	62
60	90	16
70	70	13
70	80	10
70	90	2

the sex attribute has value 1 for men and 2 for a women. All other attributes are also binary with values "no" and "yes", so, in order to create rules, the existence of each one is possible when its value is "yes" or 2.

In Table 12.7, we can see different examples of rules for various values of support and confidence. Support is an indication of how frequently an itemset appears in the dataset. Confidence demonstrates the number of times the "if—then" statements are true. Table 12.8 shows the number of Association Rules available based on various support and confidence levels.

12.5 Conclusion

This chapter provides an extended description of the main data mining techniques which can be categorized in predictive and descriptive analytics. After examining each one in detail, a literature review was contacted with a view to highlight some of the most popular cases where data mining has been used to identify epidemic outbreaks.

A real medical dataset was tested by data mining techniques to validate if the methodology can result in valuable conclusions. Classification, clustering and association rules were utilized. Valuable information was obtained from classification and Deep Learning in particular, which achieved an accuracy score of 83.38%. Clustering was unable to discriminate properly between the two cases of the dataset so it was not considering an appropriate technique for the particular project. Lastly, with association rule mining we were able to identify valuable relationships between the attributes of the dataset and spot how one attribute can impact the other regarding hepatitis.

12.5.1 Discussion

The most important challenge relates with the choice of dataset that involves many missing values. Most of the algorithms provided by RapidMiner were unable to operate on such a dataset, necessitating cleaning and preprocessing. In particular, we dealt with missing values, duplicates, data feature selection, data feature extraction and data transformation.

Classification was the most appropriate method for our dataset because the main challenge was to predict if somebody is infected by hepatitis or not. After applying seven classifiers, the Deep Learning approach achieved the highest performance with accuracy equal to 83.38% and standard deviation ranges from -3.86 to 3.86%.

Furthermore, for the application of Association rule mining, we needed to exclude all numerical values with a view to obtaining patterns extracted only from categorical ones. These results may be characterized as unreliable, because many association rules do not logically follow other given association rules. Also, this technique produces various patterns, many of which do not make sense or do not contain the class attribute. Hence, it is difficult to identify and forecast patterns and behaviors about the existence and expansion of hepatitis.

In addition, clustering presents certain weaknesses as it initially generated eight clusters while only two classes exist in the dataset. Thus, we manually adjusted the parameters, so that it created two clusters.

Clustering and association rule techniques concluded to important knowledge assumptions of our data, but the most important task was to find algorithms capable of sufficiently predicting the existence of hepatitis. So, classification is the most appropriate data mining technique for our needs.

12.5.2 Overview of Contribution

In this chapter, we investigated the issue of dealing with epidemics using data mining techniques highlighting their applications for knowledge extraction and management [41] in the domain of healthcare. First, we discussed the background, definitions, and processes of data mining. Then, we reviewed data mining techniques including predictive and the descriptive analytics. Moreover, we identified and examined the most commonly used methods, such as classification, clustering, and association rules, their advantages and drawbacks. The importance of data mining in the study and management of epidemic diseases, such as Ebola, Mumps, Measles, Cholera and Dengue fever was also highlighted. It is safe to conclude that data mining has been widely used in the healthcare and medical fields. This showcases the descriptive and predictive power of analytics which can be utilized to detect and prevent potential epidemic outbreaks.

Furthermore, we tested a real dataset with the data mining techniques in order to examine which were applicable and more efficient. Classification, clustering and association rules were applied to the hepatitis dataset with the help of RapidMiner.

12.5.3 Future Directions

There are several aspects of our research which need further exploration. First, more datasets regarding medical data can be examined with a view to improving outcomes. Furthermore, more metrics can be used in the case of classification to identify the best performing model.

In addition, the prediction of the epidemics' dissemination could be more efficient if sentiment analysis of microblogging data, such as Twitter is performed. The identification of epidemics-related posts may contribute to detection, mitigation and prediction of epidemics as well as the prevention of multiple deaths. Also, it would be more informative if we could associate geographic information with each post. Thus, the combination of classification and sentiment analysis increases the possibility of detecting epidemic outbreaks in short term.

References

1. Ibrahim, N., Akhir, N.S.M., Hassan, F.H.: Predictive analysis effectiveness in determining the epidemic disease infected area. AIP Conf. Proc. **1891**(1), 020064 (2017)
2. Suggala, R.K.: A Survey on Prediction and Detection of Epidemic Diseases Outbreaks (2019)
3. Thapen, N., Simmie, D., Hankin, C., Gillard, J.: Defender: detecting and forecasting epidemics using novel data-analytics for enhanced response. PloS One **11**(5), e0155417 (2016). https://doi.org/10.1371/journal.pone.0155417
4. Ravì, D., Wong, C., Deligianni, F., Berthelot, M., Andreu-Perez, J., Lo, B., Yang, G.Z.: Deep learning for health informatics. IEEE J. Biomed. Health Inform. **21**(1), 4–21 (2016)
5. Christaki, E.: New technologies in predicting, preventing and controlling emerging infectious diseases. Virulence **6**(6), 558–565 (2015)
6. Koukaras, P., Rousidis, D., Tjortjis, C.: Forecasting and prevention mechanisms using social media in healthcare. Adv. Comput. Intell. Healthc. **7**(2020), 121–137 (2020)
7. Leopord, H., Cheruiyot, W.K., Kimani, S.: A survey and analysis on classification and regression data mining techniques for diseases outbreak prediction in datasets. Int. J. Eng. Sci **5**(9), 1–11 (2016)
8. Zhang, S., Tjortjis, C., Zeng, X., Qiao, H., Buchan, I., Keane, J.: Comparing data mining methods with logistic regression in childhood obesity prediction. Inf. Syst. Front. J. **11**(4), 449–460 (2009)
9. Yoo, I., Alafaireet, P., Marinov, M., Pena-Hernandez, K., Gopidi, R., Chang, J.F., Hua, L.: Data mining in healthcare and biomedicine: a survey of the literature. J. Med. Syst. **36**(4), 2431–2448 (2012)
10. Tjortjis, C., Saraee, M., Theodoulidis, B., Keane, J.A.: Using T3, an improved decision tree classifier, for mining stroke related medical data. Methods Inf. Med. **46**(5), 523–529 (2007)
11. Fayyad, U., Piatetsky-Shapiro, G., Smyth, P.: From data mining to knowledge discovery in databases. AI Mag. **17**(3), 37–37 (1996)

12. Liao, S.H., Chu, P.H., Hsiao, P.Y.: Data mining techniques and applications–a decade review from 2000 to 2011. Expert Syst. Appl. **39**(12), 11303–11311 (2012)
13. Murdoch, W.J., Singh, C., Kumbier, K., Abbasi-Asl, R., Yu, B.: Definitions, methods, and applications in interpretable machine learning. Proc. Natl. Acad. Sci. **116**(44), 22071–22080 (2019)
14. Sharma, V., Kumar, A., Panat, L., Karajkhede, G., Lele, A.: Malaria outbreak prediction model using machine learning. Int. J. Adv. Res. Comput. Eng. Technol. (IJARCET) **4**(12) (2015).
15. Rovatsos, M., Mittelstadt, B., Koene, A.: Landscape Summary: Bias in Algorithmic Decision-Making. Centre for Data Ethics and Innovation (2019)
16. Bellinger, C., Jabbar, M.S.M., Zaïane, O., Osornio-Vargas, A.: A systematic review of data mining and machine learning for air pollution epidemiology. BMC Public Health **17**(1), 907 (2017)
17. Sumathi, S., Sivanandam, S.N.: Data mining tasks, techniques, and applications. In: Introduction to Data Mining and Its Applications, pp. 195–216 (2006)
18. Gheware, S.D., Kejkar, A.S., Tondare, S.M.: Data mining: task, tools, techniques and applications. Int. J. Adv. Res. Comput. Commun. Eng., **3**(10) (2014)
19. Assamnew, S.: Predicting the occurrence of measles outbreak in Ethiopia using data mining technology (Doctoral dissertation, Addis Ababa University) (2011)
20. Traore, B.B., Kamsu-Foguem, B., Tangara, F.: Data mining techniques on satellite images for discovery of risk areas. Expert Syst. Appl. **72**, 443–456 (2017)
21. Ahmed, K.P.: Analysis of data mining tools for disease prediction. J. Pharm. Sci. Res. **9**(10), 1886–1888 (2017)
22. Tzirakis, P., Tjortjis, C.: T3C: Improving a decision tree classification algorithm's interval splits on continuous attributes. Adv. Data Anal. Classif. **11**(2), 353–370 (2017)
23. Tjortjis, C., Keane, J.A.: T3: an Improved classification algorithm for data mining. Lect. Notes Comput. Sci. **2412**, 50–55 (2002)
24. Kanellopoulos, Y., Antonellis, P., Tjortjis, C., Makris, C., Tsirakis, N.: k-attractors: a partitional clustering algorithm for numeric data analysis. Appl. Artif. Intell. **25**(2), 97–115 (2011)
25. Ghafari, S.M.; Tjortjis, C. (2019). A Survey on association rules mining using heuristics. WIREs Data Min. Knowl. Discov. **9**(4)
26. Yakhchi, S., Ghafari, S.M., Tjortjis, C., Fazeli, M.: ARMICA-improved: a new approach for association rule mining. Lect. Notes AI **10412**, 296–306 (2017)
27. Ghafari, S.M., Tjortjis, C.: Association rules mining by improving the imperialism competitive algorithm (ARMICA). In: IFIP Proceedings 12th International Conference on Artificial Intelligence Applications & Innovations (AIAI 2016), vol. 475, pp. 242–254. Springer (2016).
28. Wang, C., Tjortjis, C.: PRICES: an efficient algorithm for mining association rules. Lect. Notes Comput. Sci. **3177**, 352–358 (2004)
29. Dong, L., Tjortjis, C.: Experiences of using a quantitative approach for mining association rules. Lect. Notes Comput. Sci. **2690**, 693–700 (2003)
30. Buczak, A.L., Koshute, P.T., Babin, S.M., Feighner, B.H., Lewis, S.H.: A data-driven epidemiological prediction method for dengue outbreaks using local and remote sensing data. BMC Med. Inform. Decis. Making **12**(1) (2012)
31. Tarmizi, N.D.A., Jamaluddin, F., Bakar, A.A., Othman, Z.A., Hamdan, A.R.: Classification of dengue outbreak using data mining models. Res. Notes Inf. Sci. **12**, 71–75 (2013)
32. Hamami, D., Atmani, B., Cameron, R., Pollock, K.G., Shankland, C.: Improving process algebra model structure and parameters in infectious disease epidemiology through data mining. J. Intell. Inf. Syst. 1–23 (2019)
33. Fan, Q., Yao, X.A., Dang, A.: Spatiotemporal analysis and data mining of the 2014–2016 Ebola virus disease outbreak in West Africa. In: Geospatial Technologies for Urban Health, pp. 181–208. Springer, Cham (2020)
34. Mustaqeem, A., Anwar, S.M., Majid, M.: Multiclass classification of cardiac arrhythmia using improved feature selection and SVM invariants. Comput. Math. Methods Med (2018)
35. Kirk, M.: Thoughtful Machine Learning with Python: A Testdriven Approach. " O'Reilly Media, Inc." (2017)

36. Maillo, J., Ramírez, S., Triguero, I., Herrera, F.: kNN-IS: an iterative spark-based design of the k-nearest neighbors classifier for big data. Knowl.-Based Syst. **117**, 3–15 (2017)
37. Guo, G., Wang, H., Bell, D., Bi, Y., Greer, K.: KNN model-based approach in classification. In OTM Confederated International Conference "On the Move to Meaningful Internet Systems", pp. 986–996. Springer, Berlin, Heidelberg (2003).
38. Sabbeh, S.F.: Machine-learning techniques for customer retention: a comparative study. Int. J. Adv. Comput. Sci. Appl. **9**(2) (2018)
39. Nabavi, S., Jafari, S.: Providing a customer churn prediction model using random forest and boosted trees techniques (case study: Solico Food Industries Group). J. Basic Appl. Sci. Res. **3**(6), 1018–1026 (2013)
40. Smith, L.: A Tutorial on PCSA. Department of Computer Science, University of Otago., 12–28 (2006). http://www.cs.otago.ac.nz/research/techreports.php
41. Silwattananusarn, T., Tuamsuk, K.: Data mining and its applications for knowledge management: a literature review from 2007 to 2012. ArXiv, abs/1210.2872 (2012)

Chapter 13
A Powerful Holonic and Multi-Agent-Based Front-End for Medical Diagnostics Systems

Zohreh Akbari and Rainer Unland

Abstract Despite the current hype about the use of decision support systems, especially in more demanding application areas, such systems are not yet popular in the field of medical diagnosis. The reason for this is the usual method of how a diagnosis is achieved. Basically, the process of medical diagnosis consists of two important steps. As a first step, a doctor always tries to gather as much relevant information and data as possible about the patient and their complaints by performing tests, measuring conditions, and using medical equipment. The result is a solid source of information that is used in the second step, the calculation of the medical diagnosis. The first step lays the foundation for a correct diagnosis. The better the data, the better the diagnosis. However, due to the abundance of diseases, there are many possible paths from the beginning of the first encounter with the patient to the end of the data collection. And often this data collection process is already guided by a doctor's suspicion of a particular disease (category). This implies that the two steps for a medical diagnosis are often not consecutive steps, but rather interlock. Very often, after the first step, the diagnosis is already pretty clear. Unfortunately, the state-of-the-art medical diagnostic systems can only be used after the first step has been completed. The very important first step is left to the experience, knowledge, and intuition of the medical staff to complete. That is what this chapter is about. It motivates and introduces an AI-based front-end for medical diagnostic systems that controls and guides the first step of a medical diagnosis, the so-called history and physical examination. Because of the requirements for such a front-end, we concluded that a system that combines the holonic paradigm, multi-agent technology and machine learning technology would best solve the problem at hand. As will be proved in the simulation part of the paper the proposed system is highly adaptive, scalable, flexible, reliable, and robust.

Z. Akbari · R. Unland (✉)
Institute for Computer Science and Business Information Systems (ICB), University of Duisburg-Essen, Essen, Germany
e-mail: rainer.unland@icb.uni-due.de

Z. Akbari
e-mail: zohreh.akbari@icb.uni-due.de

Keywords Decision Support Systems (DSSs) · Differential Diagnosis (DDx) · History and Physical examination (H&P) · Holonic Multi-Agent System (HMAS) · Medical Diagnostics Systems (MDSs) · Swarm Intelligence (SI)

13.1 Introduction

In today's global world, a quick and reliable medical diagnosis is of the utmost importance, as is evident not least from the recent problems with COVID-19, SARS or avian flu (for expansion/explanation of all abbreviations or acronyms in this chapter please refer to Table 13.1). Such highly contagious and fatal diseases pose a serious threat to the world if they are not promptly combated with great efficiency, accuracy, and reliability. Above all, this requires a quick and reliable medical diagnosis, regardless of where the affected person is currently in the world and whether the possible disease occurs frequently in this area of the world, since the locality is less meaningful in a highly interconnected world.

Diagnostic Decision Support Systems (DDSSs) hereafter called Medical Diagnostics Systems (MDSs) for short are a specific type of Clinical Decision Support Systems (CDSSs) that are meant to calculate from a set of collected patient-specific data, and identified signs and symptoms as input an ordered list of potential diagnoses as output. Current state-of-the-art MDSs aim to find the most promising/appropriate link between their health knowledge and the above patient- and complaint-specific data. Thus, before these systems can be used, a physician is meant to collect, derive, and investigate this specific data. Usually, this means that a so-called complaint-directed History and Physical examination (H&P) is performed. This can be seen as a mapping from the starting point (complaint) to the endpoint, which is one instance in the immense set of instances of (existing) diseases.[1] Between the starting point and the set of diseases there is an abundance of paths, each of which describes how the end point was reached from the starting point by taking actions that lead to an increase in data and knowledge about the patient and his/her complaint. This already implies that the conduction of the H&P is a highly sophisticated task, whose correct and comprehensive knowledge and data gathering is of utter importance for the finding of the correct diagnosis.

The H&P is not yet defined precisely in literature. For this paper, we define it as consisting of the following three parts (for a comprehensive description of each part please refer to [1]):

1. Chief Complaint (CC): A concise statement describing the reason for the medical encounter.
2. Medical History(MHx): Comprises all data and information of a patient's key clinical data and medical history that are related to the chief complaint, like History of Present Illness (HPI), Past Medical History (PMH), Past Surgical

---

[1] To be precise it is only a mapping to the data set that is subsequently used to identify the correct disease.

Table 13.1 The list of abbreviations and acronyms

Abb./Acr	Expansion/Explanation	Abb./Acr	Expansion/Explanation
A&P	Assessment and Plan	HQL	Holonic-Q-Learning
AI	Artificial Intelligence	MAS	Multi-Agent System
All/RXNs	Allergies/Reactions	MDP	Markov Decision Process
ANN	Artificial Neural Network	MDS	Medical Diagnostics System
CC	Chief Complaint or Chief Concern	MEDS	Medications
CDSS	Clinical Decision Support Systems	MHx	Medical History
COVID-19	Coronavirus Disease 2019	ML	Machine Learning
CT	Computed Tomography	MLB	Madelung-Launois-Bensaude
DBSCAN	Density-Based Spatial Clustering of Applications with Noise	NLP	Natural Language Processing
DDI	Drug-Drug Interaction	NN	Neural Network
DDP	Disease Description Pattern	NP	Nurse Practitioner
DDSS	Diagnostic Decision Support Systems	PA	Physician Assistant
DDx	Differential Diagnosis	PE	Physical Exam
ECG or EKG	Electrocardiogram	PMH	Past Medical History
EHR	Electronic Health Record	PSH	Past Surgical History
EMR	Electronic Medical Record	RL	Reinforcement Learning
ES	Expert System	ROS	Review of Systems
FH or FHx	Family History	SARS	Severe Acute Respiratory Syndrome
GA	Genetic Algorithm	SH or SHx	Social History
H&P	History and Physical examination	SI	Swarm Intelligence
HMAS	Holonic Multi-Agent System	SVM	Support Vector Machine
HMDS	Holonic Medical Diagnostics System	UML	Unified Modeling Language
HPI	History of Present Illness	WHO	World Health Organization

History (PSH), Medications (MEDS), Allergies/Reactions (All/RXNs), Social History (SH or SHx), Family History (FH or FHx), Review of System (ROS).[2]

3. Physical Exam (PE): Means to measure and examine important vital signs (body temperature, blood pressure, heart rate, respiration rate), perform blood tests, etc. It evaluates the body using observation, palpitation, percussion, and auscultation. Observation includes using instruments to look into your eyes, ears, nose,

---

[2] ROS is an inventory of the body systems that is obtained through a series of questions in order to identify signs and/or symptoms which the patient may be experiencing.

and throat. Comprehensive physical exams, may also include laboratory examination, radiologic studies, Electrocardiogram (ECG or EKG) interpretation, etc.

Some of the above data and information may already be available, e.g., if the patient has been a patient of the doctor for some time already or if the patient has already provided data from other doctors or medical institutions. In addition, some data is often collected by default. All this data and information can be referred to as the starting set for the further execution of the H&P process. The challenge now is to get from this starting set to the final data set in an efficient and goal-oriented manner. This walk is usually steered by performing a so-called Differential Diagnosis (DDx). This is a systematic diagnostic method of identifying the possible disease in the sense that the potential presence of a possible disease or condition can be viewed as a hypothesis that the doctor continues to recursively determine as true or false by collecting additional data and information, which either confirm or weaken or even contradict the original hypothesis. In the latter case, the physician must return to an earlier position within the path in order to choose another transition to another path for a new hypothesis.

From what was explained above it can be implied that in many, usually less complicated cases not only a final set of data and information is achieved but already a pretty stable and sound diagnosis. Only in case that none of the hypotheses of the doctor may have been verified during the H&P process a deeper analysis of the data and the overall health knowledge is necessary. While these exceptional cases are good examples of useful MDS usage, they nonetheless indicate a vulnerability in this late-stage MDS usage, namely MDS only start their work after the complete set of data and information is provided, i.e., after the H&P was finished. Since the complete H&P process is conducted outside of the control of the MDS, they depend entirely on the accuracy, completeness, and appropriateness of these inputs for a correct diagnosis. Therefore, regardless of how powerful they are in finding sound diagnoses a successful use of the MDS completely relies on the data and information gathered during the H&P. Or, to say it the other way round, only a comprehensive and intelligent data and information acquisition during the H&P process paves the way for a solid and successful use of the MDS. And that can best be achieved if the MDS already steers and guides the H&P. However, to the best of our knowledge, up to now no MDS exists that also guides the H&P. They all start with the assessment phase of a diagnosis and may provide treatment plans if a solid diagnosis is achieved. This phase is often called the Assessment and Plan (A&P). The interface between the H&P and the A&P of a MDS is crisp, namely after all data and information was gathered it is not that clear if a doctor has performed a DDx. Here, the doctor already works with hypotheses what implies some kind of assessment is already integrated into the H&P process. This interlocking of H&P and A&P can be seen as a great benefit as it can help steer the H&P process more appropriately. For this reason, the system presented in this chapter mainly focuses on the management and control of the H&P. The difference between state-of-the-art MDSs and our front-end (called the Holonic Medical Diagnostics System (HMDS)) can be seen in Fig. 13.1.

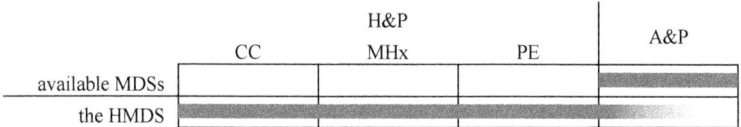

Fig. 13.1 The H&P sections supported by available MDSs and the HMDS

Since the H&P is steered by DDx, during examinations our system will in fact continuously try to improve the ongoing DDx lists (i.e., hypotheses lists). Accordingly, the current system is generally also able to produce acceptable final DDx lists and has the potential to be extended and work as a complete and independent MDS. However, at this stage, we have considered its ability in guiding the H&P as its main goal and have left the design of the necessary ML and NLP algorithms that should be added to the system to support the total coverage of A&P step, as future work. In other words, despite the fact that the system can effectively produce the final DDx in rather straightforward cases, to deal with more complicated cases it still needs to be equipped with additional well-designed ML and NLP algorithms. It should also be noted that this ability also exclusively supports the completion of assessment, and even though having the assessment (i.e., diagnosis), the general relevant treatment plan for this diagnosis can also be provided, the complete implementation of A&P includes considerations such as avoiding negative Drug-Drug Interactions (DDIs). As a result, at this stage, the system can (1) be used as a reminder for physicians and improve the diagnosis by providing immediate second opinions even on signs and symptoms that are to be controlled, or (2) be added as software extension to state-of-the-art MDSs and help them to fit well into clinical workflows. These systems are already equipped with powerful ML and NLP algorithms that are specially designed and tuned over many years for this purpose. Accordingly, especially in complicated cases, this integration would allow the state-of-the-art MDSs to exploit to the maximum their actual potential. In other words, the key to wider adoption of available MDSs is to include DSSs from the beginning of the patient encounter so that they not only cover but, especially, also guide the H&P process.

The proposed system guides the user in performing DDx directed H&Ps. To be specific, it can determine the meaningful data that is to be gathered for an error-free diagnosis (i.e., relevant signs, symptoms, medical test, etc.). Accordingly, as mentioned already, the system is meant to be used by physicians as a supportive tool especially also in more critical cases. However, as the shortage of medical doctors is worsening in many countries worldwide in recent years, if permitted by the health law of the respective country, (experienced) nurses (Nurse Practitioners (NPs)) and/or Physician Assistances (PAs) may also use this system in order to be guided through the efficient and comprehensive completion of the H&P report. This will allow doctors to treat more patients in a certain period of time, as they would just need to review and assess the H&P report. In third world countries where medical treatment facilities might be far away, the user can even be a person with some basic medical knowledge or the patient him- or herself, who may use the system in order to become aware of the possibilities and receive suggestions on finding the right experts to be contacted.

The remainder of this chapter is organized as follows. Section 13.2 provides a brief literature review and an overview about the research domain that motivates our research approach. This is rounded off by a discussion on the state-of-the-art MDSs. Section 13.3 covers the system analysis and design process. For this purpose, first the DDx domain is introduced. As this domain meets the characteristics of holonic domains and consequently our system is implemented as a Holonic Multi-Agent System (HMAS), this section also briefly discusses the underlying features and concepts of HMASs. The second subsection then describes the architecture, functionality, and self-organization of the proposed system. The Machine Learning (ML) techniques that support the functionality and self-organization of this system are then introduced in Sect. 13.4. This is followed by the presentation of the assessment simulations that monitor the diagnosis and learning abilities of the system in Sect. 13.5. Section 13.6 summarizes the importance of this study and proposes ideas for further improvements. Finally, Sect. 13.7 reviews the research motivation, approach, and results.

13.2 State of the Art

In previous decades, medical knowledge has been expanding exponentially. According to [2], the projected doubling time for medical knowledge, which was about 50 years in 1950, is now less than three months. As the trend towards an increasingly digitalized healthcare industry plays a significant role in this expansion, information technology itself can be a solution to this exponential knowledge growth and help the healthcare providers to assimilate and apply this knowledge effectively.

Since the 1950s computer scientists have aimed to support and improve healthcare systems. During these years, this field has explored a wide range of methods, from limited pioneering algorithms to the recent cognitive systems (see Fig. 13.2) (for a comprehensive review on the pioneering methods please refer to [3]). In the early 1970s researchers started to investigate the potential clinical applications of Artificial Intelligence (AI) techniques, which caused significant impact on the improvement in this field. During the 1970s most of the leading research was based on Expert Systems (ESs) [4]. In the 1980s and 90 s, systems based on fuzzy set theory, Bayesian belief networks, and Neural Networks (NN) were developed [5]. With the introduction of the agent concept in 1990 [6, 7] researchers started to combine Multi-Agent System (MAS) technology with the earlier paradigms and designed neural network agents, expert system agents, and data mining agents to tackle the scalability challenge (e.g. [8–10]). This has led to recent development of cognitive systems that rely on a number of AI methods including machine learning, neural networks, Natural Language Processing (NLP), and sentiment analysis to mimic human thought processes [11].

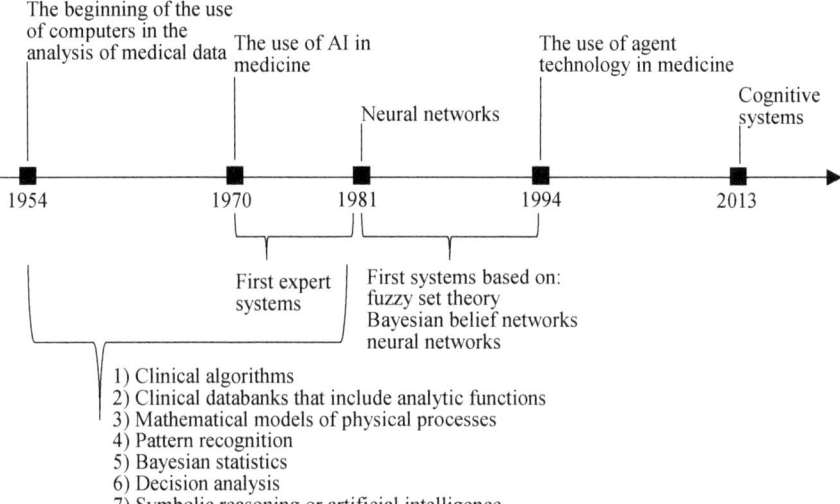

Fig. 13.2 The history of the use of computers in analyzing medical data

According to [12], several limitations in early models prevented a widespread acceptance of AI in medicine. The field also experienced periods of reduced funding and interest during both AI winters, which occurred in 1974–1980 and 1987–1993. In the early 2000s, many of the mentioned limitations were overcome. The successful application of IBM Watson DeepQA in providing evidence-based medicine responses by extracting information from Electronic Medical Records (EMRs) and other electronic resources, along with the improvement of computer hardware and software programs, caused digitalized medicine to become more readily available, and the field started to attract researchers' attention again and grew rapidly.

The book series on advanced computational intelligence in healthcare presents some of the mentioned research results in various categories such as intelligent decision support systems, Virtual Reality (VR) systems for therapeutic purposes, and biomedical informatics [13–19]. Moreover, the proceeding series of annual KES international conference on innovation in medicine and healthcare provide an overview of the latest research in the field since 2013 and may serves as an excellent reference resource for researchers [20–27].

CDSSs are outstanding examples for the usage of computers in medicine. As proposed by Robert Hayward from the Centre for Health Evidence, "Clinical decision support systems link health observations with health knowledge to influence health choices by clinicians for improved health care". Some comprehensive overviews on the CDSSs are presented in [28–30]. As suggested in [28], CDSSs can be categorized into two groups: knowledge-based and non-knowledge-based CDSSs. Knowledge-based CDSSs are rooted in early expert systems and non-knowledge-based CDSSs are based on Machine Learning (ML) techniques. The most remarkable non-knowledge-based CDSSs are based on neural networks and Genetic Algorithms (GAs) [28]. Reviews on the Artificial Neural Networks (ANNs) that are introduced for medical diagnosis purposes can be found in [31–33]. A comprehensive survey on the applications of genetic algorithms in medicine is given in [34].

Some notable examples of CDSSs can be found in Table 13.2. This table sorts these systems according to their release year. As can be seen, early CDSSs were mainly expert systems, however, recent instances are exclusively machine learning systems. As stated in [35], INTERNIST-I alerted the designers of expert systems about the challenges involved in developing expert systems. The abandonment of the development of this system, and the introduction of its successor, i.e., QMR (Quick Medical Reference), marks a change of view on the part of its developers about expert diagnostic consultant systems, which has also influenced other systems that were introduced since then. Due to this change of view of diagnostic consultants, instead of oracles, developers started to design clinician's assistants that manage and augment medical information more efficiently to support their users in reaching correct diagnoses.

As already mentioned in the previous section, an MDS is a specific type of clinical decision support system that is developed to provide an ordered list of potential diagnoses for given signs and symptoms. The physician then takes the suggested diagnoses together with the supportive information and determines which diagnoses might be relevant and which are not, and, if necessary, orders further tests to narrow down this list [28]. In fact, these systems do not aim to replace physicians but to remind them about ignored possible diagnoses. As mentioned already, the input of these systems should include not only the chief complaint but also the information about all relevant signs and symptoms that are needed for the purpose of final DDx. This implies that in order to utilize these systems a physician should first complete the patient's medical record by performing a complaint-directed H&P, which itself is also steered by DDx.

As introduced earlier, the H&P is "a critical component of a patient encounter in which information relevant to the present complaint is obtained, by asking questions about family and personal medical history and the organ systems examined in as great detail as necessary to manage the present condition or evaluate-workup-the patient" [61]. To gather this information a so-called H&P form is used that includes all already mentioned parts of the H&P. This document covers a wide range of signs and symptoms. Knowing what to include and what to leave out is largely dependent on one's knowledge and experience, and here again differential diagnosis concerns could keep the whole process focused.

As the first step in the encounter with a patient, this examination organizes the patient data. Mostly this already allows the physician to narrow down the differential diagnosis list to a few options. Indeed, quite often, upon receiving the chief complaint and slightly more information, the physician will already have an initial differential diagnosis (list) in mind to begin with, which leads to a more focused execution of the H&P. The initial assumption will in the next steps recursively and incrementally be validated, e.g., by requesting and using the results of comprehensive physical exams, also known as executive physicals. They include, depending on the actual

Table 13.2 Notable examples of CDSSs

Ref	System	Discipline / disease	Year	Category
[36]	INTERNIST-I: Rule-based ES	Internal medicine	1974	Expert systems
[37]	CASNET (Causal Associational NETworks)	Glaucoma	1974	
[38]	PIP (Present Illness Program): Medical ES	Edema	1976	
[39]	MYCIN: Rule-based ES	Infectious disease	1976	
[40]	PUFF: an ES for interpretation of pulmonary function data	Pulmonology	1983	
[41]	QMR (Quick Medical Reference)	Internal medicine	1986	
[42]	CADUCEUS: Medical ES	Internal medicine	1986	
[43]	DXplain	Internal medicine	1987	
[44]	Iliad: ES for internal medical diagnosis (teaching tool)	Internal medicine	1991	
[45]	Papnet: a commercial NN-based computer program	Cervical cancer	1991	Machine learning systems
[46]	An ANN for the diagnosis of myocardial infarction	Cardiology	1991	
[47]	ANNs for single photon emission computed tomography	Radiology	1993	
[48]	An ANN for diagnosis of acute pulmonary embolism	Pulmonology	1995	
[49]	Evolving neural networks for detecting breast cancer	Oncology	1995	
[50]	Neuroserum: an artificial neural net-based diagnostic tool	Pathology	1998	
[51]	VisualDx	Internal medicine	2001	
[52]	Isabel	Internal medicine	2002	
[53]	An ANN for diagnosis of heart disease	Heart disease (murmurs)	2006	

(continued)

Table 13.2 (continued)

Ref	System	Discipline / disease	Year	Category
[54]	Intelligible Support Vector Machines (SVMs)	Diabetes mellitus	2010	
[55]	An ANN trained with genetic algorithm	Tuberculosis	2011	
[56]	GA based system for the diagnosis of cervical precancer	Cytology	2011	
[57]	An ANN for automatic diagnosis of small bowel tumor	Small bowel tumor	2012	
[58]	An ANN for diagnosis of Coronary heart disease	Cardiology	2012	
[59]	IBM Watson	Oncology	2013	
[60]	Support vector machines for diagnosis of tuberculosis	Tuberculosis	2017	

context, laboratory tests, chest x-rays, pulmonary function testing, audiograms, full body CT (Computed Tomography) scanning, EKGs, heart stress tests, vascular age tests, urinalysis, and mammograms or prostate exams. However, this process may mean that in case of hypotheses turns out to be less likely a backtracking has to be executed. In general, this also implies, especially in more complicated cases, that the diagnosis process can become very costly. What does this mean with respect to the use of state-of-the-art MDSs in the diagnosis process?

1. The first implication from the above description of the H&P process is that, when a physician performs it and no complications occur, s(he) will reach a diagnosis already. Thus, the later use of an MDS will be of limited value since it will often only confirm what was already assumed. As a result, these systems are especially used in complicated cases where the data gathered in the H&P has not led to a definitive A&P.
2. Secondly, since the available MDSs usually only start their work after all inputs that are necessary from the point of view of the physician, they are prone to irrelevant or missing input. It is always possible that the MDS diagnosis is a misdiagnosis as it was based on less relevant and/or incomplete inputs provided in the first place because the physician may have an incorrect or no specific disease in mind. However, this is particularly unfortunate if the MDS is only used in complicated cases, since the probability that it will not provide a correct diagnosis due to only partially correct inputs is then comparatively high.

The above shortcomings, however, should not be a reason to ignore the benefits of using these systems. In fact, a system capable of undertaking the H&P can be added as a software component to the available MDS and promote the wider use of such systems by filling the gap. Accordingly, the idea of this work is to already involve clinical decision support systems from the very beginning of the patient encounter, which means to not only cover but, especially also, guide the data gathering and computation during the execution of the H&P.

The state of the art of MDSs includes IBM Watson and Isabel. According to [62], Watson is a cognitive system with the capability of understanding natural language. Healthcare was one of the first industries in which Watson was applied [63]. However, not every implementation has gone smoothly [64]. In fact, although Watson is very powerful, as discussed already above, in straightforward cases its usefulness is restricted to just confirming what was already achieved by the physicians through the execution of the H&P. To the best of our knowledge, Watson has never been involved in the initial core medical diagnosis process, but mainly in improving the diagnosis and assisting with identifying treatment options for patients who have already been diagnosed [59].

The second MDS to be considered here is Isabel [52, 65], which is an internet-delivered CDSS that is associated with the highest rates of diagnosis retrieval compared to all other similar tools [66]. The system uses a powerful natural language processing software and a set of algorithms to ensure the relevant output [67, 68]. Using Isabel clinical features are received automatically from the electronic medical records. As a result, here again, the output of the system is very much depending on the output of the H&P.

In this context, it should also be noted that available Electronic Health Record Systems (EHRSs) can capture patient's data, analyze it, and provide insights for clinicians. However, in terms of the H&P they solely provide a digital form and do not guide the user in performing a focused examination. Therefore, it is still the user who has to decide on the right questions and examinations. A few computer programs and mobile applications have been designed that aim to assist their users in performing the H&P, however they are mostly teaching tools and none of them are designed to guide the diagnosis process. Some notable examples of such applications are eH&P™ [69], Smart Medical Apps-H&P [70], Clinicals—History & Physical [71], and the History & Physical Exam pc [72].

As a result, the integration of a system that can guide the H&P into state-of-the-art MDSs can be the key to a wider adoption of these systems. Such a system will act as the missing gear which allows state of the art MDSs to fit into the clinical workflow.

13.3 Differential Diagnosis and the Holonic Medical Diagnostics System (HMDS)

13.3.1 Differential Diagnosis as a Holonic Domain

Even if during a differential diagnosis a disease may have reasonable probability, there are usually a number of other diseases whose signs and symptoms overlap with those of that disease. As a result, enough evidence and supporting information is to be provided to make sure that these diseases have significantly lower probabilities. To diagnose pulmonary tuberculosis, for instance, a group of pulmonary diseases including pneumonia, sarcoidosis, etc., should all be inspected. In many cases there might be different groups of diseases to be considered, which may even be of different granularities or abstraction levels. The differential diagnosis of chronic dyspnea is an example since it can exhibit characteristics ranging from pneumonia to depression (see Table 13.3 [73, p. 174]).

In order to deal with the high complexity of medical knowledge and data in the differential diagnosis process it seems to be reasonable to recursively divide the knowledge from top to bottom into smaller units that concentrate on smaller specific parts of the higher-level knowledge and data. This fits perfectly to how multi-agent systems are meant to work. Agents are meant to be expert on specific areas only

Table 13.3 The differential diagnosis of chronic dyspnea (shortness of breath)

System	Type	Possible diagnosis
Pulmonary	Alveolar	Bronchoalveolar carcinoma, chronic pneumonia
	Interstitial	Drugs (e.g., methotrexate, amiodarone) or radiation therapy, lymphangitic spread of malignancy, passive congestion
	Obstructive	Asthma/bronchitis/bronchiectasis, bronchiolitis obliterans, chronic obstructive pulmonary disease, intrabronchial neoplasm, tracheomalacia
	Restrictive (extrinsic)	Kyphoscoliosis, obesity, pleural disease/effusion, pneumothorax
	Vascular	Chronic pulmonary emboli, idiopathic pulmonary hypertension
Cardiac	Arrhythmia	Atrial fibrillation, inappropriate sinus tachycardia, sick sinus syndrome/bradycardia
	Myocardial	Cardiomyopathies, coronary ischemia
	Restrictive	Constrictive pericarditis, pericardial effusion/tamponade
	Valvular	Aortic insufficiency/stenosis, congenital heart disease, mitral valve insufficiency/stenosis
Gastrointestinal	Dysmotility	Gastroesophageal reflux disease/aspiration, neoplasia
Neuromuscular	Metabolic	Acidosis
	Neurogenic	Amyotrophic lateral sclerosis, muscular dystrophies, phrenic nerve palsy, poliomyelitis
Other	Anemias	Iron deficiency, hemolysis
	Deconditioning/obesity	Sedentary lifestyle
	Pain/splinting	Pleural-based malignancy
	Psychological/functional	Anxiety/hyperventilation, depression

and need to cooperate in order to solve complex problems, i.e., this technology in general has been shown to be highly appropriate for the engineering of open, distributed, and heterogeneous systems. A survey on multi-agent based DSSs for medical classification problems is presented in [74], and some notable multi-agent based MDSs are [9, 75–81].

The distinctive characteristics of the differential diagnosis process and, in particular, its recursive and backtracking-driven problem-solving approach fit very well to the principal working method of holonic multi-agent systems. Such systems combine the concepts of agents and holons.

"An agent is a computer system that is situated in some environment, and that is capable of autonomous action in this environment in order to meet its delegated objectives" [7, p. 4, 82, p. 21]. As stated in [83, p. 64], "A holon is a whole-part construct that is composed of other holons, but it is, at the same time, a component of a higher level holon". As a super-holon they appear to be autonomous wholes for the lower level while, at the same time, as a sub-holon they are a dependent part of the upper level. The organizational structure of a holonic society, or holarchy, is robust, efficient, and adaptable to environment changes [34].

The terms holon and holonic agents are used synonymously in holonic MASs. According to [84], a holonic agent may join several other holonic agents to form a super-holon. This group of agents now act as if it were a single holonic agent with the same software architecture. Accordingly, by super-holon, a composition of subordinate agents, also called sub-holons or sub-agents, are denoted. In contrast to sub-structures in Koestler's framework, in HMASs all entities are restricted to agents, and furthermore, sub-holons should always have the same structure as the super-holons [84].

So far, there have been very few attempts to apply holonic approach to medical systems. The system proposed in [85] is an MDS, however, it applies a completely different approach than that adopted in DDx. Self-organization in this system targets decision-making abilities of the system in finding the right case-based connections between the problem solvers and the decisions on finding the best diagnosis is supported by Bayesian decision-making [86]. The system introduced in [87] aims to implement a remote healthcare system and uses the holonic approach in order to make the collaboration between the remote medical entities possible. Similarly, [88] proposes a holon-based architecture for the hospital information systems and uses the holonic approach in order to manage the information flow to support the administrational needs of hospitals.

As suggested in [84], the holonic approach is well suited for domains that involve operator abstraction, hierarchical structure, decomposable problem settings, higher frequent intragroup communications, social cooperative elements, and bounded rationality. The differential diagnosis domain meets these characteristics:

1. *Operator abstraction*: In a differential diagnosis process different diseases or even different groups of diseases might be considered. As a result, actions can be of different granularity.

2. *Hierarchical structure*: Differential diagnosis is to be conducted on different levels of abstraction. They help the system to be able to react correctly in case of limited information.
3. *Decomposability*: The overall problem of diagnosing a patient's disease can be broken down into sub-problems by weighting the likelihood of the presence of possible diseases.
4. *High focus on intragroup communication*: In order to conduct a differential diagnosis, agents that represent diseases or a group of diseases that cause similar signs and symptoms normally interact more strongly and can therefore be classified into the same super-holons. Holons provide facilities for efficient intra-holonic communication, which means that the system works more efficiently if most of the communication is carried out within holons and not between different holons (inter-holonic communication).
5. *Social Elements*: In order to perform a differential diagnosis, agents need to cooperate. Cooperative elements in the domain can be implemented using holonic agents in order to model the cooperative sub-domain.
6. *Situatedness and real time requirement*: In differential diagnosis, real-time behavior is a vital issue and beside improving the preciseness of the diagnosis, the system is expected to speed up the patient encounter process. The holonic architecture allows the designer to set the requirement of bounded rationality for all members of existing super-holons in order to find the best possible action within a given resource allocation.

In short, the differential diagnostic problem can be recursively broken down into sub-problems by weighting the likelihood of the presence of possible diseases. These subproblems may induce different abstraction levels and can be of different granularities. According to the nature of the problem, the problem solvers are collaborative and those causing similar signs and symptoms need to communicate more, which is to be conducted in timely manner. Accordingly, the differential diagnoses domain clearly meets the characteristics of holonic domains.

In fact, using the holonic multi-agent approach diseases with similar signs and symptoms can be grouped together to form holons and this process can then be repeated with the resulting holons to build additional holons on higher levels of abstraction. This encapsulation then enables the implementation of the DDx, i.e., any holon that has a member which can be viewed as a hypothesis or is involved in the ongoing DDx may suggest the system to differentiate between that member and the rest of its member as they can cause very similar signs and symptoms. To this end, this holon can question the signs and symptoms associated with its members or request medical tests that are carried out for the diagnosis of those diseases. The determination of the exact data required and their order is of course a crucial task that needs to be addressed carefully (for more information please refer to [89]). The next section describes in detail how a holonic multi-agent system can be designed to implement the DDx process.

13.3.2 The Holonic Medical Diagnostics System

The holonic medical diagnostics system consists of two types of agents: comparatively simple Disease Representative Agents or DRAs as the end nodes of the holarchy and more sophisticated Disease Specialist Agents or DSAs as decision makers on the higher levels in between (Fig. 13.3). DRAs are simple atomic agents. Each DRA is an expert on a specific disease and maintains a Disease Description Pattern (DDP), i.e., the holon identifier—an array of possible signs, symptoms, and test results. In order to join the diagnosis process, these agents only need to perform pattern matching (i.e., calculating the Euclidean distance between their DDPs and the diagnosis request description pattern). DSAs are holons consisting of DRAs and/or DSAs that rely on similar signs and symptoms. Based on the holonic approach, these

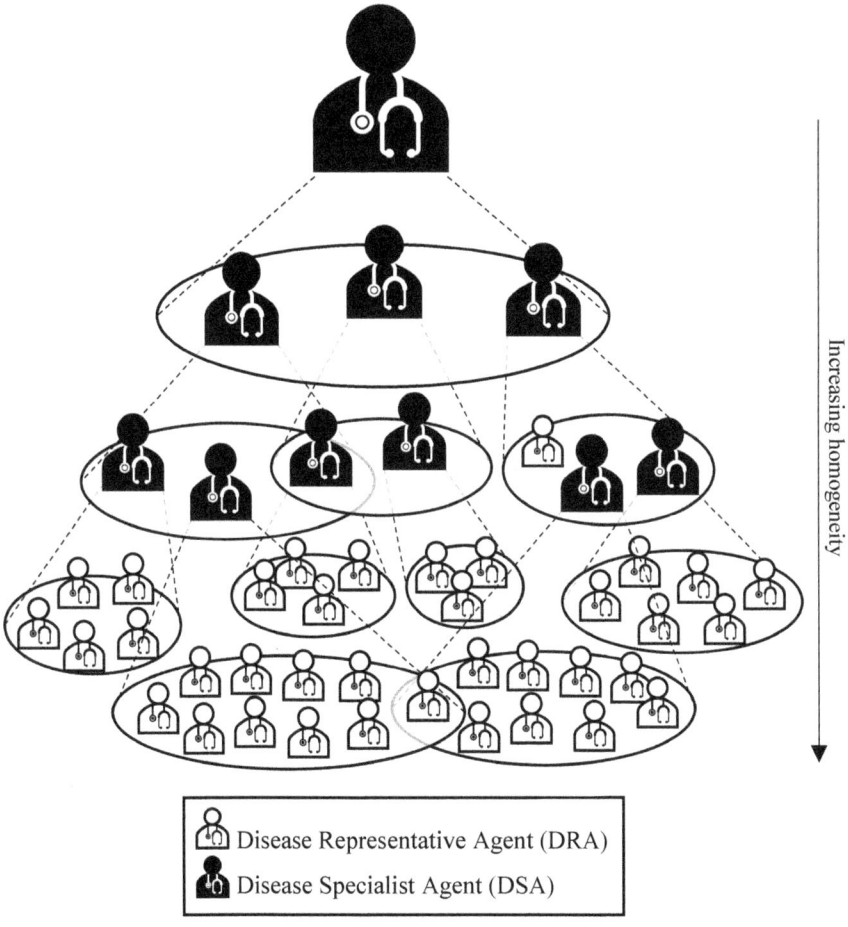

Fig. 13.3 DRAs and DSAs in the HMDS

agents, in fact, encapsulate the agents that need to have more communications for the purpose of differential diagnosis. Their holon identifier is the average of the holon identifiers of their members. The holarchy has one root, the head, which represents, as usual, also its interface to the outside world. The environment for all other holons are their super-holons.

The diagnosis request is received by the head of the holarchy and placed on its blackboard (for more information on blackboard systems, please refer to [90, 91]). Any member of this DSA, can read the messages on this blackboard. A DRA's reaction will be to send back its similarity. However, a DSA may decide to join the diagnosis process or not. The decision is made based on some statistical information about the DSA's members. In case the request is not an outlier, the head will decide to join the diagnosis process. This means that it will place the information on its blackboard, then the same process repeats recursively until the request reaches the leaves. Results and questions obtained by participating agents now flow from bottom to the top of the holarchy and are sorted on their way up according to their similarity. This implies that originally not provided relevant information might be requested from the user in a second step. Figure 13.4 demonstrates the diagnosis process in the HMDS.

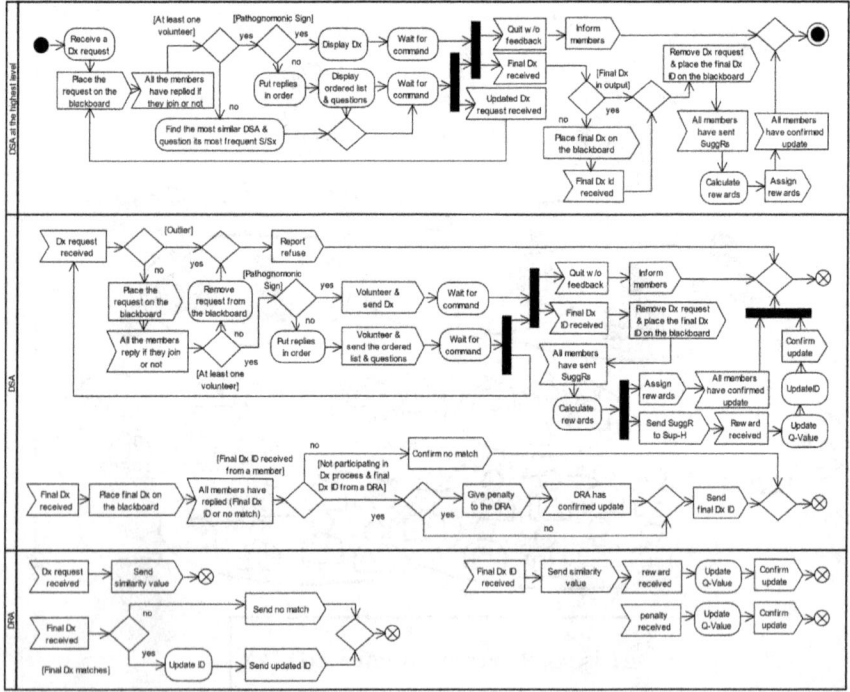

Fig. 13.4 A UML activity diagram demonstrating the diagnosis process in the HMDS

The system orders the diagnoses based on their similarity to the diagnosis request. The frequency of diseases will also be displayed as valuable hints for final diagnosis. These values may also be used to detect possible outbreaks faster. It should be noted that the system does not consider the frequency of diseases as a factor in ordering the top diagnoses, since as a CDSS one of the main goals of this system is to remind the physicians about the critical possible diseases, which could very likely be rare diseases.

As mentioned, the communication between agents is solely done via the blackboards of the DSAs. According to their types, agents in the HMDS also need to save a subset of the following data in their memory: respective signs and symptoms, a list of super-holons and their corresponding Q-values, a list of sub-holons and their corresponding Q-values, diagnosis request, intermediate results of the diagnosis process. In addition, the members of the super-holons need to have access to some of the data kept by their super-holons, and even share some information with the other members of their super-holons. With this regard, the super-holon's functionalities can best be supported by blackboard systems [89, 92].

The system performs clustering in order to build its initial holarchy and then will continuously use Reinforcement Learning (RL) for the purpose of self-organization. Both methods will be introduced in next section. However, in order to describe the self-organization process in the HMDS, it is to be noted that as for reinforcement learning, a specific Q-learning method is proposed and used in this study. Based on this method a value called the Q-value is introduced for each of the connections in the holarchy, which indicates how promising that connection is. To implement the exploration–exploitation trade-off, these values are used. The probability of exploration would be higher if the Q-value is closer to the outlier threshold in its super-holon. The agent starts with the possibility of a guided exploration, which allows an agent to join another DSA with similar interests, i.e., a DSA that has been activated with the agent during the same differential diagnosis process. In case this agent is not an outlier the super-holon will accept its membership and a connection will be granted. If not successful, the agent will then try the random possible vertical and horizontal movements in the holarchy, i.e., random exploration.

13.4 Learning in the HMDS

There are three different reasons to use machine learning in this system. As mentioned earlier, the system should build up its initial holarchy based on the holon identifiers. In addition, the system needs to update its data and reorganize its holarchy according to the feedback. To build up the initial holarchy of the system possible labeled data could have been examples of diseases and their groups together with examples of groups of diseases and their groups on higher levels. As this data is not available, unsupervised learning, namely, clustering is used for this purpose. To update the data, labeled data is available as the system receives feedback, i.e., confirmed cases of different diseases. So, supervised learning, in the form of exponential smoothing is applicable to this problem. To reorganize the holarchy, labeled data is not available. However, it can be obtained in interaction with the environment as agent's actions are rewarded. Therefore, reinforcement learning, in the form of an adapted Q-learning variant is applied for this purpose.

As mentioned, the system uses clustering, in order to establish super-holons. The Density-Based Spatial Clustering of Applications with Noise (DBSCAN) [93] is one of the best algorithms matching this goal. The key idea of this algorithm is that for each point of a cluster the neighborhood of a given radius, i.e., ε, must contain a minimum number of points. So, the clusters are detected by merging the immediate neighboring areas that exceed the given density threshold.

The algorithm is unable to detect clusters that lie too close to each other. Moreover, to detect its input parameter ε, it starts a user interaction based on some graphical representation of the data. For each point the radius that covers the given minimum number of points is calculated and then ε is set as a noise threshold. To improve this algorithm, we made two changes [94]:

1. The negative effect of large values corresponding to border points is eliminated by replacing this value for each point with the smallest radius detected that covers the point, and
2. To automatically detect parameter ε, according to the empirical rule this value has been set to mean plus three standard deviations of the new values.

The second machine learning method used in the system is exponential smoothing, which is used in order to update the disease description patterns. Every time a new case of a disease is diagnosed and then confirmed by the physician using the feedback loop, the system considers the signs and symptoms of the patient to update the corresponding disease description pattern. Using this technique, exponentially decreasing weights are assigned to the past observations and recent ones are given relatively higher weights. As a result, the smoothed disease description pattern is a simple weighted average of the current observation and the previous smoothed disease description pattern.

In the HMDS, the holarchy is in fact keeping track of the best decisions made by the system performing self-organization. This process should also be supported by an appropriate machine learning technique. Given the nature of the problem, the lack of desired input/output pairs, and the accessibility of a dynamic environment, reinforcement learning appears to be the best solution to this problem.

To use this method, the problem is to be modeled as a Markov Decision Process (MDP). MDPs are models for sequential decision-making when outcomes are uncertain [95]. An MDP is a 5-tuple (S, A, T, R, γ), where S is a set of agent-environment states, A is a set of actions the agent can take that cause state transitions based on a probability function T, R is a reward function that quantifies the reward the agent gets for taking each action, and $\gamma \in [0, 1)$ is a discount factor that controls the importance of the immediate reward versus the potential future reward. The solution to an MDP, also called a policy, is described as a function that maps states to actions. The optimal solution maximizes the expected cumulative reward.

In the above-mentioned process of self-organization, the problem is to decide how favorable it is for a holon to be a member of another holon. As the holonic architecture involves nested whole-part structures, this decision includes the evaluation of the quality of the membership of holon's direct and indirect super-holons on intermediate levels. Accordingly, describing the problem as a Markov decision process, the states are the existing holons and the actions are membership trials. Figure 13.5 illustrates how the self-organization process in HMDS has been represent modeled as an MDP. Considering the mentioned guided and random explorations (see Sect. 13.3) actions may also be added or removed from the list of available actions for each agent.

Generally, MDPs are used for homogeneous swarms solving a single problem. As the HMDS is a heterogeneous swarm with shared sub-problems, an extension of MDP introduced in [96] is suggested that is augmented by new element P, which is a

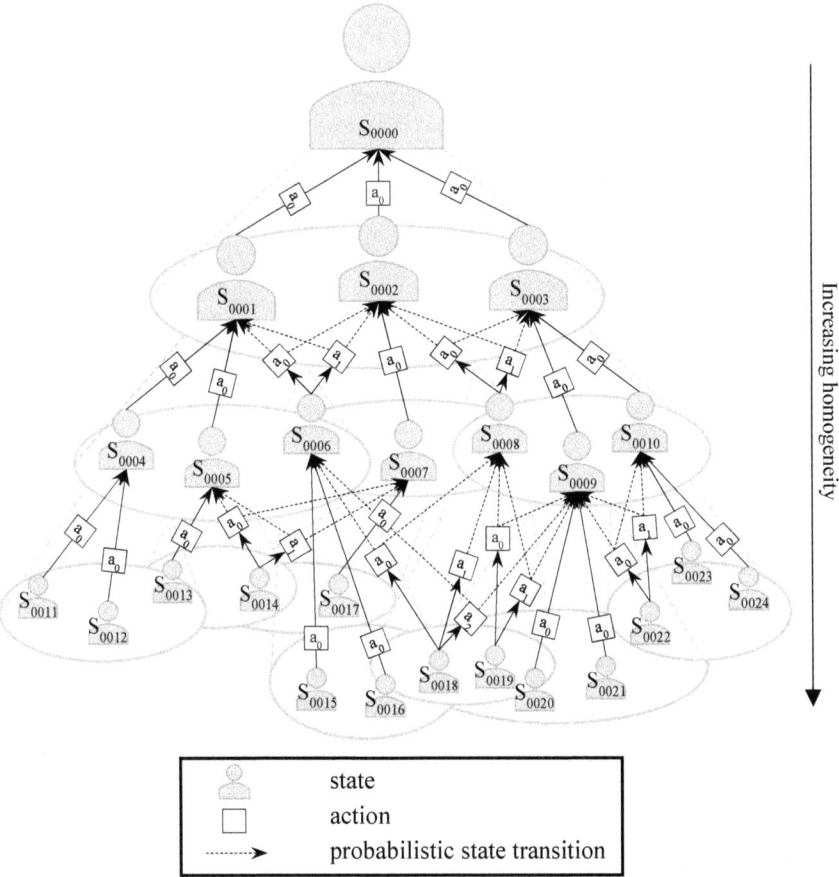

Fig. 13.5 A graphical representation of self-organization in HMDS: dashed arrows indicate probabilistic state transitions for a given action, and black arrows represent actions available in each state

set of profiles that for each state indicates its visitors' collective profile and allows the measurement of the affinity between agents—according to [83] this value describes the compatibility of two holons in working together toward a shared objective. In this representation of the problem, the optimal solution should still only maximize the reward. However, at each time step the best action will be the one that maximizes the reward as well as the affinity simultaneously. Thus, in order to update the Q-value for the estimation of optimal future values the $argmax$ function is used instead of the max function:

$$Q_{new}(s_t, a_t) \leftarrow (1 - \alpha_t) Q_{old}(s_t, a_t)$$
$$+ \alpha_t \left(R_{new}(s_t, a_t) + \gamma \underset{Q_{old}(s_{t+1}, a)}{\operatorname{argmax}} \left(Q_{old}(s_{t+1}, a) \cdot Aff(agtP, P(s_{t+2})) \right) \right) \quad (13.1)$$

For further information on this topic please refer to [96] and [89].

The Holonic-QL (HQL) is a special application of the mentioned Q-learning technique. This method was introduced to realize self-organization in the HMDS [92]. In HQL, the Q-value is in fact measuring how favorable it is for a holon to be a member, i.e., a sub-holon, of another holon. In this case, the states are the existing holons $\{h_i\}$ and $\mathfrak{h}_i$, denotes the associated actions of trying the membership in holon i:

$$Q_t(sub(h), \mathfrak{h}) \leftarrow (1 - \alpha_t) Q_{t-1}(sub(h), \mathfrak{h})$$
$$+ \alpha_t \left(R_t(sub(h), \mathfrak{h}) + \gamma \underset{Q_{t-1}(h, \sup(\mathfrak{h}))}{\operatorname{argmax}} \left(Q_{t-1}(h, \sup(\mathfrak{h})) \cdot Aff(agtP, sup(h)) \right) \right)$$
$$(13.2)$$

where,

$$\alpha_t = \frac{1}{1 + Visits_t(sub(h), \mathfrak{h})} \quad (13.3)$$

$$Aff(agtP, P(h)) = 1 - \frac{d(agtP, P(h))}{\max d(agtP, P(h))} \quad (13.4)$$

In case of a deterministic reward function, the convergence of the Q-learning method can be proven following the same simple approach as the one taken in [97], which uses a theorem on random iterative processes convergence introduced in [98, 99]. For Q-learning methods with nondeterministic reward functions such as HQL method, however, the general convergence theorem for Q-learning method presented in [100] can be adapted.

The terms feedback and reward have different definitions here. A feedback is the final diagnosis, suggested by the physician. However, a reward is a numerical value, which is calculated using a reward function that considers the feedback. As the HMDS is going to be used as a multi-user system in hospitals, the possibility of biased feedback is reduced. Moreover, the system will consider counterfactual learning. Using this method, the physician's diagnosis is given the highest selection probability, i.e., $1 - \varepsilon$, and all the others are ranked and weighted using the softmax rule. For this reason, the most common softmax method, which uses the Gibbs or Boltzmann distribution [101], is used and have been adapted to the problem as follows:

$$p(d_i) = \varepsilon \frac{e^{sim F_i/\tau}}{\sum_{j=0}^{9} e^{sim F_j/\tau}} \quad (13.5)$$

where d_i for $0 \leq i \leq 9$ is a disease in output list of the system, $sim F_i$ is the product of the similarity of d_i to the diagnosis request and the frequency of it, and τ is a positive parameter called temperature. Low temperatures cause a bigger difference in the selection probability of the diseases. ε can be defined in such a way that it grows with an increasing number of diagnoses. And if τ is defined to decrease over time, the system will initially focus primarily on the physician's inputs. However, over time, it tends to trust its own knowledge more and more.

$$\varepsilon = 1 - \frac{1}{number\ of\ diagnoses/c + 1} \quad (13.6)$$

$$\tau = 1 - \varepsilon \quad (13.7)$$

The system can then use this feedback to update the holon identifier of the DRA acting for the final diagnosis, and to calculate the rewards for the RL technique.

The term reward engineering, first coined by Daniel Dewey in [102], refers to the engineering of the environment so that reward maximization leads to desirable behavior. In the HMDS, the most inclusive holon will receive and pass the feedback to its members. This action is repeated until the feedback is announced to all DSAs, which act as the environment for their members and calculate their rewards. In other words, the HMDS has distributed environments, i.e., the highest holon receives the feedback from the outside world, however, the environment for every other holon is its super-holon, from which it receives its reward. Figure 13.6 illustrates the difference between the agent-environment interaction in Q-learning and Holonic-Q-learning.

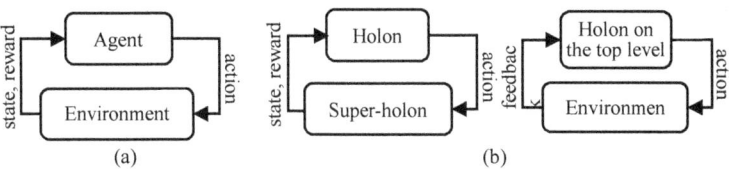

Fig. 13.6 The agent-environment interaction in **a** Q-learning **b** Holonic-Q-learning

Cooperability is the decisive factor in calculating the reward in the HMDS. The reward function is defined in such a way that the more relevant the problem is for a super-holon, the more strongly incompatibilities in this super-holon are punished. As soon as the final diagnosis is received by the head of the holarchy it will announce it on its blackboard and the members will then send back their similarity. This value is called the suggested reward ($sugg\,R_i$). Considering the distribution of these values, statistically those values that are more than three standard deviations away from the mean value are considered as outliers. And, of course, the closer they are to the mean the higher the cooperability has been. The value r^* is defined here as the maximum suggested reward. Higher values mean higher relevance for the problem. Therefore, incompatibilities should be penalized more. As a result, the difference between the reward and the r^* is directly proportional to the difference between the suggested reward and the average reward, and the proportionality constant is r^* over 3σ:

$$\frac{r^* - r_i}{r^*} = \frac{|\bar{r} - sugg\,R_i|}{3\sigma} \qquad (13.8)$$

Therefore,

$$r_i = \begin{cases} 0 & sugg\,R_i \text{ is an outlier} \\ r^*(3\sigma - |\bar{r} - sugg\,R_i|)/3\sigma & else \end{cases} \qquad (13.9)$$

As a result, if the suggested reward is very close to the average reward the final reward is also very close to the maximum reward. On the other hand, if the suggested reward is far away from the average, the final reward will be relatively low. Moreover, when the problem is relevant to the super-holon, the r^* will be higher and, therefore, incompatibilities will be penalized more. To have a uniform reward metrics, however, the reward value can be adjusted to

$$r_i = \begin{cases} 0 & sugg\,R_i \text{ is an outlier} \\ 1 - r^*\left(1 + \frac{3\sigma - |\bar{r} - sugg\,R_i|}{3\sigma}\right) & else \end{cases} \qquad (13.10)$$

so that Q-values are updated comparably.

It should be noted that a super-holon that is participating in an ongoing diagnosis process will use the reward function to calculate the rewards. However, if a super-holon, which had originally not participated in the diagnosis process, realizes that the final diagnosis matches the knowledge of one of its members, it will assign the reward -1 (penalty) to this DRA which actually had this diagnosis included in its knowledge base. This will cause the Q-value to deviate from the mean value, which will force the member to start exploring, i.e., to move away from its current location to, hopefully, a more appropriate location. This exploration is essential here as that was the reason why the diagnostic request was not received at all by the holon. To this end, DSAs that have not participated in the ongoing diagnosis process and do not include the final diagnosis as one of their members will, too, pass the final diagnosis, however, only to their DSA members so that such wrongly positioned DRAs could be punished and consequently start exploring.

13.5 Simulations

13.5.1 The Assessment of the Diagnosis Abilities

As a proof of concepts of our system we have tested the reliability of our system against several examples that were published in the literature. All the experiments were performed on Intel(R) Celeron(R) CPU 1.90 GHz with 10 GB RAM on the Microsoft Windows 10 platform and the simulations have been conducted using the GAMA platform, which is a modeling and simulation development environment for building spatially explicit agent-based simulations [103].

Case 1: Lung Cancer The first example is based on an actual H&P report, which is provided in [104] for study purposes. This report is the final H&P report, so having the chief complaint, the relevant signs and symptoms have been checked and the necessary medical tests and the final differential diagnosis list are given. In this simulation, the ability of the system in guiding the H&P is to be checked. For this reason, the chief complaint is given to the system as the diagnosis request and the reaction of the system is monitored using the actual report as a benchmark. Briefly, the H&P report includes:

- *Chief Complaint (CC):* Shortness of Breath (SOB).
- *History of Present Illness (HPI):* Chest pain, chills, cough, fever, history of breathing troubles/asthma/pneumonia/TB exposure, history of cancer in family, history with tobacco, night sweats, productive cough, vomit, weight loss, wheezing.
- *Review of Systems (ROS):* Routine with focus on anxiety, fainting, fatigue and weakness, heart palpitations and arrhythmias, change in skin color, changes in appetite.
- *Physical Exam (PE):* Normal with focus on cyanosis, edema, swollen lymph nodes.
- *Diagnostic Tests:* Blood test, CT scan.
- *Assessment and Plan:* (1) asthma (asthma tests), (2) lung cancer (X-ray / CT scan, biopsy), (3) pneumonia (blood test), (4) sarcoidosis (blood test), (5) tuberculosis (PPD: Purified Protein Derivative skin test for tuberculosis).

Providing the simulated version of the HMDS with the shortness of breath as the chief complaint, the DSA of the pulmonary diseases will be activated and the initial differential diagnosis provided by the system will be: (1) asthma, (2) COPD, (3) pulmonary edema, (4) bronchitis, (5) pulmonary embolism, (6) lung cancer, (7) sarcoidosis, (8) tuberculosis, (9) lymphoma, and (10) pneumonia (see Fig. 13.7).

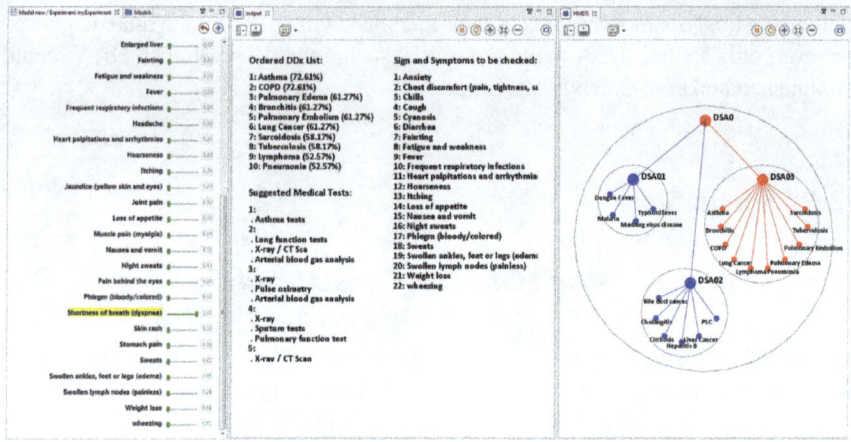

Fig. 13.7 The output of the simulated HMDS for shortness of breath

It should be noted that in reality the initial differential diagnosis list cannot be found on a H&P report, since this is actually something the physician would have in mind, according to which s(he) will start checking the signs and symptoms to improve the list. Accordingly, to assess the system with respect to its ability in finding the initial differential diagnosis list, its suggested signs and symptoms should be compared to the ones mentioned in the H&P report. The suggested signs and symptoms to be checked include: anxiety, chest discomfort, chills, cough, cyanosis, diarrhea, fainting, fatigue and weakness, fever, presence of frequent respiratory infections, heart palpitations and arrhythmias, hoarseness, itching, loss of appetite, nausea and vomit, night sweats, phlegm (bloody/colored), sweats, edema, swollen lymph nodes, weight loss, wheezing. These signs and symptoms match the ones mentioned in the HPI, ROS, and PE sections of the original H&P report (see Fig. 13.7).

After entering the value of these signs and symptoms according to their presence or absence, the final DDx list will be: (1) asthma, (2) lung cancer, (3) pulmonary edema, (4) tuberculosis, (5) sarcoidosis, (6) pneumonia, (7) bronchitis, (8) pulmonary embolism, (9) COPD, and (10) lymphoma. The suggested medical tests will include asthma tests, an X-ray/CT scan, sputum cytology, biopsy, pulse oximetry, arterial blood gas analysis, and sputum test for tuberculosis. This result matches the contents of the actual H&P report to a considerable degree and will further improve through learning (see Fig. 13.8).

Case 2: Metastatic Lung Cancer to Bile Duct Cancer The HMDS also acts well in the presence of multiple diseases at the same time, like metastasis cases. This example is extracted from a medical paper on cancer metastasis [105]. The signs and symptoms in this case included abdominal pain, coarse breath sounds, dry cough, jaundice, and shortness of breath; and the final diagnosis was metastatic lung cancer to common bile duct cancer. The suggested medical tests were blood test, CT scan, ERCP (Endoscopic Retrograde Cholangiopancreatography), biopsy. Giving these

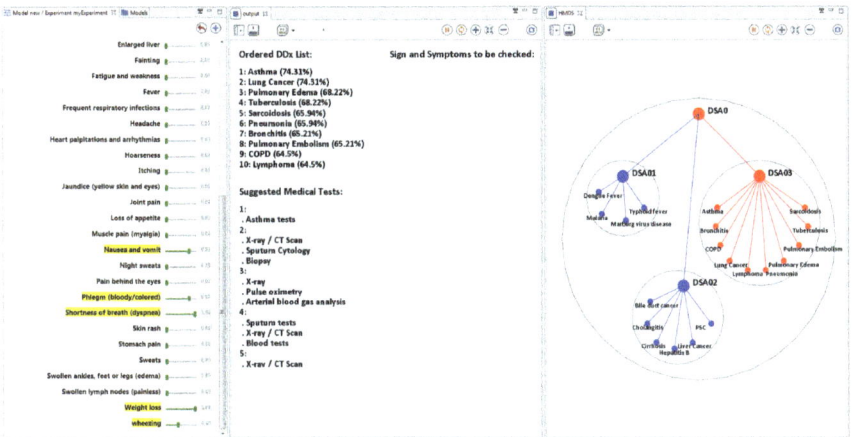

Fig. 13.8 The final output of the simulated HMDS for case 1

symptoms to the HMDS as the diagnosis request two different DSAs will be activated: the DSA of pulmonary diseases and the DSA of hepatology and gastrointestinal disorders. Their super-holon will then order the output of both members. The DDx list will include: (1) bile duct cancer, (2) cholangitis, (3) asthma, (4) lung cancer, (5) hepatitis B, (6) pulmonary edema, (7) PSC, (8) pulmonary embolism, (9) bronchitis, (10) lymphoma. It should be noted that the order of the final list is based on the similarity between the input and the DDP saved for each disease in the system. As a result, the differential diagnosis list includes the bile duct cancer as the first and the lung cancer as the fourth possible diagnosis, and therefore the possibility of metastasis can be clearly passed to the physician (see Fig. 13.9).

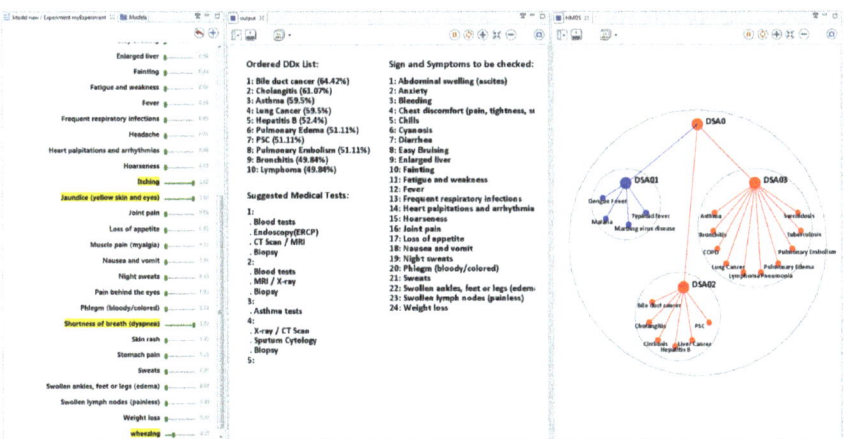

Fig. 13.9 The final output of the simulated HMDS for case 2

13.5.2 The Assessment of the Self-Organization Abilities

Case 3: The Assessment of Clustering in the HMDS As mentioned, the initial holarchy of the HMDS can be created using clustering at different levels of the holarchy. For this reason, the most common and inclusive DSA of the system accepts all the DRAs as its members, clusters them, and defines for each of the clusters (i.e., super-holons) a head. Each new DSA will then perform clustering on its members and defines new DSAs as its own members. This action is repeated recursively until no further clustering is necessary. As mentioned earlier, this step can be performed once while the system is being defined, which will speed up the system's self-organization. The system can later reorganize its architecture using reinforcement learning. This section presents a simulation with 45 diseases and 135 signs and symptoms.

Figure 13.10 illustrates the result of clustering in the HMDS. The clustering is done based on the Euclidean distances between the DDP, i.e., the holon identifier of each of the DRAs. Each DSA that solely includes DRAs has in fact grouped all those diseases that are covered by its members. It should be noted that this grouping is done in the range of only those diseases that were used in the simulation. So, there might be a slight difference between the list of diseases suggested by this simulation and the ones considered for DDx in actual clinical practice. For a complete list of diseases that should be covered in the DDx of each of the diseases please refer to [106]. As already mentioned, the holon identifier of DSAs is the average of the holon identifiers of their members. As a result, the groups formed on the higher levels can help the user to indicate the right signs and symptoms to be checked in cases where the diagnosis request is not precise enough to reach DSAs that contain DRAs.

Case 4: The Assessment of Reinforcement Learning in the HMDS In this simulation, the system covers 45 diseases in a holarchy of four levels. Here, again, a real case is used, in which the Madelung-Launois-Bensaude disease (MLB) is suggested as a new differential diagnosis of acromelic arthritis [107]. MLB is a disease that causes the concentration of adipose tissue in the proximal torso. In 2008, for the first time, some instances of this disease had been observed with distal adipose tissue that were misdiagnosed first as arthritis, which normally includes joint pain and joint swelling. The common signs and symptoms of MLB are unhealthy body fat distribution, adipose tissue (proximal upper body), fatigue, and physical deformity. The new signs and symptoms observed in distal MLB were joint pain (hands and knees) and joint swelling.

In this experiment, the new observations will be given to a version of the HMDS, which so far has not considered the MLB disease with arthritis for the reason of differential diagnosis. The system should then be able to come to the same conclusion as in [107] and add the DRA representing the MLB disease to the super-holon containing the DRA that represents arthritis. In this case, the DRA acting for MLB will be a multi-part, as it will be shared by more than one super-holon. To demonstrate the system's reactions to this new finding the user interface of the system displays the

13 A Powerful Holonic and Multi-Agent-Based Front-End ... 339

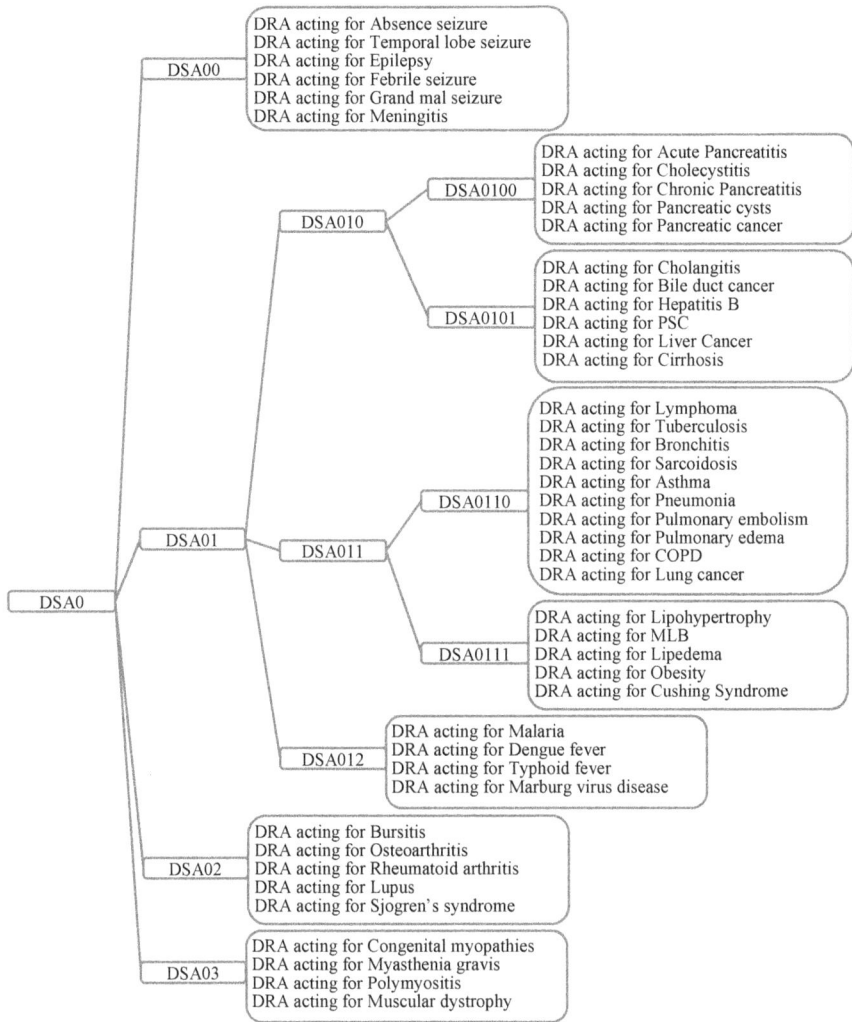

Fig. 13.10 The result of clustering in the simulated HMDS

corresponding Q-values on a specially dedicated diagram (see Fig. 13.11). Essentially, if an agent is not involved in a diagnosis process it will not receive any reward and as a result, its Q-value will remain the same during that round. As the agent participates in a diagnosis process, it will be rewarded and consequently its Q-value will be updated. In case the Q-value of any of the members of the super-holon is getting close to be a noise (close to lower three-sigma limit), the agent will start exploring new opportunities to join new super-holons. One promising approach for this agent is to try to become a member of those super-holons that were activated at

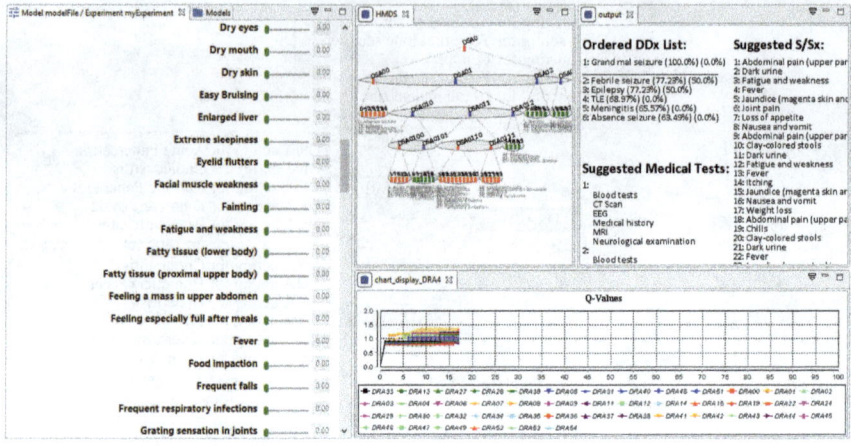

Fig. 13.11 The Q-value diagram on the user interface

the same time with its current super-holon, i.e., guided exploration. This will guarantee that the agent would have some common interests with the members of its new super-holon(s).

In this simulation, before entering the signs and symptoms of distal MLB as the diagnosis request, the system is first provided with some random diagnosis requests. As a result, it became easier to monitor the changes of the Q-values of the DRA reacting for MLB on the Q-value diagram. Figure 13.12 shows the changes in the Q-values of the different DRAs in case 4. Receiving the common instances of MLB disease, the super-holon of the DRA acting for MLB will be activated. This DSA includes the DRAs acting for the following diseases: Lipohypertrophy, MLB, lipedema, obesity, and Cushing syndrome. Entering the distal MLB instances into

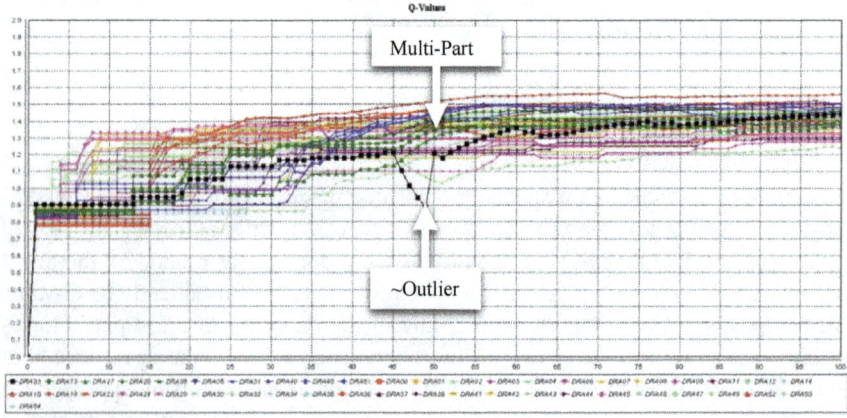

Fig. 13.12 Changes in the Q-values of the different DRAs in case 4

the system, as the DRA acting for MLB now represents a disease with signs and symptoms that are not common in its super-holon, its Q-value will get closer to the lower outlier threshold and will look for the possibility of guided exploration.

While working on distal MLB instances, the super-holon of the DRA acting for arthritis will also be activated. This super-holon includes the DRAs acting for the following diseases: bursitis, osteoarthritis, rheumatoid arthritis, lupus, and Sjogren's syndrome. It should be noted that this means that even the untrained system could have been able to suggest both diseases in its final DDx list and as a result help the physician to consider the possibility of MLB. In any case, based on the guided exploration option, the DRA acting for MLB that will eventually start looking for a chance to join some new super-holons, will try to become a member of the super-holon of the DRA acting for arthritis. Considering the holon identifier of its members, this super-holon will then check whether the DRA acting for MLB would be an outlier. Since this is not the case, it will accept this new member and, accordingly, a connection is granted. This means that from that point on, the system will consider the MLB disease as a differential diagnosis for arthritis. At this stage, the Q-value being displayed for the DRA acting for MLB will be the maximum value of the Q-values to its super-holons, which in this case is the Q-value to its new super-holon. As it can be seen from the diagram, since this value is now not close to the outlier threshold of at least one of its super-holons, the DRA will stop here its exploration.

Case 5: The Assessment of System's Behavior in Integrating a New DRA
According to the World Health Organization (WHO), "New diseases have been emerging at the unprecedented rate of one a year for the last two decades, and this trend is certain to continue" [108]. In recent years, for example, many infectious diseases have been discovered, including SARS, MERS, Ebola, chikungunya, avian flu, swine flu, Zika and, most recently, COVID-19. In order to support the diagnosis of such new diseases, the system should be able to assign DRAs to these diseases and allow them to find their right position in the holarchy.

This simulation demonstrated the system's behavior in integrating COVID-19. The DRA acting for COVID-19 is first introduced to the system as a member of the most inclusive DSA. At this stage, this DRA calculates its Euclidean distance to the rest of the members of its super-holon and then sends a membership request to the closest member. As the DRA acting for COVID-19 is not an outlier in this super-holon, the membership request will be accepted, and the DRA will become a member of this DSA. The same approach is followed by the agent until no further downward movement is possible, i.e., the new super-holon has no DSA members or the membership request from the DRA is rejected by all DSA members that have received a request. In this case the DRA acting for COVID-19 ends up in a super-holon that includes the DRAs acting for influenza and common cold. This finding is consistent with some of the diseases considered for the differential diagnosis of disease in patients screened for COVID-19, as listed in [109]. The diagnostic algorithm includes a test for the most common respiratory pathogens. Among the diseases that are considered by the simulated system, these pathogens are the cause

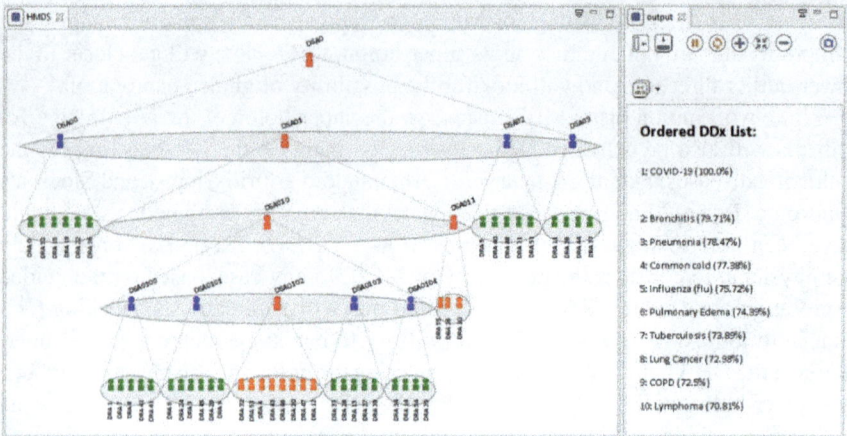

Fig. 13.13 System's output in diagnosing a COVID-19 case

for bronchitis, common cold, different types of influenza, and different types of pneumonia, that may also cause pulmonary edema.

Figure 13.13 demonstrates the output of the simulated system in diagnosing a COVID-19 case (signs and symptoms of this disease are given as input). In fact, two DSAs were activated in response to the given input and the second DSA added the rest of the mentioned diseases to the differential diagnosis list. It should be noted that the system may produce different outputs by integrating more diseases and of course through learning. However, as the system follows the logic behind the differential diagnosis process these all should contribute to its improvement.

13.6 Discussion

This study proposed a well-designed HMAS that according to the system assessments can successfully guide DDx and eventually conduct the H&P process. This system improves the state of the art of the MDSs by addressing their critical shortcoming, i.e., the lack of implementation of the ability to guide the user in providing the system with the all-encompassing input, which is the key to a flawless diagnosis. By means of this system the following advantages can be obtained as compared to available MDSs:

1. It reduces diagnostic errors by providing immediate second opinions even on signs and symptoms to be checked in the H&P.
2. It guides and facilitates filling out the H&P form at the same time.
3. It helps to tackle physician shortages by guiding nurses in preparing the H&P reports that are then to be controlled by physicians.

4. It can be added as a software component to available MDSs and provide them with the required comprehensive inputs. This integration would also allow these systems to fit into the clinical workflow, and as a result promotes the wider use of them.
5. Can offer attractive side benefits, e.g., helping us to broaden our knowledge on diseases, providing a means of more timely detection of outbreaks, and so on.

However, before the system can be used in practice, a few further issues need to be resolved. Considering the current system as a front-end for MDSs following issues are to be addressed:

1. Even though state-of-the-art MDSs are already equipped with NLP algorithms that can interpret the H&P report, it is still suggested to provide a smooth and comprehensive interface across which these two components could exchange information rapidly and reliably. This interface can also allow the system to receive learning data (i.e., feedback) from the MDS component in order to improve its performance.
2. Our current system is based on a given and considered complete ontology in only one language. Unfortunately, in reality, there are usually a large number of ontologies available for the same application area. In addition to understanding natural language in the medical field, ontology matching here, therefore, is a major challenge.
3. The system continuously displays the ongoing DDx list for transparency as it suggests the signs and symptoms to be checked or the medical tests to be conducted. The system orders the diagnoses based on their similarity to the diagnosis request and additionally displays the frequency of diseases as valuable hints for final diagnosis. With respect to the order of the questions, in practice, a physician may apply one of the following approaches: (1) probabilistic approach: starting with those diseases that are more likely, (2) prognostic approach: starting with those diseases that are fatal or seriously harmful, (3) pragmatic approach: starting with those diseases that are more responsive to treatment. Each approach has its own limitations and experienced physicians simultaneously integrate all three approaches while updating and reordering the DDx list. As the pragmatic approach mainly becomes meaningful when dealing with the final version of the DDx list, currently the system continuously applies the prognostic and when not applicable the probabilistic approach in order to avoid delay in treatment and considers some simple predefined adjustments as well. However, in both cases further detailed investigation and analysis are needed. The system should be improved to steer clear of unrelated questions as much as possible, and moreover, to be able to backtrack, i.e., abandon a candidate as soon as it determines that it cannot possibly be completed to a valid diagnosis. Furthermore, termination criterion should be addressed thoroughly to avoid simplistic approaches.

The two last mentioned issues should also be resolved if we want to expand the current system to act as a fully-fledged and independent MDS. Along with these issues, following problems are also to be solved:

1. In order to support the total coverage of A&P step the system still needs to be equipped with the necessary ML and NLP algorithms that can help the system in dealing with complicated cases. Using these algorithms, the diagnosis can also benefit from the analysis and interpretation of the latest medical findings.
2. The system, as it currently stands, is not a black box (as is the case with most machine learning systems) on the account of the fact that it is clear that its reasoning is based on the DDx of the listed possible diseases. However, text-based explanation of the reasoning and the justification (findings) can be provided and unaccepted hypotheses may also be included in final report for more transparency. Our approach is not well suited for such challenges, respectively tasks. This means that some really fundamental research is to be conducted in order to get an idea of how such an explanation component can look like and how it can be added to the system.
3. Finally, in order for such a system to be useful, e.g., in third world countries, disease treatment suggestions need to be provided. This includes considerations such as avoiding negative drug-drug interactions. Again, this is a highly complex task and may even need to automatically scan and understand relevant literature and examinations / simulations published in relevant sources.

Along with the introduction of the HMDS as a practical contribution, this study has led to some theoretical contributions to the machine learning techniques that are applicable to systems that adopt a similar approach for problem solving to the one followed in this study. What makes this system distinguishable is the way it applies the holonic approach. Oppose to available HMASs that mainly apply ML techniques to support the rather sophisticated problem-solving decision-making process, this process in our system has been kept as simple as possible and generally the position of agents is decisive for their cooperation and success. As a result, the mentioned machine learning techniques are targeting the holarchy formation, to organize and continuously reorganize the holarchy based on the environment it is dealing with in case of need.

To put it concisely, due to the complexity of the DDx and as neither the number of levels nor the number of the groups in each level of the holarchy are predefined, clustering (unsupervised learning) has been used to establish super-holons and eventually build up the initial holarchy of the system. As mentioned, DBSCAN is one of the best algorithms matching this goal, especially due to the fact that it does not require one to specify the number of clusters in the data a priori. However, in order to deploy this algorithm, we needed to eliminate its shortcomings so that could be applied to complex medical data. The algorithm is unable to detect clusters that lie too close to each other. Moreover, to detect its input parameter, it starts a user interaction based on some graphical representation of the data. As the determination of the mentioned parameter gets complicated when dealing with large and complex data such as medical data, we have suggested a small adjustment in the data that is used to determine the parameter, and proposed the use of the empirical rule to automatically detect this parameter (for more information please refer to [94]).

In this study, the self-organization problem has been expressed as a sequential decision-making problem and accordingly modelled as an MDP. In this case, the problem is to decide how favorable it is for a holon to be a member of another holon. As the holonic architecture involves nested whole-part structures, this decision includes the evaluation of the quality of the membership of holon's direct and indirect super-holons among intermediate level holons. Accordingly, describing the problem as an MDP, the states are the existing holons and the actions are membership trials.

Sequential decision-making problems that can be modeled as Markov decision processes can be solved using methods that combine dynamic programming and reinforcement learning. Many studies have been conducted in this area; however, focusing on available swarm RL algorithms provides a clear view of the areas that still need attention. Most of the studies in this area are concentrating on homogeneous swarms and to date, systems introduced as heterogeneous swarms merely include very few, i.e., two or three homogeneous sub-swarms, which either according to their capabilities address specific sub-problem of the general problem or exhibit different behaviors to reduce the risk of bias.

In this study a novel approach has been introduced that allows individuals with higher heterogeneity rates, which are even addressing different problems, to behave as a swarm when solving shared sub-problems (for more information please refer to [96]). In fact, the affinity between two agents that indicates the compatibility of agents to work together towards solving a specific sub-problem is used to design a heterogeneous swarm RL algorithm that allows heterogeneous swarms to solve sequential decision-making problems consisting of sub-problems that should be addressed by different sub-groups of its members. As a result, the affinity-based heterogeneous swarm RL essentially allows the agents that are not identical but are capable of collaboration to exhibit swarm behavior providing them with the means of sharing their knowledge and eventually dealing with problems that match their specialties. This learning method essentially allows such agents to collect information from a larger swarm and to be able to make better decisions using this broader knowledge.

It should be noted that even though the experiments have shown that the affinity-based heterogeneous swarm RL method is able to increase the performance of the heterogeneous agents solving SDMPs, this method clearly has its own limitations and is solely applicable when sub-groups of agents with significant lesser extent of heterogeneity are extractable and are in addition to that sufficiently populated to be able to exhibit meaningful swarm behavior. Regarding the suggested RL method it should also be noted that very few studies have been done on the machine learning methods that can be applied to HMASs and the research in this area is still at a very nascent stage. Notable examples of the available methods are [110] and [111]. Even though using these methods learning in each level can be influenced by the learning results, i.e., the behavior, of the holons on the other levels (inter-holonic learning data), these methods do not aim to improve the inter-holonic connections, i.e., the memberships. In contrast, the approach presented in this study in particular aims to refine the holarchy, as the position of agents in this system will greatly define their behavior.

13.7 Conclusion

COVID-19 as a new disease and the catastrophic overloading of the medical profession in many countries around the world that followed have led to a rethinking of the rules for medical services. While many countries did not allow other people than doctors to make a medical diagnosis, usually while the patient must be with the doctor, it is now considered that diagnoses might be done online and in simple cases or as a first assessment by less educated medical personal. Thus, we are just a small step away from deploying MDSs for these purposes. However, for these systems to conduct such demanding tasks in a highly reliable way it needs to be assured that the diagnoses given are based on a solid input. In the past the information and data gathering were done by a real specialist, the doctor. Now it may also be done by less educated people. This is only possible if the MDSs is already involved in the diagnosis finding from its first step, namely the execution of the H&P through a differential diagnosis. This is where our research picks up. Triggered by the fact that state-of-the-art MDSs only start their work after all relevant input was delivered, we decided to add a new front-end to those systems that executes and guides the H&P process.

After a comprehensive study of how such a system might look like and what the underlying technologies need to be, we concluded that a holonic multi-agent system that relies in its task on various machine learning technologies is the best option. The holonic structure of our system, which in the end emulates a swarm intelligence system, permits to come to guided medical diagnoses without the burden of deploying hugely computing-intense and highly complex high-level AI systems that rely on understanding the complex medical field. In contrast, our system consists of a large number of comparatively simple pattern matchers, extended by only slightly more sophisticated decision makers on the higher levels of abstraction, that draw their strength from their intense cooperation. Accordingly, the system is equipped with machine learning techniques that mainly target the holarchy formation, as the problem-solving decision-making process in this system has been kept as simple as possible and generally the position of agents is decisive for their cooperation and success.

The system applies an improved version of DBSCAN algorithm in order to build its initial holarchy. After receiving feedback, it also uses this data to update its knowledge about the diseases using exponential smoothing method. An adapted Q-learning method is also introduced in this study for the purpose of self-organization of the system.

In order to prove the applicability and reliability of our system a number of simulations on the basis of real-world cases that were published in literature were conducted. The results have been very promising and clearly suggest that our approach has great potential. However, as already mentioned in the discussion section, before the system can be used in practice, a few further issues need to be resolved. In order to use the system as a front-end for available MDSs it is suggested to provide a smooth and comprehensive interface across which these two components could exchange information rapidly and reliably. Moreover, with respect to input, the system is to be equipped with NLP and ontology matching algorithms. Concerning the output, further detailed investigation and analysis are needed to support the system in reasoning on the order of the output lists. Along with the two last mentioned issues steps towards a fully-fledged MDS also include the design of (1) additional ML and NLP algorithms for full coverage of final assessment phase, (2) an explanation component that can provide text-based explanations for the final output, and (3) a plan component that can suggest patient-specific treatment plans.

References

1. Goldberg, C.: Practical guide to clinical medicine. UCSD School of Medicine [Online]. Available: https://meded.ucsd.edu/clinicalmed/write.html. Accessed 15 March 2021
2. Densen, P.: Challenges and Opportunities Facing Medical Education. Am. Clin. Climatol. Assoc. **122**, 48–58 (2011)
3. Shortliffe, E.H., Buchanan, B.G.: Knowledge Engineering for medical decision making: A review of computer-based clinical decision aids. In Proceedings of the IEEE, Vol. 67, No. 9 (1979)
4. Open Clinical. 2017 [Online]. Available: http://www.openclinical.org/dss.html
5. Miller, R.A., Geissbuhler, A.: Clinical diagnostic decision support systems—an overview. In Clinical Decision Support Systems: Theory and Practice, Springer (1998)
6. Shoham, Y.: Agent-Oriented Programming (Technical Report STAN-CS-90-1335). Stanford University, Computer Science Department (1990)
7. Wooldridge, M.: Intelligent agents. In Multiagent systems. The MIT Press (1999)
8. Iantovics, B.L.: Agent-Based Medical Diagnosis Systems. Comput. Inform. **27**, 593–625 (2008)
9. Klüver, C., Klüver, J., Unland, R.: A Medical Diagnosis System based on MAS Technology and Neural Network," Business Process, pp. 179–191. Serv. Comput. Intell. Serv. Manag. (2009)
10. Chao, S., Wong, F.: Multi-agent learning paradigm for medical data mining diagnostic workbench. Data mining and multi-agent integration, pp. 177–186 (2009)
11. Cognitive Computing. TechTarget, [Online]. Available: https://searchenterpriseai.techtarget.com/definition/cognitive-computing. Accessed 27 October 2018
12. Kaul, V., Enslin, S., Gross, S.: History of artificial intelligence in medicine. Gastrointest. Endosc. **92**(4), 807–812 (2020)
13. Yoshida, H., Jain, A., Ichalkaranje, A., Ichalkaranje, N. (eds.): Advanced Computational Intelligence Paradigms in Healthcare - 1. Springer-Verlag, Berlin Heidelberg (2007)
14. Vaidya, S., Yoshida, H. (eds.): Advanced Computational Intelligence Paradigms in Healthcare - 2. Springer-Verlag, Berlin Heidelberg (2007)
15. Sordo, M., Vaidya, S. (eds.): Advanced Computational Intelligence Paradigms in Healthcare - 3. Springer-Verlag, Berlin Heidelberg (2008)
16. Bichindaritz, I., Vaidya, S., Jain, A. (eds.): Computational Intelligence in Healthcare 4. Springer-Verlag, Berlin Heidelberg (2010)
17. Brahnam, S., Jain, L.C. (eds.): Advanced Computational Intelligence Paradigms in Healthcare 5. Springer-Verlag, Berlin Heidelberg (2011)
18. Brahnam, S., Jain, L.C. (eds.): Advanced Computational Intelligence Paradigms in Healthcare 6. Springer-Verlag, Berlin Heidelberg (2011)
19. Maglogiannis, I., Brahnam, S., Jain, L.C. (eds.): Advanced Computational Intelligence in Healthcare-7. Springer-Verlag, Berlin Heidelberg (2020)

20. Howlett, R.J., Tsihrintzis, G., Toro, C., Virvou, M., Jain, L.: Innovation in medicine and healthcare 2013. In Proceedings of First International Conference. Impact: The Journal of Innovation Impact, vol. 6, no. 1 (2013).
21. Graña, M., Toro, C., Howlett, R., Jain, L.C. (eds.): Innovation in medicine and healthcare 2014. IOS Press (2015)
22. Y Chen, Y.-W., Torro , C., Tanaka, S., Howlett, R., Jain, L. (eds.): Innovation in medicine and healthcare 2017. Springer International Publishing (2016)
23. Chen, Y.-W., Tanaka, S., Howlett, R., Jain, L. (eds.): Innovation in medicine and healthcare 2017. Springer International Publishing (2016)
24. Chen, Y.-W., Tanaka, S., Howlett, R., Jain, L. (eds.): Innovation in medicine and healthcare 2017. Springer International Publishing (2018)
25. De Pietro, G., Gallo, L., Howlett, R.J., Jain, L.C., Vlacic, L. (eds.): Innovation in Medicine and Healthcare (KES-InMed-18)," in Intelligent Interactive Multimedia Systems and Services, pp. 171–276. Springer, Cham (2018)
26. Chen, Y.-W., Zimmermann, A., Howlett, R., Jain, J. (eds.): Innovation in medicine and healthcare systems, and multimedia. Springer, Singapore (2019)
27. Chen, Y.-W., Tanaka, S., Howlett, R., Jain, L. (eds.): Innovation in medicine and healthcare. Springer, Singapore (2020)
28. Berner, E.S.: Clinical decision support systems: theory and practice. Springer (2016)
29. Berner, E.S.: Clinical decision support systems: State of the Art," AHRQ Publication No. 09–0069-EF. Agency for Healthcare Research and Quality, Rockville, MD (2009)
30. Alther, M., Reddy, C.K.: Chapter 19: Clinical decision support systems. In Healthcare Data Analytics, Chapman and Hall/CRC 2015, , pp. 625–656 (2015)
31. Papik, K., Molnar, B., Schaefer, R., Dombovari, Z., Tulassay, Z., Feher, J.: Application of neural networks in medicine-a review, 4(3), pp. MT538-MT546, Medical Science Monitor (1998)
32. Al-Shayea, Q.K.: Artificial neural networks in medical diagnosis. Int. J. Comput. Sci. Issues **8**(2), 150–154 (2011)
33. Amato, F., Alberto, L., Peña-Méndez, E.M., Vaňhara, P., Hampl, A.H.J.: Artificial neural networks in medical diagnosis. J. Appl. Biomed. **11**, 47–58 (2013)
34. Ghaheri, A., Shoar, S., Naderan, M., Hoseini, S.S.: The applications of genetic algorithms in medicine. Oman Med. J. **30**(6), 406–416 (2015)
35. Wolfram, D.: An appraisal of INTERNIST-I. Artif. Intell. Med. **7**(2), 93–116 (1995)
36. Pople, H.E.: Presentation of the Internist system. In Proceedings of the AIM workshop. Rutgers University, New Brunswick, NJ (1976)
37. Weiss, S.: A system for model-based computer-aided diagnosis and therapy, Ph.D. Thesis. Computers in Biomedicine, Department of Computer Science, Rutgers University, CBM-TR-27-Thesis (1974)
38. Pauker, S.G., Gorry, G.A., Kassirer, J.P., Schwartz, W.B: Towards the simulation of clinical cognition: Taking a present illness by computer. Amer. J. Med. **60** (1976)
39. Shortliffe, E.H.: Computer-Based Medical Consultations: MYCIN. Elsevier, New York (1976)
40. Aikins, J.S., Kunz, J.C., Shortliffe, E.H., Fallat, R.J.: PUFF: an expert system for interpretation of pulmonary function data. Comput. Biomed. Res. **16**(3), 199–208 (1983)
41. Miller, R., Masarie, F., Myers, J.: Quick medical reference (QMR) for diagnostic assistance. MD Comput **3**(5), 34–48 (1986)
42. Winston, P.H., Prendergast, K.A.: CADUCEUS: an experimental expert system for medical diagnosis. The AI Business: Commercial Uses of Artificial Intelligence, pp. 67–80 (1986)
43. Barnett, G., Cimino, J., Hupp, J., Hoffer, E.: DXplain. An evolving diagnostic decision-support system. JAMA **258**(1), 67–74 (1987)
44. Lincoln, M., Turner, C., Haug, P., et al.: Iliad training enhances medical students' diagnostic skills. J. Med. Syst. **15**(1), 93–110 (1991)
45. De Cresce, R.P., Lifshitz, M.S.: PAPNET™ Cytological Screening System. Laboratory Medi. **22**(4), 276–280 (1991)

46. Baxt, W.: Use of an arteficial neural network for the diagnosis of myocardial infarction. Ann. Intern. Med. **115**(11), 843–848 (1991)
47. Tourassi, G.D., Floyd, J.C.: Artificial neural networks for single photon emission computed tomography. A study of cold lesion detection and localization. Invest. Radiol. **28**(8), 671–677 (1993)
48. Tourassi, G., Floyd, C., Sostman, H., Coleman, R.: Artificial neural network for diagnosis of acute pulmonary embolism: effect of case and observer selection. Radiology **194**(3), 889–893 (1995)
49. Fogel, D., Wasson, E., Boughton, E.: Evolving neural networks for detecting breast cancer. Cancer Letters, **96**(1), 49–53 (1995)
50. Costa, A., Cabestany, J., Moreno, J., Calvet, M.: Neuroserum: An artificial neural Net-Based diagnostic aid tool for serum electrophoresis. In Third international conference on neural networks and expert systems in medicine and healthcare (1998)
51. Tleyjeh, I.M., Nada, H., Baddour, L.M.: VisualDX: Decision-support software for the diagnosis and management of dermatologic disorders. Clin. Infect. Dis. **43**(9), 1177–1184 (2006)
52. Fisher, H., Tomlinson, A., Ramnarayan, P., Britto, J.: Isabel: support with clinical decision making. Pediatr. Nurs. **15**(7), 34–35 (2003)
53. Higuchi, K., Sato, K., Makuuchi, H., Takamoto, F.A.S., Takeda, H.: Automated diagnosis of heart disease in patients with heart murmurs: application of a neural network technique. J. Med. Eng. Technol. **30**(2), 61–68 (2006)
54. Barakat, N., Bradley, A.P., Barakat, M.N.H.: Intelligible support vector machines for diagnosis of diabetes mellitus. IEEE Trans. Inf Technol. Biomed. **14**(4), 1114–1120 (2010)
55. Elveren, E., Yumuşak, N.: Tuberculosis disease diagnosis using artificial neural network trained with genetic algorithm. J. Med. Syst. **35**(3), 329–332 (2011)
56. Duraipandian, S., Zheng, W., Ng, J., Low, J.J., Ilancheran, A., Huang, Z.: In vivo diagnosis of cervical precancer using Raman spectroscopy and genetic algorithm techniques. Analyst **136**(20), 4328–4336 (2011)
57. Barbosa, D.C., Roupar, D.B., Ramos, J.C., Tavares, A.C., Lima, C.S.: Automatic small bowel tumor diagnosis by using multi-scale wavelet-based analysis in wireless capsule endoscopy images. Biomedical engineering online, **11**(1) (2012)
58. Atkov, O.Y., Gorokhova, S.G., Sboev, A.G., Generozov, E.V., Muraseyeva, E.V., Moroshkina, S.Y., Cherniy, N.N.: Coronary heart disease diagnosis by artificial neural networks including genetic polymorphisms and clinical parameters. J. Cardiol. **59**(2), 190–194 (2012)
59. Saxena, M.: IBM Watson progress and 2013 roadmap, 23 February 2013 [Online]. Available: https://www.slideshare.net/manojsaxena2/ibm-watson-progress-and-roadmap-saxena/7-Watson_Healthcare_Products_1H_2013. Accessed 23 January 2018
60. Yahiaoui, A., Er, O., Yumusak, N.: A new method of automatic recognition for tuberculosis disease diagnosis using support vector machines. Biomedical Res. **28**(9) (2017)
61. Segen, J.C.: Concise dictionary of modern medicine, McGraw-Hill (2002)
62. IBM: IBM WATSON [Online]. Available: http://ibmwatson237.weebly.com/. Accessed 25 September 2020
63. IBM Watson supercomputer. TechTarget, [Online]. Available: https://searchenterpriseai.techtarget.com/definition/IBM-Watson-supercomputer. Accessed 1 November 2018
64. Herper, M.: MD Anderson Benches IBM Watson In Setback For Artificial Intelligence In Medicine. Forbes, 19 February 2017 [Online]. Available: https://www.forbes.com/sites/matthewherper/2017/02/19/md-anderson-benches-ibm-watson-in-setback-for-artificial-intelligence-in-medicine/#7d4e6da63774. Accessed 01 November 2018
65. Ramnarayan, P., Kulkarni, G., Britto, J.: ISABEL: a novel Internet-delivered clinical decision support system. In Current Perspectives in Healthcare Computing, pp. 245–256 (2004)
66. Riches, N., Panagioti, M., Alam, R., Cheraghi-Sohi, S., Campbell, S., Esmail, A., Bower, P.: The effectiveness of electronic differential diagnoses (DDX) generators: a systematic review and meta-analysis. PloS one **11**(3), e0148991 (2016)

67. Isabel Products. Isabel, [Online]. Available: https://www.isabelhealthcare.com/products?hsCtaTracking=7e5a6ff1-1381-4d02-984c-924e476167ae%257C9627ae5d-a0d7-46ad-964b-098b1a59088f. Accessed 01 November 2018
68. Bauman, D.: Isabel differential diagnosis tool achieves 98% accuracy in new study. Isabel [Online]. Available: https://www.prweb.com/releases/2017isabelaidemonstrates/03impressiveaccuracy/prweb14198903.htm. Accessed 26 September 2020
69. eH&P™ custom History & Physical Exam™. [Online]. Available: http://www.scymed.com/en/smnxab/smnxabch.htm. Accessed 26 October 2018
70. Smart Medical Apps—H&P. Smart Medical Apps, [Online]. Available: https://play.google.com/store/apps/details?id=com.smartmedicalapps.checklist&hl=en. Accessed 23 September 2020
71. Clinicals—History & physical. Medical Gear [Online]. Available: https://play.google.com/store/apps/details?id=com.smartddx.clinicals&hl=en. Accessed 23 September 2020
72. History & Physical Exam pc. Börm Bruckmeier Publishing LLC, [Online]. Available: https://play.google.com/store/apps/details?id=com.bbi.History_and_Physical_Exam_a pocketcards. Accessed 23 September 2020
73. Wahls, S.A.: Causes and Evaluation of Chronic Dyspnea. Am. Fam. Physician **86**(2), 173–180 (2012)
74. Salem, H., Attiya, G., El-Fishawy, N.: A Survey of Multi-Agent based Intelligent Decision Support System for Medical Classification Problems. International Journal of Computer Applications 123(10) (2015)
75. Lhotska, L., Marik, V., Vlcek, T.: Medical applications of enhanced rule-based expert systems. Int. J. Med. Informatics **63**(1–2), 61–75 (2001)
76. Zaidi, S.Z., Abidi, S.S., Manickam, S.: Leveraging intelligent agents for knowledge discovery from heterogeneous healthcare data repositories. Stud. Health Technol. Inform. **90**, 335–340 (2002)
77. Arus, C., Celda, B., Dasmahaptra, S., Dupplaw, D.: On the design of a web-based decision support system for brain tumour diagnosis using distributed agents. In International Conference, Web Intelligence and Intelligent Agent Technology Workshops, IEEE/WIC/ACM (2006)
78. Iantovics, B.L.: A novel diagnosis system specialized in difficult medical diagnosis problems solving. In Emergent Properties in Natural and Artificial Dynamical Systems (2006)
79. Mateo, R.M.A., Cervantes, L.F., Yang, H.K., Lee, J.: Mobile agents using data mining for diagnosis support in ubiquitous healthcare. In KES International Symposium on Agent and Multi-Agent Systems: Technologies and Applications (2007)
80. Iantovics, B.: Hybrid expert system agents. In Proceedings of the International Conference European Integration between Tradition and Modernity, Petru Maior University Press, Tg. Mureş (2007)
81. Kazar, O., Sahnoun, Z., Frecon, L.: Multi-agents system for medical diagnosis. In: International Conference on Intelligent System and Knowledge Engineering (2008)
82. Wooldridge, M.: An introduction to multi agent systems. Wiley (2009)
83. Rodriguez, S.A.: From analysis to design of holonic multi-agent systems: a framework, methodological guidelines and applications, PhD Thesis, University of Technology of Belfort-Montbéliard (2005)
84. Gerber, C., Siekmann, J.H., Vierke, G.: Holonic multi-agent systems, Technical Report DFKI-RR-99–03, German Research Centre for Artificial Intelligence (1999)
85. Unland, R.: A holonic multi-agent system for robust, flexible, and reliable medical diagnosis. In Meersman, R., Tari, Z., (eds.), OTM-WS 2003, LNCS 2889 (2003)
86. Al-Qaysi, I., Unland, R., Weihs, C., Branki, C.: Medical Diagnosis Decision Support HMAS under Uncertainty HMDSuU. In: Brahnam, S., Jain, L.C. (eds.) Advanced Computational Intelligence Paradigms in Healthcare 5, pp. 67–94. Springer, Berlin, Heidelberg (2010)
87. Ulieru, M.: Internet-enabled soft computing holarchies for e-health applications-soft computing enhancing the internet and the internet enhancing soft computing. Enhancing the Power of the Internet, pp. 131–165 (2004)

88. Moise, G., Moise, P.G., Moise, P.S.: Toward Holons-based architecture for medical systems. In IEEE/ACM International Workshop on Software Engineering in Healthcare Systems (SEHS) (2018)
89. Akbari, Z.: A Holonic Multi-Agent System for the Support of the Differential Diagnosis Process in Medicine (PhD dissertation). University of Duisburg-Essen, Essen (2021)
90. Corkill, D.D.: Blackboard systems. In AI Experts 6(9) (1991)
91. Corkill, D.D.: Collaborating software: blackboard and multi-agent systems & the future. In Proceedings of the International Lisp Conference (2003)
92. Akbari, Z., Unland, R.: A Holonic Multi-Agent System Approach to Differential Diagnosis," Multiagent System Technologies: 15th German Conference, MATES 2017, vol. LNCS **10413**, 272–290 (2017)
93. Ester, M., Kriegel, H.-P., Sander, J., Xu, X.: A density-based algorithm for discovering clusters in large spatial databases with noise. In the 2nd International Conference on Knowledge Discoverey and Data Mining (1996)
94. Akbari, Z., Unland, R.: Automated Determination of the Input Parameter of the DBSCAN Based on Outlier Detection. Artif. Intell. Appl. Innov., IFIP Adv. Inf. Commun. Technol. **475**, 280–291 (2016)
95. Puterman, M.L.: Markov Decision Processes: Discrete Stochastic Dynamic. Wiley., New York (1994)
96. Akbari, Z., Unland, R.: A Novel Heterogeneous Swarm Reinforcement Learning Method for Sequential Decision Making Problems. Mach. Learn. Knowl. Extr. **1**(2), 590–610 (2019)
97. Melo, F.S.: Convergence of Q-learning: A simple proof," Institute of Systems and Robotics. Tech. Rep **1–4**, 2001 (2001)
98. Jaakkola, T., Jordan, M.I., Singh, S.P.: On the convergence of stochastic iterative dynamic programming algorithms. Massachusetts Institute of Technology, Artificial Intelligence Laboratory, A.I. Memo No. 1441 (1993)
99. Jaakkola, T., Jordan, M.I., Singh, S.P.: On the convergence of stochastic iterative dynamic programming algorithms. Neural Comput. **6**(6), 1185–1201 (1994)
100. Watkins, C., Dayan, P.: Technical Note: Q-Learning. Mach. Learn. **8**, 279–292 (1992)
101. Sutton, R.S., Barto, A.G.: Reinforcement learning: an introduction. MIT Press (1998)
102. Dewey, D.: Reinforcement learning and the reward engineering principle. In 2014 AAAI Spring Symposium Series (2014)
103. GAMA platform. [Online]. Available: https://gama-platform.github.io/. Accessed 9 November 2018
104. University of North Carolina—School of Medicine, History and Physical Examination (H&P) examples [Online]. Available: https://www.med.unc.edu/medclerk/education/grading/history-and-physical-examination-h-p-examples. Accessed 24 January 2018.
105. Cochrane, J.: Metastatic lung cancer to the common bile duct presenting as obstructive jaundice. J. Hepatol. Gastrointest. Disord. **2**(121) (2016)
106. Medscape. WebMD, [Online]. Available: https://emedicine.medscape.com/. Accessed 28 February 2019
107. Lemaire, O., Paul, C., Zabraniecki, L.: Distal Madelung-Launois-Bensaude disease: an unusual differential diagnosis of acromelic arthritis. Clin. Exp. Rheumatol. **26**, 351–353 (2008)
108. Team, W.: Chapter 5: SARS: lessons from a new disease. World Health Organization (WHO) [Online]. Available: https://www.who.int/whr/2003/chapter5/en/. Accessed 12 December 2020.
109. Bordi, L., Nicastri, E., Scorzolini, L., Di Caro, A., Capobianchi, M.R., Castilletti, C., Lalle, E.: Centers, Differential diagnosis of illness in patients under investigation for the novel coronavirus (SARS-CoV-2), Italy, February 2020, Eurosurveillance, vol. 25, no. 8, pp. 2–5 (2020)
110. Hilarie, V., Koukam, A., Rodrigue, S.: An adaptive agent architecture for holonic multiagent system. In ACM Trans on Autonomous Adaptive Systems 3, no. 1 (2008)

111. Abdoos, M., Mozayani, N., Bazzan, A.L.: Towards reinforcement learning for holonic multi-agent systems. Intell. Data Anal. **19**(2), 211–232 (2015)

Chapter 14
Computer-Aided Detection of Depressive Severity Using Multimodal Behavioral Data

Jiaqing Liu, Yue Huang, Shurong Chai, Hao Sun, Xinyin Huang, Lanfen Lin, and Yen-Wei Chen

Abstract This chapter presents depressive severity detection using deep learning methods for automatic audio, visual and audiovisual emotion sensing. The article starts from basic methods on experimental design and data acquisition systems for computer-aided depressive severity diagnosis. Next, typical baseline behavioral features such as facial expressions and speech prosody will be introduced. From the experimental results of the baseline systems introduced in this chapter, readers can not only compare between the performance of different baseline features but also have a general understanding of computer-aided depressive severity diagnosis.

Keywords Depressive severity · Dynamic facial features · Multimodal · Emotional speech · Convolutional neural network (CNN) · Gated recurrent unit (GRU)

14.1 Introduction

Depressive tendencies is widespread in the population and can negatively impact people's daily lives in several ways. In particular, university students are at a high risk of depressive tendencies as they can face intense academic, financial, and interpersonal pressures [1] while going through a critical period of transition from adolescence to adulthood and making many important life decisions [2]. Students with

---

J. Liu · S. Chai · Y.-W. Chen
College of Information Science and Engineering, Ritsumeikan University, Shiga, Japan

Y. Huang · X. Huang (✉)
School of Education, Soochow University, Jiangsu, China
e-mail: hxy5128@163.com

H. Sun · L. Lin · Y.-W. Chen
College of Computer Science and Technology, Zhejiang University, Hangzhou, China

Y.-W. Chen
Zhejiang Lab, Research Center for Healthcare Data Science, Hangzhou, China

Y. Huang
Westlake University, Hangzhou, China

depressive tendencies may exhibit typical symptoms, such as low mood, loss of interest, and decreased energy. Such symptoms are a serious problem and are especially found among university students, as they can affect academic performance and health, and may in extreme cases lead to suicide [1].

People with depressive tendencies are screened using self-assessment questionnaires, such as the Beck's Depression Inventory (BDI) [3] and the Center for Epidemiologic Studies Depression Scale (CES-D) [4]. In this study, we define university students with depressive tendencies as those whose BDI-II and CES-D scores meet or exceed the depression assessment criteria, but do not meet the diagnostic criteria for major depressive disorder given in the DSM-5[5].

Depression, given its high incidence and negative impacts, such as impaired personal functions and social-economic burden [6–8], has become a serious social problem, worthy of our increased attention. Currently, the depression rate among Chinese university students has risen to 23.8% [2]. Previous research has shown that depressive tendencies experienced by young people may persist into adulthood and develop into depressive disorder [9, 10]. Therefore, effectively recognizing such symptoms in university students can help university mental health workers to identify and help them earlier, reducing the risk of depression.

Most existing studies on the development of automated depression diagnosis systems have attempted to extract appropriate features from clinical interview datasets (e.g., the AVEC depression dataset) [11–13], focusing their analysis on patients with clinical depression from the western culture [11–15]. However, there have been few studies on the combination of expression, action, and speech data to extract multimodal features, and in particular, there is currently no multimodal dataset based on Chinese university students with and without depressive tendencies.

In this chapter, automatic computer-aided depressive severity diagnosis will be introduced, including basic experimental design and performances of baseline audiovisual features.

14.2 Multimodal Behavioral Dataset of Chinese University Students with and Without Depressive Tendencies

Figure 14.1 gives an overview of our study. First, we created a multimodal dataset to investigate the relationship between university students with and without depressive tendencies and their observed behaviors during several behavioral experiments. The dataset comprises two components: the behavioral dataset and the screening survey results. Later (in Sect. 14.3), we will extract visual audio features from part of these data to use them to develop a model (or mapping function) for investigating the relationship between participants' behavior and their depressive severity. In this study, we use the results of screening surveys as ground truth regarding depressive severity.

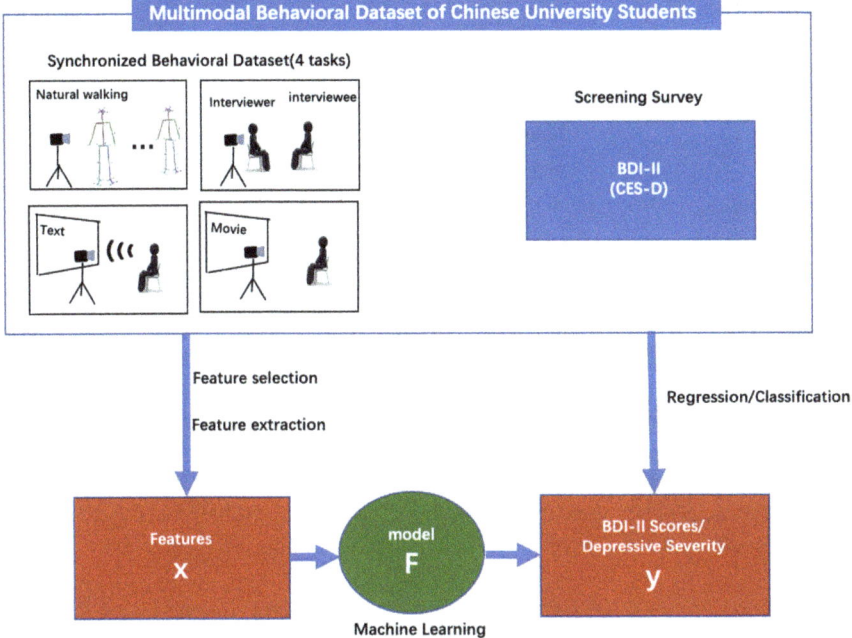

Fig. 14.1 Overview of our study into the relationship between university students' depressive tendencies and their observed behaviors

14.2.1 Collecting Survey Data

This study was reviewed and approved by Soochow University in China. In this study, we used BDI-II screening survey data as ground truth regarding depressive severity. We used two scales (BDI-II and CES-D) to increase data credibility and eliminate participants whose scores differed significantly.

Beck Depression Inventory-II The BDI is a 21-item self-reported depression metric. Each item is rated on a Likert scale with four possible answers, increasing in intensity from 0 to 3, yielding a total BDI score of between 0 and 63. In this study, we used the second BDI version, revised by Wang et al. [16]. There are four specific levels of depressive severity: 0–13 as minimal (no depression), 14–19 as mild, 20–28 as moderate, and 29–63 as severe [17]. For binary classification, 14 is the classification boundary. In this study, the BDI-II data's internal consistency was 0.88.

Center for Epidemiologic Studies Depression Scale The CES-D is a 20-item self-reported depression metric. Each item is rated on a Likert scale with four possible answers, increasing in intensity from 0 to 3, yielding a total CES-D score of between 0 and 60. The Chinese version of CES-D [18] was adopted in this study. Following the

Table 14.1 Differences in the groups' demographic and psychological characteristics

	DP ($N = 51$)	HP ($N = 51$)
Age($M \pm SD$)	18.98 ± 0.91	18.84 ± 0.83
Gender (n)		
Male	26	26
Female	25	25
BDI-II($M \pm SD$)	21.31 ± 6.72	5.45 ± 4.12
CES-D($M \pm SD$)	24.18 ± 6.82	7.53 ± 4.89

original author's recommendation [19], We set the threshold for possible depression to 16. In this study, the CES-D data's internal consistency was 0.86.

Participants were recruited by distributing and collecting questionnaires on campus. Students who met the screening criteria were invited to participate in the study through phone calls or text messages. All participants were first taken through a consent process. They were then invited to complete the BDI-II and CES-D again, and the resulting scores were used to select participants for further experimental analysis.

For the experiment, 102 participants (Chinese university students) were recruited for the study. According to their scores on standardized self-report questionnaires (BDI-II [19] and CES-D [20]), the participants were divided into two groups: depressed persons (DP) and healthy persons (HP). The DP group comprised 51 participants (26 male and 25 female): BDI-II $\geq$ 14 and CES-D $\geq$ 16, none of whom met the DSM-5 diagnostic criteria for major depressive disorder. The HP group comprised 51 participants (26 male and 25 female): BDI-II $<$ 14 and CES-D $<$ 16, none with histories of mental illness. There was no age difference between the DP and HP groups ($t(100) = 0\ 0.80, p = 0.43$). The BDI-II ($t(100) = 14.38, p < 0.001$) and CES-D ($t(100) = 14.17, p < 0.001$) scores were significantly higher in DP than in HP. Differences in the groups' demographic and psychological characteristics were presented in Table 14.1. A preliminary study of this database is referenced in [21].

14.2.2 Acquiring Behavioral Data

Next, four experimental tasks were attempted for data collection, and the data acquisition system is shown in Fig. 14.2. The four experimental tasks in this study were designed on the basis of preliminary experiments with reference to relevant studies [22–24].

In this subsection, we will introduce the multimodal data acquisition system used to build our behavioral dataset. Participants sat 2.7 m away from the display screen, which was 1.9 m × 1.06 m. A web camera (Logitech C920) was set up directly 1.2 m away in front of them to synchronously collect their expression and voice

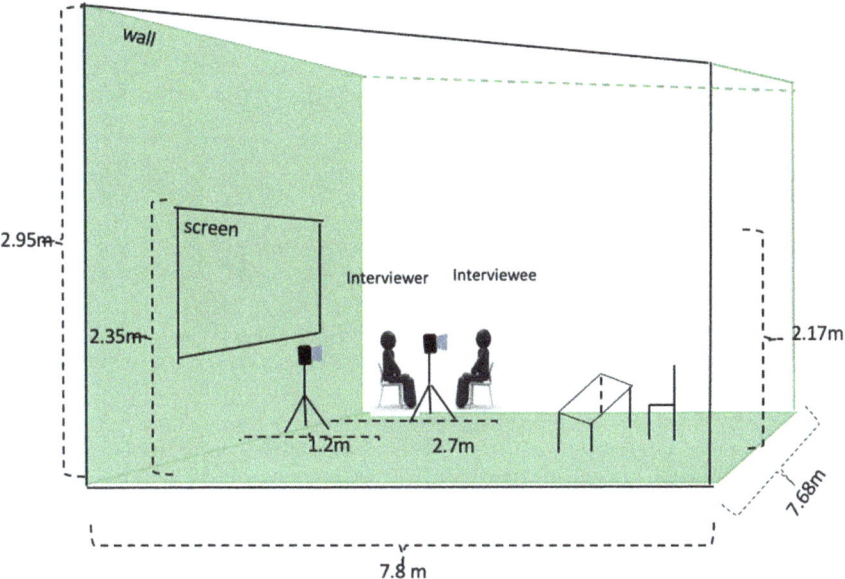

Fig. 14.2 Illustration of the data acquisition system

information at a resolution of 1920 × 1080 with a frame rate of approximately 50 frames per second.

As shown in Fig. 14.1, the experimental tasks in the behavioral database in this study comprised four tasks: natural walking, natural situational interview, reading emotional text, and freely watching emotional videos. The four experimental tasks were completed on the same day, and each participant completed all the experimental tasks in the order of Tasks 1–4 (the sequence arrangement of the four experimental tasks was adjusted and determined according to the feedback of the participants in the pre-experiment and the coherence of the whole experiment). Adequate rest time was set between tasks to reduce the interference between different tasks.

In task 2, we designed 13 questions based on the diagnostic criteria for major depressive disorder given in the DSM-5 [5] and the Hamilton Depression Rating Scale [20]. These questions were designed to elicit spontaneous speech from the participants, along with related facial expressions and actions. We also ensured that the participants were not clinically depressed during this process. Those who answered yes to fewer than five of the first nine questions were not asked the remaining questions (10–13). Table 14.2 presents 13 main topics covered during the interviews (task 2).

To facilitate the follow-up research for exploring the cross-valence stability of the interview questions, participants would be asked three types of emotional questions at the beginning of the interview. (1) Neutral question: Can you tell me something about your recent study and life? (2) Positive question: Please share with me a good

Table 14.2 List of topics covered during the interviews (task 2)

Topic	Sample questions
1	How has your mood been for the last two weeks?—Have you felt sad for most of the days?
2	What are you usually interested in?—Have you been interested in this during the last two weeks?—Have these activities brought you pleasure during this time? -Has your interest in other topics diminished?
3	Has your appetite changed at all during the last two weeks? -Has your weight changed during this time?—By how much has it increased or decreased?—Has it changed by more than 5% of your original body weight?
4	How have you slept during the last two weeks? -Did you have insomnia (such as having difficulty falling asleep, waking during the night, waking in early hours and unable to fall asleep again) or sleep too much?
5	Here, notes were made of the behavior observed during the interview, such as fidgetiness, playing with hands, hair, inability to sit still, standing during the interview, hand wringing, nail biting, hair pulling, biting of lips
6	How has your energy been over the last two weeks? -Have you always been tired?—Have you experienced back pain, headaches, or muscle pain, or heaviness in your limbs, head, or back?
7	Have you blamed yourself for anything over the last two weeks? -Have you felt guilty for most of the day during the last two weeks? -Have you felt worthless during this time?—Did it last for most of the day during the last two weeks?
8	Have you felt unable to think over the last two weeks? -Did this last for most of the day during the last two weeks? -Have you been able to concentrate on what you were doing during this time?—Did it last for most of the day during the last two weeks? -Have you felt hesitant to do something during this time? -Did it last for most of the day during the last two weeks?
9	Have you experienced any extreme thoughts or behaviors over the last two weeks, such as hurting yourself or committing suicide? -Did you act on them?
10	Have the problems you've talked about had a negative impact on your social life, studies, or daily life, giving you pain or discomfort?
11	Are these problems related to a particular substance or disease?
12	Have you ever had any psychiatric disorders (schizophrenia spectrum disorders or other psychiatric disorders)? -Were/was these/this associated with the onset of the problems you've talked about?
13	Have you had a remarkably persistent high level of emotional ego-inflation or mood irritability, or an unusually persistent increase in activity or energy most of the day more than 4 days a week?

memory and describe the scene at that time. (3) Negative question: Please share with me a sad memory and describe the scene at that time.

Task 3 was inspired by related work [25] to collect more audio information from the participants. The emotional sentences are listed in Table 14.3.

Table 14.3 List of emotional sentences. n is the number of keyframes in each sentence (task 3)

Emotional type	Sentence ID	Content written in Chinese (translate to English)	n
Positive	No. 1	盼啊!盼啊!眼看春节就快到了。 (Wish ah! Wish ah! The Spring Festival is coming soon.)	12
	No. 2	想到这,我不由得笑了起来。 (Thinking about it, I couldn't help laughing.)	11
	No. 3	在春节前,人们个个喜气洋洋,个个精神饱满。 (Before the Spring Festival, people are all beaming, and in high spirit.)	18
	No. 4	逛街的人络绎不绝,有的在买年画,有的在买年货。 (People go shopping in an endless stream, some are buying New Year pictures, some are buying New Year goods.)	20
	No. 5	有的围着火炉看电视,还有的人在打麻将打扑克等等,不一而足。 (Some were watching TV by the fire, others were playing mah-jongg and poker, and so on.)	26
	No. 6	大年三十,人们常常玩到深夜,嘴里啃着美味水果,手里燃放烟花爆竹。 (On New Year's Eve, people often play late into the night, eating delicious fruit and setting off fireworks in their hands.)	28
	No. 7	大人小孩都载歌载舞,忘情地玩个痛快。 (Adults and children are singing and dancing and enjoy themselves.)	16
Neutral	No. 1	卢沟桥位于北京广安门外永定河上,距天安门15千米 (Lugou Bridge is located on the Yongding River outside Guang'anmen Square in Beijing, 15 km away from Tiananmen Square.)	23
	No. 2	它始建于金代大定年间,历时3年建成,定名为"广利桥" (It was built in the Dading period of the Jin Dynasty, took 3 years to build, and was named "Guangli Bridge".)	22
	No. 3	又因永定河旧称卢沟河,所以广利桥俗称卢沟桥。 (Because the Yongding River was formerly known as the Lugou River, the Guangli Bridge is commonly known as Lugou Bridge.)	20
	No. 4	卢沟桥是北京地区现存的最古老的一座联拱石桥 (Lugou Bridge is the oldest existing multi-arch stone bridge in Beijing.)	21
	No. 5	明清两代都有重修,现在所见到的为1986年重修复原后的石桥 (The stone bridge was rebuilt in the Ming and Qing dynasties, and what we see now is the stone bridge that was rebuilt in 1986.)	28

(continued)

Table 14.3 (continued)

Emotional type	Sentence ID	Content written in Chinese (translate to English)	n
	No. 6	桥长266.5米, 桥面宽9.3米, 为花岗岩所修成。 (The bridge is 266.5 m long and 9.3 m wide. It is made of granite.)	24
Negative	No. 1	三十三年前的一次车祸让妈妈永远的离开了我们 (Thirty-three years ago, a car accident took my mother from us forever.)	21
	No. 2	妈妈您在另一个世界过得还好吗 (Mom, how is life with you in the other world?)	14
	No. 3	儿子好想念您呀 (Your son misses you so much!)	7
	No. 4	这么多年来, 儿子一时一刻没有忘记您那慈祥的笑容 (Over these years, your son never forgot your kind smile for a moment.)	22
	No.5	虽然您离开时我只有十三岁, 虽然生前一张照片也没留下, 可是儿子永远也忘不了您 (Although I was only thirteen when you left me, and you had not left a single picture yet, I will never forget you.)	35
	No. 6	多少次夜里梦见您的身影: 多少次梦中想您哭醒 (I have dreamed of you many times during the night and have cried for you many times in my dreams.)	20
	No.7	妈妈, 您怎么那么狠心就扔下我们不管了呢? (Mom, why did you leave us so cruelly?)	18

14.3 Computer-Aided Detection of Depressive Severity

In this section, we make a preliminary application of the multimodal dataset established in the previous section, to evaluate the feasibility of this dataset in predicting depressive severity among university students using data from Task3 as an example. Figure 14.3 shows the architecture of our proposed model. Our deep neural network model comprises three parts: (1) the subnetworks for each single modality feature extraction; (2) a gated recurrent unit (GRU) network for each audiovisual representation; (3) the final decision layer for depressive severity detection.

14.3.1 Feature Extraction

In this subsection, we will explain how we selected the baseline behavioral features, which can be used to investigate the relationship between university students with depressive severity and their observed behaviors. The baseline features are inspired by AVEC 2019 [26]. For ethical reasons, we have not published raw video images.

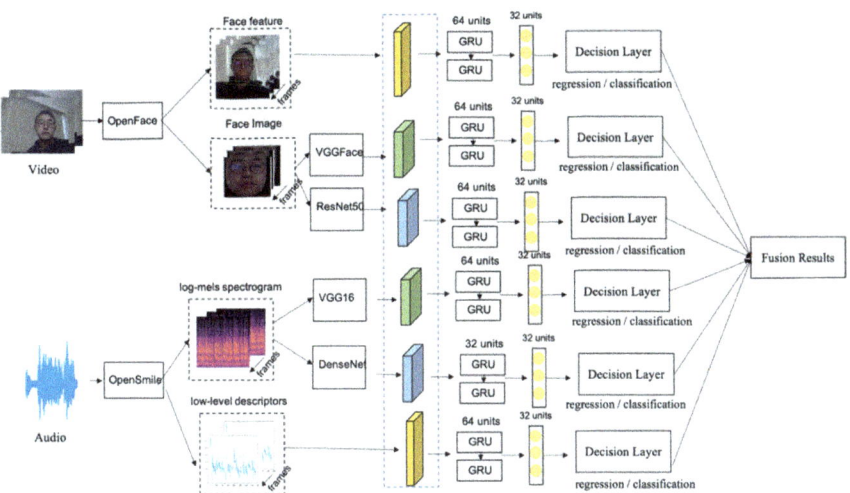

Fig. 14.3 The architecture of the proposed model. The unimodal features are extracted separately and concatenated in a decision strategy

14.3.1.1 Audio Features

The first step in analyzing the prosodic features of a person's speech is to isolate the speech from silence, other speakers, and noise. For audio features, we use the openSMILE [27] toolkit to compute the extended Geneva minimalistic acoustic parameter set (eGeMAPS) [28], which has 36 features and Mel frequency cepstral coefficents (MFCCs), including their 1st and 2nd order derivatives (deltas and double-deltas) as a set of acoustic low-level descriptors (LLDs). These low-level features (eGeMAPS and MFCCs) are also summarized over time by computing their mean and standard deviation using a sliding window of 4 s and a hop size of 1 s. The functionals of the eGeMAPS and MFCCs are represented as eGeMAPS -F and MFCCs-F, respectively.

The bags-of-words (BoW) model, which commonly used in natural language processing and information retrieval, that represents the distribution of LLDs according to a dictionary that was trained on the distribution is used as mid-level features. The codebook size is 100. To generate BoW representations, both the eGeMAPS and MFCC features are processed a summarized over a block of a 4-s length duration. The open-source toolkit oepnXBOW4 [29] is used to execute these processes. The BOW representation of the eGeMAPS and MFCC features is represented as BoW-E and BoW-M, respectively.

For deep representations, inspired by the development of deep learning (DL) in image processing, Mel-spectral images of speech instances are fed into pre-trained image recognition convolution neural networks using VGG-16 [30] and DENSENET-201[31] to extract high-level features. In particular, the audio waves are first transformed into mel-spectogram images with 80 mel-frequency bands with 4-s window width and a hop size of 1 s. Following that, the mel-spectogram images are

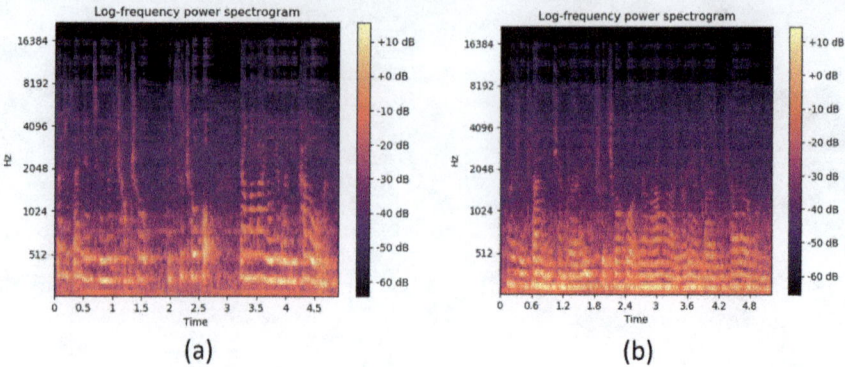

Fig. 14.4 Examples of log-mels spectrogram for depression **a** and non-depression **b**

forwarded through the networks pre-trained by ImageNet [32]. A 4096-dimensional feature vector is then extracted from the second fully connected layer in VGG-16 networks and a 1920- dimensional feature vector of the last average pooling layer of DENSENET-201 networks, respectively (Fig. 14.4).

14.3.1.2 Video Features

For low-level descriptors of visual features, we use the OPEN-FACE toolkit [33] to extract the intensities of 17 facial action units for each video frame (Fig. 14.5), along with a confidence measure. The generation of BoW representations of visual features is the same as audio features.

For deep visual representations, we employed a VGG-16 [30] network and a ResNet-50 network pre-trained with the Affwild dataset [34], which focuses on human affect understanding. In particular, the OPEN-FACE toolkit [33] is used to detect the face region and, subsequently, perform face alignment. Following that, the aligned face images are forwarded through the two pre-trained models, respectively. As a result, a 4096-dimensional deep feature vector from the VGG-16 network and

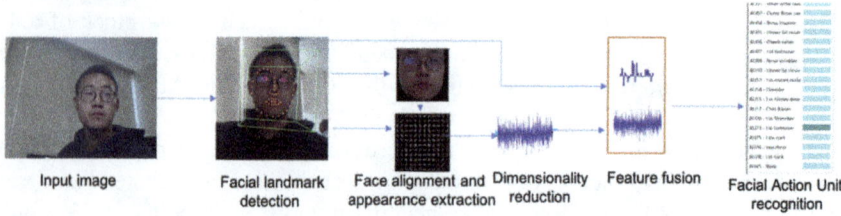

Fig. 14.5 Low-level descriptor extraction of visual features using OpenFace, including facial landmark detection, head pose and eye gaze estimation, facial action unit recognition

a 2048-dimensional deep feature vector from the ResNet-50 network are extracted for each frame.

14.3.2 Detection Model

Finally, we will introduce the baseline GRU network and a late fusion strategy to combine audio and visual modalities in this subsection.

A GRU was proposed by Cho et al. [35] to make each recurrent unit adaptively capture dependencies of different time scales. Similar to a long short-term memory unit, the GRU has gating units that modulate the flow of information inside the unit, but without separate memory cells [36]. For each audio-visual feature, we use a GRU network with two-layers, each of which has 64 nodes for their hidden layers. Next, we develop a fully connected neural network that has one hidden layer with 32 nodes; a single linear layer to map to the desired output size of one for a BDI-II score regression task and an output of four for a classification task.

We define the two tasks used in our experiments: BDI-II score regression task and depressive severity classification task. In the BDI-II score regression task, we predict participants' BDI-II scores, which ranges from 0 to 63 in our database. The loss function for the BDI-II score regression task is the concordance correlation coefficient (CCC) loss function (L_{ccc}). (L_{ccc}) can be defined as Eq. (14.1) to maximize the agreement between a true value (y) and prediction depressive symptoms degree ($\hat{y}$).

$$L_{ccc} = 1 - \frac{2p_{\hat{y}y}\sigma_{\hat{y}}\sigma_y}{\sigma_{\hat{y}}^2 + \sigma_y^2 + (\mu_{\hat{y}} - \mu_y)^2} \tag{14.1}$$

where $p_{\hat{y}y}$ is the Pearson coefficient correlation between $\hat{y}$ and y, σ is the standard deviation, and μ is a mean value.

In the classification task, we discretize the BDI-II score into 4 classes [17]: minimal (no depression) [0–13], mild [14–19], moderate [20–28], and severe [29–63]. We treat this problem as a multi-class classification problem, and cross-entropy loss is used. The cross-entropy loss can be defined as follows:

$$L_{CE} = -\sum_{i}^{n} y_i \log(p_i) \tag{14.2}$$

where y_i is the truth label, and p_i is the SoftMax probability for the ith class.

Decision fusion (late fusion) is the most commonly used method for multimodal depression severity detection. We train a regressor (or classifier) for each modality and combine the individual predictions as inputs to a fusion regressor (or classifier) to build the baseline fusion results.

Table 14.4 Distribution of our training, development, and test sets

Task		Train	Dev	Test
Regression task		72	10	20
Classification task	Minimal [0–13]	36	5	10
	Mild [14–19]	14	2	4
	Moderate [20–28]	16	2	4
	Severe [29–38]	6	1	2

As shown in Fig. 14.3, the model has been obtained as follows. First, the single feature streams are trained separately using the ground truth. Next, the output of the 8 audio single streams and 4 visual streams are used as inputs to the decision fusion.

14.4 Performance Evaluation

In this section, we report the results of our model variants described in Sect. 14.3.

14.4.1 Experimental Setup

Our novel multimodal behavioral dataset for task 3, which is described in Sect. 14.2, is used in our experiments. The dataset contains data for 102 participants. We divide the dataset into training, development, and test sets. The distribution of our training, development, and test sets is summarized in Table 14.4.

For evaluation using the test set, we use the best performing model on the development set. To handle the bias, we converted the BDI-II score labels to floating-point numbers by downscaling with a factor of 38 before training. Root mean squared error (RMSE) results are reported using the original BDI-II scale. The model is implemented using PyTorch and is trained with an ADAM optimizer.

14.4.2 Evaluation Functions

We use well-known standard evaluation metrics for depressive severity detection to evaluate regression/classification results.

We use the CCC as a measure of estimated scores (regression task), which is the common metric in dimensional depressive severity detection to measure the agreement between true BDI-II scores (y) and predicted BDI-II scores ($\hat{y}$). The CCC is formulated as follows:

$$CCC = \frac{2p_{\hat{y}y}\sigma_{\hat{y}}\sigma_y}{\sigma_{\hat{y}}^2 + \sigma_y^2 + (\mu_{\hat{y}} - \mu_y)^2} \tag{14.3}$$

where $p_{\hat{y}y}$ is the Pearson coefficient correlation between $\hat{y}$ and y, σ is the standard deviation, and μ is a mean value. This CCC is based on Lin's calculation [37]. The range of the CCC is from -1 to 1, where -1 represents perfect disagreement and 1 represents perfect agreement.

We also use the RMSE, which is defined as Eq. (14.4), as another measure for the regression task.

$$RMSE = \sqrt{\frac{\sum_i^N (y_i - \hat{y}_i)}{N}} \tag{14.4}$$

For the classification task, the accuracy (denoted as *Acc*) is defined on all test samples and is the fraction of predictions that the model obtained correctly. For *Acc*, 1 represents the best accuracy and 0 represents the worst accuracy. *Acc* is defined as follows:

$$Acc = \frac{Number\ of\ Correnc\ Predictions}{Total\ Number\ of\ Predictions} \tag{14.5}$$

14.4.3 Results

We summarized the results of using each audio feature and visual feature in Tables 14.5 and 14.6, respectively, to demonstrate the effect of each feature. CCC and RMSR are the metrics used to evaluate the results of the regression task, and Acc is the metric used to evaluate the results of the classification task. The best result for each measure is highlighted in bold.

For the regression task, the best results in terms of the CCC score from audio features were achieved with BoW-M, eGeMAPS-F, and eGeMAPS-F for negative, neutral, and positive emotional speech, respectively. The model with Res-ImageNet features achieved the best result for visual features in all three valences. These results indicate the low-level features are more useful for audio-based depression detection, whereas representations learned by deep neural networks are more powerful for visual-based depression detection. In terms of valence, the positive-emotional speech achieved the best results both in audio-based and visual-based BDI-II score regression.

The results of fusing all features (multi-modal features) are summarized in Table 14.7. Compared with Tables 14.5 and 14.6, one can conclude that the decision fusion (multi-model) outperforms any single-modal, which indicates that feature fusion may provide complementary information for depressive severity detection.

Table 14.5 The results of using each audio feature on development dataset and test dataset

Negative

Partition			Audio								
			Low-level features				Middle-level features (BoW)		High-level features (DL)		
			EGEMAPS	MFCCs	EGEMAPS-F	MFCCs-F	BoW-M	BoW-e	DNet	VGG
Dev	CCC		0.04	0.32	0.16	−0.14	**0.54**	0.10	0.26	0.31
	RMSE		23.07	10.59	12.77	17.00	9.90	10.48	11.25	**9.81**
	Acc		0.50	0.50	**0.70**	**0.70**	0.50	0.60	0.60	**0.70**
Test	CCC		−0.06	0.16	−0.03	**0.31**	−0.03	−0.19	0.20	−0.12
	RMSE		22.72	14.62	17.46	**11.37**	14.95	13.61	12.61	13.28
	Acc		0.10	0.25	0.30	**0.35**	0.25	0.30	0.25	0.25

Neutral

Dev	CCC		0.43	0.12	**0.79**	0.51	0.17	0.22	0.51	0.49
	RMSE		10.69	15.35	**5.79**	9.99	14.91	10.31	9.47	9.47
	Acc		0.60	0.50	0.70	**0.80**	0.70	0.60	0.60	0.50
Test	CCC		−0.21	0.07	0.19	−0.15	**0.29**	0.15	0.18	0.10
	RMSE		14.31	13.26	11.95	16.22	12.29	**9.96**	13.18	11.68

(continued)

Table 14.5 (continued)

Negative								
Acc	0.15	0.20	0.25	0.15	0.25	**0.30**	0.25	**0.30**
Positive								
Dev	CCC	0.36	0.24	**0.87**	0.43	0.57	0.39	0.60	0.47
	RMSE	10.94	12.47	**4.92**	11.80	9.24	9.38	8.65	9.67
	Acc	**0.60**	**0.60**	**0.60**	**0.60**	**0.60**	0.50	**0.60**	**0.60**
Test	CCC	0.16	−0.14	−0.50	**0.52**	0.27	−0.98	−0.23	0.05
	RMSE	12.32	17.50	19.23	**10.80**	12.53	12.82	13.75	12.67
	Acc	**0.35**	0.25	0.30	**0.35**	0.30	**0.35**	0.30	**0.35**

Table 14.6 The results of using each visual feature on development dataset and test dataset

Partition			Visual			
			Low-level features	High-level features (DL)		
			FAUs	Res-Affwild	ResImageNet	VGG-Affwild
Negative						
Dev		CCC	0.56	0.68	**0.72**	0.19
		RMSE	9.56	7.22	**7.02**	10.23
		Acc	**0.70**	0.60	0.60	0.50
Test		CCC	0.002	−0.06	−0.24	**0.008**
		RMSE	15.93	12.91	15.19	**11.42**
		Acc	**0.40**	0.25	0.30	0.30
Neutral						
Dev		CCC	0.65	0.47	**0.72**	0.44
		RMSE	8.33	9.20	**6.29**	8.83
		Acc	**0.70**	0.50	0.60	0.50
Test		CCC	−0.27	**−0.10**	−0.15	−0.12
		RMSE	19.79	16.84	13.74	**12.59**
		Acc	0.25	0.25	**0.30**	0.25
Positive						
Dev		CCC	0.40	0.78	**0.80**	0.39
		RMSE	9.73	6.93	**6.20**	10.04
		Acc	0.50	**0.60**	**0.60**	0.50
Test		CCC	**0.29**	−0.23	0.09	0.18
		RMSE	13.60	14.99	**10.77**	11.59
		Acc	**0.35**	0.25	0.2	0.30

14.5 Conclusions

In this chapter, we introduced a novel multimodal behavioral dataset of Chinese university students with and without depressive tendencies. We have also presented the baseline networks and their results for audio and visual features. These results indicated that low level features performed better in audio-based depression detection, whereas DL features performed better in visual-based depression detection. The prediction results in the emotional speech scenario indicated behavioral features in positive-emotional speech have more potential in depressive severity identification. In the future, there will be a better way to use the audio-visual features for depressive severity detection, which is worth researching and exploring.

Table 14.7 The results of fusing all audio and visual features (multi-modal features) on development dataset and test dataset

Negative			
	Dev	CCC	0.52
		RMSE	8.38
		Acc	0.40
	Test	CCC	−0.05
		RMSE	10.59
		Acc	0.45
Neutral			
	Dev	CCC	0.61
		RMSE	7.22
		Acc	0.60
	Test	CCC	−0.03
		RMSE	10.64
		Acc	0.55
Positive			
	Dev	CCC	0.71
		RMSE	6.32
		Acc	0.40
	Test	CCC	0.06
		RMSE	10.13
		Acc	0.50

Acknowledgements This work is supported in part by Japan Society of Promotion of Science (20J13009).

References

1. Chen, L., Wang, L., Qiu, X. H., Yang, X. X., Qiao, Z. X., Yang, Y. J., Liang, Y.: Depression among Chinese university students: prevalence and socio-demographic correlates. PloS One **8**(3), e58379 (2013)
2. Lei, X. Y., Xiao, L. M., Liu, Y. N., Li, Y. M.:Prevalence of depression among Chinese University students: a meta-analysis. PLoS One **11**(4), e0153454 (2016)
3. Setterfield, M., Walsh, M., Frey, A.L., McCabe, C.: Increased social anhedonia and reduced helping behaviour in young people with high depressive symptomatology. J. Affect. Disord. **205**, 372–377 (2016)
4. Brinkmann, K., Franzen, J.: Blunted cardiovascular reactivity during social reward anticipation in subclinical depression. Int. J. Psychophysiol. **119**, 119–126 (2017)
5. American Psychiatric Association.: Diagnostic and statistical manual of mental disorders (DSM-5®). American Psychiatric Pub (2013)
6. Hysenbegasi, A., Hass, S. L., Rowland, C. R.: The impact of depression on the academic productivity of university students. J. Ment. Health Policy Econ. **8**(3), 145 (2005)

7. Hu, T.W.: The economic burden of depression and reimbursement policy in the Asia Pacific region. Australas. Psych. **12**(sup1), s11–s15 (2004)
8. Sobocki, P., Lekander, I., Borgström, F., Ström, O., Runeson, B.: The economic burden of depression in Sweden from 1997 to 2005. Eur. Psychiatry **22**(3), 146–152 (2007)
9. Aalto-Setälä, T., Marttunen, M., Tuulio-Henriksson, A., Poikolainen, K., Lö-nnqvist, J.: Depressive symptoms in adolescence as predictors of early adulthood depressive disorders and maladjustment. Am. J. Psychiatry **159**(7), 1235–1237 (2002)
10. Liu, X.C., Ma, D.D., Kurita, H., Tang, M.Q.: Self-reported depressive symptoms among Chinese adolescents. Soc. Psychiatry Psychiatr. Epidemiol. **34**(1), 44–47 (1999)
11. Jan, A., Meng, H., Gaus, Y. F.B.A., Zhang, F.: Artificial intelligent system for automatic depression level analysis through visual and vocal expressions. IEEE Trans. Cogn. & Dev. Syst. **99**, 1–1 (2017)
12. Jan, A., Meng, H., Gaus, Y. F. A., Zhang, F., Turbzadeh, S.: Automatic depression scale prediction using facial expression dynamics and regression. In Proceedings of the 4th International Workshop on Audio/Visual Emotion Challenge (pp. 73–80). ACM (2014, November)
13. Yang, L., Jiang, D., Xia, X., Pei, E., Oveneke, M.C., Sahli, H.: Multimodal measurement of depression using deep learning models. In Proceedings of the 7th Annual Workshop on Audio/Visual Emotion Challenge (pp. 53–59). ACM(2017, October).
14. Dibeklioğlu, H., Hammal, Z., Cohn, J.F.: Dynamic multimodal measurement of depression severity using deep autoencoding. IEEE J. Biomed. Health Inform. **22**(2), 525–536 (2018)
15. Girard, J.M., Cohn, J.F., Mahoor, M.H., Mavadati, S., Rosenwald, D.P.: Social risk and depression: Evidence from manual and automatic facial expression analysis. In 2013 10th IEEE International Conference and Workshops on Automatic Face and Gesture Recognition (FG) (pp. 1–8). IEEE (2013, April).
16. Wang, Z., Yuan, C. M., Huang, J., Li, Z. Z., Chen, J., Zhang, H. Y., et al.: Reliability and validity of the Chinese version of Beck Depression Inventory-II among depression patients. Chinese Mental Health J. **25**(6), 476–480 (2011)
17. Beck, A.T., Steer, R.A., Brown, G.K.: Beck depression inventory-II. San Antonio **78**(2), 490–498 (1996)
18. Wang, X. D., Wang, X. L., Ma, H.: Manual of mental health assessment scales. Chinese Mental Health Journal(supplement) (1999)
19. Radloff, L.: The CES-D scale: a self-report depression scale for research in the general population. Applied Psychological Measurement, 1(3), 385–401(1977)
20. Hamilton, M.: Development of a rating scale for primary depressive illness. Br. J. Clin. Psychol. **6**(4), 278–296 (1967)
21. Liu, J.Q., Huang, Y., Huang, X.Y., Xia, X.T., Niu, X.X., Chen, Y.W.: Multimodal Behavioral Dataset of Depressive Symptoms in Chinese College Students–Preliminary Study. In: Chen YW. et. al. (eds) Innovation in Medicine and Healthcare Systems, and Multimedia. Smart Innovation, Systems and Technologies, vol 145, pp. 79–190. Springer, Singapore (2019)
22. McIntyre, G., Göcke, R., Hyett, M., et al.: An approach for automatically measuring facial activity in depressed subjects[C]//2009 3rd International Conference on Affective Computing and Intelligent Interaction and Workshops. IEEE, 1–8 (2009)
23. Pan, W., Wang, J., Liu, T., et al.: Depression recognition based on speech analysis[J]. Chin. Sci. Bull. **63**(20), 2081–2092 (2018)
24. Wang, J.Y.: An exploratory study on auxiliary diagnosis of depression based on speech. Doctoral Dissertation. Chinese Academy of Science, Beijing (2017)
25. Joshi, J., Goecke, R., Parker, G., Breakspear, M.: Can body expressions contribute to automatic depression analysis?. In 2013 10th IEEE International Conference and Workshops on Automatic Face and Gesture Recognition (FG) (pp. 1–7). IEEE (2013, April)
26. Ringeval F., Schuller B., Valstar M., Cummins N., Cowie R., Tavabi L., Schmitt M., Alisamir S., Amiriparian S., Messner E.-M., et al.: Avec 2019 workshop and challenge: state-of-mind, detecting depression with ai, and cross-cultural affect recognition. In Proceedings of the 9th International on Audio/Visual Emotion Challenge and Workshop, pp. 3–12, (2019)

27. Florian E., Felix W., Florian G., and Björn S.: Recent Developments in openSMILE, the Munich Open-Source Multimedia Feature Extractor. In Proc. 21st ACM International Conference on Multimedia (ACM MM). ACM, Barcelona, Spain, 835–838 (2013)
28. Florian, E., Klaus, R.S., Björn, S., Johan, S., Elisabeth, A., Carlos, B., Laurence, D., Julien, E., Petri, L., Shrikanth, S.N., Khiet, P.T.: The Geneva Minimalistic Acoustic Parameter Set (GeMAPS) for Voice Research and Affective Computing. IEEE Trans. Affect. Comput. **7**(2), 190–202 (2016)
29. Maximilian S., Björn S.: openXBOW—Introducing the Passau Open-Source Crossmodal Bag-of-Words Toolkit. Journal of Machine Learning Research (2017)
30. Karen S., Andrew Z.: Very deep convolutional networks for large-scale image recognition. https://arxiv.org/abs/1409.1556. 14 pp (2014)
31. Gao H., Zhuang L., Laurens van der M., Kilian Q.W.: Densely Connected Convolutional Networks. In The IEEE Conference on Computer Vision and Pattern Recognition (CVPR). IEEE, Honolulu, HW, 4700–4708 (2017)
32. Deng, J., Dong, W., Socher, R., Li, L.-J., Li, K., Fei-Fei, L.: ImageNet: A Large-Scale Hierarchical Image Database, In The IEEE Conference on Computer Vision and Pattern Recognition (CVPR) (2009)
33. Tadas, B., Amir, Z., Yao, C.L., Louis, P.M.: OpenFace 2.0: Facial Behavior Analysis Toolkit. In Proc. 13th IEEE International Conference on Automatic Face & Gesture Recognition (FG 2018). IEEE, Xi'an, P. R. China, 59–66 (2018)
34. Dimitrios K., Panagiotis T., Mihalis A. N., Athanasios P., Guoying Z., Björn S., Irene K., Stefanos Z.: Deep affect prediction in-the-wild: Aff-wild database and challenge, deep architectures, and beyond. Int. J. Comput. Vis. **127**(6), 907–929 (2019)
35. Cho, K., van Merrienboer, B., Gulcehre, C., Bougares, F., Schwenk, H., and Bengio, Y.: Learning phrase representations using RNN encoder-decoder for statistical machine translation. CoRR, abs/1406.1078, (2014)
36. Chung J., Gülçehre C.,Cho K., Bengio Y.: Empirical evaluation of gated recurrent neural networks on sequence modeling. CoRR, abs/1412.3555, (2014)
37. Lawrence I-Kuei L.: A concordance correlation coef- ficient to evaluate reproducibility, Biometrics, pp. 255–268 (1989)

Chapter 15
Classifying Process Traces for Stroke Management Quality Assessment: A Deep Learning Approach

Giorgio Leonardi, Stefania Montani, and Manuel Striani

Abstract Stroke management process trace classification can support quality assessment, since it allows to verify whether better-equipped Stroke Centers actually implement more complete processes, suitable to manage complex patients as well. In this paper, we present an approach to stroke trace classification based on deep learning techniques: in particular, we have tested a traditional architecture, based on Recurrent Neural Networks, as well as novel, more complex ones, which combine recurrent networks with convolutional models. Experimental results have shown the feasibility of the approach, and the superiority of composite architectures, which have led to higher accuracy values.

Keywords Classification · Deep learning · Process traces · Stroke management

15.1 Introduction

A stroke is a severe medical condition where poor blood flow to the brain can result in cell death, leading to serious risks for patient health and survival. It is estimated that, by 2025, 1.5 million European people will suffer a stroke each year [1].

Acute stroke care in hospitals is best performed in organized Stroke Units, where patient outcomes are better than those of patients managed in general medical or neurological wards [2]. The European Stroke Organisation (ESO) Stroke Unit Certification Committee, has therefore worked on the definition of evidence-based needs for acute stroke care, in order to stimulate the certification of more advanced stroke care facilities. As a result, it has introduced two certification levels: (1) ESO Stroke

---

G. Leonardi · S. Montani (✉) · M. Striani
DISIT, Computer Science Institute, Università del Piemonte Orientale, Alessandria, Italy
e-mail: stefania.montani@uniupo.it

G. Leonardi
e-mail: giorgio.leonardi@uniupo.it

M. Striani
e-mail: manuel.striani@uniupo.it

Units (SUs) and (2) ESO Stroke Centers (SCs) [3]. ESO Stroke Centers must meet all the requirements of an ESO Stroke Unit, and additionally they should provide more advanced diagnostic and therapeutic equipment, have a larger staff and have expertise on rare or complex stroke subtypes. In many countries, however, significant organizational problems are still observed not only in certified SUs, but sometimes also in SCs (see, e.g., the document in footnote[1] for the Italian situation). Therefore, a thorough analysis of medical processes is needed, in order to verify if the actual performance of a hospital is satisfactory and is coherent with its declared level.

In our previous work [4], we proposed to tackle the above needs by considering stroke management process traces (i.e., the sequences of activities actually executed on the single patients at the hospital at hand, and logged in the hospital information system). Traces can be classified (distinguishing between the SU class and the SC class), to verify if the logged activities are coherent with the level assigned to a given hospital, in a quality assessment perspective. In particular, in [4] we realized classification according to a trace similarity metric, able to take into account temporal information as well as domain knowledge [5, 6]. Results were not particularly convincing. Therefore, we also introduced a deep learning strategy [7], which proved to be more effective.

In this paper, we further investigate that research direction, by performing stroke trace classification resorting to different deep learning architectures. Specifically, we adopt both a traditional solution based on Recurrent Neural Networks, and two novel, more complex ones, based on the definition of composite architectures, which conjugate recurrent networks with the power of convolutional ones.

The paper is organized as follows: in Sect. 15.2 we introduce deep learning and present traditional deep learning architectures; in Sect. 15.3 we summarize related work about process trace classification and prediction; in Sect. 15.4, which is the core of our technical contribution, we detail our deep learning approach to stroke trace classification for quality assessment; in Sect. 15.5 we present experimental results, while Sect. 15.6 is devoted to discussion and conclusions.

15.2 Background

Deep learning architectures are able to stack multiple layers of operations, in order to create a hierarchy of increasingly more abstract *deep* features [7]. These techniques have achieved a great success in computer vision, and their adoption is gaining increasing attention in several domains, including health care (see, e.g., [8–10]).

In the following, we will introduce some background information about the main types of deep learning architectures, that will be useful to present our approach. A table of acronyms (Table 15.1) is provided below, as a useful quick reference.

---

[1] https://www.sanita24.ilsole24ore.com/art/medicina-e-ricerca/2017-04-14/stroke-unit-mercerara-strutture-e-personale-dati-lontani-dm-702015-162809.php?uuid=AEEhud5.

Table 15.1 Table of acronyms

Acronym	Definition
ESO	European stroke network
SU	Stroke unit
SC	Stroke center
CNN	Convolutional neural network
RNN	Recurrent neural network
LSTM	Long short time memory network

15.2.1 Convolutional Neural Networks

Convolutional Neural Networks (CNNs) operate by exploiting multiple convolution operators. A convolution is an operation which takes a filter and multiplies it over the entire area of the input. Convolution layers are followed by pooling (i.e., subsampling) layers, meant to further reduce dimensionality.

The convolution + pooling modules can be stacked in the network, providing progressively deeper architectures. The output of the final pooling layer is then flattened, and provided as an input to a fully connected network, outputting the class.

As an example, Fig. 15.1 presents a well-known, basic CNN architecture, known as LeNet-5 [11]. LeNet-5, a 7 layer CNN, was deployed in many banking systems to recognize hand-written numbers on cheques.

Composed of sparse connections with tied weights, CNNs have significantly fewer parameters than a fully connected network of similar size [12].

It is also possible to use kernels of varied size in a convolution layer to capture features at different levels of abstraction [13], a strategy that mitigates the problem of correctly setting the kernel size.

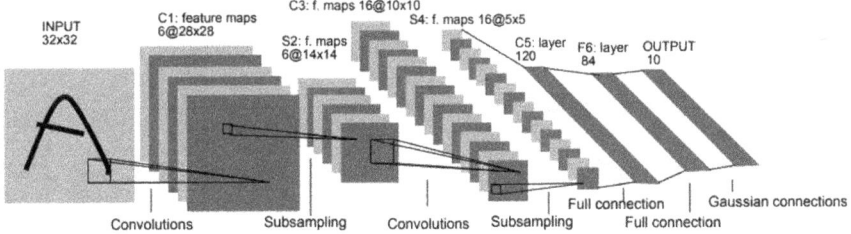

Fig. 15.1 Basic CNN architecture (LeNet-5)

15.2.2 Autoencoders

The main idea behind Autoencoders is to reduce the input into a latent space with fewer dimensions, and then try to reconstruct the input from this representation. The first step is called encoding, and the second step is the decoding phase. During encoding, by reducing the number of variables which represent the data, we force the model to learn how to keep only meaningful information, from which the input is reconstructable. It can thus be viewed as a dimensionality reduction/compression technique. Once the model achieves a desired level of performance recreating the input, the decoding part may be removed, leaving just the encoding model. This model can then be used to encode the input to a fixed-length deep features vector, which can then be provided to a classifier.

In image and time series classification, convolutional Autoencoders are often adopted [14]. In this kind of architecture, the encoding phase uses convolutional layers, followed by pooling layers, meant to further reduce dimensionality. The convolution + pooling modules can be stacked in the network, as described in the previous subsection. The decoding phase, on the other hand, uses up-sampling and convolutions.

Figure 15.2 presents a simple convolutional Autoencoder architecture. *Source* https://hackernoon.com/autoencoders-deep-learning-bits-1-11731e200694—last accessed March 10th, 2021.

An alternative Autoencoder architecture, sometimes adopted for temporal data sequences, is the Encoder-Decoder Long Short Term Memory one [15, 16]; details on Long Short Term Memory Networks are provided in the next subsection.

15.2.3 Recurrent Neural Networks

Recurrent Neural Networks (RNNs) [17] are Neural Networks specialised for processing sequential data. The idea in RNNs is to preserve the results of previous calculations with memories, i.e., with feedback connections that provide a parame-

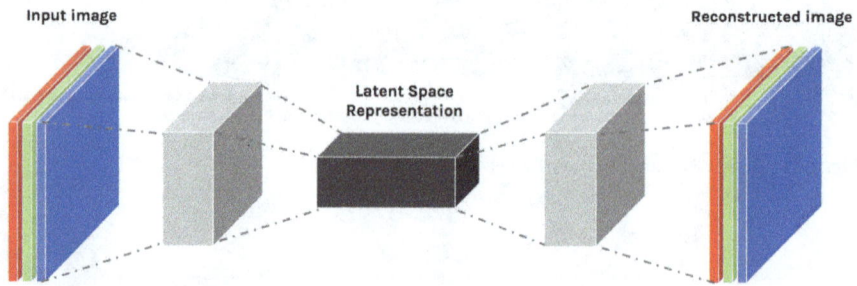

Fig. 15.2 Basic convolutional autoencoder architecture

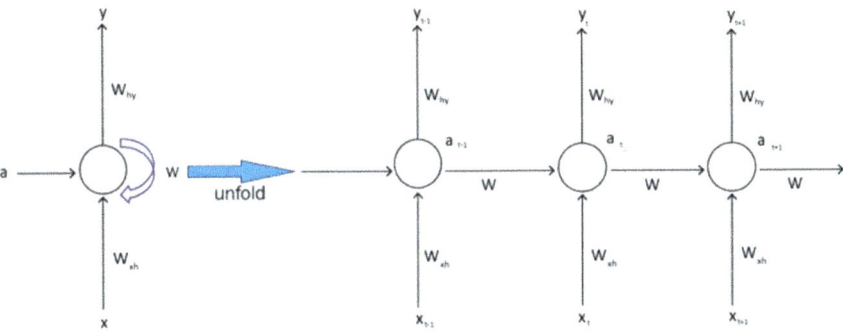

Fig. 15.3 Basic RNN architecture

ter sharing across different parts of the model. Specifically, the hidden layer in the RNNs considers both the current input and the results of the last hidden layer, unlike traditional Neural Networks where there is no dependency between the calculation results.

All RNNs have the form of a chain of repeating modules of Neural Network, as shown in Fig. 15.3 (*source* https://pub.towardsai.net/introduction-to-the-architecture-of-recurrent-neural-networks-rnns-a277007984b7—last accessed March 10th, 2021).

In order to achieve long-term memory, the RNN model requires a significant amount of model training time. Normalization (a process by which the inputs are linearly transformed to have zero mean and unit variance) can be applied to accelerate training. However, in the case of RNNs some of the inputs of the nth layer are from the $(n-1)$th layer, and are not raw inputs: as the training progresses, the effect of normalization thus reduces, causing the vanishing gradient problem [18], which can slow down the entire training process and cause saturation. The Long Short Term Memory Network (LSTM, [18]) architecture has been proposed in order to shorten the training time, and to deal with the vanishing gradient problem. The core idea in LSTMs is to introduce a cell state, more complex than the memory cell in basic RNNs, where information can be added or removed by gated structures, composed of a sigmoid Neural Network layer and a multiplication operation [18].

A basic LSTM module is shown in Fig. 15.4 [19]. The gates calculate their activations at time step t also considering the activation of the memory cell at time step $t-1$.

LSTMs can also manage long-distance dependencies in input sequences. Indeed, in LSTM networks a long-term memory can be implemented, where the information flows from cell to cell with minimal variations, keeping certain aspects constant during the processing of all inputs.

The performance of LSTMs can however be reduced due to rapid overfitting in small datasets. In order to deal with these difficulties, a dimension shuffle layer can be introduced [20]. This layer transposes the temporal dimension of the input, and reduces training time [20].

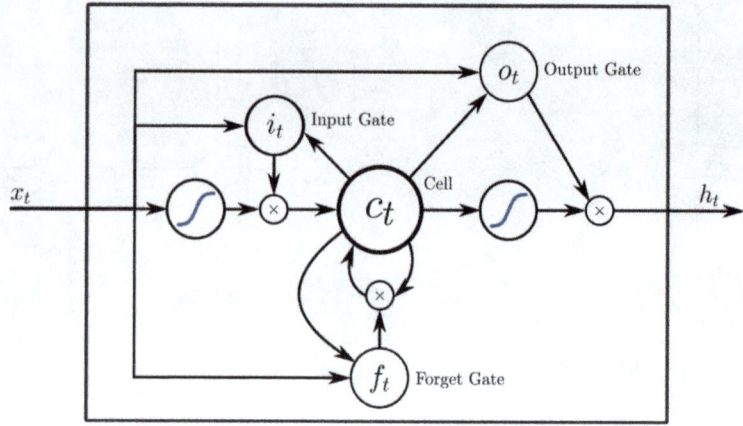

Fig. 15.4 Basic LSTM module

15.3 Related Work

Process prediction/classification [21] exploits the activities logged in process traces to make predictions about the future of a running trace (such as, e.g., the remaining time to complete the work, the next activity to be executed, the needed resources), or to classify the trace on the basis of some categorical or numerical performance properties (as in our work). Process prediction and classification can be useful both for a better planning of the needed resources, and for quality assessment, by means of the identification of non-compliances with respect of the expected performance.

In the literature, most works in this field are focused on the prediction of the next activity in a running process trace. While classical business process management approaches use an explicit model representation such as a state-transition model [22] or an Hidden Markov Model [23], a more recent research direction exploits deep learning.

In particular, several authors rely on RNNs [17], and more specifically on LSTM networks [18]. LSTMs can potentially learn the complex dynamics within the temporal ordering of input sequences; therefore, they are well suited to manage the sequential data of process activity logs.

In [24], the authors use LSTM networks to predict the type of the next activity of an ongoing process trace and the time until the next activity (its timestamp). The network architecture consists of a shared LSTM layer that feeds two independent LSTM layers specialized in predicting the next activity and in predicting times, respectively. The experiments show that the LSTM approach outperforms model-based approaches. The work in [25] proposes a different network architecture which comprises two LSTM hidden layers. An empirical evaluation shows that this approach sometimes outperforms the approach of [24] at the task of predicting the next activity. In [26] the authors combine the approach in [25] with the idea of interleaving shared and specialized layers from [24] to design prediction architectures that can handle large numbers of activity types. The paper in [27], on the other hand, is more generally devoted to classification. In this work, RNNs are used in a system designed to solve any classification problem (including next activity prediction) based on activity sequences.

In [28] the authors propose to predict the next activity using a multi-stage deep learning approach. In this approach, after having mapped each activity to a feature vector, the authors reduce the input dimensionality by extracting n-grams and applying a hash function; then, the input is passed through two Autoencoder layers. The transformed input is finally processed by a feed-forward Neural Network responsible for the next activity prediction.

A different approach [29] relies on CNNs [12]. In particular, in [29] the authors resort to an architecture [13] that uses kernels of varied size in a convolution layer to capture features at different levels of abstraction, as discussed in Sect. 15.2: such architecture processes information at different scales and then aggregates them to efficiently extract relevant features. The authors have obtained better results in predicting the next activity with respect to LSTM architectures in their experiments.

Overall, our approach is thus inserted in a very active research panorama, which is recently focusing on promising deep learning solutions.

15.4 Deep Learning Process Trace Classification for Quality Assessment

Inspired by existing literature contributions, we have tested a deep learning approach for stroke trace classification, in a quality assessment perspective.

In order to adopt deep learning, process traces have to be converted to numerical vectors. In our work, we have covered this task by implementing and testing three different techniques. The first and simpler one resorts to a hash function, that converts each activity into an integer. The second alternative is more semantic, and borrowed from the area of natural language processing. It exploits word2vec [30], an algorithm that uses a Neural Network to learn word associations from a large corpus of text. It represents each distinct word as a numerical vector, such that the cosine similarity between two vectors indicates the level of semantic similarity between the words represented by those vectors. Finally, the third approach resorts to GloVe [31], an unsupervised learning algorithm for obtaining vector representations for words, where training is performed on aggregated global word-word co-occurrence statistics from a corpus.

Converted traces have then been provided in input to different architectures.

In particular, motivated by the successful examples described in Sect. 15.3 (see, e.g. [24, 25]), we have first defined and tested an LSTM-based architecture, depicted in Fig. 15.5. It exploits a dimension shuffle block, as described and motivated in Sect. 15.2. The actual LSTM block is then composed of 256 units with $tanh$ activation

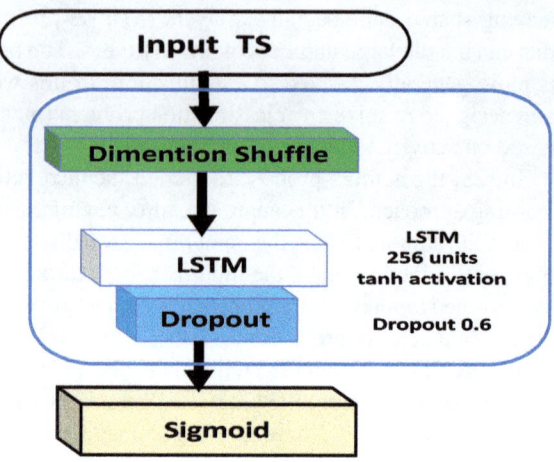

Fig. 15.5 LSTM-based classification architecture

function and is followed by a dropout layer, which randomly forces a fraction of the input units to be ignored at each update during training time, to help prevent overfitting [32]. The final layer is a sigmoid layer.

Besides the classical architecture described above, we also propose two novel, more complex solutions, able to combine convolutional modules with LSTMs, with the aim of taking advantage of the strengths of both. Defining composite architectures is an approach that has proved helpful in the medical domain, as reported, e.g., in [33].

Specifically, in **Architecture 1** (see Fig. 15.6) we have adopted two convolutional modules in series. Each module uses three convolutions with kernels of sizes 1, 3, and 5, and a further parallel path which implements a 3 max-pooling operation (see also [13]). This convolutional branch is in parallel to an LSTM branch, built as the one described in Fig. 15.5. In this way, the two branches perceive the input in two different views. The two branches are then concatenated. The final layer is a sigmoid layer.

In **Architecture 2**, on the other hand, we have placed a convolutional module as the one described above in series with two parallel branches; the first branch contains another analogous convolutional module, while the second one exploits LSTM. In this way, an already compressed input is provided to the LSTM branch, in order to reduce computation time. In this case dimension shuffle is not applied. The two branches are then concatenated, and a sigmoid layer completes the architecture. Placing the convolutional module before the two parallel branches has two advantages. First, it reduces the input vector's length. This becomes relevant when reaching the LSTM layer, which during training constitutes the most computationally expensive part of the network. Second, convolution extracts local information from neighboring input points, a first step towards learning temporal dependencies. Then, the LSTM layer is responsible for capturing both short and long-term dependencies. This architecture is shown in Fig. 15.7.

All parameters were set experimentally, as explained in Sect. 15.5.

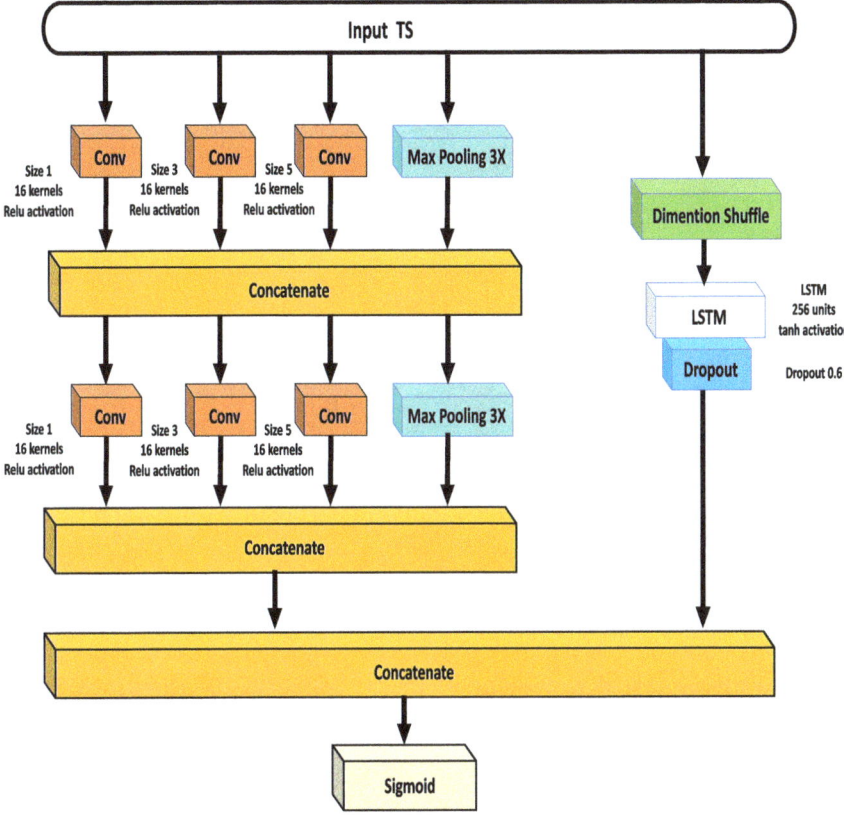

Fig. 15.6 Composing CNN and LSTM: architecture 1

15.5 Experimental Results

Our dataset was comprised of 5013 process traces, composed by a number of activities ranging from 10 to 25 (16 on average). In particular, 2629 traces were generated in a SC, while 2384 were generated in a SU.

The deep learning approach was realized and tested by means of the tool TensorFlow.[2]

Tests were run on a machine with the following characteristics: AMD Ryzen 7 3800X processor, with 32 Gb of DDR4 ram, and NVidia Geforce GTX 960 GPU.

For our experiments, we divided our datasets in two parts: 70% of the data where used for training, and 30% for test. On training data, we performed a 10 fold cross validation, in order to choose the parameter values that give the lowest cross validation average error.

In the tables below, we report results on test set, at 40 epochs.

---

[2] https://www.tensorflow.org/.

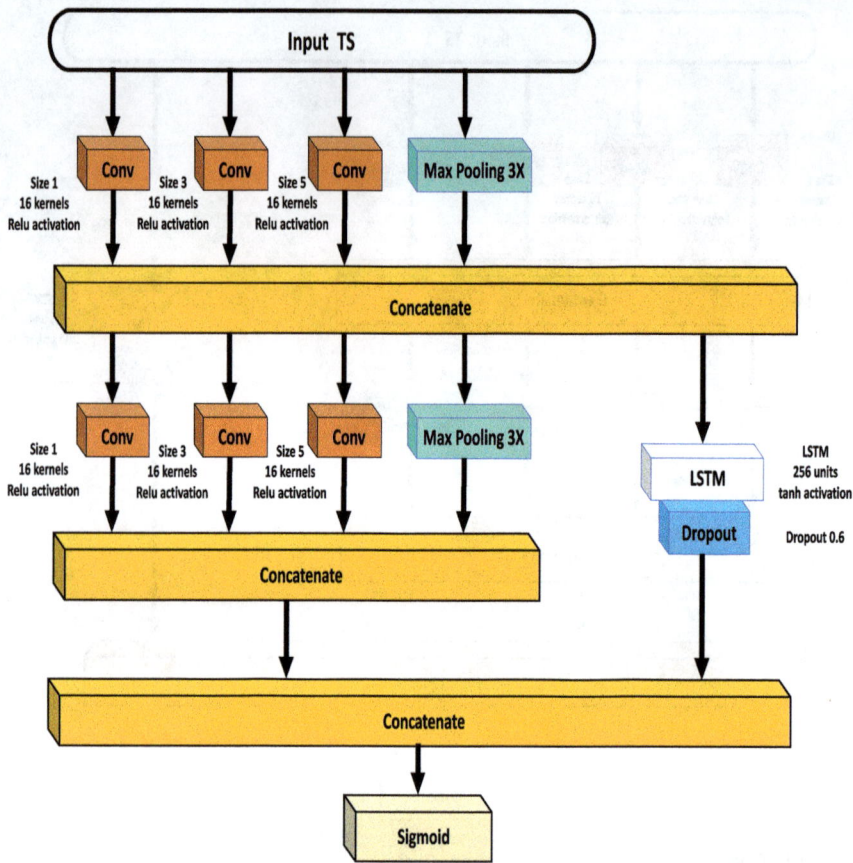

Fig. 15.7 Composing CNN and LSTM: architecture 2

Table 15.2 shows the results in terms of precision (average over the two classes), recall (average over the two classes), K-statistics and accuracy for the LSTM-based architecture in Fig. 15.5, distinguishing among the three different trace to vector conversion approaches we described in Sect. 15.4 .

As it can be observed, results are not particularly convincing: specifically, when hashing conversion is used, accuracy reaches a value of 67%, paired to a k-statistics value approximable with 0. The situation does not improve when pre-processing the traces by means of word2vec or GloVe.

Tables 15.3 and 15.4 presents the results of classification by means of Architecture 1 (see Fig. 15.6) and Architecture 2 (see Fig. 15.7), respectively. As it can be observed, results are basically in line with the ones of Table 15.2.

Following the suggestion of medical experts, we thus made a second experiment. In this case, we separated the SC class and the SU class into two subclasses each, in order to distinguish between traces generated on particularly complex patients, and

Table 15.2 Experimental results obtained by the LSTM-based architecture (Fig. 15.5)

Conversion	Precision	Recall	K-stat	Accuracy
Hash	0.45	0.67	0.00	0.67
word2vec	0.43	0.66	0.00	0.65
GloVe	0.28	0.52	0.00	0.52

Table 15.3 Experimental results obtained by architecture 1 (Fig. 15.6)

Conversion	Precision	Recall	K-stat	Accuracy
Hash	0.62	0.67	0.02	0.68
word2vec	0.68	0.66	0.30	0.67
GloVe	0.68	0.68	0.34	0.65

Table 15.4 Experimental results obtained by architecture 2 (Fig. 15.7)

Conversion	Precision	Recall	K-stat	Accuracy
Hash	0.60	0.67	0.03	0.68
word2vec	0.67	0.66	0.33	0.67
GloVe	0.68	0.62	0.33	0.72

Table 15.5 Experimental results obtained by the LSTM-based architecture on SC patients

Conversion	Precision	Recall	K-stat	Accuracy
Hash	0.43	0.66	0.00	0.65
word2vec	0.43	0.67	0.01	0.66
GloVe	0.42	0.66	0.00	0.64

traces generated on simpler patients. Such a distinction was made by experts referring to: (i) clinical data and patient's characteristics, available in the hospital information system (such as, e.g., the presence of co-morbidities), and (ii) the presence of specific activities in the trace (such as procedures for managing uncommon and problematic stroke types) or of repeated diagnostic/monitoring steps (such as frequent Computer Assisted Tomographies, to monitor the evolution over time of a particularly critical situation).

Classification outcomes remained stable for the LSTM-based architecture, as shown in Table 15.5, which refers to the SC patients (details for the SU ones, that did not improved in this case either, are not reported).

On the other hand, classification outcomes improved significantly within the SC traces, resorting both to Architecture 1 and Architecture 2. Moreover, as it can be observed from Tables 15.6 and 15.7, accuracy improvement was never weaker when substituting the hashing conversion with the use of word2vec or GloVe, suggesting that a more semantic approach, able to take into account the content of the whole

Table 15.6 Experimental results obtained by architecture 1 (Fig. 15.6) on SC patients

Epochs	Precision	Recall	K-stat	Accuracy
Hash	0.72	0.73	0.33	0.76
word2vec	0.74	0.73	0.31	0.76
GloVe	0.73	0.73	0.40	0.79

Table 15.7 Experimental results obtained by architecture 2 (Fig. 15.7) on SC patients

Epochs	Precision	Recall	K-stat	Accuracy
Hash	0.68	0.68	0.32	0.75
word2vec	0.74	0.73	0.30	0.79
GloVe	0.74	0.74	0.35	0.78

trace and the relations between activities, can represent an added value towards data interpretation and classification.

Instead, results did not improve much within the SU class patients (and are therefore not reported).

15.6 Discussion and Conclusions

In this paper, we have proposed a set of deep learning approaches to stroke trace classification. The first approach relies on a classical LSTM solution, while the more complex ones are composite architectures conjugating LSTM with CNNs.

The rather poor results obtained in our first experiments, where we considered all available traces, improved significantly for the composite architectures when focusing on the SC class. These further experiments allowed us to distinguish between more complex patients and simpler ones; the outcomes suggest that two types of processes are actually carried out in SCs, depending on the patient condition—which makes sense from the medical viewpoint; however, an analogous improvement was not observed when working within the SU traces. We thus make the hypothesis that SUs are much more heterogeneous than SCs, and more affected by organizational problems, which may limit their capacity to apply the right protocol to the right patient. Further tests will be needed to support this claim.

Our experiments also showed that the combination of convolutional and recurrent modules, as in Architecture 1 and Architecture 2, can lead to better distinguish between complex and simple SC patients, capturing the distinctive features of process traces in a finer way than the traditional LSTM approach. In the future, we will perform additional analyses, in order to check if this trend is confirmed (and possibly reinforced) at larger numbers of epochs, and in order to verify whether one of the two composite architectures performs better than the other, or if the choice of a semantic conversion technique such as GloVe or word2vec has a positive impact on results (as it seems to be so far).

Since deep learning methods operate as black boxes, and it can difficult to provide a meaning for the abstracted *deep* features, or to justify misclassification, in our future work we will also consider the issue of explainability. To this end, we will investigate whether it is possible to adapt a knowledge-based strategy, as the one we adopted in [34].

Last but not least, we also believe that further improvements of classification results might be obtained by resorting to a trace abstraction technique, such as the one described in [35, 36]. Such an approach can hide irrelevant details, that could lead to misclassification, while keeping the most important information in the trace. This research direction will be considered in our future research as well.

References

1. Bejot, Y., Bailly, H., Durier, J., Giroud, M.: Epidemiology of stroke in europe and trends for the 21st century. La Presse Medicale **45**(12, Part 2), e391–e398 (2016) (QMR Stroke)
2. Kjellstrom, T., Norrving, B., Shatchkute, A.: Helsingborg declaration 2006 on european stroke strategies. Cerebrovasc. Dis. **23**, 229–241 (2007)
3. Ringelstein, E.B., Chamorro, A., Kaste, M., Langhorne, P., Leys, D., Lyrer, P., Thijs, V., Thomassen, L., Toni, D.: European stroke organisation recommendations to establish a stroke unit and stroke center. Stroke **44**(3), 828–840 (2013)
4. Leonardi, G., Montani, S., Striani, M.: Process trace classification for stroke management quality assessment. In: Watson, I., Weber, R.O. (eds), Proceedings of Case-Based Reasoning Research and Development—28th International Conference, ICCBR 2020, Salamanca, Spain, June 8–12, 2020, volume 12311 of Lecture Notes in Computer Science, pages 49–63. Springer (2020)
5. Montani, S., Leonardi, G.: Retrieval and clustering for business process monitoring: results and improvements. In: Diaz-Agudo, B., Watson, I., (eds), Proceedings of International Conference on Case-Based Reasoning (ICCBR): Lecture Notes in Artificial Intelligence 7466, page 269–283, p. 2012. Springer, Berlin (2012)
6. Montani, S., Leonardi, G.: Retrieval and clustering for supporting business process adjustment and analysis. Inf. Syst. **40**, 128–141 (2014)
7. LeCun, Y., Bengio, Y., Hinton, G.E.: Deep learning. Nature **521**(7553), 436–444 (2015)
8. Faust, O., Hagiwara, Y., Hong, T.J., Lih, O.S., Acharya, U.R.: Deep learning for healthcare applications based on physiological signals: a review. Comput. Methods Progr. Biomed. **161**, 1–13 (2018)
9. Striani, M., Leonardi, G., Montani, S.: Deep learning for haemodialysis time series classification. In: Proceedings of KR4HC/ProHealth and TEAAM workshops, LNCS (to appear). Springer (2019)
10. Sani, S., Wiratunga, N., Massie, S., Cooper, K.: KNN sampling for personalised human activity recognition. In: Aha, D.W., Lieber, J., (eds), Proceedings of Case-Based Reasoning Research and Development—25th International Conference, ICCBR 2017, Trondheim, Norway, June 26–28, 2017, volume 10339 of Lecture Notes in Computer Science, pages 330–344. Springer, 2017
11. LeCun, Y., Bottou, L., Bengio, Y., Haffner, P.: Gradient-based learning applied to document recognition. In: Proceedings of the IEEE, pages 2278–2324 (1998)

12. Alom, M.Z., Taha, T.M., Yakopcic, C., Westberg, S., Sidike, P., Nasrin, M.S., Hasan, M., Van Essen, B.C., Awwal, A.A.S., Asari, V.K.: A state-of-the-art survey on deep learning theory and architectures. Electronics **8**(3) (2019)
13. Szegedy, C., Liu, W., Jia, Y., Sermanet, P., Reed, S.E., Anguelov, D., Erhan, D., Vanhoucke, V., Rabinovich, A.: Going deeper with convolutions. In: IEEE Conference on Computer Vision and Pattern Recognition, CVPR 2015, Boston, MA, USA, June 7–12, 2015, pages 1–9. IEEE Computer Society (2015)
14. Wen, T., Zhang, Z.: Deep convolution neural network and autoencoders-based unsupervised feature learning of EEG signals. IEEE Access **6**, 25399–25410 (2018)
15. Chu, K.L., Sahari, K.S.M.: Behavior recognition for humanoid robots using long short-term memory. Int. J. Adv. Robot. Syst. **13**(6), (2016)
16. Mehdiyev, N., Lahann, J., Emrich, A., Enke, D., Fettke, P., Loos, P.: Time series classification using deep learning for process planning: a case from the process industry. Procedia Comput. Sci. **114**, 242–249 (2017)
17. Pascanu, R., Gülçehre, Ç., Cho, K., Bengio, Y.: How to construct deep recurrent neural networks. In: Bengio, Y., LeCun, Y. (eds) Conference Track Proceedings 2nd International Conference on Learning Representations, ICLR 2014, Banff, AB, Canada, April 14–16, 2014 (2014)
18. Hochreiter, S., Schmidhuber, J.: Long short-term memory. Neural Comput. **9**(8), 1735–1780 (1997)
19. Greff, K., Srivastava, R.K., Koutník, J., Steunebrink, B.R., Schmidhuber, J.: LSTM: A search space odyssey. IEEE Trans. Neural Netw. Learn. Syst. **28**(10), 2222–2232 (2017)
20. Karim, F., Majumdar, S., Darabi, H., Chen, S.: LSTM fully convolutional networks for time series classification. IEEE Access **6**, 1662–1669 (2018)
21. Breuker, D., Matzner, M., Delfmann, P., Becker, J.: Comprehensible predictive models for business processes. MIS Quarterly **40**, 1009–1034 (2016)
22. Le, M., Gabrys, B., Nauck, D.: A hybrid model for business process event prediction. In: Bramer, M., Petridis, M. (eds) Research and Development in Intelligent Systems XXIX, Incorporating Applications and Innovations in Intelligent Systems XX: Proceedings of AI-2012, The Thirty-second SGAI International Conference on Innovative Techniques and Applications of Artificial Intelligence, Cambridge, England, UK, December 11–13, 2012, pages 179–192. Springer (2012)
23. Lakshmanan, G.T., Shamsi, D., Doganata, Y.N., Unuvar, M., Khalaf, R.: Markov prediction model for data-driven semi-structured business processes. Knowl. Inf. Syst. **42**(1), 97–126 (2015)
24. Tax, N., Teinemaa, I., van Zelst, S.J.: An interdisciplinary comparison of sequence modeling methods for next-element prediction. CoRR, abs/1811.00062 (2018)
25. Evermann, J., Rehse, J.R., Fettke, P.: Predicting process behaviour using deep learning. Decis. Support Syst. **100**, 129–140 (2017)
26. Camargo, M., Dumas, M., González Rojas, O.: Learning accurate LSTM models of business processes. In: Hildebrandt, T.T., van Dongen, B.F., Röglinger, M., Mendling, J. (eds), Proceedings of Business Process Management—17th International Conference, BPM 2019, Vienna, Austria, September 1–6, 2019, volume 11675 of Lecture Notes in Computer Science, pages 286–302. Springer (2019)
27. Hinkka, M., Lehto, T., Heljanko, K., Jung, A.: Classifying process instances using recurrent neural networks. In: Daniel, F., Sheng, Q.Z., Motahari, H. (eds) Business Process Management Workshops - BPM 2018 International Workshops, Sydney, NSW, Australia, September 9–14, 2018, Revised Papers, volume 342 of Lecture Notes in Business Information Processing, pages 313–324. Springer (2018)
28. Mehdiyev, N., Evermann, J., Fettke, P.: A multi-stage deep learning approach for business process event prediction. In: Loucopoulos, P., Manolopoulos, Y., Pastor, O., Theodoulidis, B., Zdravkovic, J. (eds) 19th IEEE Conference on Business Informatics, CBI 2017, Thessaloniki, Greece, July 24–27, 2017, Volume 1: Conference Papers, pages 119–128. IEEE Computer Society (2017)

29. Di Mauro, N., Appice, A., Basile, T.M.A.: Activity prediction of business process instances with inception CNN models. In: Alviano, M., Greco, G., Scarcello, F. (eds), Proceedings of AI*IA 2019—Advances in Artificial Intelligence—XVIIIth International Conference of the Italian Association for Artificial Intelligence, Rende, Italy, November 19-22, 2019, volume 11946 of Lecture Notes in Computer Science, pages 348–361. Springer (2019)
30. Mikolov, T., Chen, K., Corrado, G., Dean, J.: Efficient estimation of word representations in vector space. In: Bengio, Y., LeCun, Y. (eds) Workshop Track Proceedings 1st International Conference on Learning Representations, ICLR 2013, Scottsdale, Arizona, USA, May 2–4, 2013 (2013)
31. Pennington, J., Socher, R., Manning, C.D.: Glove: Global vectors for word representation. In: Moschitti, A., Pang, B., Daelemans, W. (eds), Proceedings of the 2014 Conference on Empirical Methods in Natural Language Processing, EMNLP 2014, October 25–29, 2014, Doha, Qatar, A meeting of SIGDAT, a Special Interest Group of the ACL, pages 1532–1543. ACL (2014)
32. Srivastava, N., Hinton, G.E., Krizhevsky, A., Sutskever, I., Salakhutdinov, R.: Dropout: a simple way to prevent neural networks from overfitting. J. Mach. Learn. Res. **15**(1), 1929–1958 (2014)
33. Roy, S., Kiral-Kornek, I., Harrer, S.: Chrononet: a deep recurrent neural network for abnormal EEG identification. In: Riaño, D., Wilk, S., ten Teije, A. (eds), Proceedings of Artificial Intelligence in Medicine—17th Conference on Artificial Intelligence in Medicine, AIME 2019, Poznan, Poland, June 26–29, 2019, , volume 11526 of Lecture Notes in Computer Science, pages 47–56. Springer (2019)
34. Leonardi, G., Montani, S., Striani, M.: Deep feature extraction for representing and classifying time series cases: towards an interpretable approach in haemodialysis. In: Proceedings of the 33rd International Florida Artificial Intelligence Research Society Conference, FLAIRS: Miami, p. 2020. AAAI Press, Florida (2020)
35. Montani, S., Leonardi, G., Striani, M., Quaglini, S., Cavallini, A.: Multi-level abstraction for trace comparison and process discovery. Expert Syst. Appl. **81**, 398–409 (2017)
36. Montani, S., Striani, M., Quaglini, S., Cavallini, A., Leonardi, G.: Semantic trace comparison at multiple levels of abstraction. In: Aha, D.W., Lieber, J. (eds), Proceedings of Case-Based Reasoning Research and Development—25th International Conference, ICCBR 2017, Trondheim, Norway, June 26–28, 2017, volume 10339 of Lecture Notes in Computer Science, pages 212–226. Springer (2017)

Chapter 16
Synergy-Net: Artificial Intelligence at the Service of Oncological Prevention

Ruggiero Bollino, Giampaolo Bovenzi, Francesco Cipolletta, Ludovico Docimo, Michela Gravina, Stefano Marrone, Domenico Parmeggiani, and Carlo Sansone

Abstract In recent years the constant development of diagnostic techniques has contributed to improving the prognosis of many diseases. Among all, oncological diseases remain those in which a correct and early diagnosis can not only significantly improve the patient's quality of life but also impact the effectiveness of the therapy itself. Artificial Intelligence can provide valuable aid to this need through the development of predictive models to support the physicians in the diagnosis of the disease. The project "Synergy-Net: Research and Digital Solutions in the Fight Against Oncological Diseases", born from the collaboration between the Department of Medical and Advanced Surgical Sciences of the University of Campania "L. Vanvitelli", the National Informatics Inter-University Consortium (National Informatics

---

R. Bollino · F. Cipolletta
Bollino IT S.p.A., Via delle Industrie 31, 80147 Naples, Italy
e-mail: ruggiero@bollino.com

F. Cipolletta
e-mail: f.cipolletta@bollino.com

L. Docimo · D. Parmeggiani
DAMSS, Università della Campania "L.Vanvitelli", P.zza L. Miraglia 2, 80138 Naples, Italy
e-mail: ludovico.docimo@unicampania.it

D. Parmeggiani
e-mail: domenico.parmeggiani@unicampania.it

G. Bovenzi · M. Gravina · S. Marrone (✉) · C. Sansone
University of Naples Federico II, Via Claudio 21, 80125 Naples, Italy
e-mail: stefano.marrone@unina.it

G. Bovenzi
e-mail: giampaolo.bovenzi@unina.it

M. Gravina
e-mail: michela.gravina@unina.it

C. Sansone
e-mail: carlo.sansone@unina.it

G. Bovenzi · C. Sansone
CINI, Laboratorio ITEM "C.Savy", Via Cintia 21, 80125 Naples, Italy

© The Author(s), under exclusive license to Springer Nature Switzerland AG 2022
C.-P. Lim et al. (eds.), *Handbook of Artificial Intelligence in Healthcare*, Intelligent Systems Reference Library 211, https://doi.org/10.1007/978-3-030-79161-2_16

Inter-University Consortium), Lab ITEM "C. Savy" and Bollino IT S.p.A., aims at the realisation of a technological platform to support the early oncological diagnosis based on the integration of an interoperable communication and clinical data management system leveraging AI. The project has a deeply interdisciplinary nature (lung cancer, breast cancer, colorectal cancer, gastrointestinal carcinomas, prostate cancer, thyroid cancer and malignant skin tumours), which requires the collaboration of very different professionals, including general practitioners, specialist doctors, radiologists, surgeons, pathologists, molecular biologists and oncologists, as well as the support of a team of researchers for aspects related to machine learning and expert system development in health care. The core of the project consists in the creation of a Computer-Aided Detection/Diagnosis (Computer-Aided Detection/Diagnosis) system that, based on Machine Learning and Deep Learning techniques, assists the operator in the analysis of screening data such as anamnestic information, blood tests, instrumental and diagnostic images. The assistance to the operator is achieved by suggesting the portions of information (e.g. regions in an X-ray image) on which to focus more attention. The use of the system will help the physician in the development of increasingly personalised diagnostic and therapeutic strategies, meeting the criteria of tailored therapy/surgery, a desirable objective of any cancer prevention program.

Keywords Artificial intelligence · Early diagnosis · Oncological diseases · CAD system · Machine learning · Deep learning

Abbreviation

AI	Artificial Intelligence
AUC-ROC	Area Under the Receiver Operating Characteristic Curve
BCC	Basal Cell Carcinoma
CAD	Computer-Aided Detection/Diagnosis
CBIR	Picture Archiving and Communication Systems
CINI	National Informatics Inter-University Consortium
CLD	Color Layout Descriptor
CNN	Convolution Neural Network
CT	Computed Tomography
CV	Cross Validaion
D-CNN	Deep Convolution Neural Network
DC	Dominant Colour
DCE-MRI	Dynamic Contrast Enhanced Magnetic Resonance Imaging
DICOM	Digital Imaging and Communications in Medicine
DL	Deep Learning
FN	False Negative
FP	False Positive
GI	Gastrointestinal

HMMD	Hue-Min-Max-Difference
HSV	Hue-Saturation-Value
IoU	Intersection over Union
k-NN	k-Nearest Neighbors
MAP	Mean Average Precision
ML	Machine Leaning
MRI	Magnetic Resonance Imaging.
NB	Narrowband
NBI	Narrow Band Imaging
NN	Neural Network
P	FPrecision
PACS	Picture Archiving and Communication Systems
PET	Positron Emission Tomography
R	Recall
R-CNN	Region CNN
ROC	Area Under the Receiver Operating Characteristic Curve
ROI	Regions of Interest
SCC	Squamous Cell Carcinoma
SCD	Scalable Color Descriptor
SEN	Sensitivity
SPECT	Single-Photon Emission Computed Tomography
SSD	Single-Shot Detector
SVM	Support-Vector Machine
TP	True Positive
US	UltraSound
UV	Ultraviolet
WHO	World Health Organization
WLR	White Light Reflectance
YOLO	Only-Look-Once

16.1 Introduction

The budget for cancer research has gradually increased over the past years. Despite this, prevention and early diagnosis still remain the most important phases in cancer cure. World Health Organization (World Health Organization) cancer screening guidelines suggest different procedures for different types of cancer, among which mammography for breast [55], pap-test for cervix [1], etc. Focusing on imaging techniques, although they improved the prognosis over the last decades, their use also comes with some drawbacks [30], among which it is worth to mention i) the huge amount of time associated with their analysis (especially true for techniques rich in data, such that DCE-MRI) and ii) the intra-inter operator variability (namely the generation of a different report by the same operator about the same examination in two different time instant, or the generation of a different report by the different operators about the same examination in the same time instant).

To face these problems in recent years physicians started making use of tools designed to assist in the detection of cancerous lesions and, sometimes, also in the evaluation of a complete diagnosis [10]: these instruments are known as Computer-Aided Detection and Diagnosis (Computer-Aided Detection/Diagnosis) systems and, supported by an appropriate and proved medical validity, are widely used in the analysis of complex medical investigations both for the extension of data to be taken into account (World Health Organization—Computed tomography—Positron Emission Tomography) and for an intrinsic uncertainty of the data due to the scanning process (such as UltraSound scans—UltraSound). CAD systems analyse data using strict mathematical patterns, according to well-defined and deterministic algorithms. This characteristic allows to remove the difficulties due to inter- and intra-observer variability and to reduce the effort needed to perform the analysis by limiting the amount of data the physician have to focus on. Mathematics features behind the deductions (both in the detection and in the diagnosis phase) allow evaluating sensitivity and specificity of such instruments in a precise and strict way, showing objective improvement in these parameters [11].

With the aim of fully supporting the physician, a typical CAD system usually provides both lesion detection and diagnosis. This need has increasingly prompted the design of semi-automatic or fully automatic systems since it has been shown that these tasks can be addressed in a *pattern recognition* framework with the use of suitable features and classifiers. For this reason, a lot of new features have been designed by domain experts to improve classification results. This was the case until a Deep Convolution Neural Network (Deep Convolution Neural Network or simply Convolution Neural Network) won the 2012 Large Scale Visual Recognition Challenge [21], a popular open-source contest in which participants have to correctly classify images to one of the 1000 classes. From that moment on, an increasing interest stated to be paid by researches on the study and on the application of CNN in several contexts, giving rise to new CNN architectures, training and optimization strategies able to compete with, and in some cases surpass, humans in many tasks [3].

Researches agree that CNN success is in their hierarchical architecture that makes them able to autonomously learn how to extract features, from a low to a high-level, that describe salient characteristics of the input data better when compared to hand-engineered ones. Several studies demonstrated that this stands for a wide number of different applications, particularly for those domains lacking effective expert-designed features [22]. One of the drawbacks of using Deep Learning approaches is related to their need for huge amounts of training sample (w.r.t. non-deep ones) when it comes to training a model from scratches. This can be particularly critic for domains in which collecting a large number of samples is difficult, expensive and time-consuming, such in biomedical image processing. To face this problem, several works make use of "Transfer Learning", a term that refers to transfer knowledge learnt in a task to another one by pre-training an AI model on a huge dataset (e.g. ImageNet [8]) before performing a fine-tuning (re-train) of some of the layers (usually last ones) to adapt the network to the new classification task, while preserving as past learnt knowledge as possible. Thanks to this, in recent years several researchers started developing machine learning based CAD for helping physicians with different cancers, including breast [33], brain [5], bowel [23], etc.

16.2 Synergy-Net

The Synergy-Net project aims in developing a Computer Aided Diagnosis (Computer-Aided Detection/Diagnosis) system, i.e. a computer-aided medical diagnosis system intended to support physicians in the early diagnosis for different tumours. The aim of such a system is not to replace the human operator, but to support they by reducing the amount of data to be analysed, assisting in this analysis, or simplifying accessing the data. The overall system is therefore designed to take into account the needs associated with processing medical data (including imaging, anamnestic, genetic, etc.). The reason why we decided to design such a system is that one of the problems associated with the early diagnosis of oncological diseases (especially when based on biomedical images) is the large amount of data to be analysed. Several studies [15, 43, 47] have shown that this amount of work can have a significant impact on the results of the analysis, as attention and critical thinking skills tend to be inexorably reduced as stress and the amount of information analysed per unit of time increase. Broadening the number of physicians involved in the analysis phases may result in a limited improvement, since the presence of different experiences, although presenting undoubted advantages, often results in a high intra-operator variability (the same operator reports differently the same examination, if analysed in different moments and psycho-physical conditions) and inter-operator variability (two different operators, with comparable experience, report differently the same examination analysed in the same conditions) [42, 46]. These difficulties become even more relevant when the pathologies under examination are of an oncological nature, since, to date, early diagnosis remains the most effective tool for improving the prognosis.

Born from the collaboration between the Department of Medical and Advanced Surgical Sciences of the University of Campania "L. Vanvitelli", the National Informatics Inter-University Consortium (National Informatics Inter-University Consortium) Lab ITEM "C. Savy" and Bollino IT S.p.A., the Synergy-Net project is designed to support the early oncological diagnosis based on the integration of an interoperable communication and clinical data management system leveraging AI. The project has a deeply interdisciplinary nature (lung cancer, breast cancer, colorectal cancer, gastrointestinal carcinomas, prostate cancer, thyroid cancer and malignant skin tumours), which requires the collaboration of very different professionals, including general practitioners, specialist physicians, radiologists, surgeons, pathologists, molecular biologists and oncologists, as well as the support of a team of researchers for aspects related to machine learning and expert system development in health care. As a CAD, it should be able to support the operator in the aforementioned ways. Based on the experience maturated over the years by the partners, during the design and the development of the Synergy-Net project we took into account for the following aspects and challenges:

- One of the biggest challenges remains the reduction of the amount of data to be analysed. On this regards, in a previous work [32] we designed a Deep Learning (Deep Learning) based approach for lesion segmentation. The idea is to pre-identify and select the most-suspect Regions of Interest (Regions of Interests) to be submitted for the medical opinion. This allows to reduce the amount of data that the physician has to analyse, allowing them to focus attention only on certain areas;
- Another important aspect to be taken into account is that medical images are more than pictures. This is particularly critic for imaging procedures involving several acquisitions, for example before and after the use of a contrast agent. In this case, a CAD intended to support the physician in the study of such data must be able to extrapolate the information content associated with all the temporal acquisitions. Being able to take into account for this characteristics makes the Computer-Aided Detection/Diagnosis (and thus the physician) to consider all the crucial information associated with a lesion while removing the (possibly) noisy data resulting from the repeated acquisitions. An example for this has been realised for breast Dynamic Contrast Enhanced Magnetic Resonance Imaging (Dynamic Contrast Enhanced Magnetic Resonance Imaging), where we developed [14] a Convolutional Neural Network (Convolution Neural Network) able to perform the lesion malignancy assessment based on only three acquisitions, independent from the number of acquired pre and post contrast series;
- Among all the types of noise that could affect medical images, motion artefacts are probably the most problematic. This issue is related to the patient's moments during image acquisition. The difficulty for the patient to remain still is unavoidable, as it is due to often uncontrollable factors such as breathing, pain, uncomfortable positions, long acquisition times etc. It is therefore important to verify whether implemented AI-based algorithms are robust to such inevitable events. To quantify this aspect, we performed a statistical analysis of the impact that motion artefacts have on AI-bases lesion segmentation and classification systems. Results suggest that approaches based on Deep Learning techniques tend to be more robust to such artefacts when compared to non-DL ones [12];
- In addition to supporting diagnosis, a CAD should also be able to assist the physician in retrieving historical information from archives. Indeed, medical centres make use of archiving systems, known as Picture Archiving and Communication Systems (Picture Archiving and Communication Systems), able to store large quantities of images, but designed to provide access to them on the basis of certain metadata (e.g. gender, age, pathology, etc.). One of the real use cases is instead associated with the physician's need to quickly access reports and images of a previously reported case. This operation is often non-trivial given the number of patients analysed on average per day. In order to meet this need, an example-based image retrieval system (Picture Archiving and Communication Systems, Content Based Image Retrieval) has been developed designed to allow a physician

to access all historical reports that resemble the case under examination in terms of morphology, texture, etc. [13];
- In the medical domain reproducibility of the results is really important. Unfortunately, the use of Artificial Intelligence (and in particular of deep learning) makes reproducibility not trivial to pursue. The reasons behind this problem are mostly due to the randomness associated with optimisation algorithms and GPU libraries. To face this problem, in a previous work [29] we showed that it is possible shit the reproducibility problem from a purely numerical problem to a statistical one, by defining reproducibility intervals on a statistical basis.

These aspects and experience guided the design and the development of the Synergy-Net project. As a result, the Synergy-Net architecture consists of several modules interacting with each other to provide the required functionalities. Next sections will describe each of the Synergy-Net components, starting from those directly associated with the analysis of medical images by means of AI techniques.

16.2.1 Medical Imaging and AI

As mentioned above, the Synergy-Net system is configured within the Computer Aided Diagnosis (Computer-Aided Detection/Diagnosis), i.e. computerised systems supporting the medical diagnosis. In general, CAD systems can work on images, on tabular data (e.g. clinical, anamnestic, etc.), on time series (e.g. electroencephalogram et similia), or on a combination of these. In the case of the Synergy-Net project, the data analysed are purely image/video and tabular data. Of the two, biomedical images are those that require a preliminary stage for their representation in terms of features that can be assimilated by an expert system.

Medical imaging refers to the process by which the structure of the human body can be explored from the outside through the formation of images. Medical images are divided into planar and tomographic images. Planar images are able to represent the part of the body under examination on a flat, two-dimensional surface, while tomographic images correspond to sections (layers) of the human body, offering the possibility of reproducing its structure three-dimensionally. Examples of planar images are X-rays, mammograms, ultrasound scans and scintigraphy, while positron emission tomography (Positron Emission Tomography), single-photon emission computed tomography (single-photon emission computed tomography), computed tomography (Computed tomography) and magnetic resonance imaging (World Health Organization) are tomographic images. In addition to the three spatial dimensions provided by tomographic techniques, the temporal dimension is also added, allowing the evaluation of spatial dynamics. DCE-MRI is a clear example of tomographic imaging with the addition of the temporal dimension (thus a 4D volume, as illustrated in Fig. 16.1). It involves the injection of a contrast agent into a vein, i.e. a special paramagnetic substance that is distributed in the vessels and organs, accentuating tissue and vascularisation differences and allowing the visualisation of lesions in the organ under

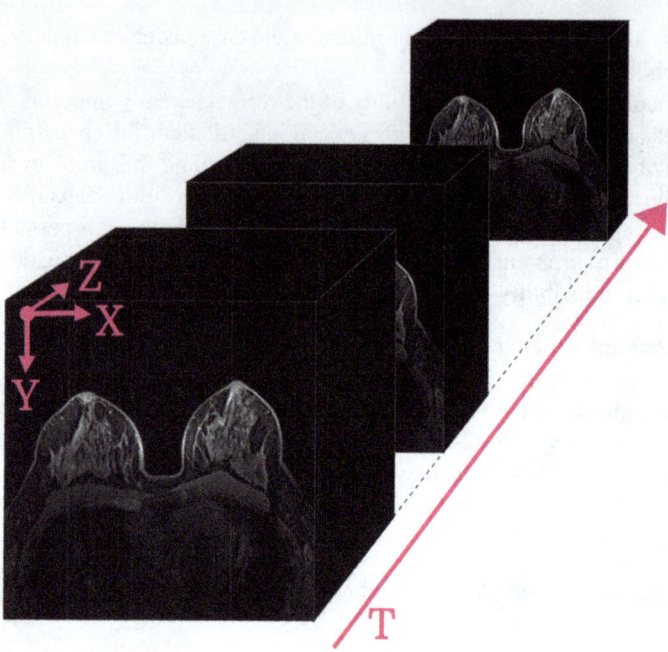

Fig. 16.1 Illustrative example of a breast DCE-MRI. The arrow indicates the volumes acquired at different times

examination. Magnetic resonance imaging with contrast agent is one of the most widely used screening techniques for the diagnosis of tumours, particularly in the breast, as the dynamics of the contrast agent allows morphological and physiological analysis of tissue vascularisation.

A digital image consists of a two-dimensional, usually square, matrix of elements called pixels. In tomographic images, however, the pixels correspond to the volume elements that make up the layers (or slices) of the body. For this reason, they are commonly known as voxels (short for volumetric pixels). Digital medical images conform to the Digital Imaging and Communications in Medicine (Digital Imaging and Communications in Medicine) standard to enable them to be transferred, stored and processed by computer systems. In particular, a DICOM file has a part containing information about the patient's data, the protocol used and the size of the image matrix, and a part containing the values of the pixels or voxels that make up the image or volume. This implies that tomographic images provide much more information than planar images, allowing the morphological and functional study of the body part and/or organ under examination. However, the large amount of data available makes the analysis of this type of image very complex and time-consuming: in fact, even an expert radiologist could easily make a mistake by not recognising a lesion or not investigating it with subsequent analyses. As described in the previous section, Computer-Aided Detection and Diagnosis (Computer-Aided Detection/Diagnosis) systems are widely used in the analysis of tomographic images both to handle the large amount of available data and the complex nature of the investigation. To this aim, a typical CAD system consists of a sequence of independent steps (or modules) each intended to perform a given processing on the input data, with the aim of implementing an automatic (or semi-automatic) analysis. The most common modules are as follows:

- *Digitisation module.* This module is needed to acquire and archive medical images. As already mentioned, medical images are stored using the Digital Imaging and Communications in Medicine standard, which allows them to be processed and stored by a computer system;
- *Image Pre-processing Module* [12]. This module includes a series of preliminary elaborations with the aim of improving the quality of medical images by reducing the noise introduced during the actual acquisition, mainly caused by the patient's movements. An example of this is the motion correction performed with DCE-MRI;
- *Organ Segmentation module.* Segmentation is the process of dividing an image into Regions of Interest (Regions of Interests). This module is needed to identify only the portion of the image related to the organ of interest. For example, in the case of breast MRI, the acquired images not only contains breast tissue but also what is around it, i.e. other organs and the air outside the body. For this reason, in order to have a better analysis, it is important to have the system focus only on the organ to be analysed, ignoring what is not of interest;
- *Lesion Detection/Segmentation Module.* Once the organ of interest has been identified, the next stage is the detection of lesions within it. On this regards, it is necessary to clarify the difference between lesion detection and segmentation. By lesion detection we mean the identification of a region of the image where the lesion resides, while lesion segmentation coincides with the process of determining the pixels related to the lesion. In short, lesion detection determines an area around the lesion, whereas lesion segmentation identifies the lesion with the precision of a single pixel;
- *Lesion Classification module.* The lesion classification module performs the staging of the lesions identified by the previous module. In particular, a lesion is automatically classified as benign or malignant (or classified according to a different scale) by a system capable of analysing its physiological and morphological characteristics.

The Synergy-Net system operates on this same idea, implementing one or more of the described stages as needed by the study under analysis.

16.2.2 The Synergy-Net Architecture

The Synergy-Net system can be schematised as consisting of three main components: Front-End Interface, Artificial Intelligence Models, Orchestrator (Fig. 16.2).

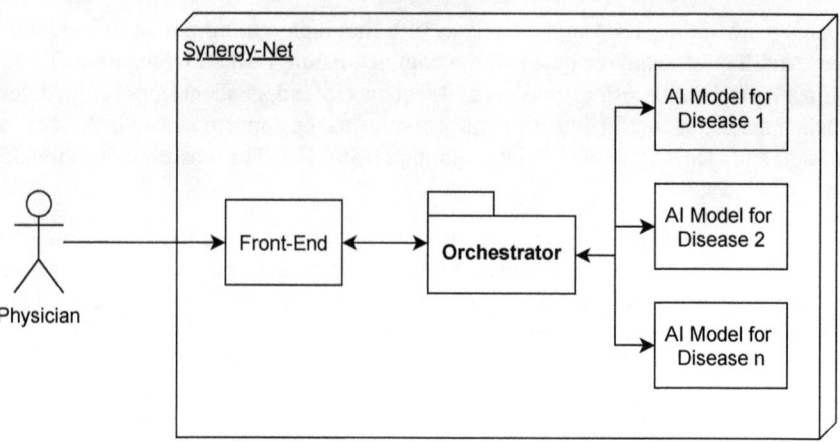

Fig. 16.2 High-level architecture of the Synergy-Net system

16.2.2.1 Front-End

The Front-End is the interface through which the physician accesses the system functions. In particular, following an authentication phase, the physician is able to:

- Upload data to be analysed (e.g. one or more images)
- View uploaded data
- Process the uploaded data (e.g. lesion segmentation/classification)
- View additional information about the processing performed.

During the data-gathering stage, the physician can also use the Front-End interface to provide feedback on the processing performed. In particular, after a segmentation procedure, for each Regions of Interest (Region of Interest) produced by the system, the physician can:

- mark whether they is satisfied with the Regions of Interest obtained, rating it as "excellent", "good", "sufficient", "insufficient".
- In the event of a "good" or inferior result, the physician may mark in a free text field the reasons which led them to this judgement.
- In the event of a "sufficient" or "insufficient" result, the physician may enter (draw) the Regions of Interest he/she would have liked to see at the output.
- If the physician considers that the Regions of Interest identified by the system is a false positive (Regions of Interest that should not be produced by the system), he/she shall be able to label it as such.
- In the event that the physician argues that the system has not produced a Regions of Interest when needed, they can insert (draw) it, also indicating its characteristics.
- In any case, the physician have access to an additional text field to indicate, if any, notes related to the overall result obtained for the image under analysis.

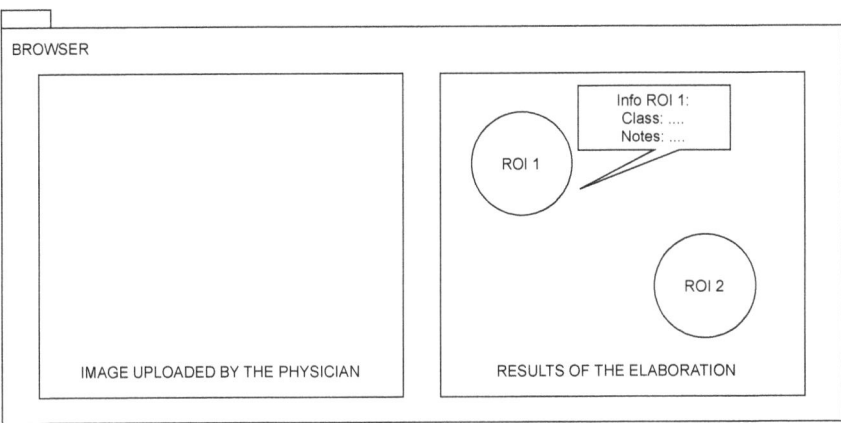

Fig. 16.3 Example front-end mock-up for the Synergy-Net project

Similarly, after a classification, for each produced output associated with a Regions of Interest previously indicated by the physician or produced by the segmentation phase, the physician can indicate:

- whether they are satisfied with the result obtained, evaluating it as "correct", "wrong pathology", "wrong";
- In case of "wrong pathology", the physician can indicate the correct pathology (chosen from a predefined set, different for each pathology);
- In case of "wrong" result, the physician can insert the reasons that led them to this assessment.

The functions remain unchanged if the classification does not refer to a Regions of Interest but to the whole image (Fig. 16.3). During the operational phase, the front-end will allow the physician to select the patient's data to be analysed by AI models, receiving the results on the same interface and modalities used during the data gathering.

16.2.2.2 AI Models

Given the different characteristics of the data and of the desiderata related to the different pathologies considered within the Synergy-Net project, the system provides an Artificial Intelligence (Artificial Intelligence) model for each <Investigation, Task> pair (e.g. <Mammography, Classification>, <Mammography, Segmentation>, <Nevoscopy, Classification>, etc). The models are built in Python and accessible via a call of the type "output = Pathology(Image, Task)". For example, in the case of <Nevoscopy, Classification>, the function to be call is "output = skinCancer(Image, Classification)" where

- *skinCancer* is the name of a Python function;
- *Image* is the image to be analysed (e.g. numpy array containing the image uploaded by the physician);
- *Classification* is a value indicating the task required (e.g. '1')
- *output* is an .xml file containing the result of the processing.

Each of the AI models will have specific characteristics that the input data must respect for correct processing (e.g. size of the numpy containing the image to be processed).

16.2.2.3 Orchestrator

The orchestrator is the module responsible for interfacing the user (the logged-in physician) with the desired AI model. In particular, the orchestrator

- Prepares the input data in a manner consistent with what is required by the AI modules (e.g., encode the image uploaded by the physician into a numpy array of a size consistent with what is required by the AI model);
- Calls the Python function for the functionality requested by the physician;
- Displays the results produced by the processing system.

16.2.2.4 Regions of Interest Communication Protocol

All the aforementioned modules communicate with each other by means of XML files describing Regions of Interests. This choice has been made to provide a unified, simple and interoperable representation and communication methodology. The structure of a generic XML file associated to each processed image is reported in Fig. 16.4.

16.2.3 Synergy-Net: Analysed Tumours

Eight oncological diseases are analysed by means of artificial intelligence techniques within the Synergy-Net project: liver cancer, gastric cancer, melanoma, prostate cancer, thyroid cancer, colon rectum cancer, breast cancer and lung cancer (Fig. 16.5).

These pathologies differ not only in their clinical characteristics but also in the instrumentation used (Fig. 16.6) and in the tasks that it is possible/desired to perform in an automated manner using artificial intelligence techniques (Fig. 16.7). Two macro-tasks can be identified:

1. Semantic segmentation, i.e. the identification (pixel-based or ROI-based) of portions of tissue with suspicious and/or attention-worthy characteristics;

16 Synergy-Net: Artificial Intelligence at the Service of Oncological Prevention

```xml
<Image>
     <ROI>
          <Id>A01</Id>
          <Description>Suspect mass in left breast</Description>
          <Coordinates>15,50,18,90</Coordinates>
          <Source>Physician</Source>
          <Label>Ductal Cancer</Label>
          <Confidence>95,7</Confidence>
          <Notes>Notes from physician</Notes>
     </ROI>
     <ROI>
          <Id>A01</Id>
          <Description> Suspect mass in right breast </Description>
          <Coordinates>80,5,88,30</Coordinates>
          <Source>AI</Source>
          <Label>No Cancer</Label>
          <Confidence>98,2</Confidence>
          <Notes> Notes from AI </Notes>
     </ROI>
</Image>
```

Fig. 16.4 Example of an XML file used for the regions of interest communication protocol

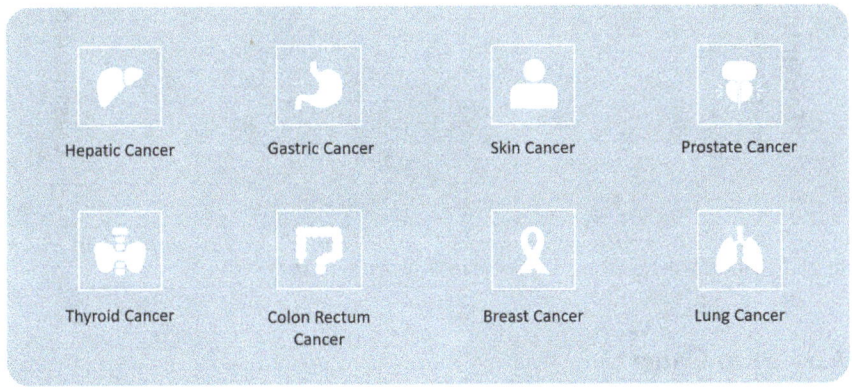

Fig. 16.5 Oncological pathologies analysed withing the Synergy-Net project

2. Classification, i.e. the prediction of the associated oncological risk and/or staging of the neoplastic lesion.

Given the different nature of the organs involved, the possible pathologies and the diagnostic instrumentation used, each pathology requires a different approach to achieve the desired objective. Next sections detail the work (done or in progress) for each of them, excluding the liver cancer for which the available data has not allowed for a suitable analysis.

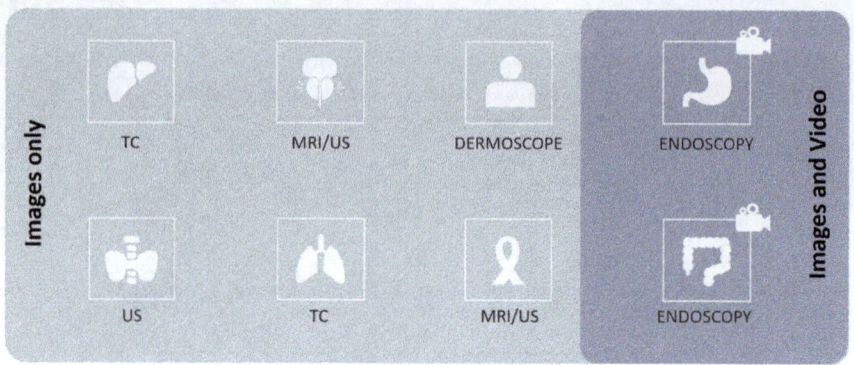

Fig. 16.6 Different type of medical imaging for different types of tumours/tissues

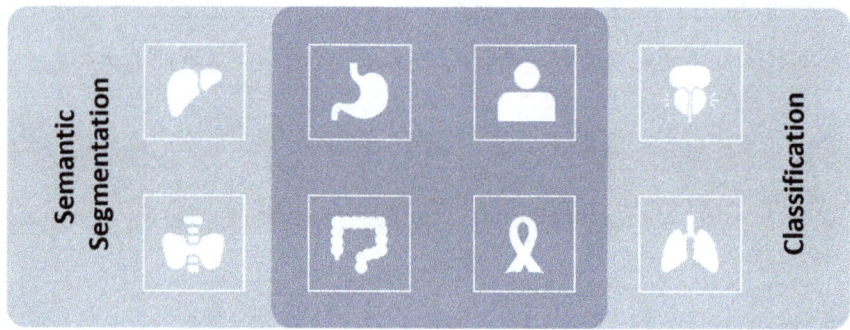

Fig. 16.7 Different desiderata and different tools to obtain them

16.3 Skin Cancer

Supporting the early diagnosis of skin cancer is crucial for the sake of any kind of treatment or surgery. The skin cancers can be roughly divided into two categories: melanoma and non-melanoma. The most common skin cancer belongs to the category of non-melanoma tumours with 2 and 3 million new diagnoses each year. More in details, non-melanoma skin cancers usually develop in the outermost layer of skin (epidermis), with the basal cell carcinoma (basal cell carcinoma) and squamous cell carcinoma (squamous cell carcinoma) representing the most common types. Melanoma, the most serious type of skin cancer, develops in the cells (melanocytes) that produce melanin—the pigment that gives to skin its color. The exact cause of all melanomas isn't clear, but exposure to ultraviolet (ultraviolet) radiation from sunlight or tanning lamps and beds appears to be linked to melanoma occurrence. Skin cancer diagnosis is a non-trivial challenge since the risks of this disease is usually underestimated. Although skin cancer has several distinguishing characteristics, people tend not to consult a physician for skin exam. However, the early diagnosis is the key factor in treatment success.

Nowadays, detection of melanoma is strongly improved by means of novel approaches to support the visual inspection such as total body photography, dermoscopy, automated diagnostic systems and reflectance confocal microscopy. Dermoscopy is the most spread method for skin cancer detection. It consists of a non-invasive, in-vivo technique and it is performed by means of a manual instrument called dermatoscope. The procedure allows examination of skin structures and patterns not visible to the naked eye [2, 28, 31]. An interesting aspect of such a technique is the possibility of the images to be digitised for storage, far transmission or sequential analysis. Thanks to this feature dermatologists have begun to incorporate novel imaging techniques into diagnostic algorithms. The automatic skin cancer diagnosis techniques are traditionally based on computer vision applications that implement one or more of the following approaches:

Geometry analysis: like all the tumour forms, the growth of the lesion has an irregular pattern which, in the case of skin tumour forms, leads to asymmetry in the shape. It is important, therefore, to rely on powerful descriptors such as area, perimeter, convexity, the major/minor-axis' length and angle, compactness, elongation, eccentricity (also known as ellipticity), roundness (or circularity) and sphericity [2, 18].

Color analysis: the tonality of the skin when a tumour grows may change in a discriminant way. Therefore, automatic approaches may benefit from colour analysis. This descriptors are mainly histogram derived considerations and require the choice of a colour space such as RGB, Hue-Saturation-Value (Hue-Saturation-Value), YCrCb, and the novel Hue-Min-Max-Difference (Hue-Min-Max-Difference). Colour analysis is performed with colour descriptors, such as the Scalable Color Descriptor (Scalable Color Descriptor), defined by a fixed colour space quantization, the Haar transform encoding, the dominant colour (dominant colour), that quantifies the distribution of the salient colours in the image, Color Layout Descriptor (Color Layout Descriptor) that captures the spatial layout of the dominant colours and so on [27, 49, 51].

Texture analysis: texture, like colour, is a powerful low-level descriptor in skin tumour classification. Computer Vision literature is plenty of textural descriptors that can be roughly divided into local or global approaches operating in space or frequency domain [27, 49].

However, the extraction of descriptive characteristics should be developed by domain experts who need to rely on robust segmentation methodology.

While newer hand-crafted features are continuously proposed by domain experts, in the last years several studies have been conducting to exploit deep learning approaches for skin cancer detection. More in details, deep Convolutional Neural Networks (Convolution Neural Networks), composed of different convolutional layers stacked in a deep architecture, have obtained wide popularity thanks to their ability to autonomous learn compact hierarchical features that best fit the specific input domain.

Convolutional Neural Networks (Convolution Neural Networks) are machine learning models borrowed from traditional Neural Networks (Neural Networks). Such architectures share most of the features: they are both made of neurons, usually organized in layers stratified to create a feed-forward network in which the output of a layer is the input of next one. However, while traditional Neural Networks operate on the features designed and extracted by a domain expert, Convolution Neural Networks use a hierarchy of convolution operations to autonomously design the features that better model the problem under analysis. Although this characteristic gives to Convolution Neural Networks a great representational ability, it also comes with a huge number of parameters to learn. Despite the efforts made to design increasingly compact networks, Convolution Neural Networks tend to strongly focus on the input dataset (also know as overfit behaviour) when the training phase is limited to few training instances. The solution would be to provide a large number of input instances but, when these are not easily available, especially in medical domain. A valid solution is to transfer the knowledge learned by a previous trained Convolution Neural Network (also on a different domain) to the new input domain. More in details, the pre-trained Convolution Neural Network is the starting point to train a model for the new task with a proper amount of available training data. The knowledge transfer technique is also known as *Transfer Learning* and can be obtained by following two approaches:

Fine-Tuning: consists in training the Convolution Neural Network by using as starting point the weights of the same network pre-trained on a different domain. To adapt the network to the specific task to solve, the last few layers of the pre-trained Convolution Neural Network (usually called fully connected layers) should be modified to handle the different number of classes. Since the first network's layers usually learn general features, their weights are not updated during the training.

Feature-Extraction: uses the pre-trained Convolution Neural Network to extract the features from the input images by relying on the output of the first convolutional layers. As a consequence, no further training is required and for each image a feature vector is obtained. The extracted features are then used as input for different models, such as traditional Machine Leaning approaches, or for a mapping function in a novel and bigger vectorial space. This approach is strongly promoted because the knowledge of the pre-trained network is able to efficiently map the instances for several tasks (also for very different domains).

Both the approaches aim to reduce the computational burden of training a network from scratch. However, only the Feature-Extraction approach also performs a space transformation that may help to index a bunch of images efficiently relying on visual peculiarity not easy to catch up with handcrafted features.

Several studies have been proposed in literature exploiting deep learning approaches for skin cancer diagnosis. Codella et al. [7] proposed to use a pre-trained network called AlexNet [21] as a feature-extractor to map the images in a bigger feature-space (4096 features). The vectors in the new space were used to train a Support-Vector Machine (Support-Vector Machine) model.

Pomponiu et al. [34] proposed to apply data augmentation to obtain a bigger number of images. This feeding approach consisted in applying affine transformations to the input images during the training phase with the aim of improving generalization behaviour. The authors also changed the classification model with a weaker k-Nearest Neighbors (k-Nearest Neighbors) model.

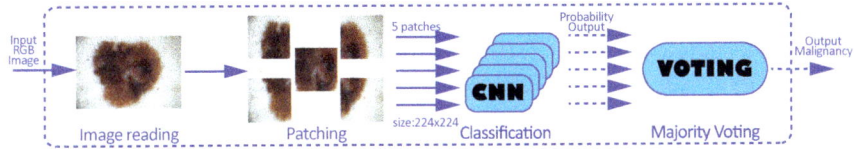

Fig. 16.8 Proposed approach for the skin cancer diagnosis within the Synergy-Net project

A novel deep learning approach proposed by Haenssle et al. [16] consisted of using a more complex pre-trained network called GoogLeNet Inception-v3 [45]. To adapt the network to the skin cancer detection task, while handling the limited amount of data, fine tuning is exploited.

In Synergy-Net project the implemented methodology proposes to improve the outcome of the automatic diagnoses approaches by using an ensemble of pre-trained deep convolutional neural networks and a suitable voting strategy (Fig. 16.8).

The approach consists of four main stages organised as follows:

Image Reading: Since there are several tools and cameras for dermoscopy that can provide digital images suitable for computer vision aided analysis, it is required a suitable read, conversion and representation format able to be compliant with the subsequent steps. The formats accepted are JPEG, BMP, PNG, DICOM, NIFTI and the image is, therefore, converted into RGB matrices.

Patching: The whole image is divided into five patches extracted from the four corners and form the centre. Each patch is, then, resized to the squared size of 224×224 to be compliant with the input of the subsequent stage (the input of the neural network).

Classification: Each patch undergoes a neural network to create an ensemble classification of the same lesion with five points of view. The result is obtained with a pre-trained Alexnet [21] fine-tuned on our dataset. The output of this stage for each image is a five elements vector representing the probability of each patch to belong to malignant melanoma.

Voting: The five element vector is, therefore, combined to produce an ensemble decision by applying a weighted majority voting. The most probable class (malignant/non-malignant) is returned.

The dataset was collected and labelled by experienced dermatologists. It consists of 200 patients (77 female and 123 male subjects) with several images per patient as described in Table 16.1. The table also shows the four different skin lesions included in the dataset and the relative considered classes. Lesions belong to patients with age from 1 to 100 years old and are from different part of the body.

The images composing the dataset have different resolution ranging from a minimum of 1999x1333 pixel to a maximum 5184x3456 and three RGB channels.

The proposed Convolution Neural Network has been evaluated using the high-level neural networks API Keras (Python 3.6) with TensorFlow 1.6 as back-end. Python scripts have been executed on a physical server hosted at University of Naples

Table 16.1 Dataset composition

Lesion	Patients	Male	Female	Images	Class
Nevus (Mole)	23	13	10	24	(B) Benignant
Angioma	27	14	13	27	(B) Benignant
Seborrheic Keratosis	50	32	18	51	(B) Benignant
Melanoma	100	64	36	107	(M) Malignant
Total	200	123	77	209	$\frac{B}{M} = \frac{102}{107}$

Table 16.2 Proposed approach variants comparison. AUC median values (obtained with a 10-folds CV)

Augmentation	SubPatch	Voting	Area under the receiver operating characteristic curve (%)
Yes			84.1
	Yes	OR	55.28
	Yes	Majority	60.91
Yes	Yes	OR	83.63
Yes	Yes	Majority	**87.27**

The best result is reported in bold

Federico II HPC center[1] equipped with 2 × Intel(R) Xeon(R) Intel(R) 2.13GHz CPUs (4 cores), 32 GB RAM and a Nvidia Titan Xp GPU (Pascal family) with 12GB GRAM.

The solutions proposed in literature have been developed by strictly implementing the design published in their works and evaluated on the same set of data and configuration of cross-validation (fixing the seeds of the pseudo-random generators). To face the size limitation of the training dataset a data augmentation approach has been applied. Spatial affine transformation such as Left/Right flip, Top/Bottom flip, 90 degrees rotations has been applied.

Finally, in order to train the proposed models, a cross-entropy loss has been minimized and the performance has been evaluated in 10-fold cross-validation considering the median values of the Area Under the Receiver Operating Characteristic (Area Under the Receiver Operating Characteristic Curve) Curve or Area Under the Receiver Operating Characteristic Curve.

Table 16.2 reports the results of the approach implemented for Synergy-net project obtained by varying the training stage (with or without the augmentation). The impact of patches extraction strategy has been also evaluated by considering the baseline approach, consisting in feeding the CNN with whole image.

---

[1] http://www.scope.unina.it.

Table 16.3 Our approach compared with the literature proposals. AUC median values (obtained with a 10-folds CV)

Approach	Metodology	Area under the receiver operating characteristic curve (%)
Haenssle et al. [16]	Inception-v3 (FineTuning)	55.68
Pomponiu et al. [34]	Alexnet (FeatureExtraction) + kNN	76.41
Codella et al. [7]	Alexnet (FeatureExtraction) + SVM	78.06
Haenssle et al. [16] + Augmentation	Inception-v3 (FineTuning)	80.91
Codella et al. [34] + Augmentation	Alexnet (FeatureExtraction) + SVM	84.54
Proposed Approach	Ensamble of Alexnet (FineTuning)	**87.27**

The best result is reported in bold

To evaluate the effectiveness of the proposed approach, the results were compared with those obtained by applying the approaches described in [7, 16, 34] using a 10-fold Cross Validation (Cross Validation) ensuring that the lesions from the same subject are always included in the same Cross Validation fold, to obtain a reliable and fair evaluation. Since Table 16.2 clearly shows that a form of augmentation improves the model to generalise the problem and thus improves the final result, the solutions proposed in literature that did not already apply this approach are evaluated using the augmentation technique introduced for Synergy-net project . Results are reported in Table 16.3, showing that even if literature proposals are in the best condition, our solution achieves the best classification results in terms of AUC.

As part of the project, the data acquisition is currently going on providing novel data with the aim of retraining the model and further validating the insights. Moreover, future works will be focused on investigating the data fusion of geometrical, textural and deep features to provide a more robust machine learning approach in skin lesion diagnosis.

16.4 Lung

According to the World Health Organization (World Health Organization), the lung cancer is one of the most frequent diseases, causing the death estimated for nearly 1.59 million people per year [40]. It is strictly associated with the consumption of tobacco products, showing an increase of 2% per year in its worldwide incidence. Cancer screening guidelines [48] recommends annual screening with low" dose Computed Tomography (Computed tomography) for high" risk groups to reduce cancer mortality. Indeed, still today early diagnosis is considered the key to reduce mortality and increase the chances for a successful treatment.

Over the years, Computed tomography imaging has demonstrated great potential in cancer detection, providing information about the presence and the stage of a tumour. From a technical perspective, it is a radiological technique that uses computer-processed combinations of multiple X-ray measurements taken from different angles to provide a series of sectional images (slices) of the body allowing to distinguish the various organs and tissues based on their density.

CT images are analysed to determine exactly where to perform a biopsy procedure, to guide certain local treatments (cryotherapy, radiofrequency ablation, etc.) or to assess whether a cancer is responding to treatment or not. As a consequence, there is a rising interest among the researchers to develop lung cancer diagnosis and detection methods that are based on CT images analysis. However, CT image analysis is a long and tedious task, strongly affected by human error due to the fatigue in making annotations. Therefore, several studies exploit Deep Learning (Deep Learning) to propose solutions that automatically detect and diagnose lung tumours. Indeed, as happened for other biomedical imaging procedures, in recent years deep learning approaches have gained popularity also in lung CT analysis, outperforming previous state-of-art machine learning techniques in lesion detection.

Given Deep Learning characteristics, some authors analysed the exploitation of Convolution Neural Networks also in lung Computed tomography imaging. In particular, one of the most useful tasks is the detection of suspicious Region of Interest (Regions of Interest) as a box around a portion of tissue. For example, in [9] a Region CNN (Region CNN) has been used for nodule segmentation. The idea was to use an Region CNN, supported by a pre-trained VGG backbone, to perform the nodule detection slice-by-slice. Then, to reduce the number of false positives, a 3D-Convolution Neural Network is used to classify the previously extracted 3D patches into nodule or non-nodule. A similar approach has also been used in [24], with authors proposing a Masked Region CNN, with a pre-trained ResNet101 architecture used as a backbone. More recently, in [6] the authors proposed the use of a 3D-UNet to catch more information from the context of one slice for detection. Also in that case, a support network has been used to perform false positives reduction.

The flip side of the coin is that, usually, training a deep learning based solutions require a large set of Computed tomography images, appropriately annotated by expert physicians. Unfortunately, image labelling is an excessively time-consuming procedure that is almost impossible to be performed during the classic screening procedures. This problem is commonly addressed by crowd-sourced annotation, dataset sharing, etc. However, this is not possible with medical imaging since this type of data contains very sensitive information, making its sharing subject to rigid procedures. The situation is even more complex in the case of lung CT imaging, since the use of different scanners, acquisition protocols, etc., make the public availability of some datasets useless.

Nonetheless, in literature there are some deep learning based approaches that showed impressive performance in lung cancer detection on publicly available datasets, such as the one made available for the LUng Nodule Analysis (LUNA[2]) competition. As Convolution Neural Networks proved to be able to learn features that are prone to be transferred between different tasks, the solution proposed for Synergy-Net project aims to analyse whether it is possible to use a network trained on the LUNA dataset to detect lung cancer on a dataset having different characteristics. As a case of study, the recent U-Net solution proposed in [6] is used, since it represents one of the most effective, yet simple, solutions so far proposed for the LUNA challenge.

Lung cancer detection consists in the localisation of damaged tissue, resulting in the definition of a Region Of Interest (Regions of Interest) that should be further investigated. Each Computed tomography scan involves the acquisition of a set of images (slices), reconstructing the portion of the body under analysis.

As aforementioned, the CNN-based solution presented in [6] for lung nodule segmentation is adapted for nodule detection. More in details, lung cancer detection is performed customizing both pre-processing and post-processing steps, in order to make the considered dataset compatible with the one (LUNA) used to train the model. The proposed solution can be summarised in three main stages:

- **Data preparation**, consisting in the application of a set of transformations on input images with the aim of making them compatible with the involved Convolution Neural Network input;
- **Nodule segmentation**, that produces a segmentation mask for each lung nodule;
- **Bounding box definition** that adapts Convolution Neural Network output to cancer detection task.

The last stage is needed as the approach proposed in [6] performs a pixel-wise segmentation, while the aim is to generate a box-shaped Regions of Interest.

The dataset was collected and labelled by experienced pulmonologist. It consists of 43 patients (14 with benign pathology, 21 with primary tumor malignancy, 15 with metastases, and 1 with bordeline diagnosis). The dataset differs from the one used for the LUNA competition since:

- The series were acquired with scanners from different manufacturers;
- There are series with and without contrast;
- Series are acquired with different Computed tomography kernel;
- Series have various Slice Thickness and Pixel Spacing.

These differences make the proposed analysis more realistic, allowing to assess whether it is possible to use a pre-trained lung Computed tomography lesion detector a dataset different from the one used for the training.

The Data Preparation step aims in making the Computed tomography images compatible with the considered CNN input. More in details, the Computed tomography scans used for image acquisition present different resolutions, resulting in slices with diverse pixel spacing. As a consequence, the voxels in different CT acquisitions represent volumes of unequal size. Moreover, traditional Convolution Neural

---

[2] https://luna16.grand-challenge.org/.

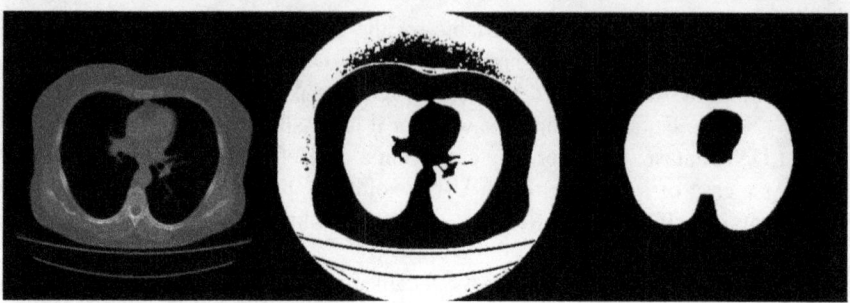

Fig. 16.9 Data pre-processing. From the original middle slice (on the left), a rough lung mask (middle) is extracted by using the k-means algorithm with k = 2. This mask is refined by means of morphological operation. Finally, only the central biggest region is preserved, obtaining the final lung mask

Networks are not scale invariants since they could not be able to detect different sized features, especially if they weren't in the training set. Thus, it necessary to have volumes with an isotropic resolution in order to use the CNN properly. To this aim, each Computed tomography series is re-sampled with a bi-linear interpolation to have a spacing of 1 mm in every direction x, y, z, as this is the pixel spacing of original training data.

A chest Computed tomography acquisition includes different organs, resulting in the need for a lung segmentation module. To this aim, the lungs are segmented by using the properties of the Hounsfield Scale: each voxel in the Computed tomography series is clipped to a maximum value of 4096 and to a minimum value of -1024, and then normalized in [0–1] before using the central slice to derive the threshold to use for distinguishing the pixel belonging to the lung tissue from the others. K-means algorithm, with $k = 2$, is used to determine the aforementioned threshold. The result of Data Preparation step is a binary lung mask, including only lung parenchyma. This mask is further refined by considering only the largest regions obtained and applying dilation and erosion operations on them. Figure 16.9 shows the procedure described in this step.

The obtained maks is used to extract the lung voxels. These are then inserted (centred) into an empty volume of 384x288x384 pixel to match the size of the data used to train the considered network.

In [6] the authors perform nodule segmentation involving a 3D U-shaped Convolution Neural Network (3D UNet). Although a CT acquisition is a 3D volume, the segmentation is conducted slice by slice in a 3D manner. The involved Convolution Neural Network takes a 3D volume as input working with a stack of 11 slices in order to provide the segmentation mask for the 6th (central) slice. In this way, the features extracted from the slice and its context are exploited improving network performance. The output of this step is a nodule segmentation mask that define the outline of the cancer in each Computed tomography acquisition.

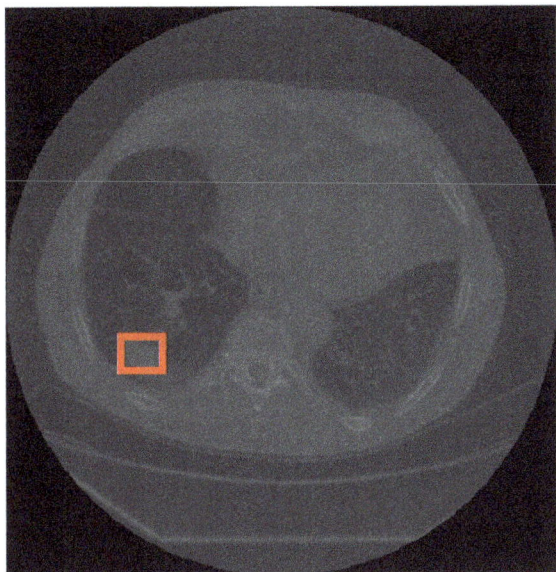

Fig. 16.10 An example of bounding box for a detected nodule

The Bounding Box Extraction step processes the segmentation masks in order to get the bounding boxes for each nodule detected. As results of the re-sampling operation described in the previous step, new slices are created between two original ones. Thus, the produced segmentation also refers to these new slices. The main idea to solve this problem is to aggregate new slices with old ones obtaining more candidates for each original slice. The candidates are then combined together as follows:

- candidates are grouped for each original slice;
- a mask is generated for each original slice by considering the union of all candidate slices;
- the pixel-wise cancer probability is normalised by dividing it to the number of candidates;
- a bounding box is extracted for each connected component whose probability is given by the mean of the probability of the pixel in the final mask.

An example of the results is reported in Fig. 16.10.

Experiments are implemented in PyTorch and performed on on a physical server hosted at University of Naples Federico II HPC center[3] equipped with 2 × Intel(R) Xeon(R) Intel(R) 2.13 GHz CPUs (4 cores), 32 GB RAM and a Nvidia Titan Xp GPU (Pascal family) with 12 GB GRAM. The performance of the proposed methodology are evaluated in terms of True Positive (True Positive), that is the number

---

[3] http://www.scope.unina.it.

Table 16.4 Results of the proposed methodology on a private dataset

Metric	Value
TP	203
FN	130
SEN	0.61
F1	0.63

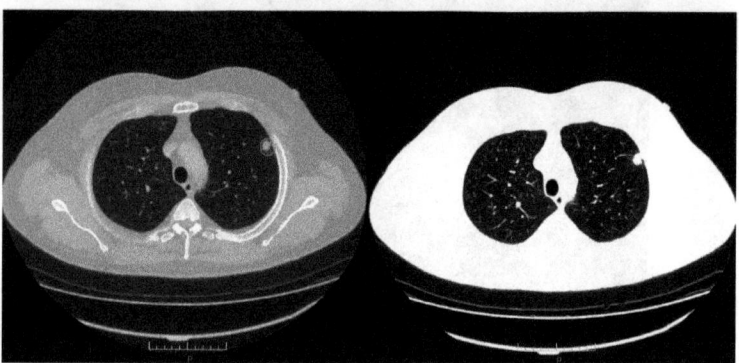

Fig. 16.11 Missing annotation is an important problem that afflicts ct images: on the left there a ground truth for a slice, on the right a missing annotation for the nodule in same position of the one on the left, for the next slice. The methodology described in this work is capable to find the nodule on the right. Quantitative performance evaluation is influenced by this phenomenon

of correct detected nodules, False Negative (False Negative), namely the number of mis-detected nodules, Sensitivity (Sensitivity) that measures the proportion of positives that are correctly identified, defined as $\frac{TP}{TP+FN}$ and the harmonic mean of the precision and the recall (F1), defined as $2 \cdot \frac{precision \cdot recall}{precision+recall}$ Table 16.4 shows the results of the described solutions.

Despite results are encouraging, it is worth noting that the presented results need to be cross-validated by visual analysis since CT images can be affected by lack of annotation [24] due to possibility of human error in CT exploration procedure. An example of this issue is presented in Fig. 16.11, confirming that the explored solution is able to detect nodules that have not been annotated by the physicians.

Experimental results on the dataset collected with the Synergy-net project demonstrated that the analyzed methodology could be a powerful tool to assist physicians in the diagnosis and the detection of lung cancer.

16.5 Colon Rectum Cancer

Colon rectum cancer is one of the leading causes of death worldwide. Colorectal polyps are important precursors to the cancers, which may develop if the polyps are left untreated. In order to detect polyps in their early stage and remove them before they deteriorate to cancer cells, doctors need to visualize the gastrointestinal (gastrointestinal) tract directly.

Colonoscopy is the gold-standard screening test for colorectal cancer reducing the risk of death through the detection of tumours at an earlier stage as well as through the removal of precancerous adenomas, namely polyps made up of tissue that looks much like the normal lining of colon, but shows different characteristics if looked at under the microscope. In some cases, a cancer can start in the adenoma. As a consequence, certain polups, including smaller polyps, flat polyps and polps in the left colon, may be missed during colonoscopy. There are two independent reason why a polyps may be missed during colonoscopy: (1) it was never in the visual field or (2) it was in the visual field but not recognized. Several hardware innovations have sought to address the first problem by improving visualization of the colonic lumen, for instance by providing a larger, panoramic camera view. However, the problem of unrecognized polyps within the visual field has been more difficult to address, since it requires the physician to be extremely vigilant with the aim of avoiding errors.

In recent years, several studies have been conducting to provide solutions for automatic polyp detection in colonoscopy. More in details, recent proposed works exploit deep learning (Deep Learning) approaches in the implementation of systems for polyps detecton and classification in colonoscopy images. In 2016 Ribeiro et al. [38] explored Convolution Neural Networks for colonic polyp classification investigating different network configurations obtained by varying filter sizes for filtering operations and strides for overlapping patches. In 2017 Zhang et al. [52] proposed using a pre-trained Convolution Neural Network, CaffeNet [20], trained on non-medical source domain as feature extractor and used support vector machine for the classification of colorectal polyps. In the same year, Yuan et al. [50] proposed a Convolution Neural Network based algorithm to detect polyp automatically in colonoscopy videos. In the proposed algorithm, the frames from a real-time colonoscopy video database were first pre-processed using edge detection and morphology operations. Then each connected component (edge contour) was extracted as one candidate patch. After that, a Convolution Neural Network with AlexNet [21] architecture was adopted to classify each candidate into with polyp or non-polyp class. In 2018, Zheng et al. [54] introduced a unified, real-time polyp detection based on Only-Look-Once (Only-Look-Once) [36] convolutional neural network (Convolution Neural Network). The model was pre-trained in non-medical images and then trained with three public colonoscopy datasets. Polyp detections were then performed on narrowband (narrowband) imaging endoscopy. The performance and rapidity of the Only-Look-Once algorithm during the training and test stages had the potential to help endoscopists localize colorectal polyps during endoscopy.

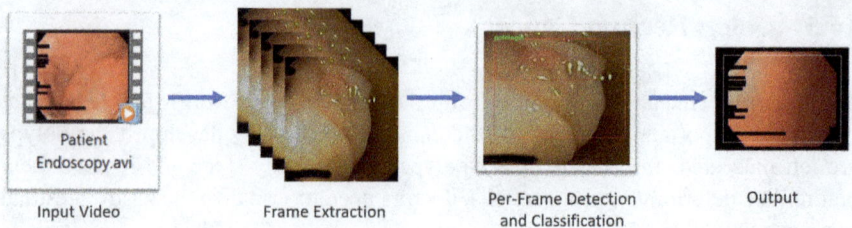

Fig. 16.12 Designed pipeline for the analysis of the colon rectum cancer

In 2019 Qadir et al. [35] introduced a new polyp detection framework to improve polyp detection performance in colonoscopy videos and integrate temporary information. This frame could be used with any object detector. The proposed method made a final decision for the situation at hand, combining temporal video analysis and individual frame analysis. The proposed method was tried with Single-Shot Detector (Single-Shot Detector) [26] used with MobileNet [19] backbone and Faster R–Convolution Neural Network [37] used with a Inception-Resent [44] backbone.

Liu et al. [25] implemented Single Shot Detection (Single-Shot Detector) [26] with three feature extractors InceptionV3 [45], ResNet-50 [17], and VGG16 [41]. Authors used public datasets and compared their model with other polyp detection methods. They also added a few layers to Single-Shot Detector [26], so their model showed increased accuracy and comparable results.

Zheng et al. [53] proposed a deep learning algorithm for automatic polyp detection and polyp localization in colonoscopy videos. This method first performs a segmentation and localization process such as U-Net [39]. The subsequent process uses optical flow to monitor the polyps. Finally, a regression model and a well-trained CNN are used to overcome the failure caused by movements. This algorithm had the highest scores in both the polyp detection and polyp localization task in the MICCAI 2018 Endoscopic Vision Challenge on Gastrointestinal Image Analysis.

Detection of tumors, nuclei, or lesions plays the most crucial role in diagnosing the disease in the medical image analysis. The purpose of the object detection system provides strong support for object segmentation, differentiation between malignant and benign tumors, or the detection of tumors or lesions. By using localization in fully automatic end-to-end applications, a detailed analysis of medical images can be done without human intervention. To this aim, the implemented solution within Synergy-Net project consists in two main modules for lesion detection and classification respectively (Fig. 16.12).

The lesion detector is based on a Single-Shot Detector (Single-Shot Detector) [26], since it takes one shot to detect multiple object present in an image. Single-Shot Detector [26] has two components: a backbone model and Single-Shot Detector head. Backbone model usually is a pre-trained image classification network used as a feature extractor while the Single-Shot Detector head is just one or more convolutional layers added to this backbone whose outputs are interpreted as the bounding boxes and classes of objects in the spatial location of the final layers activations. The lesion detector aims to identify suspicious, or potentially neoplastic, tissues. The network used as backbone is VGG16 [41], a very well known convolutional neural network, pretrained on Imagenet dataset[8].

Lesion classification module aims to categorize the suspicious tissues in different diseases. More in details, AlexNet [21] is used for distinguish the lesion among different classes. To handle the small dataset size, the involved Convolution Neural Network is pretrained on Imagenet dataset [8] and fine tuning is exploited to adapt the network to the specific task to solve.

The dataset was collected by an experienced gastroenterologist that defined the regions of interest (suspicious tissues) and provided their classification. It consists of 43 patients (27 with low-grade dysplasia, 13 with high-grade dysplasia and 13 with hyperplastic cancer), with a different number images.

Performance are evaluated in a 10 fold cross validation, ensuring that the lesions from the same subject are always included in the same Cross Validation fold. In the lesion detection module mean average precision (mean average precision) is used as evaluation metric. More in details, the detector make predictions in terms of bounding boxes for each element in the image. For each predicted bounding box the overlap with the ground truth bounding box is measured in terms of intersection over union (intersection over union) as shown in Fig. 16.13.

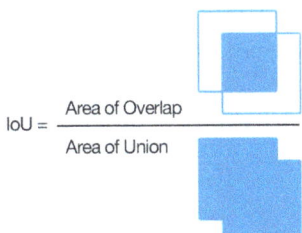

Fig. 16.13 Intersection over union (IoU) computation

Since the IoU is in 0–1 range, a threshold is selected, classifying a prediction as True Positive (True Positive) if the IoU exceeds the threshold and as a False Positive (False Positive) otherwise. Precision (FPrecision) and recall (recall) are then computed measuring the percentage of correct predictions (Eq. 16.1) and the validity of the predictions (Eq. 16.2) respectively.

$$P = \frac{TP}{TP + FP} \qquad (16.1)$$

$$R = \frac{TP}{TP + FN} \qquad (16.2)$$

The MAP is the mean of the average precision (mean average precision), that is the area under the precision-recall curve. Table 16.5 shows the result of the lesion detector module considering two different thresholds for intersection over union.

The performance of lesion classification module is evaluated in terms of accuracy, that is the ratio of correctly predicted observation to the total observations. Table 16.6 shows the confusion matrix for the classification task, allowing the visualization of the performance. Each row of the matrix represents the instances in a predicted class, while each column represents the instances in a correct class.

Figure 16.14 shows the output of the implemented system: the lesion detection module identifies the suspicious, or potentially neoplastic, tissue and the classifier provides the diagnosis. The proposed solution for Synergy-net project aims to perform an automatic polyp detection in colonoscopy by processing images acquired during the exam. However, it can be used to the implementation of a real-time system operating during the exam itself. Since the colonoscopy often consists in the acquisition of videos, each frame can be treated as a different image to be processed.

Table 16.5 Lesion detection module performance obtained by variyng the threshold with a 10-folds cross validation

Threshold	MAP
0.3	0.734
0.5	0.484

Table 16.6 Confusion matrix for the classification task. Each row of the matrix represents the instances in a predicted class, while each column represents the instances in a correct class

	Low-grade dysplasia	High-grade dysplasia	Hyperplastic cancer
Low-grade dysplasia	20	3	0
High-grade dysplasia	0	13	0
Hyperplastic cancer	2	1	11

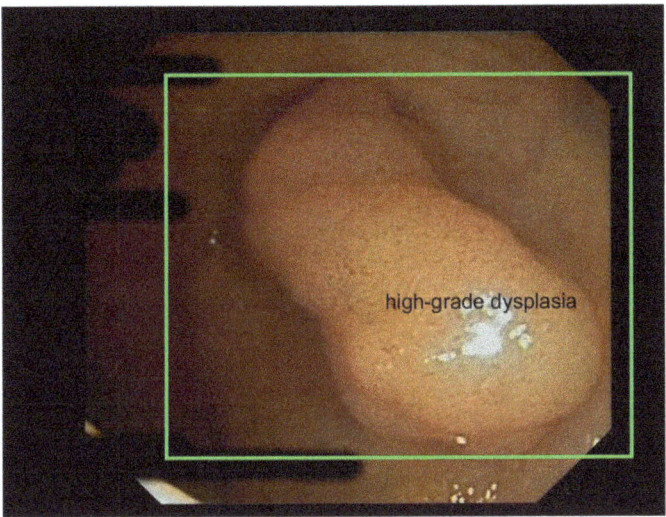

Fig. 16.14 An example of the output of the implemented system: the lesion detection module identifies the suspicious, or potentially neoplastic, tissue and the classifier provides the diagnosis

16.6 Breast Cancer

The breast cancer worldwide number of cases has significantly increased since the 1970s. This phenomenon is partly due to modern lifestyles, with recent studies showing that tumours are mostly an environmental rather than a genetic disease, being the results of factors like pollution, smoking, nutrition, radiation, stress, and traumas. Tumours grow and expand without evident signs, coming out with symptoms only at an advanced stage of the disease. For this reason, early detection is the key factor to improve breast neoplasm prognosis.

Nowadays, mammography and Dynamic Contrast Enhanced-Magnetic Resonance Imaging (Dynamic Contrast Enhanced Magnetic Resonance Imaging) are gold standard or screening for early stage breast cancer. Unfortunately, Dynamic Contrast Enhanced Magnetic Resonance Imaging is very expensive (w.r.t. mammography) and its long acquisition time also limits the number of patients that can be analysed per day. Thus, within the Synergy-net project the aim is to develop a method that guide the choice of performing also a Dynamic Contrast Enhanced Magnetic Resonance Imaging acquisition by analysing the mammography of a patient.

This task is still ongoing. The main difficulties are in the data collection, since there is the need to have patients (for different types of tumours) who underwent both mammography and Dynamic Contrast Enhanced Magnetic Resonance Imaging. The data collection is expected to be completed shortly and a first proof-of-concept of the proposed approach should be available by the end of the year 2021, thanks to the wide past experience we have for this organ and imaging technique.

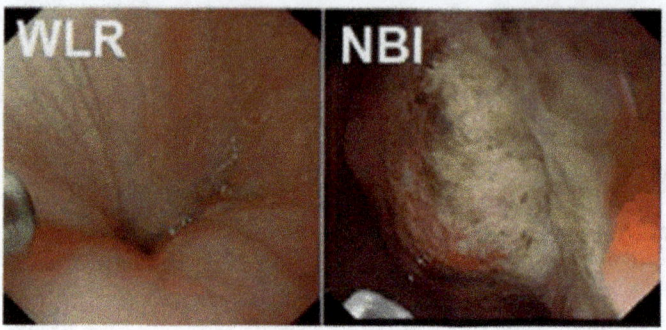

Fig. 16.15 Example of a white light reflectance (white light reflectance) and of a narrow band imaging (narrow band imaging) image (*Source* [4])

16.7 Gastric Carcinoma

The analysis of gastric carcinoma involves the use of images obtained by digestive endoscopy (gastroduedonoscopy) with the aim of performing pre-cancerous lesions early diagnosis. In particular, the aim is to establish the presence of pre-cancerous lesions by considering both diagnostic images and anamnestic/clinical data of patients.

For each patient, we acquire four White Light Reflectance (White Light Reflectance) and four Narrow Band Imaging (Narrow Band Imaging) images (Fig. 16.15 taken at 4 well-defined locations (for a total of 8 images for each patient) and anamnestic/clinical information. All lesions are proven by histopathological report, on a scale of 1–5 representing the degree of tissue malignancy. The anamnestic/clinical data associated to the patient are collected by means of a form, filled in partly by the patient and partly by the physician, before performing the endoscopic examination.

This task is still ongoing. The main difficulties are in the data collection that had to be interrupted due to the COVID-19 emergency. We are working to start the data gathering agian, but at the moment it is not possible to estimate the ETA.

16.8 Thyroid Cancer

Thyroid analysis is mainly performed by ultrasound imaging (thyroid ultrasonography) and hematochemical analysis (thyroid factors). Although the ultrasound analysis has the enormous advantage of being cheap (in relation to other biomedical imaging examinations) and non-invasive, it has on the other hand two major problems:

- Inter-operator variability consisting in different reporting of the same study by two different operators

- Intra-operator variability, consisting in different reporting of different studies (of the same patient) by the same operator.

The problem is related to the fact that, by its nature, ultrasound has a very strong operator-dependent component, which is not only related to the instrumental settings, but also to the specific positioning of the probe. Intra-operator variability, in particular, can result in a different analysis of the thyroid districts. Given the enormous preventive potential of thyroid ultrasound, the goal of the Synergy-Net project is to provide a positioning system, based on artificial intelligence, that helps operators to always position the probe in extremely similar positions. To this aim, the system autonomously identifies some anatomical regions to be used as a reference, such as the esophagus, the carotid artery, and so on. However, the overall system is still in the design phase in order to achieve a system with a higher capacity for generalization.

16.9 Prostate Cancer

As for other oncological pathologies, the diagnosis of prostate carcinoma can be obtained only after the analysis of the tissue, taken by biopsy. Given the position of the organ, the biopsy is typically assisted by ultrasound images and the standard procedure consists in taking different portions of tissue from different areas, since it is not possible to identify a-priori suspicious tissues. Since the described procedure is highly invasive, The objective identified for the Synergy-net project is to analyze biomedical images in order to guide the operator in the identification of tissues that are most suspicious. On the one hand, the number of biopsy retrievals while on the other hand is minimized, while, on the other hand the probability of acquiring tissues containing the neoplastic cells is maximized. To this aim, different types of data should be taken into account, including Dynamic Contrast Enhanced-Magnetic Resonance Imaging (Dynamic Contrast Enhanced Magnetic Resonance Imaging), ultrasound images and information related to patient age, familiarity with the disease.

This task is still ongoing. The main difficulties are in the data collection that experienced several delays due to the COVID-19 emergency. Despite this, the data collection is expected to be completed in few months and a first proof-of-concept of the proposed approach should be available by early 2022.

16.10 Conclusions and Future Perspectives

In this chapter we have introduced and described "Synergy-Net: Research and Digital Solutions in the Fight Against Oncological Diseases", an ongoing project aiming at the realisation of a technological platform to support the early oncological diagnosis based on the integration of an interoperable communication and clinical data management system leveraging AI. Due to its deeply interdisciplinary nature, the

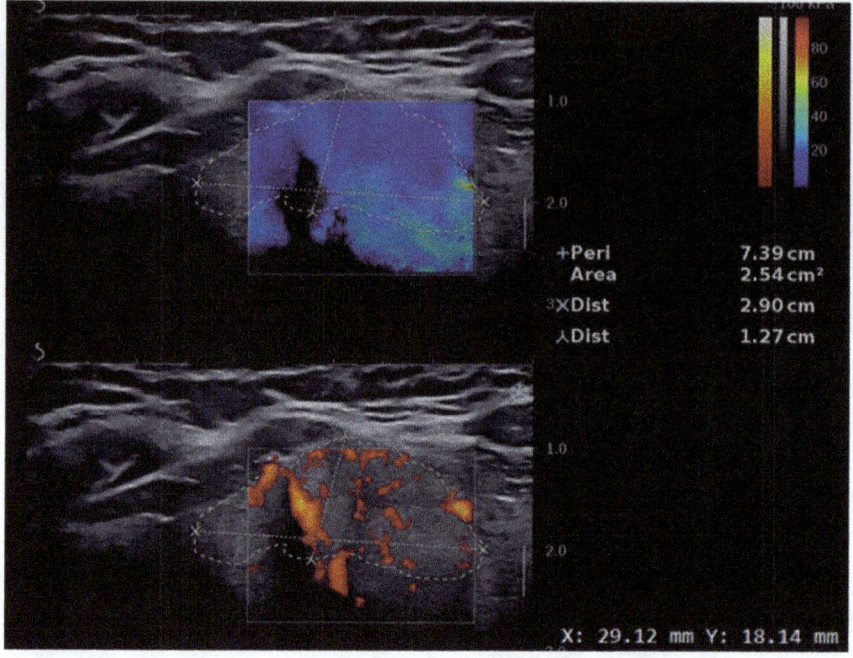

Fig. 16.16 Example of an elastosonography UltraSound image of the breast

Synergy-Net system has been designed as a modular CAD where each module cooperates with the others, under the guidance of an orchestrator, to provide the required computation.

This interdisciplinary nature allowed to work in parallel on different organs, exploiting common architectures, solutions and ideas while designing ad-hoc solutions. The flip side of the coin is that the project progresses are not aligned, mostly due to different need (e.g. conditions that need to be meet for involving a patient) and desiderata. This has been further complicated by the ongoing COVID-19 emergency. The result is that while the design of AI-bases algorithm for some organs is completed (or almost completed), for other organs we are still in the data collection stage.

Despite this, while working to complete also ongoing tasks, we are also already planning future steps. Two are the main ideas we are working on. The first is to leverage modern Elastosonography US imagining (Fig. 16.16 as a low-cost and side effects free methodology for early diagnosis of oncological diseases for all the tumorus considered in the Synergy-Net project.

The second idea is to provide an integrated prevention trough data fusion techniques with the aim of simultaneously analyze information from multiple sources, in order to provide an integrated tool built on the medical knowledge of each specialist

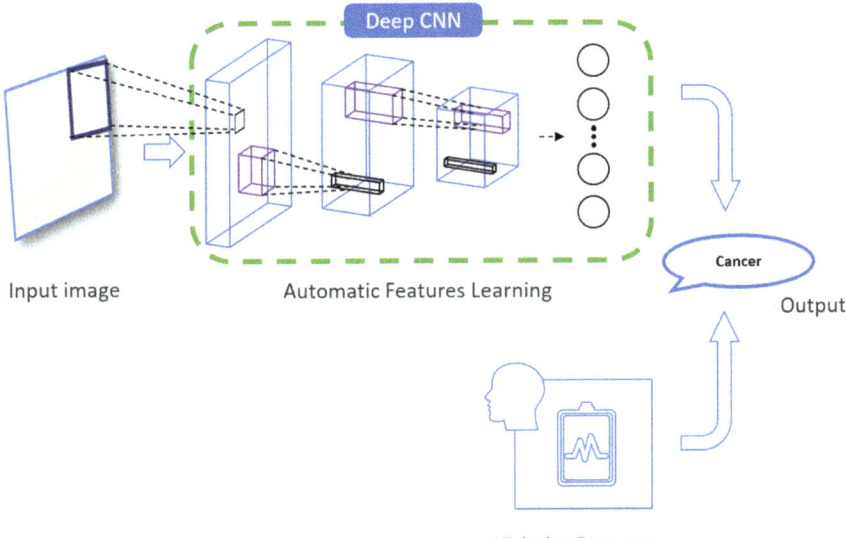

Fig. 16.17 Illustration of the described integrated prevention system

(Fig. 16.17. This will be further improved by the use of DNA sequencing tests, aimed at finding correlations between mutations and imaging anomalies, leading to cancer.

Acknowledgements This work is part of the "Synergy-net: Research and Digital Solutions against Cancer" project (funded in the framework of the POR Campania FESR 2014-2020—CUP B61C17000090007). We thanks professor G. Argenziano (director of Dermatology Unit), professor M. Santini (director of Thoracic Surgery Unit), professor E. Procaccini (director of Breast Unit), professor V. Napolitano (director of Endoscopy Unit), professor M. Romano (director of Gastroenterology Unit), professor M. De Sio (director of Urology Unit) and professor G. Docimo (director of Thyroid Surgery Unit) from Universitá della Campania "L.Vanvitelli" for providing data, giving insights and useful discussions. We also thanks Ernesto de Rosa (Bollino.IT) for the support and effort pushed to sustain the Synergy.Net project.

References

1. Arbyn, M., Anttila, A., Jordan, J., Ronco, G., Schenck, U., Segnan, N., Wiener, H., Herbert, A., Von Karsa, L.: European guidelines for quality assurance in cervical cancer screening—Summary document. Ann. Oncol. **21**(3), 448–458 (2010)
2. Argenziano, G., Soyer, H.P., Chimenti, S., Talamini, R., Corona, R., Sera, F., Binder, M., Cerroni, L., De Rosa, G., Ferrara, G., et al.: Dermoscopy of pigmented skin lesions: results of a consensus meeting via the internet. J. Am. Acad. Dermatol. **48**(5), 679–693 (2003)
3. Assael, Y.M., Shillingford, B., Whiteson, S., De Freitas, N.: Lipnet: End-to-end sentence-level lipreading. arXiv:1611.01599 (2016)
4. Bergholt, M.S., Zheng, W., Ho, K.Y., Yeoh, K., Huang, Z.: Raman endoscopy for objective diagnosis of early cancer in the gastrointestinal system. J. Gastroint. Dig. Syst. **S1**, 008 (2013)

5. Chan, T.: Computer aided detection of small acute intracranial hemorrhage on computer tomography of brain. Comput. Med. Imaging Graph. **31**(4–5), 285–298 (2007)
6. Cheng, G., Xie, W., Yang, H., Ji, H., He, L., Xia, H., Zhou, Y.: Deep convolution neural networks for pulmonary nodule detection in CT imaging (2019)
7. Codella, N., Cai, J., Abedini, M., Garnavi, R., Halpern, A., Smith, J.R.: Deep learning, sparse coding, and SVM for melanoma recognition in dermoscopy images. In: International Workshop on Machine Learning in Medical Imaging. pp. 118–126. Springer (2015)
8. Deng, J., Dong, W., Socher, R., Li, L.J., Li, K., Fei-Fei, L.: Imagenet: a large-scale hierarchical image database. In: 2009 IEEE Conference on Computer Vision and Pattern Recognition, pp. 248–255. IEEE (2009)
9. Ding, J., Li, A., Hu, Z., Wang, L.: Accurate pulmonary nodule detection in computed tomography images using deep convolutional neural networks. In: International Conference on Medical Image Computing and Computer-Assisted Intervention, pp. 559–567. Springer (2017)
10. Doi, K.: Computer-aided diagnosis in medical imaging: historical review, current status and future potential. Comput. Med. Imaging Graph. **31**(4–5), 198–211 (2007)
11. Fenton, J.J., Taplin, S.H., Carney, P.A., Abraham, L., Sickles, E.A., D'Orsi, C., Berns, E.A., Cutter, G., Hendrick, R.E., Barlow, W.E., et al.: Influence of computer-aided detection on performance of screening mammography. New England J. Med. **356**(14), 1399–1409 (2007)
12. Galli, A., Gravina, M., Marrone, S., Piantadosi, G., Sansone, M., Sansone, C.: Evaluating impacts of motion correction on deep learning approaches for breast DCE-MRI segmentation and classification. In: International Conference on Computer Analysis of Images and Patterns, pp. 294–304. Springer (2019)
13. Gravina, M., Marrone, S., Piantadosi, G., Moscato, V., Sansone, C.: Developing a smart PACS: CBIR system using deep learning. In: 2020 25th International Conference on Pattern Recognition (ICPR). IEEE
14. Gravina, M., Marrone, S., Piantadosi, G., Sansone, M., Sansone, C.: 3TP-CNN: radiomics and deep learning for lesions classification in DCE-MRI. In: International Conference on Image Analysis and Processing, pp. 661–671. Springer (2019)
15. Griffith, C.D., Mahadevan, S.: Inclusion of fatigue effects in human reliability analysis. Reliabi. Eng. Syst. Safety **96**(11), 1437–1447 (2011)
16. Haenssle, H.A., Fink, C., Schneiderbauer, R., Toberer, F., Buhl, T., Blum, A., Kalloo, A., Hassen, A.B.H., Thomas, L., Enk, A., et al.: Man against machine: diagnostic performance of a deep learning convolutional neural network for dermoscopic melanoma recognition in comparison to 58 dermatologists. Ann. Oncol. **29**(8), 1836–1842 (2018)
17. He, K., Zhang, X., Ren, S., Sun, J.: Deep residual learning for image recognition. In: Proceedings of the IEEE Conference on Computer Vision and Pattern Recognition, pp. 770–778 (2016)
18. Henning, J.S., Dusza, S.W., Wang, S.Q., Marghoob, A.A., Rabinovitz, H.S., Polsky, D., Kopf, A.W.: The cash (color, architecture, symmetry, and homogeneity) algorithm for dermoscopy. J. Am. Acad. Dermatol. **56**(1), 45–52 (2007)
19. Howard, A.G., Zhu, M., Chen, B., Kalenichenko, D., Wang, W., Weyand, T., Andreetto, M., Adam, H.: Mobilenets: efficient convolutional neural networks for mobile vision applications. arXiv:1704.04861 (2017)
20. Jia, Y., Shelhamer, E., Donahue, J., Karayev, S., Long, J., Girshick, R., Guadarrama, S., Darrell, T.: Caffe: Convolutional architecture for fast feature embedding. In: Proceedings of the 22nd ACM international conference on Multimedia, pp. 675–678 (2014)
21. Krizhevsky, A., Sutskever, I., Hinton, G.E.: ImageNet Classification with Deep Convolutional Neural Networks. In: Advances in Neural Information Processing Systems, pp. 1–9 (2012)
22. Le, Q.V., Zou, W.Y., Yeung, S.Y., Ng, A.Y.: Learning hierarchical invariant spatio-temporal features for action recognition with independent subspace analysis. In: CVPR 2011, pp. 3361–3368. IEEE (2011)
23. Li, B., Meng, M.Q.H., Lau, J.Y.: Computer-aided small bowel tumor detection for capsule endoscopy. Artif. intell. Med. **52**(1), 11–16 (2011)

24. Liu, M., Dong, J., Dong, X., Yu, H., Qi, L.: Segmentation of lung nodule in CT images based on mask R-CNN. In: 2018 9th International Conference on Awareness Science and Technology (iCAST), pp. 1–6. IEEE (2018)
25. Liu, M., Jiang, J., Wang, Z.: Colonic polyp detection in endoscopic videos with single shot detection based deep convolutional neural network. IEEE Access **7**, 75058–75066 (2019)
26. Liu, W., Anguelov, D., Erhan, D., Szegedy, C., Reed, S., Fu, C.Y., Berg, A.C.: SSD: Single shot multibox detector. In: European Conference on Computer Vision, pp. 21–37. Springer (2016)
27. Manjunath, B.S., Ohm, J.R., Vasudevan, V.V., Yamada, A.: Color and texture descriptors. IEEE Trans. Circ. Syst. Video Technol. **11**(6), 703–715 (2001)
28. Marghoob, A.A., Swindle, L.D., Moricz, C.Z., Negron, F.A.S., Slue, B., Halpern, A.C., Kopf, A.W.: Instruments and new technologies for the in vivo diagnosis of melanoma. J. Am. Acad. Dermatol. **49**(5), 777–797 (2003)
29. Marrone, S., Olivieri, S., Piantadosi, G., Sansone, C.: Reproducibility of deep cnn for biomedical image processing across frameworks and architectures. In: 2019 27th European Signal Processing Conference (EUSIPCO), pp. 1–5. IEEE (2019)
30. Marrone, S., Piantadosi, G., Fusco, R., Petrillo, A., Sansone, M., Sansone, C.: Automatic lesion detection in breast DCE-MRI. In: Image Analysis and Processing (ICIAP), pp. 359–368. Springer, Berlin Heidelberg (2013)
31. Menzies, S., Ingvar, C., McCarthy, W.: A sensitivity and specificity analysis of the surface microscopy features of invasive melanoma. Melanoma Res. **6**(1), 55–62 (1996)
32. Piantadosi, G., Marrone, S., Galli, A., Sansone, M., Sansone, C.: DCE-MRI breast lesions segmentation with a 3TP U-net deep convolutional neural network. In: 2019 IEEE 32nd International Symposium on Computer-Based Medical Systems (CBMS), pp. 628–633 (2019)
33. Piantadosi, G., Marrone, S., Fusco, R., Sansone, M., Sansone, C.: Comprehensive computer-aided diagnosis for breast T1-weighted DCE-MRI through quantitative dynamical features and spatio-temporal local binary patterns. IET Comput. Vision **12**(7), 1007–1017 (2018)
34. Pomponiu, V., Nejati, H., Cheung, N.M.: Deepmole: Deep neural networks for skin mole lesion classification. In: 2016 IEEE International Conference on Image Processing (ICIP), pp. 2623–2627. IEEE (2016)
35. Qadir, H.A., Balasingham, I., Solhusvik, J., Bergsland, J., Aabakken, L., Shin, Y.: Improving automatic polyp detection using CNN by exploiting temporal dependency in colonoscopy video. IEEE J. Biomed. Health Inf. **24**(1), 180–193 (2019)
36. Redmon, J., Divvala, S., Girshick, R., Farhadi, A.: You only look once: unified, real-time object detection. In: Proceedings of the IEEE Conference on Computer Vision and Pattern Recognition, pp. 779–788 (2016)
37. Ren, S., He, K., Girshick, R., Sun, J.: Faster R-CNN: towards real-time object detection with region proposal networks. arXiv:1506.01497 (2015)
38. Ribeiro, E., Uhl, A., Wimmer, G., Häfner, M.: Exploring deep learning and transfer learning for colonic polyp classification. Comput. Math. Methods Med. **2016** (2016)
39. Ronneberger, O., Fischer, P., Brox, T.: U-net: convolutional networks for biomedical image segmentation. In: International Conference on Medical Image Computing and Computer-Assisted Intervention, pp. 234–241. Springer (2015)
40. Serj, M.F., Lavi, B., Hoff, G., Valls, D.P.: A deep convolutional neural network for lung cancer diagnostic. arXiv:1804.08170 (2018)
41. Simonyan, K., Zisserman, A.: Very deep convolutional networks for large-scale image recognition. arXiv:1409.1556 (2014)
42. Singh, K., Bønaa, K., Solberg, S., Sørlie, D., Bjørk, L.: Intra-and interobserver variability in ultrasound measurements of abdominal aortic diameter. The Tromsø study. Eur. J. Vascular Endovascular Surgery **15**(6), 497–504 (1998)
43. Stec, N., Arje, D., Moody, A.R., Krupinski, E.A., Tyrrell, P.N.: A systematic review of fatigue in radiology: is it a problem? Am. J. Roentgenol. **210**(4), 799–806 (2018)
44. Szegedy, C., Ioffe, S., Vanhoucke, V., Alemi, A.: Inception-v4, inception-ResNet and the impact of residual connections on learning. In: Proceedings of the AAAI Conference on Artificial Intelligence, vol. 31 (2017)

45. Szegedy, C., Vanhoucke, V., Ioffe, S., Shlens, J., Wojna, Z.: Rethinking the inception architecture for computer vision. In: Proceedings of the IEEE Conference on Computer Vision and Pattern Recognition, pp. 2818–2826 (2016)
46. Tiderius, C.J., Tjörnstrand, J., Åkeson, P., Södersten, K., Dahlberg, L., Leander, P.: Delayed gadolinium-enhanced MRI of cartilage (DGEMRIC): intra-and interobserver variability in standardized drawing of regions of interest. Acta radiologica **45**(6), 628–634 (2004)
47. Waite, S., Kolla, S., Jeudy, J., Legasto, A., Macknik, S.L., Martinez-Conde, S., Krupinski, E.A., Reede, D.L.: Tired in the reading room: the influence of fatigue in radiology. J. Am. Coll. Radiol. **14**(2), 191–197 (2017)
48. Wender, R., Fontham, E.T., Barrera Jr, E., Colditz, G.A., Church, T.R., Ettinger, D.S., Etzioni, R., Flowers, C.R., Scott Gazelle, G., Kelsey, D.K., et al.: American cancer society lung cancer screening guidelines. CA: Cancer J. Clin. **63**(2), 106–117 (2013)
49. Yu, H., Li, M., Zhang, H.J., Feng, J.: Color texture moments for content-based image retrieval. In: Proceedings of International Conference on Image Processing. vol. 3, pp. 929–932. IEEE (2002)
50. Yuan, Z., IzadyYazdanabadi, M., Mokkapati, D., Panvalkar, R., Shin, J.Y., Tajbakhsh, N., Gurudu, S., Liang, J.: Automatic polyp detection in colonoscopy videos. In: Medical Imaging 2017: Image Processing. vol. 10133, p. 101332K. International Society for Optics and Photonics (2017)
51. Zalaudek, I., Argenziano, G., Soyer, H., Corona, R., Sera, F., Blum, A., Braun, R., Cabo, H., Ferrara, G., Kopf, A., et al.: Three-point checklist of dermoscopy: an open internet study. Br. J. Dermatol. **154**(3), 431–437 (2006)
52. Zhang, R., Zheng, Y., Mak, T.W.C., Yu, R., Wong, S.H., Lau, J.Y., Poon, C.C.: Automatic detection and classification of colorectal polyps by transferring low-level CNN features from nonmedical domain. IEEE J. Biomed. Health Inform. **21**(1), 41–47 (2016)
53. Zheng, H., Chen, H., Huang, J., Li, X., Han, X., Yao, J.: Polyp tracking in video colonoscopy using optical flow with an on-the-fly trained CNN. In: 2019 IEEE 16th International Symposium on Biomedical Imaging (ISBI 2019), pp. 79–82. IEEE (2019)
54. Zheng, Y., Zhang, R., Yu, R., Jiang, Y., Mak, T.W., Wong, S.H., Lau, J.Y., Poon, C.C.: Localisation of colorectal polyps by convolutional neural network features learnt from white light and narrow band endoscopic images of multiple databases. In: 2018 40th Annual International Conference of the IEEE Engineering in Medicine and Biology Society (EMBC), pp. 4142–4145. IEEE (2018)
55. Zoorob, R., Anderson, R., Cefalu, C.A., Sidani, M.A.: Cancer screening guidelines. Am. Fam. Phys. **63**(6), 1101 (2001)

Chapter 17
New Insights on Implementing and Evaluating Artificial Intelligence in Cardiovascular Care

S. Dykstra, J. White, and M. L. Gavrilova

Abstract Artificial Intelligence is increasingly prevalent in our day-to-day lives, delivering paradigm shifts in how we function as a society. However, relative to other industries, the adoption of artificial intelligence in healthcare has progressed slowly. This chapter is focused on describing the unique challenges faced by personalized care delivery using multi-domain data patient health information. It discusses validated solutions for data management and Machine Learning approaches for combining the value of these complementary yet disparate data resources for patient-specific risk prediction modelling.

Keywords Artificial intelligence · Risk prediction modelling · Cardiovascular health · Deep learning · Electronic health records · Personalized care

17.1 Introduction

Artificial Intelligence (AI) is increasingly prevalent in our day-to-day lives, delivering paradigm shifts in how we function as a society. However, relative to other industries, the adoption of AI in healthcare has progressed slowly [1]. While machine learning (ML) techniques have mitigated the burden of numerous human tasks, such as drawing boundaries on diagnostic images, few algorithms have been implemented that meaningfully contribute intelligence to healthcare decision making (i.e. Artificial Intelligence). Accomplishing this requires broader consideration of complementary and contextual health information for the individual patient. Such data resources remain heavily compartmentalized across a complex healthcare landscape

---

S. Dykstra
Stephenson Cardiac Imaging Centre, Calgary, Canada

J. White
Libin Cardiovascular Institute of Alberta, University of Calgary, Calgary, Canada

M. L. Gavrilova (✉)
Biometrics Technologies Laboratory, University of Calgary, Calgary, Canada
e-mail: mgavrilo@ucalgary.ca

and present numerous challenges for their practical use in point-of-care decision support.

Expanded use of electronic health record (EHR) systems, designed to catalogue care across large patient populations, has led to sustained growth in ML-based risk prediction studies using this data [2]. However, awareness of key challenges surrounding the solitary use of this data have emerged, particularly for disease-focused tasks where bespoke data that is more reflective of disease phenotype(s) and patient health status are required. For example, in the field of cardiovascular medicine, patient-reported health markers (PRHM) and disease phenotype are now recognized to provide critical context for patient-specific risk modelling [3]. Through this awareness, focused interest surrounding the combined use of EHR, PRHM and raw diagnostic imaging data for the collective delivery of personalized care has emerged [4].

This chapter is focused on describing the unique challenges faced by personalized care delivery using multi-domain data patient health information. It will discuss validated solutions for data management and candidate ML approaches for combining the value of these complementary yet disparate data resources for patient-specific risk prediction modelling.

17.1.1 Artificial Intelligence and Machine Learning

AI is not a single technology; rather it is a broad collection of algorithms, methodologies, and approaches that collectively aim to mimic human cognitive function. ML is the collection of algorithms that allow a machine to learn using source data how it should perform a task, without being explicitly told how to do so. This is a key step towards AI's goal of mimicking human intelligence. As to properly mimic human intelligence algorithms need to be able to learn from data, just as humans learn by example.

Machine learning is classically described by the following statement: "A computer is said to learn from experience E with some class of tasks T and performance measure P if its performance at tasks in T, as measured by P improves with experience E" [5]. Simply put, this means that machine learning is the process of improving measured performance on a task through repeated attempts of completing that task. How performance is both measured and defined is foundationally important to this process and will be discussed further on in the chapter. At this point it is most relevant to understand that there are three main categories of machine learning algorithms: supervised learning, unsupervised learning, and reinforcement learning. For the purposes of delivering personalized risk prediction modelling, the most commonly encountered algorithms belong to supervised learning, an approach where models are trained to predict outcomes for de-novo cases through learning the association of input features and labelled outputs in a set of training cases. Predictions made are scored against these ground truth labels and iterative adjustments made to improve scores with successive attempts. This is accomplished using a cost function that describes how well a prediction is performing relative to its ground truth. Model optimization then becomes a task aimed at minimizing this cost function. The repeated process of feeding case examples and iteratively adjusting the model to minimize its cost function(s) is called training, and is how the algorithm learns underlying patterns of a dataset associated with an outcome. Following training, it is recommended to then validate an algorithm on data that was not used during its training. While this chapter will dominantly focus on supervised machine learning based algorithms, unsupervised learning is an alternative technique used when training datasets contain no labels and therefore the output is not known. The goal of these algorithms is to deduce innate structures or patterns that exist within the input data. The most common forms of unsupervised learning belong to dimensionality reduction or clustering techniques, these being aimed at exposing relationships within source data that may provide novel or relevant insights into potential use or value. Finally, reinforcement learning algorithms are a class of ML approaches that learn from interaction with their environment. Similar to how a child first learns to pass food to their mouth (by trial and error), model feedback is provided as a reward or penalty based on whether the action was correct or incorrect. This feedback is then used to adapt the model with the aim of maximizing reward. Reinforcement learning algorithms are rare in comparison to supervised and unsupervised learning methods, particularly for risk prediction modelling. This is due to the complex nature of creating an environment in which the model can interact and gain relevant feedback. For a full introduction to ML we recommend the following textbooks: *Machine Learning* by Mitchell [5], *The Elements of Statistical Learning: Data Mining, Inference, and Prediction* by Hastie et al. [6], *Deep Learning* by Goodfellow et al. [7], and *Advances in Data Science: Methodologies and Applications* by Phillips-Wren et al. [8].

Throughout this chapter, we will refer to examples of ML-based risk prediction models and algorithms with a focus on applications to cardiovascular care. We may appear to use the terms ML and AI interchangeably. However, we re-emphasize that AI is focused on mimicking human cognition, while ML are those tools used to accomplish this goal. In the context of personalized cardiovascular delivery, successful implementation of AI is anticipated to require an assemblance of ML algorithms in the context of a supportive framework that integrates these tools into the clinical workflow. To date the vast majority of progress and research in this field has focused on development and validation of isolated ML-based algorithms with limited implementation of AI-based care pathways.

17.1.2 Relevance of Artificial Intelligence to the Future of Cardiovascular Care Delivery

There is a general belief that AI will soon become a foundational component of cardiovascular practice and will deliver anticipated benefits from personalized care. In the context of our current discussion, we can describe personalized care as the capacity of machine-generated algorithms to optimize health benefits from clinical decisions through the integration of multi-domain, patient-specific data.

In the field of cardiovascular medicine, ML-based applications first emerged offering the capacity to assist clinicians in more efficiently interpreting diagnostic tests. This has been most apparent in the fields of electrocardiography (signal processing) [9] and diagnostic imaging (image processing) [10], while recent applications have emerged for the interpretation of phonocardiograms from digital stethoscopes [11]. ML-based techniques have been used for over a decade to automate the preliminary interpretation of 12-lead electrocardiograms, markedly improving the efficiency and inter-observer reproducibility of this test [9]. In diagnostic imaging, rapid growth has been seen for ML-based image analysis techniques across the fields of magnetic resonance imaging (MRI) [12], cardiac computerized tomography (CT) [13], nuclear imaging [14, 15], echocardiography [16] as well invasive coronary angiography [17]. While promoted as an emergence of AI in cardiovascular medicine, these tools have predominantly delivered discrete solutions for automating tasks otherwise manually performed by physicians.

ML-based solutions that target clinical decision making (i.e. AI-assisted care) in cardiovascular care are now emerging. Relevant examples using diagnostic test data include HeartFlow® Planner, a cloud-based service where ML-based modelling is performed from cardiac CT images to predict how the delivery of a coronary stent will improve blood flow down an obstructed vessel [18]. Tools such as these are focused on unlocking the value of single-domain diagnostic health data. Similar efforts can be appreciated from administrative or EHR-abstracted data with models focused on the prediction of heart failure re-admission [19], new-onset atrial fibrillation [20], patient mortality and prolonged length of stay [21]. Despite success of ML-based prediction modelling from singular data domains, few studies or commercial implementations have pursued multi-domain modelling pathways aimed at leveraging unique and complementary value of both diagnostic data (disease phenotype) and electronic health information (patient phenotype). It is through the bridging these independently valued data resources that optimal personalized care delivery is anticipated to be realized. This has proven challenging. As is the focus of this chapter, the implementation of AI tools in healthcare requires successful completion of three critical stages: data capturing, model development and clinical integration. The challenges faced within each of these stages are inherently amplified through a need to leverage multi-domain data resources. Thus, it is important to develop innovative solutions to deliver a scalable foundation upon which institutions can deliver personalized care.

Throughout this chapter we will describe our views on how these challenges should be resolved. We will draw on the development and ongoing implementation of a clinical service integrated personalized medicine initiative called the Cardiovascular Imaging Registry of Calgary (CIROC) at the Libin Cardiovascular Institute of the University of Calgary. CIROC is a prospective patient engagement-focused initiative for the routine capture of health data resources for development of AI-based risk models.

17.1.3 Implementing AI Within Institutional Healthcare Environments

There are three broadly relevant stages for the implementation of AI to deliver personalized cardiovascular care, these being (1) Data Capture and Management, (2) Model Development and Validation, and (3) Clinical Integration and Support. Each of these stages present unique challenges that, while commonly influenced by a specific task or aim, share themes that can be collectively discussed.

Data Capture and Management is a quintessential stage of ML-based tool development across all industries, however, must consider unique challenges and requisites in the healthcare setting [22]. While healthcare institutions share common mandates for consolidative data management, multi-domain resources remain inherently siloed, particularly with respect to diagnostic testing data. While the EHR has delivered unprecedented value for consolidating contextual health information (e.g. diagnostic codes, laboratory data, clinical notes and medications), secondary access to this resource is restricted to administrative and research purposes, presenting barriers for data usage destined for commercial tool implementation. As such, strategic consideration of appropriate data sharing agreements and the capacity to access similar data resources in clinical practice must be incorporated at this stage. Diagnostic test data is not commonly housed by EHR systems rather is summarized in an aggregate form (e.g. text reports). Raw diagnostic test data (e.g. images, ECG waveforms) or quantitative outputs of image processing (e.g. detailed image or waveform analyses) are archived on institutional servers in identified form. Upon definition of a desired model application or task, environmental surveys of available data resources should be accompanied by input from key opinion leaders to ensure the relevant inclusion of contextual health information. Comprehensively characterizing the location, accessibility, format, and privacy-related concerns of source data is then critically important prior to engaging in model development. Finally, the value of establishing a secure, institutionally-approved environment for the iterative collection of multi-domain data resources, subject matching, de-identification, cleansing and ultimate migration of consolidated resources to the modelling environment cannot be over-emphasized.

Model Development and Validation is the iterative stage of testing strategies aimed at achieving optimal model performance from available data resources. We will discuss unique challenges for risk prediction modelling using health datasets, particularly with respect to missing data and lack of performance metrics for clinical care. However, it is important to monitor for unseen bias and maximize generalizability of models intended for use in clinical environments. Expanding concern exists surrounding the introduction of training cohort bias in models that may affect important, potentially life-changing decisions [23]. There is also emerging concern that bias can be unknowingly introduced to AI models through lack of attention to equity, diversity and inclusion (EDI) within the development team [24]. To mitigate these concerns, we postulate that efforts must be undertaken at this stage to maximize model exposure to broadly representative populations, acknowledge limitations where present, and train development teams in EDI to recognize bias. Early pursuit

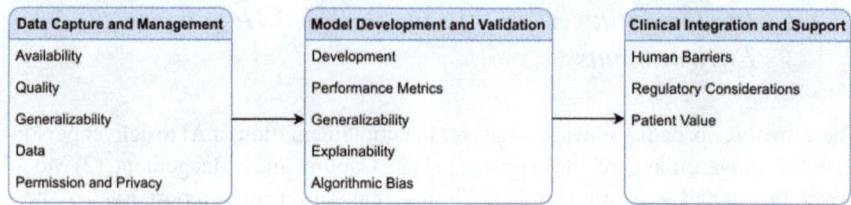

Fig. 17.1 Overview of the key areas within data, modelling, and clinical implementation that currently present challenges to the adoption of Artificial Intelligence in healthcare

of sufficiently large and diverse external validation datasets to confirm generalizability of model performance is strongly recommended (although often challenging to identify), preferably from unique practice regions [25].

Clinical Integration and Support is often the least discussed, yet most critical stage of AI implementation in healthcare. Typically necessitating support from institutional innovation teams and/or commercial vendor partners, this requires careful and strategic management of issues related to regulatory compliance, clinical data access and migration, user interface design, clinical workflow, change management, and technical support. Of these, regulatory compliance for AI/ML-based healthcare products is rapidly evolving and requires ongoing surveillance. In January 2021, the FDA announced its AI/ML-based software as a Medical Device (SaMD) Action Plan [26]. This outlined a plan towards a tailored regulatory framework for AI/ML SaMD that encourages a patient-centered approach for incorporation of AI in healthcare. This will aim to promote transparency surrounding algorithm use as well as efforts to reduce bias. Finally, the need to document real-world performance and monitor this across unique environments was acknowledged. These elements should therefore be considered early during the planning and development of clinical tools designed to deploy AL/ML-based models in practice. Specific challenges related to the construction and maintenance of these systems will be discussed in more detail (Fig. 17.1).

17.2 Data Capture and Management

"You can have data without information, but you cannot have information without data". In this quote by author and programmer Daniel Keys Moran, we are reminded that not all data provides us value; however data is foundational to both knowledge and wisdom. In this light, prediction models are only as good as the data made available to them during training. ML algorithms cannot learn patterns associated with an outcome if the data provided has little relevance to that outcome, is too noisy, or is provided in too small a quantity to adequately learn these patterns.

The majority of tools embedded across hospital environments were designed to support the administration of healthcare, not gather insights relevant for personalized care delivery. This remains evident by the way data elements are both captured and organized by institutional EHR platforms, frequently nuanced by institutional- and site-dependent adaptations that make data normalization uniquely challenging. User interactions with these systems are often inconsistent and biased by clinician preference, commonly resulting in high rates of missing data. Diagnostic test data faces a unique host of challenges in both raw (source) and aggregate (reported) form: raw data commonly biased by manufacturer or acquisition preferences while reported data frequently plagued by poor standardization and text-based descriptions. Finally, access to multiple data repositories is notoriously challenging and requires careful consideration of data permissions (i.e. informed patient consent), particularly for model development [27]. Overall, this generates unique and valid concerns regarding both the development and institutional deployment of AI models using multi-domain patient health data. We will discuss these challenges and describe validated approaches to their management.

17.2.1 Data Availability

Healthcare organizations generate large amounts of data relevant to individual patient health and the understanding of health trajectories. The primary consumers of this data are healthcare professionals (e.g. physicians, nurses, allied health professionals), healthcare administrators (of clinics or hospitals), and financing institutions supporting the other two (e.g. payers). However, secondary use of this data for the monitoring and improvement of healthcare delivery is also sought by societal organizations (e.g. American Heart Association, American College of Cardiology). Supporting this network requires a multi-dimensional system which stores and manages a wide variety of data, including patient reported health measures (PHRMs), clinical notes, medical investigation results (including diagnostic imaging and laboratory results), and hospital administrative data. As most medical record systems have become digitized, they are collectively known as electronic health records (EHRs). While a critical repository for aggregate data generated throughout a patient's journey, it is important to recognize that the EHR does not store source data of diagnostic tests, rather only summary interpretations of these tests. Source data is often retained, however is spread across an assemblance of vendor-neutral archival systems (e.g. Picture Archiving and Communication System (PACS), and vendor-specific software platforms: the latter often in the hundreds across any given institution. With rapidly expanding interest surrounding the use of source data to develop deep-learning prediction algorithms, as well as desire to contextualize these models through EHR data, unique challenges surrounding data availability are becoming apparent.

There are several key data domains relevant to personalized healthcare delivery. Patient reported outcome measures (PROMs) are patient-derived estimates of current health status and provide unique contextual information regarding their symptoms, habits (i.e. smoking and alcohol consumption) and overall quality of life [28]. While falsely assumed to be routinely captured by clinical interactions, these features require dedicated and standardized tools in order to consistently deliver these variables for risk prediction modelling. EHR data, the second key domain, is often confused with administrative health data. The latter is a coded summary of care performed that is used for tracking healthcare resource use: the former is clinical documentation of that care. While both are used for prediction modelling, administrative data is considered more appropriate for population-level predictions, while EHR data is more appropriate for patient-level predictions. While EHR systems continue to strive towards data standardization surrounding care documentation, this is acknowledged with their primary mandate to support administrative operations. Therefore, while the occurrence and results of a laboratory test may be readily available, the nuances of patient health status and care decisions surrounding these results may not be apparent. Finally, diagnostic source data is now considered an invaluable data domain for the delivery of personalized care. Beyond the summary report of tests (often text-based) that are delivered to the EHR, source image or waveform data can be leveraged to deliver deeper insights into disease phenotype. For example, deep learning algorithms have now been used to predict if a patient currently in a normal heart rhythm is experiencing atrial fibrillation, a common cause of stroke, from a 12-lead ECG source data [29]. These resources are commonly available but are stored to disparate servers across institutions. Data may be stored in proprietary formats and often without pre-established mechanisms for batch de-identification or migration. Overall, PROMs, EHR and Diagnostic source data each represent invaluable data assets for the delivery of personalized healthcare. With this, bespoke and targeted efforts must be undertaken by institutions to ensure their consistent capture, migration and accessibility.

The Proposed Approach The CIROC Registry was launched in January 2015 with pre-defined goals of accessing three discrete health data domains: (1) Patient reported health measures (PRHMs), (2) Electronic Health Information (EHI) from the institutional EHR (aggregate clinical records, discharge summaries, procedural and diagnostic test reports, laboratory results and medication lists) and Provincial administrative databases (Discharge Abstract Database (DADs), National Ambulatory Care Registry System (NACRS), Physician Claims database, and Vital Statistics Alberta), and iii) Diagnostic testing data. While subsequently expanded to include cardiac CT, cardiac catheterization, 12-lead ECG and Holter data, our foundational platform was focused on capturing diagnostic data from cardiac MRI to establish accurate and comprehensive descriptions of disease phenotype. To date, this Registry has successfully captured matched data resources for >15,000 unique encounters. Automated retrieval and matching of all three data domains were achieved through tailored solutions, as shown in Fig. 17.2. PRHMs were captured through the custom development of a tablet-based application to engage patients at time of arrival for diagnostic testing. This served two purposes: (1) automated consent deployment for the abstraction of

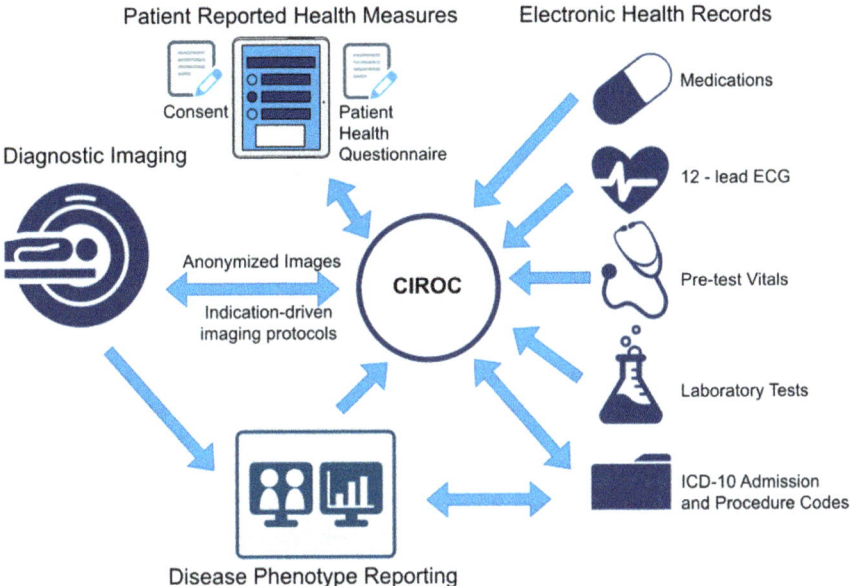

Fig. 17.2 Schematic overview of the data collection processes within CIROC. Data is collected from patient reported health measures, diagnostic images and reports, and the electronic health records

multi-domain data for risk prediction modelling, and (2) deployment of a standardized patient health questionnaire. Data abstraction from the EHR and administrative databases were achieved through custom scripts developed in partnership with the health institution's data warehouse team. A processing script was constructed for iterative data extraction from 10 institutional data repositories, a process that is updated for each patient every 3-months to capture changes in health status. Finally, diagnostic test data was collected through the development of data migration and custom reporting tools. Relevant to data availability, this ensured consistent imaging protocols were performed by technologists, raw image data was routinely transferred to a dedicated DICOM node for de-identification and labelling, and all clinical tests were interpreted using standardized reporting templates and both tabular and text data migrated for de-identification and matching.

17.2.2 Data Quality

While data volume is revered across technology industries, greater emphasis on data quality is required in healthcare settings. While inherently justified by desires to inform important, health-impacting decisions, data quality also influences model design to maximize generalizability across unique healthcare environments. Despite broader use of EHRs and digital archival systems, substantial variability remains surrounding the practice of medicine that supplies their data. Differences exist in how individual users code patient interactions through to how institutions instruct and document care. A recent systematic review identified that ML model performance for the prediction of hospital readmission was only modestly improved through the use of EHR data versus administrative data (used for tracking diagnoses and procedures), on average increasing c-statistic by only 0.03–0.04 [30]. Commonly, ML-based risk models from EHR data only marginally outperform well-executed Cox-based models [31, 32]. These observations highlight the need to pursue data resources that are tailored to address clinical questions and recognize may not be provided from the EHR.

In this context, source diagnostic data provides unique value through expanded complexity and relevance to disease phenotype. However, unique challenges exist surrounding the quality of this data for consideration by ML models. Aggregate data in the form of diagnostic test reports must be assessed for standardization of clinical interpretations. Despite advancements in natural language processing (NLP) and its application to healthcare [33, 34], dictated or free-text reports remain inferior to discreetly coded data elements provided through structured standardized reporting architectures. The quality of quantitative data elements must be considered for all manually executed measures, and consistency in use of automated processing tools known. Finally, source data quality can vary substantially and be strongly influenced by patient characteristics (e.g. poorer quality among sicker patients), hardware manufacturer, and software versions. While often beyond the control of data science teams, partnered efforts in clinical environments must be undertaken to systematically assess, standardize and optimize the quality of data planned for use in ML models. These provide expanded responsibility for institutions and clinical services to cultivate data resources well suited to the delivery of personalized medicine, rather than simply harvesting readily available resources.

The Proposed Approach In the CIROC Registry we aimed to maximally influence, and craft data resources tailored to execute our planned risk models. We recognized two data domains where this could be achieved: (1) PRHMs and (2) Diagnostic test performance and interpretation. PRHMs are deployed for all subjects at time of arrival with mandatory response fields to avoid missing data. To maximize quality of diagnostic tests we introduced tools aimed at (1) standardizing imaging protocols that were displayed to technologists based on their coded reasons for referral, (2) reporting disease features using a standardized interface that provided natural language generation for reports, and (3) coding image quality at time of image interpretation. All physicians were trained in standard operational procedures (SOPs) for test measurements at the beginning of the Registry enrollment period. Through this process contextual patient health information and disease phenotypic data were routinely captured, standardized, and consistently coded. Efforts were concurrently made to standardize manufacturer settings of imaging hardware between hospitals and compare image quality and measurements in a set of 100 healthy control subjects, serving as reference values. EHR data abstraction scripts were then confirmed for accuracy using manual review of medical records for diagnostic, procedural and medication related variables.

17.2.3 Data Generalizability

Data generalizability is the measure of how transferable and standardized a dataset is. In the context of our current discussions, it is a measure of how easily a trained model could be deployed at another institution, and how similar its performance would be in that setting. This concept is related to the idea of model generalizability, which will be discussed later. For example, most patient demographic data is highly generalizable, with a patient's age and sex being stored in years and male/female, respectively. Almost every healthcare institution could therefore receive this data and directly compare, integrate, and combine it with their own. Highly specific data elements can also be generalizable. We can use the example of left ventricular ejection fraction (LVEF) from a very specific test: cardiac magnetic resonance imaging (CMR). LVEF is a measurement of the percentage of total blood volume pumped out of the left ventricle in a single beat, and is a valuable assessment of cardiac health. How this value is calculated is not highly standardized by the Society for Cardiac Magnetic Resonance (SCMR) [35]. By providing widely-accepted guidelines or standard operating procedures (SoPs) that dictate how to derive this variable, we obtain a standardized data definition that can accompany this variable, improving its generalizability to unique clinical settings. In contrast, other variables encountered in clinical practice may be loosely defined or strongly influenced by local practice bias. For example, "reason for referral" in diagnostic testing is highly unstandardized. An identical patient could be referred as "Known cardiac sarcoidosis, evaluate for inflammation and fibrosis" or simply "Assess function". This text field is therefore not well generalizable and of lower value for modelling.

Medicine has developed data standardization protocols or ontologies in an effort to standardize the administration of healthcare. These efforts have greatly improved the generalizability of administrative health data while increasingly offering layered or hierarchical data structures. The reporting of disease classification and procedural events are structured using the International Classification of Diseases (ICD) coding system [34]. This is a standardized set of codes that are used to classify patients based on known disease states and track relevant procedures. With this standardized information, healthcare institutions can compare patient populations and contextualize clinical outcomes using a standardized ontology. While ICD codes are highly consistent, they are still subject to differences in institutional practice. The standard practice is coding by chart reviews, manually identifying appropriate ICD codes from EHR-based documentations, such as admission and discharge summaries. Therefore, different institutes and different coders may have their own operating procedures, leading to some variations in which codes are applied and how often they are applied. Ontologies have also been developed for diagnostic test data, the most commonly engaged system being Systematic Nomenclature of Medicine—Clinical Terms (SNOMED-CT) [36]. Despite value for improving the quality of administrative health data, comprehensive standardization of individual patient health records remains poorly achieved between health providers.

The lack of data generalizability and interoperability between health providers [37, 38] has catalyzed unique approaches to improve this landscape. Fast Healthcare Interoperability Resources (FHIR) is a standard for describing how medical data should be stored and contains an application programming interface (API) for exchanging and accessing medical data [37]. Created by Health Level Seven International (HL7) with the goal to facilitate interoperation between legacy healthcare systems, FIHR provides an alternative to document-centric approaches by directly exposing discrete data elements as services. It allows for basic elements of a patient's EHR (including history, hospital admissions, diagnostic reports, and medications) to be accessed and manipulated independently, creating a structured and usable data resource. Therefore, although legacy data silos may be poorly structured for the adoption of ML and AI, new standards are being created to help develop a data rich environment, one that is highly generalizable and an ideal area for AI development.

The Proposed Approach In our setting CIROC routinely captures 90 PROM variables, 500 EHR variables, 250 cardiac imaging variables in addition to raw source diagnostic test data (cardiac images and ECGs). While our local team appreciates access to these resources, we recognized need to evaluate the capacity of other centers to reproduce our work and gain value from developed risk models. While risk models are provided a wide spectrum of variables upon which to identify those of greatest importance to model performance, we then maximize generalizability by generating a parsimonious version of the optimal model. This is achieved by developing a restricted model exposed only to the top variables that have been identified to be clearly defined through an international standard, and are consistently available in routine clinical practice. This practice ensures that our developed ML-models are not only robust in performance, but of clinical value in real-world clinical settings.

17.2.4 Missing Data

Despite expanding emphasis on data quality, healthcare information systems are notorious for missing data given high variability in clinical practice, variable adherence to standardized care pathways, and lack of user input consistency. In prior studies assessing EHR systems, the reported missing data rates have ranged from 20 to 80% [39]. Many foundational issues underlie the challenge of missing data, but time and cost constraints, reporting errors, and lack of appropriate data management tools are contributory. Laboratory testing measures are commonly missing across clinical practice cohorts due to variability in surveillance intervals, these commonly influenced by illness severity. In data collected from the intensive care units at three separate hospitals for the prediction of sepsis (PhysioNet 2019 Challenge), they found patient demographics (age and sex) and vital signs (blood pressure, O^2 saturation) were highly complete, averaging around 95% complete, compared to laboratory values averaging between 1 and 25% complete [40]. One of the main reasons for the discrepancies is that demographics and vital signs are consistently reported and acquired at admission. Laboratory results are instead mainly done as required by the clinical severity of disease. This can create issues where certain patients have multiple measurements of the same test over the same time period in which another patient only has a single test. How to standardize these time-series results becomes an important question for the EHRs and ML modelling. For patient care, excessive laboratory tests are unnecessary and just incur a greater cost for no benefit, indicating that missing data is not always a bad sign. It highlights the need for better standardization and normalization of clinical data when it is being considered for ML based solutions, specifically for data that is measured irregularly and variably between patients.

Missing data poses a challenge for machine learning based algorithms. The majority of algorithms cannot accommodate missing data in the training set, requiring that data be pre-processed and missing data needs to be corrected before a model can be trained. Common approaches include: reanalyzing and collecting missing data, removing patients with missing data, or imputing the missing data. Typically in healthcare one cannot go back and get a measurement from the patient (especially in retrospective studies) and many patients have missing data, so removing all patients with missing data greatly reduces the size of your dataset, limiting the information available to the model and its generalizability. Therefore imputation is the most common method, which is simply using an algorithm to estimate the missing values.

There are a wide variety of imputation techniques that have been developed to estimate missing data. The simplest and most common are column-based approaches, which use summary statistics including the mean and median values to fill in missing data. This method does not take into consideration other features within the dataset that might be able to contribute to a more accurate estimation of the missing values. More complex imputation methods (including k-nearest neighbour (KNN) imputation [41], multivariate imputation via chained equations (MICE) [42], and multiple imputation using additive regression [43]) all use different techniques to incorporate each patient's stored data to estimate the missing variables, leading to a much better approximation than column-based summary statistics. For a more in depth summary into common multiple imputation methods refer to Li et al. [44].

While imputation has provided a method for dealing with missing data in healthcare, it is important to understand the assumptions being made when imputing as it can have considerable effects on the developed models performance and generalizability. Data can be missing for three reasons: (1) missing at completely random (MCAR), indicating that whether a data point is missing is completely unrelated to observed and unobserved data; (2) missing at random (MAR), indicating whether a missing data point can be explained by the observed data; or (3) missing not at random (MNAR), meaning that missingness is dependent on the unobserved values.

Because a user cannot usually determine the actual reason for missingness, imputation assumes the data is MAR, specifically that the observed values can explain the missing values. This introduces inherent bias into the imputed data based on the observed data. When in healthcare, many of the reasons for missing data MNAR, as hospital policy and clinical decision making, all might play a role in why a certain variable was not captured. Although it has been argued that removing all patients with missing data is therefore the safer approach, it is actually making a stricter assumption; that any data point missing is missing completely at random. To limit this bias, imputation is only performed if the level of missing data is below a certain threshold. This threshold then determines which variables can be imputed, and which need to be removed from your data, before modelling can proceed. The selection of this threshold is arbitrary and generally determined model to model based on the domain knowledge of the missing variable, and the potential reasons for why it is missing. In practice, the goal should always be to collect as high quality, and highly generalizable data as possible. Once you have the highest quality data, one can decide how to approach missing data, while identifying the assumptions and biases introduced by each method.

The Proposed Approach We routinely evaluate missing data rates of all collated data resources (PROM, EHR, and diagnostic test data). Variables with high missing rates are flagged and attempts made to identify underlying reasons behind missing values, working with our clinical collaborators and institutional data warehouse managers to determine if data quality can be improved. To address missing time-series variables (e.g. standard laboratory test values) data definitions are first considered to assess if alternate variable criteria may be sufficient for a given model, such as time from target date (e.g. expanding variable eligibility from within 1-month to within 3-months of a patient visit). Target variable completion rates are dependent on perceived capacity for imputation modelling to address missingness. In general, we routinely consider imputation for variables with missingness rates below 15%. Above this threshold careful consideration of value towards the model, reasons for observed missingness, and capacity to correct missingness in clinical practice (e.g. real-world deployment) is considered. Imputation is performed on a model-to-model basis, evaluating the pros and cons of each method in context of the clinical question and the type of missing data. This practice ensures that each model has been carefully considered along with potential biases introduced by imputation, as well as allowing us to optimize both the threshold and method. Overall, we strive to solve the data missingness problem, by collecting as high quality data as possible, and then following practices that are transparent and lead to high generalizability.

17.2.5 Data Permission and Privacy

As AI becomes more prevalent in healthcare, there are growing concerns about patient health data privacy. As our previous sections highlighted, a major determinant of growth in this field will be the ability of health data to be accessed, shared, and combined across both institutional systems and between institutions. How this data is handled is critically important due to the regulation and laws surrounding patient privacy. Data privacy protection is regulated by law with: the Health Insurance Portability and Accountability Act (HIPAA) in the US, the Personal Information Protection and Electronic Documents Act (PIPEDA) in Canada, and the General Data Protection Regulation (GDPR) in the EU. Each of these Acts while slightly different, all set standards for data security, data usage, and an individual's right to their data. The most recent of these, the GDPR, is specifically aimed at protecting the fundamental rights of individuals and emphasizes accountability and transparency in patient data.

Before AI can provide meaningful change in the healthcare sector, we must address regulatory requirements surrounding data security and privacy. In terms of security we can define 3 distinct levels of secure data: (1) anonymous data, in which technical safeguards have been used to completely remove the risk of re-identification, (2) de-identified data, in which direct and indirect identifiers have been removed but the underlying data structure could facilitate re-identification through access to other databases, (3) pseudonymous data, in which identifiers have been replaced with artificial identifiers linked to protected health information (PHI) using a separately held decoder. Only anonymous data is exempt from HIPAA/PIPEDA/GDPR security requirements, but is limited by the type of modelling that can be performed. It is only appropriate only for isolated tasks, which do not involve any validation cohorts, and cannot be iteratively developed by following patients over time. This limits the ability for prospective studies, as previous data cannot be linked to the follow-up data, not allowing for the following patient outcomes. ML is built on principles of iterative modelling, and removing the ability to retrain models once further information has been gained will greatly limit the potential of AI based tools, which can learn in real time. The concept of iterative model development and deployment is one of the biggest reasons ML based models are predicted to create a paradigm shift in healthcare [1]. This is where pseudonymous data comes in, as it is stored without protected health information, but can be re-linked to a patient, and updated iteratively using the decoder. This allows for data to be stored securely, without PHI when developing the model, but the data repository can be continually updated by linking the patient when new data and outcomes have been acquired.

In the context of regional regulations, AI based tools must consider methods that allow for transparency in how patient data is being used. One of the primary aims of the GDPR was to increase the transparency on personal data usage and increase the EU citizens control in regards to how their data is used. This has serious implications for personalized medicine. These regulations stipulate that patients must have provided their informed consent for any secondary use of health data. Patients under the GDPR also have the right to: have their data removed at any time, review and make valid corrections to their health data, know why and how their data is being used, and access their data. Many of these are currently impossible in a traditional ML setup, and will have a significant impact on how data needs to be collected, stored, and used for precision medicine. ML risk prediction models use a patient's data to learn the underlying patterns that result in clinical outcomes and once the model is trained, it is not simple to identify how the patient's data was specifically used, let alone remove a patient's data on request. To remove a patient's data the only approach would be to completely retrain and redeploy the entire model, which would have a serious impact on already developed and deployed ML models. Both patient privacy and security need to be considered at the very beginning of AI development, ensuring proper management strategies are employed to ensure the development of sustainable tools that can improve clinical decision making and patient care.

The Proposed Approach Construction of the CIROC registry was an exercise in "precision healthcare by design". By recognizing that AI based solutions require a-priori and purposeful collection of high-quality data, and that patients should be given transparent control over use of this data for model development, our framework was engineered to adhere to evolving regulatory requirements. This is visualized in Fig. 17.2. Upon arrival for diagnostic testing each patient is provided a tablet-based application that informs the patient of our institution's desire to use their health data for risk prediction modelling and obtains informed electronic consent for this purpose (electronic copy sent to patient through secure institutional email). This consent permits access to the patient's EHR and source diagnostic testing data for 10 years prior to, and 10-years following date of consent. Once consented, identified patient health data is extracted from relevant institutional data repositories and transferred to a central secure server housed within the healthcare institution. Following data matching, all data resources are de-identified using a common, patient-specific unique identifier and stored to a "pseudonymized data server" accessible to the research team. This common unique identifier is provided within a decoder accessible to the identified data server for iterative updating of future encounters and patient health information. This architecture delivers an iteratively updated, multi-domain data warehouse for initiative-consented patients with strict adherence to regional privacy and security regulations.

In this section we highlighted dominant challenges surrounding healthcare data and its management in the context of personalized medicine. We emphasized that, while the healthcare industry collects a large amount of data, significant efforts must be undertaken to understand its quality, availability and appropriate handling.

17.3 Model Development and Validation

As outlined in the previous section, many proof-of-concept ML models for personalized healthcare are emerging, demonstrating very promising results. From assisting in diagnostic tasks (automatic classification of skin lesions [45] and detection of cardiac arrhythmias [46]) to predicting relevant health outcomes (30-day hospital readmission [47] and in-hospital moratlity [48]), we can anticipate expanding focus on the adoption of AI in healthcare [1]. In this section we will provide a brief overview of how a model is developed and validated, while highlighting current limitations of these practices specific to the healthcare industry. Note that, while model selection is a very important aspect of the ML process, we do not highlight it in this chapter. In ML it is common to train a variety of models, and compare their performance, selecting the best model in terms of performance and how it can be used clinically. We instead focus on the challenges of model development and how selecting the best model can be challenging in the healthcare domain.

17.3.1 Model Development

Very briefly, ML modelling follows several standard procedures: (1) collect and clean data, (2) train model using iterative learning algorithms, (3) internally validate model, and (4) evaluate model performance on an external dataset. Throughout this section we will describe each step in detail, highlighting the challenges associated with each step. Most of the methodologies we indicate here directly relate to classification tasks commonly seen in diagnostically-focused tools (models designed to diagnose disease), or to risk prediction models that group patients according to varying levels of risk (low, moderate, high). In-depth discussion of types of ML models, and their specific use cases within healthcare is outside of the scope of this chapter (see Bohr and Memarzadeh [49] for an in-depth review). Rather, we aim to introduce basic principles of ML modelling and their associated challenges in healthcare applications.

Collected data typically needs to be cleaned, imputed, and generally reduced in dimensionality via feature selection or expert domain knowledge before it can be used for modelling. While summated in a single sentence, this is the most time consuming process of developing ML-based tools for healthcare applications due to the many challenges highlighted in Sect. 17.2. Once an adequate dataset has been prepared, model development can begin. Internal (locally available) data is commonly split into a training set and validation set. The validation set can be held separate to the training data or can be split from the same data using k-fold cross validation (see Fig. 17.3). The training set is used to train a selected machine learning model while the validation data is used to evaluate its performance. Using classification as an example, this model can be a function that predicts if a patient has a given disease or not. We use the training set to optimize this prediction function through a process called "learning", this consisting of providing training examples to the model which then predicts if they have the disease or not. We then score the model's performance by comparing each prediction to the labelled (ground truth) data. An optimization function then adjusted parameters of the model in an effort to improve performance on the training data. This process is repeated iteratively, providing updates to the prediction model until a performance threshold is met, or once the model is no longer improving. In this example, we want the model to learn general patterns in our training data that associated a set of patient features to presence of disease. We can then apply the trained model to the validation data set, this coming

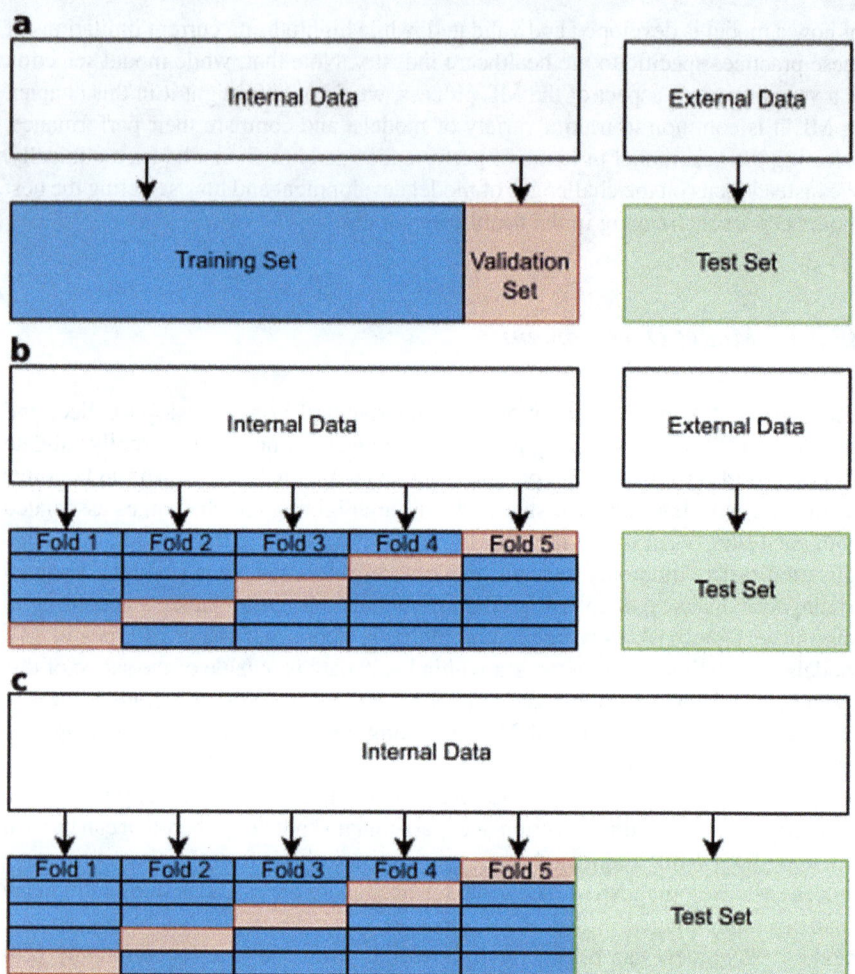

Fig. 17.3 Common methodologies for training, validating, and testing machine learning models. Blue backgrounds indicate training data, red backgrounds indicate validation data, and green backgrounds indicate testing data. **a** Holdout validation, a single split within the internal data where models are validated on a single dataset, and then evaluated for generalizability on external data. **b** Fivefold Cross validation. The internal data is split into 5 folds, with each fold being the validation cohort, for training on the other 4 folds. Models are internally validated on their average performance over the 5 folds, with the best model being tested for generalizability on the external data. **c** Internal Validation. When no external data is available, the internal data can be split in training data (typically validated using fivefold cross validation) and then an optimistic measure of generalizability can be tested on the held out internal test set

from the same patient population but not provided to the model during training. The model's hyperparameters (parameters used within the algorithm to control the learning process, and not the parameters learned during training) can then be adjusted based on the performance of the model on the validation set and the process repeated until optimal performance is achieved. Once a model has been fully optimized it should be exposed to an external test data set. The performance of the model on this external data provides an actual measure of real-world performance that can be expected from the trained model, and can be seen as an estimate of its clinical applicability. However, as previously mentioned, it can be challenging to acquire such external datasets. Therefore, a common approach is to create a separate holdout set from the initial data, there-by establishing separate training, validation, and test datasets from a single Centre's data resources. This approach must be accompanied by acknowledgement that a true estimate of the model's generalizability in real world clinical practice has not been established. Lack of this external validation is anticipated to present barriers to regulatory approval for widespread clinical adoption.

In situations where only small datasets are available, studies may forgo a holdout test set and use internal validation as an estimate of model performance. This is typically done by averaging performance over the k-folds performed during cross validation. The performance estimated from internal holdouts is generally biased and is thought of as an optimistic measure of the model's performance. A recent systematic review of studies focused on AI based diagnostic image analysis, highlighted that only 6% of the 516 studies performed appropriate external validation [50]. Indeed, until data sharing agreements become more common in healthcare, it will be very challenging for a model's true value to be elucidated across institutions due to limited ability to perform external validation. This is a serious concern for how well models can be optimized and become clinically relevant given that internally validated models struggle to generalize to external test data [51]. Figure 17.4 shows a flow chart of the model development process.

The Proposed Approach ML modelling is complex, and the exact process used for each study relies on the amount and type of data available, the clinical context of the proposed model, and early achieved model performance. Each model being sought from the CIROC registry follows key development steps as summarized above (Fig. 17.4). Once a clinical question has been presented, definitions surrounding

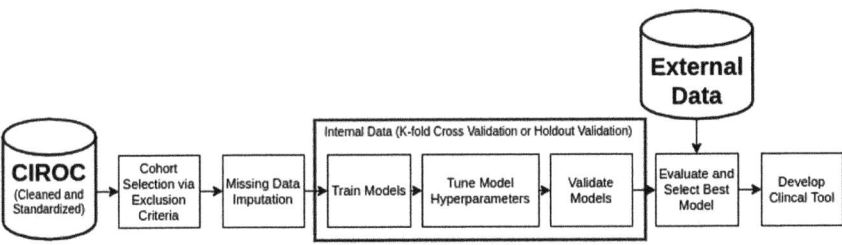

Fig. 17.4 Flow-chart depicting the standard model development process within the CIROC registry

desired outcomes are established followed by careful consideration of patient cohorts to be included or excluded. Key opinion leaders are sought to establish if bespoke data resources should be considered beyond our core (standard) data model, such as raw diagnostic source data. The availability, quality and format of each data element is then catalogued and a data cleaning plan developed. Once a final dataset is curated, decisions regarding the number and structure of models required to achieve the desired outcome are wire-framed with consideration of alternate approaches. Consideration is typically given to ensemble-based approaches. Decisions regarding appropriate model architecture and splitting are driven by review of available data resources. Modelling is engaged with iterative consideration of impact of techniques on model generalizability and explainability. Upon optimal model completion an attempt is always made to develop a parsimonious model highly achievable across unique clinical settings, and to evaluate performance using an external dataset.

17.3.2 *Model Performance Metrics May not Reflect Clinical Applicability*

Selecting ML models most valuable for clinical practice is challenging. The most commonly used metrics to evaluate a model's performance are accuracy and area under the receiver operator characteristic curve (AUC). Although widely used, these metrics can be problematic when assessing performance in certain healthcare settings [52]. Healthcare data is typically imbalanced (diseases and clinical outcomes are rare), which can affect how well a model learns. If a model is developed to maximize classification accuracy for a rare event, it may appear to perform well when predicting that most patients will be event free. This will provide a high accuracy score since the large majority of patients are event free. Instead standard healthcare models typically report a model's sensitivity (the ability of the model to correctly identify those with the disease, equivalent to true positive rate) and specificity (ability to correctly identify those without the disease) as they more accurately describe how well a model performs for patients in both the groups. Whether a model should retain better specificity versus sensitivity is dependent upon the clinical scenario and its intended clinical application. The receiver operating characteristic curve (ROC), which is a plot of sensitivity versus false positive rate (1-specificity), can be used to help evaluate overall performance of models as it allows a graphical representation of the trade-off between sensitivity and specificity. This allows for decision thresholds to be created for models that involve selecting patient treatment options, permitting for a level of certainty in the clinical decision-making process. AUC is by far the most commonly reported metric in ML for healthcare-based models, as it provides a simple numeric rating of diagnostic test accuracy, and is non-parametric (unaffected by abnormal distributions) within the population.

While commonly used, AUC is not intuitive to clinicians, patients, or health care providers. For example, what does an AUC of 0.8 mean when trying to apply a prediction to an individual patient's care? Previous studies have shown that diagnostic tests are best understood in terms of gains and losses to individual patients [53], and that screening tests are looking for concrete numbers that show the efficacy of screening strategies (e.g.. Number needed to screen: the number of patients that need to be screened for a given duration to prevent one death or one adverse event) [54]. AUC provides a summary across all decision thresholds, even some which may be clinically irrelevant, and therefore even two models with an identical AUC may have different performance in clinically relevant situations. This means that selection by AUC may not always choose the most relevant model [52]. The AUC also treats specificity and sensitivity as equally important, which is not always the case in healthcare. For example, poor sensitivity on a cancer diagnosis model could lead to a missed cancer diagnosis, delayed treatment, and death; whereas poor specificity just means an unnecessary further test, but no harm to the patient. AUC also has known issues with extrapolation (where very few data points can create an AUC where a majority of this area is from a region of the ROC that contains no clinical data) and that it does not account for disease prevalence within the patient population [52].

Healthcare desires performance metrics that are easy to comprehend and express while incorporating costs attributed to misclassification and accounting for disease prevalence. Currently, machine learning is dominated by AUC to determine best models, without considering the contextual and clinical uses of these models. Therefore one of the biggest challenges facing the adoption of ML models in personalized medicine is bridging the gap between ML specialists and clinicians, and understanding both should be involved in the process of model development and evaluation.

The Proposed Approach Using the CIROC registry, our goal is the creation of models and tools that have real-world clinical value. To this end, we have expanded the common metrics reported in our centre to include ones with clinical interpretability. With a focus on providing models that are highly predictive, but remain interpretable, transparent, and can aid in clinical decision making. We provide a variety of metrics including: Net Reclassification Index and Net Benefit metrics (methods that accounts for the different consequences of correct and incorrect diagnosis) [52, 55] as well as patient-oriented summary measures (which reflect the benefit of performing a diagnostic test based on knowledge of disease prevalence) in order to provide a clinically relevant summary of our developed ML models. These include the metrics: Number needed to predict, and Number needed to diagnose (estimating the efficacy of our developed models compared to traditional approaches) [56, 57]. Overall CIROC was designed to allow for the inclusion of clinicians an in the development process of our models, to ensure that we our data resources are being used to create models that can answer specific clinical questions. Our goal is the creation of tools that improve patient outcomes by aiding in the clinical decision making process, not just models that have a high AUC score.

17.3.3 Model Generalizability and Explainability

A majority of AI based approaches currently being explored for healthcare delivery will face challenges when migrated towards clinical implementation. The reason for this is that, while individual studies have shown strong model performance and are beginning to report more clinically relevant performance metrics [58], many are still trained using only single center data [50]. This can create key "blind spots" in the model where it can make incorrect decisions due to lack of generalizability. Since many complex ML based models do not provide transparent explanation for the decisions they make, these erroneous errors can lead to a lack of trust in the model. If physicians do not trust a model, or cannot understand the reasoning behind a model's decision, it will be challenging to adopt in clinical practice [59].

Model generalizability is a measure of how well a model performs on unseen data. This can be quite hard to predict, and to get a good estimate of real-world performance, high quality data from other institutes is required as an external validation dataset. Even with high quality data, the inherent differences in the data can affect how well a model generalizes, as site-specific practices and technological differences (including software, acquisition methods, and timing of data capture) can lead to very different measurements of the same data [60]. Different centres and geographical regions may also have significantly different patient populations, with differences in disease prevalence, rate of common comorbidities, and patient outcomes. Therefore it is important to develop methodologies and standards for implementing models into clinical care that will be as transferable as possible. Many specific features may capture the underlying pattern of disease, but if these features are not commonly reported by other sites, a developed model will not have widespread clinical applicability. Even with models designed for clinical reproducibility, it might be necessary to perform local retraining of a developed model. If a ML model is to be deployed prospectively, a centre could use the historic data, to retrain the developed algorithm. This would allow the model to capture inherent site-specific patterns within the data which will be more appropriate for the new population. For simpler modelling tasks, it has been shown that the generalization issue can be overcome by using large heterogeneous training data curated from multiple centres [25].

Model explainability goes hand in hand with model generalizability. If tools are provided that help users understand the decision making process, it can be easier to interpret where and why the model may be making an error. Most ML models do not provide inherent explainability [61], unlike the current gold standards in healthcare. In survival analysis (predicting the time to event) the Cox Proportional Hazard Model (CPH) is the most commonly used risk prediction model due to its interpretability. Each feature in the developed model is provided a regression coefficient, which can be directly assessed as the estimated hazard (increase in risk) a patient would experience given a unit change for a given feature. Therefore it is easy to understand both for patients and clinicians, and clear in how it is deciding which patients are at high risk. Because of the clear interpretability it is still the most commonly used model, even though machine learning based random survival methods (including random survival forests and survival based neural networks) are showing improved predictive performance [62, 63]. ML has developed methods in which to help explain the decisions made by complex models, but they currently fall below the inherent explainability of many statistical models. The two common approaches to model explainability in ML are variable importance (VIMP) [64] and Shapely Additive Explanations (SHAP) [65]. VIMP entails replacing a feature with a randomly generated feature, and calculating the change in performance. Whichever feature when replaced causes the biggest performance loss is the most important feature. Although useful in feature selection and identifying possible new predictor variables, it does not provide a direct estimate of hazard and does not provide patient specific estimates. SHAP is a more recent approach, which uses game theory to provide a better picture of what features are important for each patient, in each outcome. It was first proposed in 2017, and is a novel approach at feature importance, giving an importance value for each feature for each prediction. Unlike hazard estimates, and VIMP, SHAP is a patient specific technique, which provides variable importance for each patient allowing clinicians and patients transparency on the decision making process. Although a promising technique, it has yet to show clinical impact, but it indicates that the field has recognized the need for more transparency in model decision making, and only through better interpretability tools will ML modelling find its way into clinical practice.

The Proposed Approach Measuring and evaluating model generalizability is a complex task. Sourcing large external datasets is time consuming, expensive and challenged by data privacy regulations. While seeking appropriate external validation datasets, when unavailable we assess model generalizability using an internal holdout test set, recognizing the limitation of this estimate. Further growth of international collaboration and good data practices will be a focal point for CIROC in the future. To help evaluate our models clinical performance, we routinely use VIMP and SHAP to provide model transparency. We commonly report VIMP metrics, and routinely compare them to the gold standard model predictions. By implementing both models on the same dataset, we can identify where the models deviate, and study those patients to try and further understand the model decision making process. Further implementation of SHAP, allows for individual patient assessment, and directly indicates which variables were predictive for individual patients. Further studies are needed to evaluate how SHAP estimates can be used and implemented into clinical practice.

17.3.4 Algorithmic Bias and Equity, Diversity and Inclusion

A growing concern in healthcare is the concept of algorithmic fairness, ensuring that the models we create do not inherit biases that may be present within the training data [66]. Recently ML algorithms have been shown to learn societal biases, with a risk of unintended and unethical results in minority subgroups [67]. For example, a hospital mortality model varied in performance based on the patient's ethnicity due to underlying bias within the training data [68] and a skin lesion classifier algorithm that was trained on predominately fair skinned patients, which underperformed when tested on skin of colour [45]. The main reason for the failure of these models is once again due to a lack of proper training data, as it did not contain enough examples of the minority class. Therefore when introduced into the real world, the models can have unintended consequences. Model bias can appear in a variety of ways but commonly is due to the fact that models are trained via optimization algorithms, which inherently will select features that represent the majority class, as that is the easiest target to improve performance. If the sample of the minority class is small, the model might not even have enough data in order to learn the underlying if a different underlying pattern exists, leading to poor performance in that subgroup, that could be ignored if not detected in model development. Finally, there might be unobserved characteristics of the minority class that link features to the outcome, causing unlearnable noise in the outcome. These all lead to algorithmic unfairness, and need to be carefully monitored for when developing ML based models. To help reduce algorithmic bias, the focus again relies on the quality of data, and understanding the distribution of potential subgroups (age, sex, ethnicity, and socioeconomic class) within the clinical population of interest. If small subgroups do exist within the training or clinical population, sub-analysis should be performed to validate the models performance on each subgroup to ensure that developed tools are fair and not learning unwanted biases from the data.

There is also growing evidence that algorithmic bias can be introduced to AI models due to a lack of attention to equity, diversity, and inclusion (EDI) within the development team [69]. Some consider algorithmic unfairness as a failure of model development, due to not enough consideration, on the use cases of the model being developed. Although efforts have begun, to create tools and methods that can evaluate fairness in AI models [70], the model itself cannot learn the nuances of the social context into which it will be deployed. Algorithmic fairness becomes a serious issue, when potential AI tools are fully automated to make medical decisions. Who decides what level of algorithmic bias is acceptable for implementation into clinical practice and should these decisions be made without an expert who understands the society context? Many of these questions have led to the realization that the field of AI does not encompass society's diversity [71], and suggestions that further diversifying the AI community (specifically teams developing AI tools for healthcare), will lead to better models and evaluators that are better equipped to deal with identifying and eliminating potential bias. A team that encompasses diverse ages, genders, races, geographies, classes, and physical disabilities will have a better perspective on areas where these biases can be introduced, and more be likely able to engage these communities to help influence change in the data collection process. As ML and AI are further integrated in the healthcare delivery, there will need to be close monitoring of how developed tools are implemented in the workplace, and how machines and humans can work best together, while trying to limit potential bias.

The Proposed Approach We chose to carefully consider sex, age, ethnicity, and socio-economic class as critical factors that may affect the generalizability of our developed models. To accomplish this we capture comprehensive patient questionnaires within our PROMs allowing us to contextualize models to each of these patient characteristics. In each model, we can assess the influence of these potential variables to determine if biases or performance variations exist within the developed models. While the population of CIROC is 40% non-Caucasian (6% indigenous), we recognize that some models may be limited by these subgroups, and special considerations need to be taken into account for these models in clinical deployment. In order to further address algorithmic bias, all aspects of team recruitment, development, and support maintain rigorous standards for raising awareness and addressing equality issues in the workplace. In following these EDI recommendations we believe we give ourselves the best chance to catch equality issues during model development, and allow further engagement in potential solutions to underrepresented minorities within CIROC.

17.4 Clinical Integration and Support

So far we have highlighted the more technical reasons (data and model development) on why AI has been slow to gain clinical adoption. In this section we aim to provide an overview of the least discussed stage of AI deployment, but in fact the most challenging. How AI models will be integrated into clinical practice and how they are to be supported throughout their lifecycle will pose significant challenges to current healthcare procedure and regulations. Even with a highly effective algorithm, which has been trained on an optimal data source and passes all the generalizability and bias tests, it still has to get past key human barriers. These new tools will need support from institution and commercial partners, requiring the management of regulatory compliance, clinical data and access, usability, and technical support. With an increased focus on models that can be shown to improve patient care.

17.4.1 Human Barriers

As previously highlighted, a key limitation in many modern ML models is that they do not provide transparency or explainability behind their decision making process. Even if they are based on sound mathematical principles, and outperform a traditional statistical model, the clinician using the software needs to be able to trust and understand the model's results, especially in the healthcare industry, where certain treatments or disease diagnoses can have potentially life altering consequences. Given that healthcare models need to deal with risk of underlying bias, the ability to use inappropriate features, and the extreme consequences, model explainability allows for system verification. If users can catch errors and understand why the error was made, they can better work with industry partners and development teams to improve future models. In terms of performance, it is already becoming common for ML algorithms to be outperforming experts in image analysis [45, 72] and outperform the traditional risk prediction models [62, 63]. Therefore implementing these models would augment the physician's ability to decide on the best treatment or management options for each patient individually. Studies have shown that AI based tools work best when integrated into a clinicians practice, and not designed to replace the clinicians [73]. The reason for the slow adoption can partially be attributed to the barrier between ML and clinical practice, as most ML experts have no experience in clinical workflow, just as many clinicians lack the basics of ML principles. Along with the highlighted need for data accessibility, as many of these models require data that is not commonly available in clinical practice, there also needs to be a shift in the educational aspects of healthcare, where clinicians (the actual users of the developed models) have a basic understanding the principles behind AI and ML. With this background they can more easily understand, readily contribute, and provide feedback during the active development of clinical tools. Allowing them to help push for the changes needed in the technical and logistical aspects of patient care to implement better models.

The Proposed Approach CIROC is an institutional initiative, bringing together administration, clinicians, researchers, and industry partners in order to develop and implement a platform that can improve clinical decision making through the development of better data resources and precision medicine. It's the collaboration of these groups that allow for the model developers to understand the logistical and technical barriers that this tool will face in clinical practice. Our focus is therefore on developing models that can be used to augment the day to day workflow, by providing analysis tools that can save time, or risk models that estimate a patient's risk while clearly providing the logic behind the models decision. These tools will allow clinicians to more effectively make decisions surrounding patient care providing real value in healthcare. To foster collaboration between clinicians, our development team provides monthly learning sessions focused on ML principles and algorithms, and attend weekly case reviews/journal clubs. In this way the users of CIROC can better understand the day to day workflow within the centres that provide the data for CIROC and can build tools that are targeted to specific needs. These sessions also keep clinicians in the know of what cutting edge models are being developed, and what's possible in the field of AI. In this way we address the education and integration gaps that typically can limit AI deployment.

17.4.2 Regulatory Considerations and Demonstrating Patient Value

Another fundamental step in implementing AI into clinical practice relies on the updating of current regulatory practices, as they were not designed with AI in mind, and currently limit the capacity of what tools can be developed and put into clinical practice. These regulations are trending in the right direction with the FDA releasing the AI/ML-based software as a Medical Device (SaMD) Action Plan in January, 2021 [26]. This action plan is focused on making sure that safe and effective AI based technologies reach patients and healthcare providers. It highlights five key areas that are being approached to properly regulate AI, but ensure that it can be applied to clinical care. First, they are developing a tailored regulatory framework for AI/ML based SaMD, which relies on a predetermined change control plan. This framework allows the agency to embrace the iterative nature of ML, while still regulating it to ensure its safety and effectiveness. This is a major step forward in the adoption of AI intelligence in healthcare; the current regulations limited the ability to retrain developed models, which had been previously approved. This brings up concerns over concept drift, which is the idea that your model was trained at a single static time point, but the relationship between features and outcomes might change over time. In healthcare this could be due to a new preventive approach being applied at the institution, or a change in prevalence rates over time. Either of these could lead to model degradation, as the training data is no longer representative of the population it is being applied to. A focus on developing a regulatory framework that allows predetermined changes sets the stage for algorithms that can be periodically retrained optimizing potential benefit. Second, the action plan highlights that there should be a harmonization of standards in what is to be known as the Good Machine Learning Practice (GMLP), which aims to provide consistency to the requirements and expectations of developed SaMD. Ideally this will incorporate better data management and storage criteria, to improve the overall generalizability of healthcare data and models. Third, it is focused on developing patient-centered approaches that incorporate model transparency to both clinicians and patients. The developer will be required to explain to its users how the algorithms function and utilize individual patient's information. Fourth, the plan emphasizes a need for improved methods to evaluate and address algorithmic bias. Finally, developed tools will need to show and maintain real-world performance. Allowing modifications to SaMD devices based on the collection and monitoring of real-world clinical data. This will allow manufacturers to adjust the models based on this data to mitigate risk, while gaining insight into thresholds and performance metrics that are most critical to clinical care. Which is an important change, as many AI algorithms in other domains have shown a tendency to deteriorate over time [74]. Overall this plan highlights many of the challenges previously describe, which indicates that the regulatory framework currently limiting AI's adoption is being replaced with one that will embrace and push for further AI influence.

Another limiting factor is the ability for AI to show that it can provide a real-world value. Researchers are inherent preoccupied with how well did there model score, but not how much value did this model provide for patients, clinicians, and hospitals. These models need to show how they can improve the clinical workflow, in a meaningful. An example of where this was not the case, was the implementation of computer-aided diagnosis for mammography in 1998, it was found to significantly increase patient recall rate, without improving patient outcomes [75]. Therefore, increasing greatly increasing hospital costs, and requiring more patient visits without providing a net benefit to the patient. There is a required mentality shift when developing models for the healthcare domain, with methods and tests of clinical utility used as part of the model performance. This again will depend on bringing together administrators, industry partners, clinicians, and scientists, to ensure the right questions are being asked and put into context for everyone involved. With a focused effort to show how newly developed models will actually impart real-world value, the continued adoption of AI algorithms will remain slow.

The Proposed Approach Our platform has been designed to align with all of the fundamental aims of the FDA's action plan. Through the pseudonymous data server, we can aim to provide a secure environment in which model can be developed. Taking advantage of the new regulations, we can plan to ensure model performance remains stable over time, by iteratively providing the newly collected data, which can account for concept shift. We strive to abide by the highest standards of Good Machine Learning Practice, and will aim to be a part of the growing community supporting the initiative, with a focus on creating high quality data resources. Through the use of pseudonymous data, and the development of more advanced explainability tools, we will be able to direct inform patients on how their data is being used by the model. Because our models are developed within a multi-disciplinary team, our models are developed with the mindset of how this model is going to affect clinical workflow, and ensure it is providing real-world value.

17.5 Chapter Summary

AI is poised to play an increasingly prominent role in healthcare delivery. With increasingly large and complex medical data being routinely captured a shift towards data-driven decision making and personalized care is anticipated. In this chapter we described that the translation of promising research techniques into effective clinical tools is uniquely challenging in healthcare, and that barriers regarding data access, quality and generalizability must be acknowledged and managed. Following this, focus on the delivery of impactful tools that can be feasibly integrated into real-world clinical environments must be undertaken with particular attention paid to gaining physician trust. The framework required to successfully execute this part of an overarching commitment that must be undertaken by healthcare institutions to facilitate data access, promote data quality, and encourage innovative technology development in partnership with data science teams and commercial partners. Increasingly, this framework must consider direct engagement of patients in both the sourcing and meaningful use of health data to successfully achieve these goals.

Acknowledgements The authors would like to acknowledge thank the National Sciences and Engineering Research Council of Canada for partial support of this research in the form of the NSERC Discovery Grant #10007544 and NSERC Strategic Planning Grant #10022972. Authors also are very appreciative of help and advice received from our colleagues at the Biometric Technologies

Laboratory and Stephenson Cardiac Imaging Centre, with special note of thanks to Dr. Alessandro Satriano.

References

1. Davenport, T., Kalakota, R.: The potential for artificial intelligence in healthcare. Future Healthcare J. **6**, 94–98 (2019)
2. Rong, G., Mendez, A., Bou Assi, E., Zhao, B., Sawan, M.: Artificial intelligence in healthcare: review and prediction case studies. Engineering **6**, 291–301 (2020)
3. Rumsfeld John S., et al.: Cardiovascular health: the importance of measuring patient-reported health status. Circulation **127**, 2233–2249 (2013)
4. Leopold, J.A., Loscalzo, J.: The emerging role of precision medicine in cardiovascular disease. Circ. Res. **122**, 1302–1315 (2018)
5. Mitchell, T.M.: Machine Learning. McGraw-Hill (1997)
6. Hastie, T., Tibshirani, R., Friedman, J.H.: The elements of statistical learning: data mining, inference, and prediction (2009)
7. Goodfellow, I., Bengio, Y., Courville, A.: Deep Learning. MIT Press (2016)
8. Phillips-Wren, G., Esposito, A., Jain, L.C.: Advances in Data Science: Methodologies and Applications, Book. Springer (2020)
9. Mincholé, A., Camps, J., Lyon, A., Rodríguez, B.: Machine learning in the electrocardiogram. J. Electrocardiol. **57**, S61–S64 (2019)
10. Erickson, B.J., Korfiatis, P., Akkus, Z., Kline, T.L.: Machine learning for medical imaging. Radiographics **37**, 505–515 (2017)
11. Kevat, A., Kalirajah, A., Roseby, R.: Artificial intelligence accuracy in detecting pathological breath sounds in children using digital stethoscopes. Respir. Res. **21**, 253 (2020)
12. Leiner, T., et al.: Machine learning in cardiovascular magnetic resonance: basic concepts and applications. J. Cardiovasc. Magn. Reson. **21**, 61 (2019)
13. Singh, G., et al.: Machine learning in cardiac CT: basic concepts and contemporary data. J. Cardiovasc. Comput. Tomogr. **12**, 192–201 (2018)
14. Uribe, C.F., et al.: Machine learning in nuclear medicine: Part 1—Introduction. J. Nucl. Med. **60**, 451–458 (2019)
15. Zukotynski, K., et al.: Machine learning in nuclear medicine: Part 2—Neural networks and clinical aspects. J. Nucl. Med. Off. Publ. Soc. Nucl. Med. **62**, 22–29 (2021)
16. Davis, A., et al.: Artificial intelligence and echocardiography: a primer for cardiac sonographers. J. Am. Soc. Echocardiogr. **33**, 1061–1066 (2020)
17. Hampe, N., Wolterink, J.M., van Velzen, S.G.M., Leiner, T., Išgum, I.: Machine learning for assessment of coronary artery disease in cardiac CT: a survey. Front. Cardiovasc. Med. **6** (2019)
18. Tesche, C., et al.: Coronary CT angiography–derived fractional flow reserve. Radiology **285**, 17–33 (2017)
19. Mortazavi Bobak J. et al.: Analysis of machine learning techniques for heart failure readmissions. Circ. Cardiovasc. Qual. Outcomes **9**, 629–640 (2016)
20. Shaan, K., et al.: Performance of atrial fibrillation risk prediction models in over 4 million individuals. Circ. Arrhythm. Electrophysiol. **14**, e008997 (2021)
21. Thorsen-Meyer, H.-C., et al.: Dynamic and explainable machine learning prediction of mortality in patients in the intensive care unit: a retrospective study of high-frequency data in electronic patient records. Lancet Digit. Health **2**, e179–e191 (2020)
22. Kelly, C.J., Karthikesalingam, A., Suleyman, M., Corrado, G., King, D.: Key challenges for delivering clinical impact with artificial intelligence. BMC Med. **17**, 195 (2019)
23. Parikh, R.B., Teeple, S., Navathe, A.S.: Addressing bias in artificial intelligence in health care. JAMA **322**, 2377–2378 (2019)

24. Cowgill, B., et al.: Biased programmers? Or biased data? A field experiment in operationalizing AI ethics (2020). https://doi.org/10.2139/ssrn.3615404
25. Chilamkurthy, S., et al.: Deep learning algorithms for detection of critical findings in head CT scans: a retrospective study. Lancet **392**, 2388–2396 (2018)
26. FDA, U.: Proposed regulatory framework for modifications to artificial intelligence/machine learning (AI/ML)-based software as a medical device (SaMD) (2021)
27. Adibuzzaman, M., DeLaurentis, P., Hill, J., Benneyworth, B.D.: Big data in healthcare—The promises, challenges and opportunities from a research perspective: a case study with a model database. In: AMIA Annual Symposium Proceedings, vol. 2017, pp. 384–392 (2018)
28. Field, J., Holmes, M.M., Newell, D.: PROMs data: can it be used to make decisions for individual patients? A narrative review. Patient Relat. Outcome Meas. **10**, 233–241 (2019)
29. Attia, Z.I., et al.: An artificial intelligence-enabled ECG algorithm for the identification of patients with atrial fibrillation during sinus rhythm: a retrospective analysis of outcome prediction. Lancet Lond. Engl. **394**, 861–867 (2019)
30. Mahmoudi, E., et al.: Use of electronic medical records in development and validation of risk prediction models of hospital readmission: systematic review. BMJ **369**, m958 (2020)
31. Steele, A.J., Denaxas, S.C., Shah, A.D., Hemingway, H., Luscombe, N.M.: Machine learning models in electronic health records can outperform conventional survival models for predicting patient mortality in coronary artery disease. PLOS ONE **13**, e0202344 (2018)
32. Spooner, A., et al.: A comparison of machine learning methods for survival analysis of high-dimensional clinical data for dementia prediction. Sci. Rep. **10**, 20410 (2020)
33. Demner-Fushman, D., Chapman, W.W., McDonald, C.J.: What can natural language processing do for clinical decision support? J. Biomed. Inform. **42**, 760–772 (2009)
34. Young, I.J.B., Luz, S., Lone, N.: A systematic review of natural language processing for classification tasks in the field of incident reporting and adverse event analysis. Int. J. Med. Inf. **132**, 103971 (2019)
35. Kramer, C.M., et al.: Standardized cardiovascular magnetic resonance imaging (CMR) protocols: 2020 update. J. Cardiovasc. Magn. Reson. **22**, 17 (2020)
36. Lee, D., de Keizer, N., Lau, F., Cornet, R.: Literature review of SNOMED CT use. J. Am. Med. Inform. Assoc. JAMIA **21**, e11–e19 (2014)
37. Miller, A.R., Tucker, C.: Health information exchange, system size and information silos. J. Health Econ. **33**, 28–42 (2014)
38. Hajek, A.M.: Breaking down clinical silos in healthcare. Front. Health Serv. Manage. **29**, 45–50 (2013)
39. Chan, K.S., Fowles, J.B., Weiner, J.P.: Review: electronic health records and the reliability and validity of quality measures: a review of the literature. Med. Care Res. Rev. **67**, 503–527 (2010)
40. Reyna, M.A., et al.: Early prediction of sepsis from clinical data: the PhysioNet/computing in cardiology challenge 2019. Crit. Care Med. **48**, 210–217 (2020)
41. Troyanskaya, O., et al.: Missing value estimation methods for DNA microarrays. Bioinform. Oxford Engl. **17**, 520–525 (2001)
42. van Buuren, S., Groothuis-Oudshoorn, K.: Mice: multivariate imputation by chained equations in R. J. Stat. Softw. **45**, 1–67 (2011)
43. Harrell, F.E.: Hmisc: Harrell Miscellaneous library for R statistical software (2004)
44. Li, P., Stuart, E.A., Allison, D.B.: Multiple imputation: a flexible tool for handling missing data. JAMA **314**, 1966–1967 (2015)
45. Esteva, A., et al.: Dermatologist-level classification of skin cancer with deep neural networks. Nature **542**, 115–118 (2017)
46. Hannun, A.Y., et al.: Cardiologist-level arrhythmia detection and classification in ambulatory electrocardiograms using a deep neural network. Nat. Med. **25**, 65–69 (2019)
47. Bayati, M., et al.: Data-driven decisions for reducing readmissions for heart failure: general methodology and case study. PLOS ONE **9**, e109264 (2014)
48. Mansoor, H., Elgendy, I.Y., Segal, R., Bavry, A.A., Bian, J.: Risk prediction model for in-hospital mortality in women with ST-elevation myocardial infarction: a machine learning approach. Heart Lung **46**, 405–411 (2017)

49. Bohr, A., Memarzadeh, K.: The rise of artificial intelligence in healthcare applications. Artif. Intell. Healthc. 25–60 (2020). https://doi.org/10.1016/B978-0-12-818438-7.00002-2
50. Kim, D.W., Jang, H.Y., Kim, K.W., Shin, Y., Park, S.H.: Design characteristics of studies reporting the performance of artificial intelligence algorithms for diagnostic analysis of medical images: results from recently published papers. Korean J. Radiol. **20**, 405–410 (2019)
51. Bleeker, S.E., et al.: External validation is necessary in prediction research: a clinical example. J. Clin. Epidemiol. **56**, 826–832 (2003)
52. Halligan, S., Altman, D.G., Mallett, S.: Disadvantages of using the area under the receiver operating characteristic curve to assess imaging tests: a discussion and proposal for an alternative approach. Eur. Radiol. **25**, 932–939 (2015)
53. Spiegelhalter, D., Pearson, M., Short, I.: Visualizing uncertainty about the future. Science **333**, 1393–1400 (2011)
54. Rembold, C.M.: Number needed to screen: development of a statistic for disease screening. BMJ **317**, 307–312 (1998)
55. Calster, B.V., et al.: Evaluation of markers and risk prediction models: overview of relationships between NRI and decision-analytic measures. Med. Decis. Mak. Int. J. Soc. Med. Decis. Mak. **33**, 490–501 (2013)
56. Linn, S., Grunau, P.D.: New patient-oriented summary measure of net total gain in certainty for dichotomous diagnostic tests. Epidemiol. Perspect. Innov. **3**, 11 (2006)
57. Larner, A.J.: Number needed to diagnose, predict, or misdiagnose: useful metrics for non-canonical signs of cognitive status? Dement. Geriatr. Cogn. Disord. Extra **8**, 321–327 (2018)
58. Shah, N.H., Milstein, A., Bagley, P., Steven, C.: Making machine learning models clinically useful. JAMA **322**, 1351–1352 (2019)
59. Asan, O., Bayrak, A.E., Choudhury, A.: Artificial intelligence and human trust in healthcare: focus on clinicians. J. Med. Internet Res. **22** (2020)
60. Marcus, G.: Deep learning: a critical appraisal. ArXiv180100631 Cs Stat (2018)
61. Emmert-Streib, F., Yli-Harja, O., Dehmer, M.: Explainable artificial intelligence and machine learning: a reality rooted perspective. WIREs Data Min. Knowl. Discov. **10** (2020)
62. Miao, F., Cai, Y.-P., Zhang, Y.-X., Li, Y., Zhang, Y.-T.: Risk prediction of one-year mortality in patients with cardiac arrhythmias using random survival forest. Comput. Math. Methods Med. (2015)
63. Ching, T., Zhu, X., & Garmire, L.X.: Cox-nnet: an artificial neural network method for prognosis prediction of high-throughput omics data. PLOS Comput. Biol. **14**, e1006076 (2018)
64. Ishwaran, H., Kogalur, U.B., Blackstone, E.H., Lauer, M.S.: Random survival forests. Ann. Appl. Stat. **2**, 841–860 (2008)
65. Lundberg, S.M., Lee, S.-I.: A unified approach to interpreting model predictions. Adv. Neural Inf. Process. Syst. **30**, 4765–4774 (2017)
66. Crawford, K., Calo, R.: There is a blind spot in AI research. Nat. News **538**, 311 (2016)
67. Barocas, S., Selbst, A.D.: Big data's disparate impact. Calif. Law Rev. **104**, 671–732 (2016)
68. Chen, I., Johansson, F.D., Sontag, D.: Why is my classifier discriminatory? **12** (2018)
69. Panch, T., Mattie, H., Atun, R.: Artificial intelligence and algorithmic bias: implications for health systems. J. Glob. Health **9** (2019)
70. Kleinberg, J., Ludwig, J., Mullainathan, S., Rambachan, A.: Algorithmic fairness. AEA Pap. Proc. **108**, 22–27 (2018)
71. Freire, A., Porcaro, L., Gómez, E.: In: Measuring Diversity of Artificial Intelligence Conferences. ArXiv200107038 Cs (2020)
72. Lakhani, P., Sundaram, B.: Deep learning at chest radiography: automated classification of pulmonary tuberculosis by using convolutional neural networks. Radiology **284**, 574–582 (2017)
73. Sayres, R., et al.: Using a deep learning algorithm and integrated gradients explanation to assist grading for diabetic retinopathy. Ophthalmology **126**, 552–564 (2019)

74. Lu, J., et al.: Learning under concept drift: a review. IEEE Trans. Knowl. Data Eng. 1–1 (2018). https://doi.org/10.1109/TKDE.2018.2876857
75. Lehman, C.D., et al.: Diagnostic accuracy of digital screening mammography with and without computer-aided detection. JAMA Int. Med. **175**, 1828–1837 (2015)

CPSIA information can be obtained
at www.ICGtesting.com
Printed in the USA
LVHW011702270921
698835LV00002B/158